FIRST RESPONDER

Third Edition

J. David Bergeron

Gloria Bizjak

Contributing Editor
University of Maryland
Maryland Fire and Rescue Institute

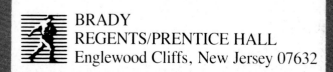

BRADY
REGENTS/PRENTICE HALL
Englewood Cliffs, New Jersey 07632

Library of Congress Cataloging-in-Publication Data

BERGERON, J. DAVID, 1944–
    First responder / J. David Bergeron ; Gloria Bizjak contributing
editor.—3rd ed.
    p.m.
    "A Brady book."
    Includes index.

    ISBN 0–89303–733–8 (pbk). ISBN 0–89303–226–3 (annotated
        instructor's ed. : pbk.)
    1. Medical emergencies. I. Bizjak, Gloria. II. Title.
    [DNLM: 1. Emergencies. 2. Emergency Medical Technicians.
    3. First Aid. WX 215 B496f]
    RC86.7.B47 1991
    616.02'52—dc20
DNLM/DLC
for Library of Congress   90–14359
                                                  CIP

Editorial/production supervision: Tom Aloisi
Acquisition editor: Natalie Anderson
Interior design: Howie Petlack, A Good Thing, Inc.
Cover design: Bruce Kenselaar
Cover photo: George Dodson
Interior design: Howie Petlack, A Good Thing
Prepress buyer: Mary McCartney
Manufacturing buyer: Ed O'Dougherty

 © 1991, 1987, 1982 by Prentice-Hall, Inc.
A Simon & Schuster Company
Englewood Cliffs, New Jersey 07632

Printed in the United States of America

10 9 8 7 6 5 4 3

ISBN 0-89303-733-8

Prentice-Hall International (UK) Limited, *London*
Prentice-Hall of Australia Pty. Limited, *Sydney*
Prentice-Hall Canada Inc., *Toronto*
Prentice-Hall Hispanoamericana, S.A., *Mexico*
Prentice-Hall of India Private Limited, *New Delhi*
Prentice-Hall of Japan, Inc., *Tokyo*
Prentice-Hall of Southeast Asia Pte. Ltd., *Singapore*
Editora Prentice-Hall do Brasil, Ltda., *Rio de Janeiro*

Notice

It is the intent of the Authors and the Publisher that this textbook be used solely as part of a formal First Responder course taught by a qualified instructor in the field. The care procedure presented here represent accepted practices in the U.S.; however, they are not offered as a standard of care. It is difficult to ensure that all the information is accurate and the possibility of error can never be entirely eliminated. The Authors and the Publisher disclaim any liability or responsibility for injury or damage to persons or property which is incurred as a consequence, directly or indirectly, of the use and application of any of the contents of this book. It is the reader's responsibility to know and follow local care protocol as provided by the medical advisors directing the system to which he or she belongs. Also, it is the reader's responsibility to stay informed of emergency care procedure changes.

Please note that many if not all of the photographs contained in this book are taken of actual emergency situations. As such, it is possible that they may not accurately depict current, appropriate, or advisable practices of emergency care. They have been included for the sole purpose of giving general insight into real-life emergency settings.

To the Student

A workbook for this text is available through your college bookstore under the title *Workbook for FIRST RESPONDER, 3rd Edition,* by J. David Bergeron. If it is not in stock, ask the book store manager to order you a copy. If your course is being offered off-campus, ask your instructor where you may obtain a copy. The workbook can help you with course material by acting as a tutorial and study aid.

■ Contents

1 THE FIRST RESPONDER   1

2 THE HUMAN BODY   19

3 PATIENT ASSESSMENT   49

4

BREATHING—THE AIRWAY AND PULMONARY RESUSCITATION 83

4A

AIDS TO RESUSCITATION (OPTIONAL) 113

5 CIRCULATION— CARDIOPULMONARY RESUSCITATION (CPR) 119

6 TWO-RESCUER CPR 145

7 BLEEDING AND SHOCK 153

11 SPLINTING 249

12 INJURIES—3: SKULL, SPINE, AND CHEST 271

16 SPECIAL PATIENTS 371

17 GAINING ACCESS TO PATIENTS 387

POST-TEST

■ Scansheets

■ Anatomy and Physiology Plates

■ Preface

The biggest change in First Responder-level care has developed due to concerns about rescuer safety. Specifically, these concerns have dealt with the need to better protect prehospital emergency care personnel from infectious diseases during the rendering of care. Even though incidence of such infection is low, it is still a major concern; a concern that supports the first responsibility of a First Responder—personal safety.

More specifically, attention is now focused on the infectious diseases because of the HIV virus and AIDS. Avoidance of direct contact with patient blood and body fluids is now a standard procedure because of AIDS. This emphasis is a part of the Third Edition and its workbook. However, AIDS alone is not the reason. Other infectious diseases are considered and combined with all aspects of personal safety to reinforce the concept of a safe rescuer.

Basic life support procedures remain essentially the same in this edition with the exception of the introduction of the pocket face mask with one-way valve as a standard piece of equipment for *all First Responders*. The mouth-to-mask method of rescue breathing is now considered the primary method used during pulmonary resuscitation and CPR. Again, it is the concern about infectious diseases that has led to this change.

There are other changes in First Responder-level care found in this text and the workbook. As predicted when First Responder training began, changes would be few from year to year. Most of the changes found in this edition are minor. Some are optional, such as blood pressure determination and oxygen therapy. In a few cases, care procedures have changed because methods that are easier to perform are beginning to replace old "tried and true" ones. The single splint method of caring for lower leg fractures is an example; however, the two-splint method is also included in the text.

There are some subtle instructional changes found in this edition; however, the major changes are obvious. Color photographs and art add a new dimension to learning, being part of a new design that improves both readability and study mechanics. Note, too, the additional attention given to glossary terms and their placement in the margins for more emphasis and easier access. Terminology, symptoms, signs, and care procedures receive emphasis with the new design.

The Learning Package

The textbook and workbook remain the major elements of the learning package. For the instructor, a new Annotated Instructor's Edition (AIE) is available containing a special introduction and teacher's notes that are found in the text margins next to relative materials. The AIE and the revised instructor's manual allow for the instructor to quickly focus in on essential materials when preparing for class and also provide ideas for instruction. The ideas are not limited to those of the author. The instructional guides that are found in the AIE and the Instructor's Manual are based on the ideas and concerns of First Responder instructors in EMS Systems, industrial training programs, and the military. Such sharing of information is essential for effective training.

Visual aids in the form of a set of presentation slides, Atlas of Injury slides, and anatomy acetate transparencies are available from the publisher. Each allows for improved instruction and enrichment. A new excitement for both instructor and students is now possible with the addition of video tapes to the publisher's training package. A whole new approach to lecture time and skills practice is possible using these tapes and their lesson plans.

The learning package offers a great variety of choices to the instructor and his or her students. The traditional approach is possible, with many options for enrichment. Non-traditional approaches can be developed from the learning package to meet the needs of a specific student or group of students. In either case, a new adventure in learning is certain to be part of the outcome.

J. David Bergeron

■ Acknowledgments

I wish to thank all the individuals and EMS professionals who have helped to make this textbook a successful tool for the teaching of First Responders.

The EMS professionals who reviewed the manuscript and provided information and guidance did an outstanding job on this edition. A very special thanks goes to the following individuals.

Bill Miller, Training Supervisor
Public Safety Training Academy
Pittsburgh, PA 15206

Wayne Hutchinson
Delaware State Fire School
Dover, DE 19901

Jim Paturas
Bridgeport Hospital
Bridgeport, CT 06610

Ben Blankenship
North Little Rock Fire Department
North Little Rock, AR 72114

Sgt. Mark Whitley
Illinois State Police Academy
Springfield, IL 62707

Kevin Krause, BS, EMT-P
New York State Disaster and
    Preparedness Commission
Albany, NY

John Doran
Connecticut Police Academy
Meriden, CT 06450

Bill Wetter, MS, EMT-P
Jefferson City Police Department
Louisville, KY 40245

Bill Locke, EMT-P
Moraine Park Technical College
EMS Education
Fondulac, WI 54395

James G. Stevens, Jr.
Maryland Fire and Rescue Institute
University of Maryland
College Park, MD

Jeannie O'Brien, RN, REMT-P
Tacoma Community College
Gig Harbor, WA 98335

Allan Braslow, PhD
Alexandria, VA 22304

MaryBeth Michos
Maryland Fire & Rescue Training
Rockville, MD 20850

Mike & Debbie Fagel
Aurora, IL 60506

Ellie Sorrel
Florida Fire & Rescue Training
Gainesville, FL 32601

Danny Beck
Office of EMS
Phoenix, AZ 85004

Chief Ricky Davidson
Shrevesport Fire Department, Division of EMS
Shrevesport, LA 71101

Gerald M. Dworkin, BS, EMT-A
Life Saving Resources
Dumfries, VA 22026

Gary Denault, EMT-I-D
Denault EMS Training Institute
Leland, IL 60531

Eileen Foster
Baltimore Department of Health
Westminster, MD 21157

Doug Stevenson, EMT-P
Houston Community College, Houston, TX
    77021

Jason T. White, Training Coordinator
Missouri Bureau of EMS
Jefferson City, MO 65102

Donald J. Gordon
University of Texas-HSC
San Antonio, TX 78284

Sue Barnes
Ohio Emergency Medical Services Agency
Columbus, OH

Mary Ann Talley, BSN, MPA
University of Alabama, EMS Training
    Program
Mobile, AL 36615

Jon Anderson
Office of Fish and Wildlife
Essex Junction, VT 05452

J. David Barrick, EMS Training Officer
Newport News Fire Department
Newport News, VA 23602

Paul H. Coffey
Director First Responder & Basic EMT
    Training
MA Dept. of Public Health, Office of EMS

John Clair
New York State EMS
Saratoga Springs, NY 12866

Jolene R. Whitney, BLS Coordinator
Bureau of EMS
Salt Lake City, Utah 84116-0660

Lou Jordan, PA
President of Emergency Training Associates
Baltimore, MD 21221

Rodger L. Ames
Arvada Fire Protection District
Arvada, CO 80003

Charles Garoni
University of Texas-H.S.C.
San Antonio, TX 78284

Dan Morabito, MICT-IC
EMS Director Memorial Hospital
Abilene, KS 67410

Ken Threet
Department of Health
Division of EMS
Helena, MT 59620

John Rasmussen
Greenville Technical College
Greenville, SC 29606

James R. Miller
Prince Georges County Fire
    Department—AEMS Bureau
Brentwood, MD

Gary W. Fulton
Division of EMS Training
Indiana University of Pennsylvania
Indiana, PA 15705

Gus Pappas
Training Department, Fort Totten
Bayside, NY 11359

Michael Greene, EMTA
Emergency Medical Training Associates Olympia,
    WA 98502
Olympia, WA 98502

Kenneth E. Gagnon
Lakeland College, EMT Training Program
Mattoon, IL 61938-8001

Leona Rowe, NAEMT-P
EMS Educational Services
Laurel, MD 20707

David A. Tomasino
MATC South Campus, EMT Training Program
Oak Creek, WI 53154

Judy Gaffron
Division of EMS
Nashville, TN 37247-0701

Diana Van Wormer, Paramedic Instructor
Northeast Metro Technical College
White Bear Lake, MN 55110

Gary McClanahan
Johnson County MED-ACT
Overland Park, KS 66210

Thomas McCarrier
Mid-State Technical College
Stevens Point, WI 54481

Linda Abrahamson, EMT-P, EMT-I/C
Lexington, IL 61753

Captain Stan Irwin
City of Leon Valley Fire Department
San Antonio, TX 78238

Phil Fontanarosa, M.D.
Akron City Hospital, Dept. of Emergency
    Medicine
Akron, Ohio 44309-2090

In addition to those persons who supplied medical, technical, and instructional information, I would like to thank everyone who helped to turn the manuscript into a book. Natalie Anderson was the Senior Editor. She continued the Brady tradition of support for EMS training, wanting only the best for today's First Responders.

The Senior Production Editor for the Third Edition was Tom Aloisi, the same person who worked so hard on the Second Edition. Tom's dedication is greatly appreciated. His skills at editing and coordinating all the aspects of production are remarkable. Tom's expert help ensured a continuity of quality for this edition.

Bill Thomas was the Copy Editor. This is a difficult job, done expertly by Bill. Howard Petlack provided the new design for the textbook, making it more suitable for a new decade. The new color artwork is the result of the special effort given to this project by John Smith and the artists at Network Graphics. Each consideration given to style, form, and color helped to improve the book.

George Dodson is the country's leading EMS photographer. His hard work has produced interesting and instructionally sound visuals for this text. He was assisted by Gloria Bizjak and her many friends and associates at the Maryland Fire and Rescue Institute, University of Maryland, College Park. As usual, this team's work proved to be outstanding.

■ Introduction

Learning to Be a First Responder

First Responder programs were developed to provide highly trained individuals with the skills necessary to begin assessing and caring for patients at the scene of injury or illness. In many areas of the nation, First Responders now are able to reach patients in less than ten minutes from the onset of the emergency. This quick response and the quality care rendered save thousands of lives each year.

Even though the First Responder concept has been around for over a decade, the majority of programs in full operation are less than five years old. First Responder programs are growing in number and complexity each year. This commitment to the First Responder concept has allowed the First Responder to become an important part of emergency services in the United States. Other nations also are developing similar programs.

The first two editions of this textbook were used by several hundred thousand students as part of their training. This new edition has taken what was found to be successful in the first edition and adds some new topics and concepts that have recently become a part of most First Responder courses.

You are about to begin your training to become a First Responder. Most likely, your training will take place in a course that follows the guidelines set by your local emergency medical services system (EMS System). Your course might be a state- or company-designed course. The vast majority of these courses are based on the guidelines originally developed as the forty-hour First Responder Course by the U.S. Department of Transportation (DOT).

Who is the authority for your course? Your instructor. Things are always changing in emergency services. Year-old memoranda and even new textbooks may not be 100 percent up to date. Your instructor keeps informed of changes in procedures, requirements, and responsibilities. Should you have any questions about sources saying different things, ask your instructor. If this text takes one approach to an emergency situation and your instructor takes a different approach, follow your instructor. We ask you to do this, not to please your instructor, but because a textbook cannot be changed on a daily basis.

REMEMBER: As a First Responder, you are considered to be part of the EMS System. The care you provide must follow your state and local guidelines.

Objectives

At the beginning of each chapter, you will find a list of objectives. These objectives tell you what you should be able to do by the end of the chapter.

The objectives used in this text are called behavioral objectives (also called performance objectives). This means that the objectives state the things you should be able to do that can be measured by you and by others.

When you read the chapter objectives, note how they are worded. Terms such as list, define, label, and apply are used. The objectives will tell you very specifically what you need to be able to do. You will not be told to understand or to know. Instead, you will be told to be able to do something that will give you and your instructor a way of seeing if you really do know and understand the materials found in each chapter.

Using This Textbook

The first three chapters of this book are critical to becoming a First Responder. Chapter 1 will define the role of a First Responder. This chapter requires careful study since it will be difficult to know what you need to learn in the rest of the course without first knowing the skills and responsibilities of a First Responder. Chapter 2 and Chapter 3 help you to see the human body in terms of injuries and medical emergencies. Before you can help patients, you will need to develop a head-to-toe approach to the human body. Unless you take great care in learning these first three chapters, you will not be able to fill the role of a First Responder.

As you study each chapter in this book, you should:

1. Go over the list of objectives found at the beginning of the chapter.
2. Make sure that you understand all the objectives before reading the chapter.
3. Read the chapter, keeping the list of objectives in mind.
4. Give special consideration to any illustrations, charts, and lists emphasized in the text.
5. After reading the chapter, go back over the list of objectives and see if you can accomplish each objective in the list.
6. Go back over the sections of the chapter that deal with the objectives that you could not meet.

You will find that the list of objectives will act as self-tests for you when you finish your reading. You will know what questions you cannot answer for any given chapter.

Medical Terms and Pronunciation

As you read through this text, you will find two types of terms used. The first type will be common, everyday terms, such as chest. You will also see terms from medicine and anatomy, such as thoracic. When a medical term is used for the first time, a pronunciation guide will be given. Therefore, when you see the word thoracic used for the first time, you will see the following:

thoracic (tho-RAS-ik)

Capitalized letters indicate the portion of the word that is emphasized. Practice saying these words and try to use them in conversations with your instructor and fellow students.

Having a large vocabulary of medical terms is not very important for First Responders. In emergency situations, telling the emergency squad that the patient has chest pains is as meaningful as saying the patient has pains in the thorax. Telling an emergency medical technician (EMT) that the patient may have a fractured right thigh bone will have as much meaning as saying a fractured right femur. There are some terms that you must learn and use. These will be noted in each chapter.

It is important that you can recognize and define many terms taken from medicine and anatomy, even though you will not use these terms in oral or written reports. Other members of the emergency care team may use these terms when conversing with you. As part of your continuing education as a First Responder, you will run into these terms in articles and reports. For these reasons, you should not ignore anatomical and medical terms.

Levels of Learning

All First Responders need the same knowledge and skills. However, while you are learning, it might be useful for you to know what is considered to be basic information and techniques. A **1st** has been placed next to all basic information and skills when they are presented in this text. Is this all you need to learn? No, see the objectives for each chapter.

After a given amount of material has been presented in a chapter, you will see a   inserted in the text. This means that you would do well to stop at that point and consider what you have just finished. If you did not understand a section or feel that you do not know the section very well, you should go back over that section before continuing with your reading.

In addition to the objectives, each chapter has a list of skills. Knowing the steps to a certain procedure will be part of the chapter. However, being able to do the procedure will not come from this text or your lecture sections. Laboratory practice sessions and field sessions will be needed to perfect these skills.

How to Study

Every person is unique. Since you are a little different from every other student, how you study will be a very personal thing. There are some standard recommendations that you might find helpful. First of all, you must follow the directions given by your instructor and the directions given in this text. If you take off on your own, you could spend too much time on minor points and not enough time on what is critical knowledge for a First Responder.

Be sure to take notes during your training. You should have class notes, reading notes, and notes from any practical situations that are part of your First Responder's course.

If possible, have your own place to study, removed from other activities. This will keep away distractions and help prevent some poor past habits of studying that waste time. Study by yourself until you are able to meet all the chapter objectives. Too often, students try to study together. Educational research has proven that this does not work.

If you do not understand something presented in class or in this text, see your instructor. Your fellow students may not understand any more than you do. They also lack the experience your instructor will have.

After you have studied and feel that you can meet all the objectives, then do meet with fellow students. Studies have shown that people remember things for a longer period of time if they have the opportunity to talk about their studies. If you have found that reading is not your best way of learning, then these meetings will be very important. You will soon see that being able to communicate with others is an important part of the task of a First Responder. Even if you have been trained in dealing with the public, you will still need practice in communicating the new information you will be using in this course.

When you study from this textbook, you should:

1. Takes notes on the statements that apply to the chapter objectives.
2. Keep a list of page numbers to go with objectives.
3. If you are allowed to keep your text, mark important items in your book.
4. After finishing your reading and before checking back on the list of objectives, be sure to go back over all illustrations, charts, and lists in the chapter.

Responsibility

It has been said that the responsibility for teaching is the teacher's and the responsibility for learning is that of the student. It is your responsibility to learn what your instructor teaches. As a First Responder, it will be your responsibility to know all local and state requirements and regulations as they deal with First Responders and the services that they perform.

In addition to the above responsibilities, as a First Responder you will be expected to stay up-to-date in both information and skills. After completing your training, it is recommended that you set aside 30 minutes to an hour each week to review part of a chapter in this text, some of your lecture notes, or some other source of First Responder information. Your local or state emergency services director will be able to tell you what you will need in terms of updated bulletins and continuing education.

It is doubtful that you would be taking this course unless you had the attitude of a professional, so nothing need be said about motivation and your responsibilities to those who are providing you with this First Responder's course. All that remains to be said in this introduction is good luck and enjoy your entry into the world of emergency care services.

CHAPTER 1

The First Responder

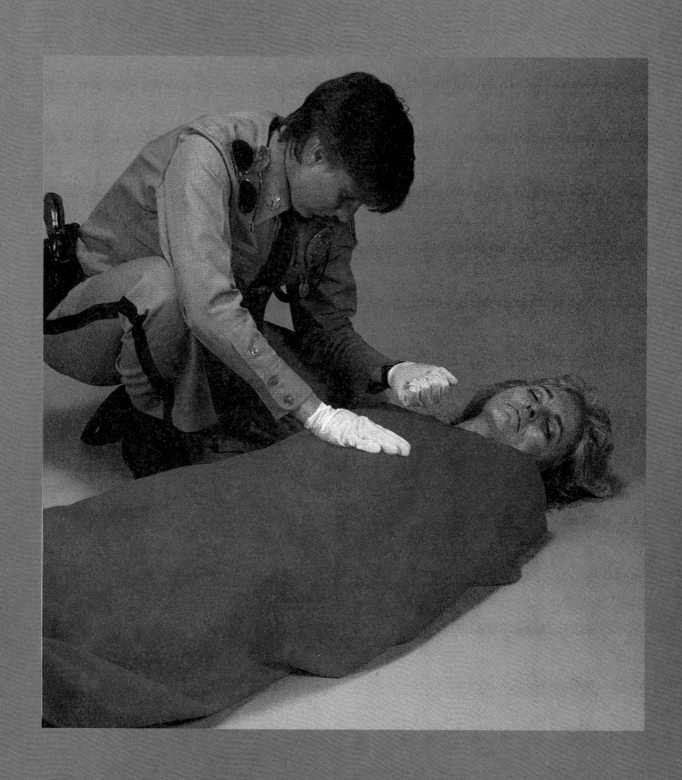

■ OBJECTIVES

By the end of this chapter, you should be able to:

1. Define *Emergency Medical Services System* (EMS System). (p. 2)
2. Define *First Responder*. (p. 4)
3. State the primary concern of the First Responder at an emergency scene. (p. 4)
4. List the four major duties of the First Responder that apply directly to patients. (p. 6)
5. List those activities that fall under the heading of First Responder responsibilities. (p. 6)
6. Define *emergency care*. (p. 6)
7. Describe the desirable traits of a First Responder. (pp. 7–8)
8. State how the concept of negligence applies to First Responder-level emergency care. (pp. 9–10)
9. Relate First Responder responsibilities to the standard of care and the Good Samaritan laws. (p. 9)
10. Define *informed consent*. (pp. 12, 14)
11. Distinguish between actual and implied consent. (pp. 12, 14)
12. Define *abandonment*. (p. 11)
13. List the medical equipment, basic tools, and supplies used by the typical First Responder. (pp. 14–15)

THE EMERGENCY MEDICAL SERVICES SYSTEM

The EMS System

Millions of lives are saved each year by medical care. The advances made in medicine during the last 50 years are startling. Accurate methods of detecting illness, complex medical procedures, elaborate equipment, and new wonder drugs are used by a highly trained health care team to provide the best of care for patients. In the last century, most patients entering hospitals died. Today, we fully expect the vast majority of those people who are hospitalized to recover and lead normal lives.

If hospitals stood by themselves, waiting for patients to come to them, many of the individuals saved each year would die before reaching medical care. A sudden, severe illness or an injury-producing accident could cause death to occur before the patient arrived at the hospital. Modern medicine tries to prevent such deaths by extending care out to the patient. This care begins at the emergency scene and continues during transport to the medical facility. After transport, an orderly transfer to the emergency department staff ensures continued care. This professional-level care is accomplished by a chain of human resources, linked together to form the Emergency Medical Services System (EMS System).

Emergency Medical Services System—the chain of human resources and services linked together to provide continuous prehospital emergency care.

The base for the EMS System is the hospital or medical facility. Physicians, nurses, allied health workers, and other members of the health care team stand ready to supply total patient care. The emergency department begins the extension of services to the patient. Emergency Medical Technicians (EMTs), working from well-equipped emergency vehicles, are an extension of the hospital's emergency department. In some situations, industrial EMTs, nurses, and others are also part of the team, providing care before the EMS System's EMTs arrive.

Often, patients need immediate care before the EMTs reach the scene. Usually, the first people to reach the patient are not trained in emergency care. In most localities, too few individuals are trained in first aid and

The EMS System—Prehospital Care

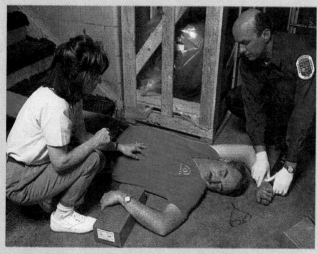

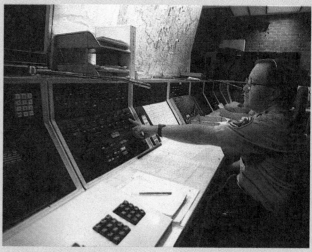

FIRST RESPONDER A person trained to provide initial care for patients suffering injury or sudden illness. Most First Responders are members of law enforcement agencies or the fire service; however, industry, governments, and the private sector have trained First Responders. The typical First Responder can assess patients, provide basic life support, and render the care that is necessary to prevent medical and injury-related problems from becoming a threat to survival.

EMS DISPATCHER An individual at the local emergency communications center who is trained to gather information about accidents and sudden illnesses. The dispatcher can alert the necessary services and pass on the information needed for a professional response. In some localities, the dispatcher is able to offer basic care instructions to the caller.

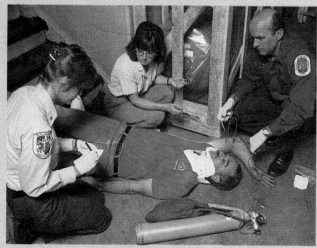

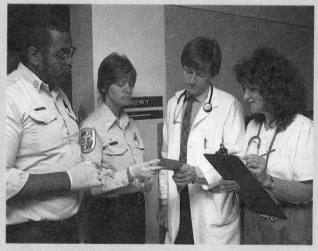

EMERGENCY MEDICAL TECHNICIAN (EMT) The basic EMT (EMT-A) has completed the Department of Transportation National Standard Training Program or its equivalent and is certified by a state emergency medical services board or other authorized agency. The EMT can assess patients, provide basic life support, render special splinting procedures, stabilize possible spinal injuries, administer oxygen, and employ special techniques for patients in shock. The EMT-Intermediate has received additional training so that he or she can initiate intermediate or advanced life support. The paramedic (EMT-P) is certified in special procedures of advanced life support.

EMERGENCY DEPARTMENT STAFF The specially trained physicians, nurses, physician's assistants, and allied health personnel who communicate with EMTs in the field and receive the patient at the hospital. They take care of the patient's immediate needs, acting as an extension of all the hospital's services.

basic life support. The American Red Cross and the American Heart Association (AHA) have successfully trained many people, but, unfortunately, not enough citizens have taken advantage of these training programs. Those trained in basic first aid and basic life support have saved many lives by providing life-saving care before the EMS System could arrive. The problem is that there are not enough people who can provide the care that is needed.

In addition to the lack of people able to provide care at the scene, there is a problem in terms of the level of care that can be provided. Individuals trained in first aid can be of significant help in providing certain types of care before EMS personnel arrive; however, their training in patient assessment and certain types of care is limited. Complicated medical emergencies and serious injuries such as those seen in automobile accidents require more highly trained individuals to be the first to provide care.

The lack of people trained to the level necessary to provide care before the EMTs arrive is the weakest link in the chain of the EMS System. It is believed that the training of First Responders will help correct this problem.

The First Responder

First Responder—a member of the EMS System who has been trained to render first care for a patient and to help EMTs at the emergency scene.

1st First Responders are part of the EMS System. They are trained to reach patients, find out what is wrong, provide emergency care, and, only when necessary, move patients without causing further injury. These individuals are usually the first trained personnel to reach the patient.

A First Responder may be a law enforcement officer, a member of the fire service, a company or union employee, or a private citizen who volunteers to help the EMS System. In all cases, a First Responder is trained and has successfully completed a First Responder course. In time, all police officers and firefighters should be trained to the First Responder level. Industry needs to have many of its employees trained as well. Truck drivers, known for their willingness to help at the scene of highway accidents, could save many lives if they were trained to the First Responder level. Of course, the more private citizens who are willing to be trained as First Responders, the stronger the EMS System will become.

Since the beginning of First Responder training programs, hundreds of thousands of people have completed formal courses, with many of these people going on to provide essential care. In most areas of the United States, First Responders are now an important daily part of the EMS System. The care they have provided has reduced suffering, prevented additional injuries, and saved many lives.

Roles and Responsibilities

1st Your primary concern as a First Responder at an emergency scene is *personal safety*. The desire to help those who are in need of care may make you forget to consider the hazards at the scene. You must make certain that you can safely reach the patient and that you will remain safe while providing care.

Part of a First Responder's concern for personal safety must be the proper protection from infectious diseases. As a First Responder assessing or providing care for patients, you must avoid direct contact with patient blood, body fluids, membranes, wounds, and burns. Personal protection from possible contact with infectious agents may require the use of:

- Approved latex or vinyl gloves
- Pocket face masks with one-way valves for rescue breathing procedures (see page 92)
- Protective eyewear such as goggles or face shields to avoid contact with droplets during certain care procedures (for example, assisting with childbirth)

- Face masks to avoid contact with airborne microorganisms
- Gowns or aprons to avoid being splashed by blood or body fluids or having direct contact with contaminated items

Typically, you will need no more than latex or vinyl gloves in most care situations; however, all the items listed above should be on hand for the rendering of safe care. More will be said about infectious diseases and personal protection in Chapter 13.

First Responders who are in law enforcement or the fire service may find that they are required to carry out certain duties before attempting to provide patient care. If this applies to you, always follow your department's standard operating procedures.

1st The EMS System responds to an emergency scene to provide care for the patient. As a First Responder, **you are part of the EMS system.** Your activities at the scene and the care you provide until more highly trained personnel arrive will help to save lives, prevent additional injury, and give comfort to patients.

Before care begins for someone, that person is a victim. Once you start to carry out your duties as a First Responder, the victim becomes a patient. Your presence at the scene means that the EMS System has begun its first phase of care. True, the patient may need a physician at the hospital

FIGURE 1–1.   The EMS system.

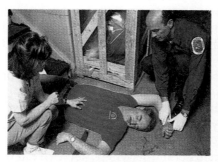

First Responder

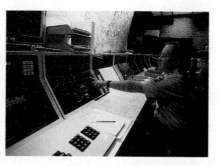

EMS Dispatcher

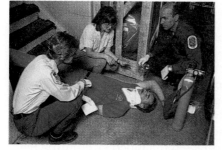

EMT's

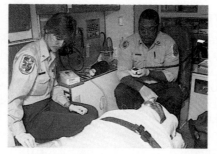

Transport

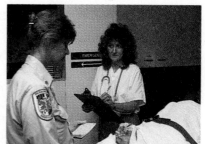

Transfer

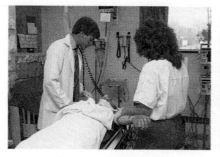

Emergency Department

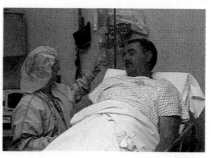

Appropriate Services

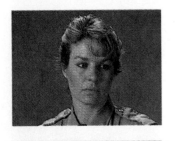
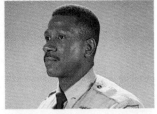
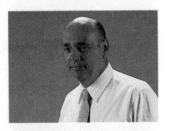
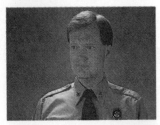
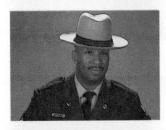
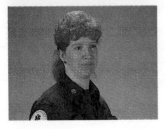

FIGURE 1–2.
First responders.

Emergency care—the prehospital assessment and basic care for the sick or injured patient. The physical and emotional needs of the patient are considered and attended to during care.

to survive, but the patient's chances of reaching the hospital alive are greatly improved because a First Responder has initiated emergency care.

1st As a First Responder, you have four main patient-related duties to carry out at the emergency scene. These duties are:

1. Safely gain access to the patient, using simple hand tools when necessary.
2. Find out what is wrong with the patient and provide emergency care using a minimum amount of equipment.
3. Lift or move the patient, only when required, and do so without causing additional injury.
4. Transfer the patient and patient information to more highly trained personnel when they arrive at the scene.

1st As a First Responder, your responsibilities at the emergency scene may include any or all of the following:

- Control an accident scene in order to protect yourself and the patients, and to prevent additional accidents.
- Make certain that the EMS System dispatcher is alerted so more highly trained personnel can come to the scene. Should the police, fire department, rescue squad, power company, or others be needed at the scene, you must make certain that the dispatcher is aware of this need.
- Gain access to patients, whether they are surrounded by a crowd, trapped in a vehicle, or inside a building.
- Find out what is wrong with a patient by gathering information from the scene, bystanders, and the patient, and by examining the patient.
- To the best of your ability, provide emergency care to the level of your training.
- Judge when safety or care requires you to move or reposition patients and do so using techniques that minimize possible injury.
- Gain help from bystanders and control their activities.
- Provide for an orderly transfer of patients and patient information to more highly trained personnel.
- Help more highly trained personnel when they arrive at the scene, working under their direction.

Emergency Care

Most students entering a First Responder course are not sure what "emergency care" means. At the First Responder level, emergency care deals with both illnesses and injuries. Emergency care can be providing emotional support to someone who is frightened because of an accident. In life-threatening emergencies, you may be required to start basic life support measures. The care you provide may keep a patient from going into shock and possibly dying. In extreme situations, you may have to breathe for a patient (pulmonary resuscitation), or breathe for him and keep his blood circulating (cardiopulmonary resuscitation—CPR).

Emergency care includes caring for cuts, bruises, burns, fractures, and internal injuries. Sometimes this care will be very simple, requiring skills you may already have upon entering your First Responder course. Other times, this care can be very complicated, and may save the patient's life or prevent the loss of an eye or a limb.

First Responder emergency care also deals with illnesses. As part of your training, you will learn to recognize and manage heart attacks, strokes, problems due to excess heat and cold, respiratory illnesses, diabetic coma, insulin shock, childbirth, poisonings, and drug abuse. You will learn how emotional support and physical care skills can be combined to help the patient until more highly trained personnel arrive.

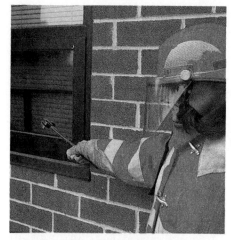
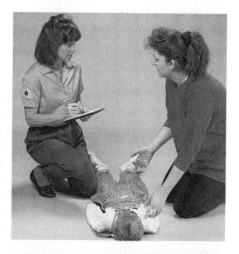
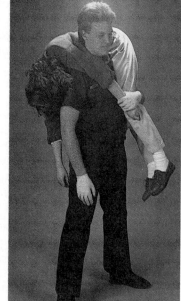
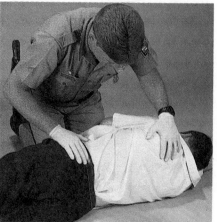
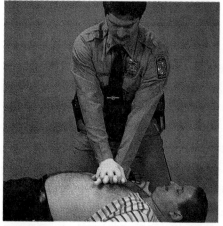

FIGURE 1–3. Main duties at the emergency scene.

First Responder Traits

To become a First Responder, you must be willing to take on additional duties and responsibilities. It takes hard work and study to become a First Responder. This effort does not end with your course, since you will have to keep your skills in emergency care methods sharp and up to date (you may be required to be recertified periodically).

If you want to be a First Responder, you have to be willing to deal with people. Individuals who are sick or injured are not at their best. You must be able to overlook rude behavior and unreasonable demands, realizing that patients may act this way because of illness or injury. Dealing with people is one of the hardest things we do. To do so in a professional manner is sometimes very difficult.

To be a First Responder, you must be honest and realistic. When helping patients, you cannot tell them they are OK if they are sick or hurt. You cannot tell them that everything is all right. They know that something is wrong. Telling someone not to worry is foolish. When an emergency occurs, there is truly something to worry about. Your conversations with patients can help them to relax, if you are honest. By telling patients that you are trained in emergency care and that you will help them, you ease fears and gain their confidence. Letting patients know that additional help is on the way also helps them to relax.

There are limits to what you can say to a patient. Telling a patient that her child is dead or a loved one is seriously injured will not help the patient. When rendering emergency care, more tact may be necessary. By saying that someone is taking care of the loved ones, you may be able to set the patient at ease. Remember, people under the stress of illness or injury often cannot tolerate any additional stress.

Being a First Responder requires that you control your own feelings at the emergency scene. You will have to learn to become involved with caring for patients, while at the same time controlling your emotional reactions to injury or serious illness. Patients do not need sympathy and tears. They need your professional care.

Providing First Responder-level care requires you to admit that accidents and other emergency scenes will affect you. You may have to speak with other EMS care providers or a specialist within the EMS System to resolve the stress and emotional problems caused by providing care (see Chapter 19).

As a First Responder, you have to be a highly disciplined professional at the emergency scene. Watch your language in front of patients and by-standers. Do not make comments about patients and the horror of an accident. Concentrate on patients and avoid unnecessary distractions. Something as simple as smoking a cigarette at the scene shows that you are not willing to discipline yourself to the level required to provide First Responder-level care.

No one can demand that you change your life-style in order to be a First Responder. However, since you may be called on to provide care almost anywhere at any time, there are a few things you should consider. Your appearance has a lot to do with gaining patient confidence. Putting on a clean shirt before running out to the store may not seem to be a reasonable request. Having one less drink at a party may sound unimportant. But the significance of such actions may prove to be very important if you have to provide care at an accident.

To be a First Responder, you must keep yourself in reasonably good physical condition. If you are unable to provide needed care because you cannot bend over or cannot catch your breath, then all your training is worthless.

When you complete your training and become a First Responder, you are someone special, filling a very important need in your community.

FIGURE 1–4.
Take a professional approach when providing care.

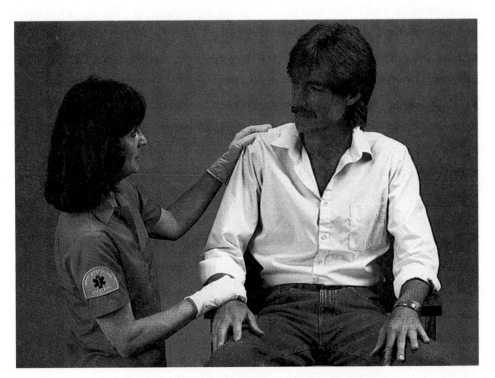

LEGAL ASPECTS OF FIRST RESPONDER CARE

Standard of Care

1st Most of us have heard about people being sued because they stopped to help someone at an accident. Successful suits of this type are not very common. Each state has established guidelines to allow emergency care to be given without the care provider having to worry about being sued. However, these laws require that a certain **standard of care** be provided. **1st** What is considered to be the standard of care is based on laws, administrative orders, and guidelines published by the EMS System and other emergency care organizations and societies. This standard of care allows you to be judged based on what is expected of someone with your training and experience, working under similar conditions.

Your First Responder course follows guidelines proposed by the U.S. Department of Transportation (DOT) or another authority that has studied what is needed to provide the standard of care required at the First Responder level. You will be trained so that you can provide this standard of care. If the care you provide is not up to this standard, you may be sued and held liable for your actions.

NOTE: Keep written notes of what you do at the emergency scene. You may be called on to provide this information at a later date. If your EMS System requires you to complete forms, submit reports, or sign patient transfer papers, do so at the proper time. You must be able to show that you provided the standard of care.

Standard of care—the care expected based on the provider's training and experience, taking into account the conditions under which the care is rendered.

Immunity

1st **Good Samaritan laws** have been developed in most states to protect individuals who help people needing emergency care. If your state has a Good Samaritan law, you will be granted immunity (protection from civil liability) if you act in good faith to provide care to the level of your training, to the best of your ability.

You will be trained to deliver the standard of care expected of First Responders. Your instructor will explain any differences in the laws of your state.

The other factor you must consider is how the Good Samaritan laws of your state affect your immunity if you are a paid provider of emergency care. In some states, special laws apply to paid providers, while the Good Samaritan laws apply only to volunteers. Again, your instructor or local EMS System can provide you with the needed information.

Good Samaritan laws—a series of state laws designed to protect certain care providers if they deliver the standard of care in good faith, to the level of their training and to the best of their abilities.

Negligence

1st The basis for most lawsuits involving prehospital emergency care is negligence. This is a term often used to indicate that you did not do what was expected, or that you did something carelessly. From a legal standpoint, negligence is a more complicated concept. As a First Responder, you could be sued for negligence if *all* the following occurred while you were providing care:

1. You (the First Responder) had a duty to provide care or decided for yourself to assume the responsiblity to provide care.

Negligence—at the First Responder level, negligence usually is a failure to provide the expected standard of care, leading to additional injury of the patient.

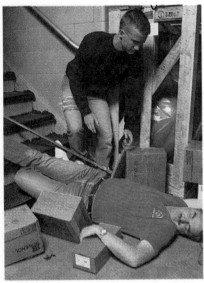

Duty to Act

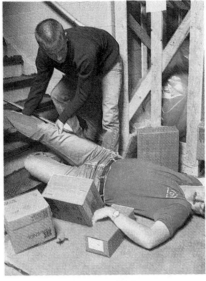

Improper Care

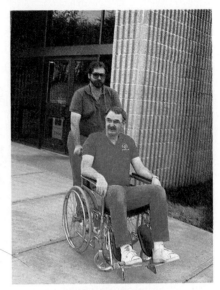

Injury Results

FIGURE 1–5. A negligent rescuer is one who has a duty to act, does not provide the standard of care, and causes the patient harm.

2.   Care for the patient was not provided to the standard of care.
3.   The patient was injured in some way as a result of this improper care.

   First Responders in the police and paid fire service have a **duty to act.** This means that they are required, at least while on duty, to provide care according to their department's standard operating procedures. In some localities, this duty to act may also apply to paid First Responders when they are off duty.

   The duty to act is not so clear in the case of volunteer First Responders. While on duty, these volunteers also may have a duty to act when at an emergency scene. What is expected when they are off duty is unclear because many states do not have specific laws concerning First Responders. Most laws provide direction for physicians and nurses only, while some legislation deals with allied health specialists and EMTs. Several states are now in the process of considering more specific laws for their EMS Systems.

   Since the laws governing the duty to act vary from state to state, and what is implied in laws that cover the emergency services also varies, your instructor or local EMS System will tell you the specifics as to when you are required to respond and provide care. Your duties will be spelled out, considering your level of training and your safety at the emergency scene.

   A First Responder is part of the EMS System, and might be considered to have a duty to act once help is offered to a patient. If care is offered and then accepted by the patient, it could be assumed that the First Responder has accepted a duty to act. A court might decide that this meets the first requirement for negligence in cases where the standard of care was not met and the patient suffered injury due to this improper care.

   The second condition for negligence would be applicable if the care was substandard for the First Responder's level of training and experience under the conditions of the emergency scene. The same would apply if the care rendered was above the level of training. In either case, the care provided was not the standard of care.

   Finally, if the first two points are established, the suit for negligence may be successful if the patient was injured (damaged) in some way due directly to the inappropriate actions of the First Responder. This is a complex legal problem, made more difficult by the fact that the damage can be physical, emotional, or psychological.

Physical damage is the easiest to understand. For example, if a First Responder moved a patient's fractured leg before applying a splint and the standard of care states that the First Responder should have suspected a fracture and splinted the limb, then the First Responder may be negligent if this action worsened the existing injury.

The same case becomes much more involved when the patient claims that the First Responder's inappropriate action caused emotional or psychological problems. The court could decide that the patient has been damaged and establish the third requirement for negligence.

Inappropriate care does not always involve splinting, bandaging, or some other physical skill. If you tell an injured or ill patient that he or she does not need to be seen by EMTs or other more highly trained personnel, you could be negligent if:

1. You had a duty to act.
2. The patient accepted your care.
3. The standard of care stated that you should have alerted or had someone alert the EMS dispatcher and request an EMT response.
4. The delay in care caused complications that led to additional injury.

1st REMEMBER: A requirement for the proof of negligence is the failure of the First Responder to provide care to the recognized standard of care. There is no guarantee that you will not be sued, but a successful suit is unlikely if you provide care to this standard.

Abandonment

1st Once you stop to help someone who is sick or injured, you have legally begun care. You now have a duty to provide care bound by the standard of care. If you leave the scene before more highly trained personnel arrive, you have *abandoned* the patient and are subject to legal action under specific laws of abandonment. Since you are not trained in medical diagnosis or how to predict the stability of a patient, you should not leave the patient if someone with training equal to your own arrives at the scene. The patient may develop more serious problems that would be better handled by two First Responders.

Abandonment—to leave a sick or injured patient before equal or more highly trained personnel can assume responsibility for care.

Some legal authorities consider abandonment to include the failure to turn over patient information during the transfer of the patient to more highly trained personnel. You must inform these providers of the facts that you gathered, the assessment made, and the care rendered.

PATIENT RIGHTS—CONSENT

1st Refusal of Care

Adults, when conscious and clear of mind, have the right to refuse your care (refusal of service). Their reasons may be based on religious grounds. They may base their decision on a lack of trust. In fact, they may have reasons that you find senseless. For whatever reasons, competent adults may refuse care. You cannot force care on them, nor can you legally restrain them until EMTs arrive. Your only course of action is to try to gain their confidence through conversation.

The courts recognize implied refusal of care. In other words, the patient does not have to speak to refuse your care. If the patient shakes his head to signal "no," or if he holds up his hand to signal you to stop, the patient has refused your help. Should the patient pull away from you, this may be viewed as refusal of care.

I, _____ hereby refuse aid

and/or transport by _____

Date: _____ Time: _____

I, _____ have refused to

transport the patient because _____

Date: _____ Time: _____

FIGURE 1–6.
A standard release form.

When your services are refused:

- Do *not* argue with patients.
- Do *not* question their reasons if they are based on religious beliefs.
- Do *not* touch patients. If you do, this could be considered to be assault and battery or a violation of their civil rights.
- Stay calm and professional. Any added stress to patients because of your actions could cause serious complications.
- Make certain that dispatch is alerted, even if patients have stated they do not want anyone's help.
- Talk with the patients. Let them know that you are concerned. Tell them that you respect their right to refuse care, but that you think they should reconsider your offer to help.
- When possible, have a neutral witness to your offer to help, your explanation of your level of training, why you think care is needed, and the patient's refusal to accept your care. If your EMS System provides you with release forms, ask the patients to please read and sign the form. Make certain that you ask patients if they understand what they have read before signing the form. Have a witness to any signing of forms.

A parent or legal guardian can refuse to let you treat a child. If the reason is fear or lack of confidence, simple conversation may change the individual's mind. In cases involving children, if the adult takes the child from the scene before EMTs arrive, you *must* report the incident to the EMTs or to the police. Some states have special laws protecting the welfare of children. In these states, such information may have to be passed on to the courts in order to find out if the child eventually received needed care.

1st **Actual Consent**

Actual consent—informed consent by a rational adult patient, usually in oral form, to accept emergency care.

An adult patient, when conscious and clear of mind, can give you **actual consent** to provide care. In First Responder care, this consent is usually oral. To qualify as actual consent, the patient must be making an informed decision. You need to tell the patient that you are a First Responder, trained in emergency care. You must tell the patient:

1. Your level of training.
2. Why you think care may be necessary.
3. What you are going to do.
4. If there is any risk to the care you offer or risk related to refusing care.

■ SCAN 1-2.

Legal Aspects of First Responder Care

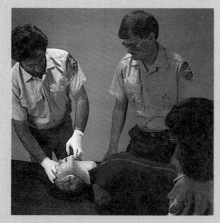 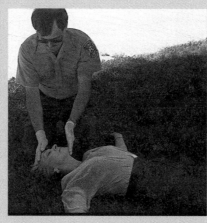 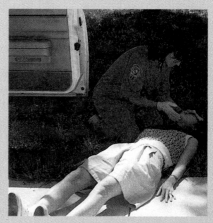

STANDARD OF CARE   Every First Responder is trained to provide the minimum accepted care. In similar situations, the care provided by two different First Responders having the same experience should be equal.

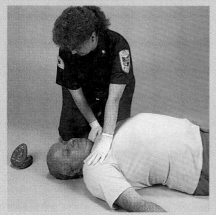 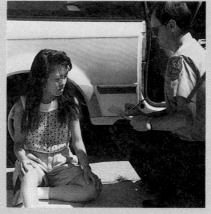 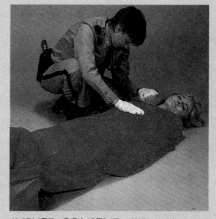

DUTY TO ACT   Some First Responders have a duty to help victims of an emergency.

ACTUAL CONSENT   The conscious, mentally competent adult must grant informed consent. She may refuse care.

IMPLIED CONSENT   When the adult is unable to give actual consent the law assumes that she would.

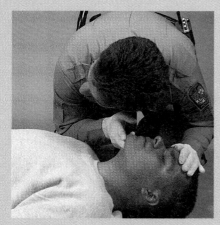 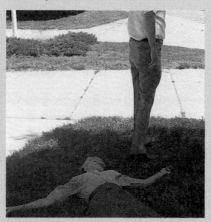 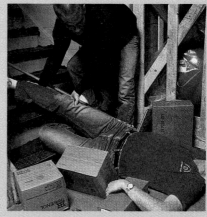

IMMUNITY   In some states, protection from liability is granted if the rescuer acts in good faith to deliver the standard of care.

ABANDONMENT   Once care is initiated, the rescuer assumes responsibility until relieved by equally or more highly trained personnel.

NEGLIGENCE   If there is a duty to act, the care is improper, and injury results, the rescuer may be liable.

Informed consent—actual consent given by a rational adult after being informed of the provider's training and what care procedures are to be done. Risks and options may have to be discussed.

Having this information allows the patient to provide you with **informed consent.**

There are occasions when a child refuses care, but a parent or guardian consents to you providing care. Legally, you have received actual consent to care for this patient. Of course, gaining the child's confidence and easing any fears should be part of your care.

1st Implied Consent

In emergency situations where a patient is unconscious, confused, or so severely injured that a clear decision cannot be made, you have the right to provide care based on **implied consent.** The law assumes that the patient, if able to do so, would want to receive treatment.

Implied consent—a legal position that assumes that an unconscious or badly injured adult patient would consent to receiving emergency care. This form of consent may apply to other types of patients (for example, mentally ill).

A form of implied consent is used in most states when a minor is involved and the parents or guardians are not on the scene and cannot be reached quickly. The law assumes that they would want care to be provided for their child. This is called **minor's consent.** The same holds true in cases of mentally or emotionally disturbed or retarded individuals. It is assumed that their parents, legal guardians, or family would give consent.

Minor's consent—a form of implied consent used when a minor is seriously ill or injured and the parents or guardians cannot be reached quickly.

PATIENT RIGHTS—CONFIDENTIALITY

You should not provide care for patients and then speak to your friends, family, and other members of the public (including the press and media) about the details of your care. You should not name the individuals who received your care. If you speak of the accident, you should not relate specifics about what a patient may have said, any unusual aspects of behavior, or any descriptions of personal appearance. To do so invades the privacy of the patient. Your state may not have specific laws stating the above, but most individuals in emergency care feel very strongly about protecting the patient's right to privacy.

NOTE: Patient confidentiality does not apply if you are asked to provide information to the police or to testify in court. You may be asked to repeat what patients tell you, call out, or tell others while under your care. You should maintain notes about each incident to which you respond.

EQUIPMENT, TOOLS, AND SUPPLIES

Most First Responders carry very little in the way of equipment, tools, and supplies. Even if you are provided with an emergency care kit, you may find yourself providing care when you do not have the kit. The typical First Responder course includes how to use items found at the emergency scene and how to make items for emergency use.

The DOT has recommended that First Responders know how to use, and carry whenever possible, the following items:

- Triangular bandages
- Roller-type bandages
- Universal dressings/gauze pads
- Occlusive dressings (for airtight seals)
- Adhesive tape
- Bandage shears

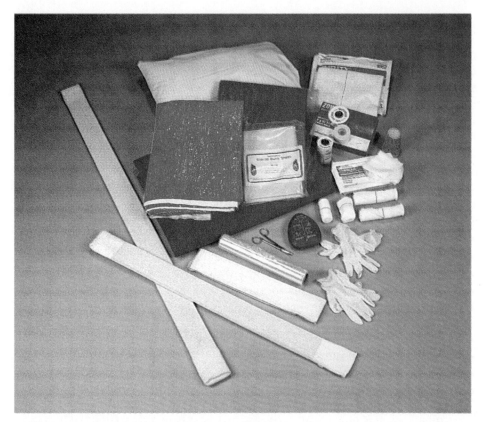

FIGURE 1–7. Medical care equipment and supplies.

- Eye protector (paper cup or cone)
- Stick (for tourniquet)
- Blanket
- Pillow
- Upper extremity splint set
- Lower extremity splint set

You may be required to know how to use or make and use other items. Your instructor may add to the above list, including those items needed for personal safety (see p. 4).

In some localities, First Responders are expected to take blood pressure. In these areas, the kit would include a blood pressure cuff and stethoscope. A few areas of the country have First Responders provide oxygen when appropriate. The First Responders in these areas are provided with oxygen delivery systems.

The DOT has suggested that all First Responders be able to use the following tools and equipment for gaining access to patients:

- Jack
- Jack handle
- Pliers
- Rope
- Screwdriver
- Hammer
- Knife
- Gloves, goggles or faceshield, and other necessary protective clothing

Your course may include other items.

FIRST RESPONDER SKILLS

In addition to learning facts and information, you will be required to perform certain skills as part of your First Responder training. These skills vary somewhat from course to course. The list below is an example of the skills learned by the typical First Responder. You are not expected to memorize this list. Read through the list and check off each skill as you learn it in your course.

As a First Responder, you should be able to:

- Assess and control the scene of a simple accident
- Gain access to patients in cars by way of doors and windows
- Gain access to patients in buildings by way of doors and windows
- Evaluate a scene in terms of safety and possible cause of accident
- Gather information from patients and bystanders
- Properly use all items of personal safety
- Conduct a primary and secondary patient survey, including the patient interview
- Determine vital signs (pulse, breathing, relative skin temperature)
- Determine diagnostic signs
- Relate symptoms and signs to specific illnesses and injuries
- Open a patient's airway, provide airway care, and perform pulmonary resuscitation for adults, infants, children, and neck breathers
- Utilize a pocket face mask with one-way valve to provide ventilations
- Detect cardiac arrest and perform one- and two-rescuer cardiopulmonary resuscitation (CPR)
- Control bleeding by using direct pressure, direct pressure and elevation, pressure dressings, pressure points, and tourniquets
- Detect shock (including allergy shock) and care for patients who develop shock
- Detect and provide care for closed injuries and open injuries, including face and scalp wounds, nosebleeds, eye injuries, neck wounds, chest injuries (including rib fractures, flail chest, and penetrating chest wounds), abdominal injuries, and injuries to the genitalia
- Carry out basic dressing and bandaging techniques
- Detect and care for possible fractures, dislocations, sprains, and strains of the extremities, using soft splints
- Detect and care for possible fractures, dislocations, sprains, and strains of the extremities, using commercial and noncommercial rigid splints
- Detect and care for possible injuries to the cranium and face (skull)
- Detect and care for possible injuries to the neck and spine
- Detect and care for possible heart attacks, strokes, congestive heart failure, seizures, diabetic coma, and insulin shock
- Care for cases of poisoning
- Classify and provide care for first-, second, and third-degree burns
- Detect and care for smoke inhalation
- Detect and care for heat exhaustion, heat stroke, heat cramps, frostnip, frostbite, freezing, and hypothermia
- Assist a mother in delivering her baby
- Provide initial care for the newborn
- Detect and care for drug abuse and alcohol abuse patients
- Perform nonemergency and emergency patient moves when required
- Perform triage at a multiple-patient emergency scene
- Work under the direction of EMTs to help them provide patient care, doing what you have been trained to do

In some systems that have very special needs, all or any of the following may be required:

- Determine blood pressure
- Use a bag-valve-mask resuscitator (ventilator)
- Deliver oxygen when appropriate, modifying techniques when the patient has a chronic obstructive pulmonary disease (COPD)
- Apply or assist in the application of a traction splint
- Apply or assist in the application of a rigid cervical or extrication-collar
- Assist in securing a patient to a long spine board or other device used to immobilize the patient's spine

SUMMARY

The emergency medical services system (EMS System) is a chain of human services established to provide care to the patient at the scene and during transport to the hospital emergency department. The weakest link in this chain is the care provided by those who arrive before the EMTs. It is believed that First Responders will help solve this problem. **First Responders are part of the EMS System.**

First Responders are usually the first trained personnel to arrive at the emergency scene. Their primary concern is their own **personal safety.** Patient assessment and care cannot begin unless the scene and the rescuers are safe.

First Responders have four main duties, including **gaining access to the patient, finding out what is wrong with the patient and providing emergency care, moving patients (when necessary),** and **transferring the patient and patient information** when more highly trained personnel arrive at the scene.

As a First Responder, you may be called upon to **control the scene, call the EMS system dispatcher, gain access to patients, determine what is wrong with patients, care for patients, move patients (when necessary), obtain help from bystanders, transfer patients and patient information,** and **assist EMTs.**

First Responder **emergency care** deals with both **injury** and **illness.** Care can range from emotional support to basic life support measures.

First Responder responsibilities are very demanding. You will have to maintain your skills and keep up to date. You will have to be able to deal with people, knowing what to say and what not to say to patients. Patients need you to perform as a professional.

In many states, specific laws have been written to allow you to provide emergency care to patients without fear of successful civil legal action being taken against you. **Good Samaritan laws** may provide most First Responders with immunity. You are protected if you **act in good faith,** providing the First Responder **standard of care to your level of training and to the best of your abilities.**

A First Responder might be found **negligent** if he has a duty to provide care, does not provide care to the standard of care, and the inappropriate care causes injury (damage) to the patient.

When you stop to provide care for a patient, you have responsibility for the patient until someone more highly trained takes over this responsibility. If you start to treat a patient and then leave the scene, you can be charged with **abandonment.**

A patient can refuse your care. You must have **actual consent** from a conscious, clear-thinking adult patient. This consent is usually oral. It must be **informed consent,** with the patient knowing your level of training and what you are going to do.

In cases when the patient is unable to give consent, you may care for the patient under the law of **implied consent.**

Implied consent also applies to children (minor's consent) and emotionally or mentally disturbed or retarded patients when their parents or legal guardians are not present.

Patients have a right to their privacy. First Responders must respect **patient confidentiality.**

A SPECIAL NOTE

Warnings emphasizing infection control appear in this chapter and throughout the book. As a First Responder, you must be aware of the potential dangers that exist when providing care. You will not be able to tell which patient carries potentially fatal microorganisms. Every patient care situation will require you to use the universal precautions recommended by the U.S. Department of Health and Human Services/Centers for Disease Control (CDC), U.S. Department of Labor/Occupational Safety and Health Administration (OSHA), U.S. Fire Administration (USFA), and National Fire Protection Association (NFPA) subcommittee on Infection Control Programs.

You must avoid contact with infectious agents and prevent the spread of these agents. Personal protective equipment must be worn when providing care. Approved, safe ventilation devices must be used for rescue breathing. Also, you must follow your local EMS System's guidelines for removing gloves, washing your hands and other skin surfaces, disposing of gloves and soiled linen, disposing of soiled dressings, and disinfecting re-usable equipment. Make certain that you receive any required immunizations against vaccine-preventable diseases and that you always follow all specific follow-up procedures after possible exposure to infectious agents.

CHAPTER 2

The Human Body

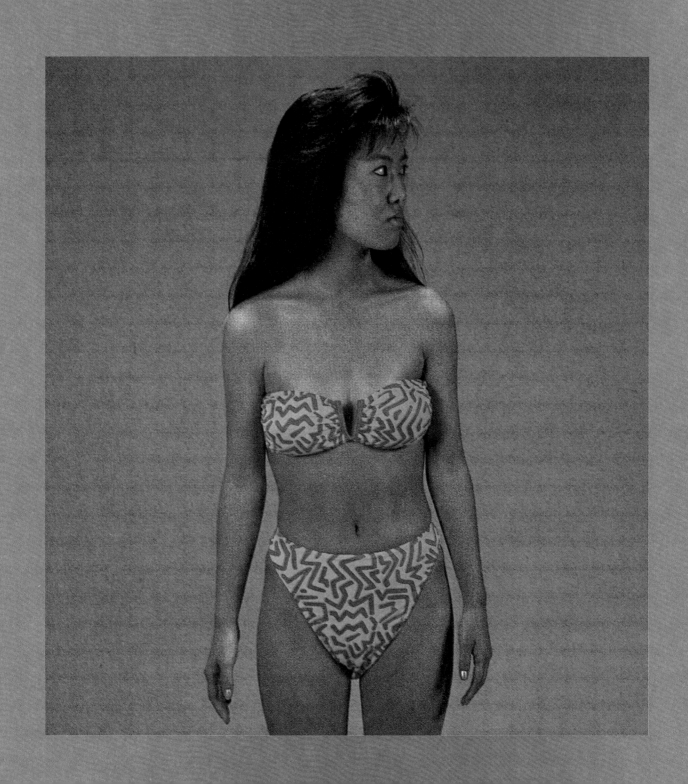

■ OBJECTIVES

By the end of this chapter, you should be able to:

1. State one of the ways in which First Responders must be able to apply their knowledge of anatomy. (p. 21)
2. Name two types of structures that are found in every location in the body. (p. 21)
3. Describe the anatomical position. (p. 21)
4. Define and properly apply the terms anterior, posterior, midline, medial, lateral, patient's right, and patient's left. (Optional terms: proximal, distal, superior, inferior) (p. 21)
5. Use common terminology to list the five major regions of the body and the subdivisions of each region. (p. 23)
6. Name and locate the four major body cavities. (pp. 24–25)
7. Identify the four abdominal quadrants. (p. 25)
8. Match given body functions to specific body systems. (p. 26)
9. Locate on your own body the anatomical position of the heart, lungs, diaphragm, stomach, liver, gallbladder, pancreas, spleen, small intestine, large intestine, kidneys, and urinary bladder. (pp. 26–31)

SKILLS

You should practice applying the knowledge gained in this chapter until you can look at another person's body and mentally determine the position of the major organs of the chest and abdomen.

OVERVIEW OF THE HUMAN BODY

The Head-to-Toe Approach

Students beginning training in First Responder and emergency care courses are often a little worried about having to learn human anatomy. Relax. You will not be learning very many new terms or structures. You might be a little surprised to find where some structures are located, since few of us have an accurate idea of the exact location of all of our body structures. As a First Responder, you will not need to be as precise as medical personnel are when they consider the human body. However, you will need to know the basic body structures and their locations.

No one will be asking you to take a stethoscope and outline the borders of the heart. You know, generally, where the heart is located in the chest. We will show you some quick ways to be more specific about the location of the heart when we study CPR, or cardiopulmonary resuscitation (KAR-de-o-PUL-mo-ner-e re-SUS-si-ta-shun).

You probably know the general location of the lungs. You may be a little off in locating the stomach and the liver. Odds are you will be less accurate in locating the uterus (womb), and even less accurate in locating the ovaries. The main thing to keep in mind as you begin your studies is that you know all these structures exist and you have a general idea of where they are located.

Do not become too concerned with trying to learn a lot of medical terminology. A head is still a head and feet are still feet. Most of the terms relating to human anatomy are so important to us that they have been a part of our vocabulary for years. Brain, eyes, ears, teeth, heart, lungs, liver, stomach, bladder, and spinal cord are all valid terms in emergency medicine.

You will learn a few new terms. You will also take a few terms that you may have heard before (such as carotid artery) and make these terms as much a part of your vocabulary as heart and lung.

1st To be a First Responder you must be able to look at a person's body and know the major internal structures and the general location of these structures. Your concern is not how the body looks dissected, or how the body looks on an anatomical wall chart. You must be concerned with living bodies and knowing where things are located as you look from the outside.

1st You know about blood vessels and nerves. As you look at any region of the body, **remember:**

- For our purposes, blood vessels go everywhere in the body, to every structure.
- For our purposes, nerves go everywhere in the body, to every structure.

When you look at an arm, you must see something that is alive and part of a living organism. You know that an arm is made of muscles, bones, blood vessels, nerves, and other tissues. When you assess injuries, *never* forget that there could be internal bleeding and that damaged nerves may be causing pain, loss of feeling, or even loss of function.

Directional Terms

1st The following is a set of very basic terms to use when referring to the human body:

Anatomical (AN-ah-TOM-i-kal) *position*—Consider the human body, standing erect, facing you. The arms are down at the sides with the palms of the hands facing forward. References to all body structures are made when the body is in the anatomical position. This is very important when considering the bones and blood vessels in the arm.

Right and Left—Always make reference to the **patient's right** and **patient's left.** Even though you may think this is very simple, many students find this to be difficult. Practice until you can use these terms correctly every time.

Anterior and posterior—**Anterior** refers to the **front** of the body and **posterior** indicates the **back** of the body. For the head, the face is considered anterior, while all the remaining structures are posterior. The rest of the body can be easily divided into anterior and posterior by following the side seams of your clothing.

Midline—An imaginary vertical line can be used to divide the body into right and left halves. Anything toward the midline is said to be **medial,** while anything away from the midline is said to be **lateral.** Remember the **anatomical position,** which places the thumb on the lateral side of the hand and the little finger on the medial side.

Anatomical position—the body is standing erect, facing the observer. The arms are down at the sides and the palms of the hands face forward.

Anterior—the front of the body or body part.

Posterior—the back of the body or body part.

Medial—toward the midline (vertical center) of the body.

Lateral—away from the vertical midline of the body.

Superior—toward the top of the body or body part.

Inferior—away from the top of the body. Toward the feet or the lower border of a body part.

There are other directional terms that can be useful. **Superior** means toward the top of the head, as in "the eyes are superior to the nose." **Inferior** means toward the feet, as in "the mouth is inferior to the nose." You cannot say something is superior or inferior unless you are comparing at least two structures. The heart is not superior, it is superior to the stomach. Since you are using the anatomical position for all your references to the body, any medical professional will know what you mean when you say a wound is just above the eye. For this reason, superior and inferior may be optional terms in your course.

Proximal and **distal** also may be optional terms in your course. These two terms are often used incorrectly and should be avoided unless you are certain of their correct usage. If we limit our discussion to the anatomy a First Responder must know, most medical professionals only use proximal

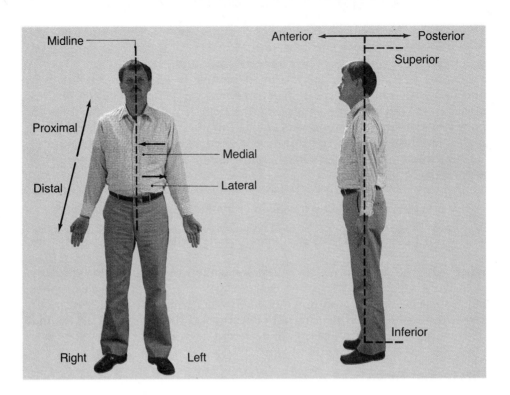

FIGURE 2–1. Directional terms.

and distal in reference to the arms and legs. To use proximal and distal, there must be a point of reference and two structures to be compared. The structure closest to the point of reference is said to be proximal, while the structure farthest away is distal. It helps to think that the close structure is in the *prox*imity of the reference, while the far structure is some *dist*ance away.

The most commonly used points of reference are the shoulder joint and the hip joint. Thus, the elbow is said to be proximal when compared to the wrist, which is distal. The knee is proximal when compared to the ankle. Trying to remember all this in an emergency situation could lead to some confusion. Since you will be talking to medical professionals on the scene, many First Responder courses consider these terms to be optional.

Most First Responders do not deal with accidents and medical emergencies on a daily basis. Unless they review and use the terms, they find the terminology becoming less useful with time. Be aware that medical and rescue personnel are trained to take your information. They will not be confused if you say front, back, above, and below. *Do not* let terminology stand in the way of clear communication with EMTs, paramedics, doctors, and other medical professional. *Do* take great care when using right and left, and medial and lateral.

NOTE: In an emergency, if you are not certain about the correct usage of a medical term, use the common term. You may seriously damage your credibility by using the wrong medical term, or you may delay the EMTs as they try to determine the actual meaning of what you have said.

Summary

All references made to body structures consider the body to be in the **anatomical position.** Always use **patient's right** and **patient's left.** Use an imaginary vertical **midline** as a point of reference. **Medial** means toward the midline, while **lateral** means away from the midline. **Anterior** refers to the front and **posterior** refers to the back.

1st Body Regions

The human body can be divided into five regions. These regions have the common, everyday names of head, neck, trunk, upper extremities (arms and hands), and lower extremities (legs and feet). Later in this text, you will be asked to study some specific areas within each of these regions. For example, you will have to understand the pelvic girdle and how the legs join the trunk of the body so that you can relate certain injuries to specific types of accidents. For now, in order to begin your new approach in viewing the body, start with the simplest of subdivisions:

Head

Cranium–housing the brain
Face
Mandible (MAN-di-b'l)—the
   lower jaw

Neck

Trunk

Chest—known as the **thorax**
   (THO-raks)
Abdomen—extending from the
   lower ribs to the pelvic girdle
Pelvis—protected by the bones
   of the pelvic girdle

Upper Extremities

Shoulder joint
Upper arm
Elbow
Forearm
Wrist
Hand

Lower Extremities

Hip joint
Thigh
Knee
Lower leg
Ankle
Foot

   Thorax, mandible, and cranium may not be used in most daily conversations, but all the other terms are already part of your vocabulary. The significant thing is to begin looking for these simple subdivisions each time you

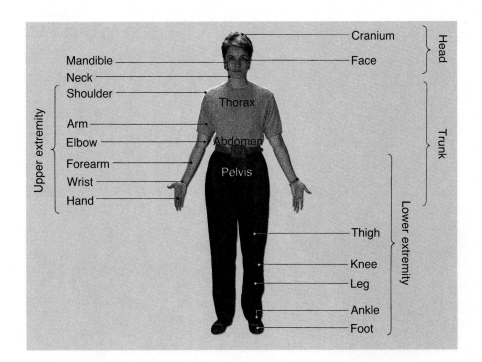

FIGURE 2–2. Body regions.

consider possible diseases and injuries. As stated earlier, more specifics will be covered throughout this text.

1st Body Cavities

There are four major body cavities, two anterior and two posterior. Housed in these cavities are the vital organs, glands, blood vessels, and nerves.

Anterior Cavities

- *Chest cavity*—Also known as the **thoracic (tho-RAS-ik) cavity.** It is enclosed by the rib cage, protecting the lungs, heart, great blood vessels, part of the windpipe (trachea) and part of the esophagus (e-SOF-ah-gus) (the tube leading from the throat to the stomach). The lower border of the chest cavity is the **diaphragm** (DI-ah-fram), a dome-shaped muscle used in breathing. The diaphragm separates the thoracic cavity from the lower anterior cavity. It is important to know the location of the diaphragm (see Figure 2–4).
- *Abdominopelvic* (ab-DOM-i-no-PEL-vik) *cavity*—The anterior body cavity below the diaphragm. There are two portions of the abdominopelvic cavity: abdominal and pelvic. If you study more anatomy on your own, you will see this term, but most people use the terms **abdominal cavity** and **pelvic cavity.**

  Abdominal cavity—This cavity extends from below the lower ribs to the region protected by the pelvic bones. The stomach, liver, gallbladder, pancreas, spleen, small intestine, and most of the large intestine can be found in this cavity. The abdominal cavity, unlike the other body cavities, is not surrounded by bones. If you consider all the organs in this cavity and the lack of this bony protection, it is easy to see why blows to the abdomen can cause severe injury.

  Pelvic Cavity—Protected by the bones of the pelvic girdle, this cavity houses the urinary bladder, portions of the large intestine, and the internal reproductive organs.

Posterior Cavities

- *Cranial cavity*—This is the braincase of the skull, housing the brain and its specialized membranes.

Thoracic cavity (tho-RAS-ik)—the anterior body cavity that is above (superior to) the diaphragm. The *thorax* (THO-raks).

Diaphragm (DI-ah-fram)—the dome-shaped muscle of breathing that separates the chest cavity (thorax) from the abdominal cavity.

Abdominal cavity—the anterior body cavity that extends from the diaphragm to the region protected by the pelvic bones.

Pelvic cavity—the anterior body cavity surrounded by the bones of the pelvis.

FIGURE 2–3. Body cavities.

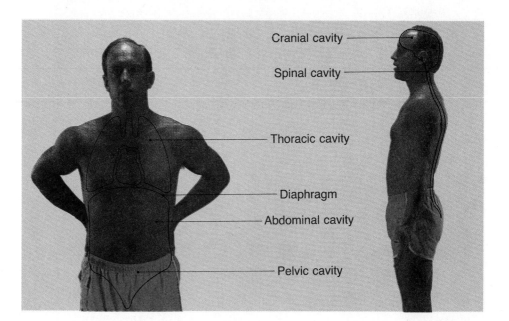

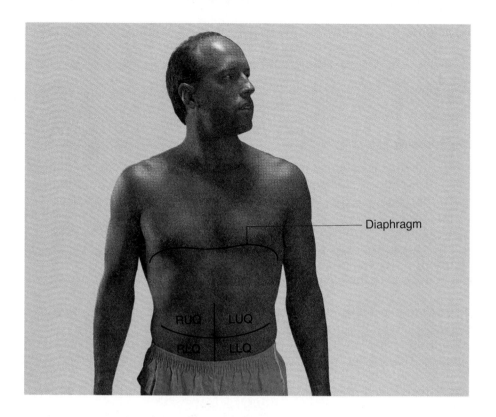

FIGURE 2–4. Abdominal quadrants.

- *Spinal cavity*—This cavity runs through the center of the backbone, protecting the spinal cord and its specialized membranes.

1st Abdominal Quadrants

The abdomen is a large body region and the abdominal cavity contains many vital organs. In other body regions, bones may be used for reference, such as counting the ribs or using a bump or notch on a bone. This is not the case when trying to be specific with the abdomen. The navel or umbilicus (um-BIL-i-kus) is the only quick point of reference available for the First Responder. To improve this situation, the abdominal wall has been divided into four quadrants (see Figure 2–4). These quadrants are the:

Abdominal quadrants—the four major regions of the abdomen that are used to provide quick points of reference.

Right Upper Quadrant (RUQ)—containing most of the liver, the gallbladder, and part of the large intestine.

Left Upper Quadrant (LUQ)—containing most of the stomach, the spleen, and part of the large intestine.

Right Lower Quadrant (RLQ)—containing the appendix and part of the large intestine.

Left Lower Quadrant (LLQ)—containing part of the large intestine.

NOTE: "Right" and "left" refer to patient's right and patient's left.

Some organs and glands are located in more than one quadrant. As you can see from the above list, the large intestine is found, in part, in all four quadrants. The same is true for the small intestine. Part of the stomach can be found in the right upper quadrant. The left lobe of the liver extends into the left upper quadrant. Pelvic organs are included in these quadrants, with the urinary bladder being assigned to both lower quadrants.

The kidneys are a special case. They are not part of the abdominal cavity, being located behind the cavity's membrane lining. Consider one kidney to be RUQ and the other to be LUQ. However, do not let this abdominal classification make you think that the kidneys are in the abdominal cavity.

The location of the kidneys makes them subject to injury from blows to the mid-back. Any pain or ache in the back may involve the kidneys.

Body Systems

Knowing the body systems and their functions can prove to be of value to the First Responder. However, most training courses do not have the time to go into great detail in terms of anatomy and physiology. Throughout the text, specific anatomy and some basic functions will be covered as they apply to injury, disease, and the First Responder-level care.

Remembering the different body functions can be useful when trying to determine the extent of injury or the nature of a medical emergency. The following lists the major body systems and their primary functions:

- *Circulatory system*—moving blood, carrying oxygen and foods to the body's cells and removing wastes and carbon dioxide from these cells.
- *Respiratory system*—exchanging air to bring in oxygen and expel carbon dioxide. This oxygen is placed into the bloodstream while carbon dioxide is being removed.
- *Digestive system*—digesting and absorbing food and removing certain wastes.
- *Urinary system*—removing chemical wastes from the blood and helping to balance water and salt levels of the blood.
- *Reproductive system*—producing all structures and hormones needed for sexual reproduction. Sometimes classified with the urinary system as the genitourinary (Jen-e-to-U-re-NER-e) system.
- *Nervous system*—controlling movement, interpreting sensations, regulating body activities, and generating memory and thought.
- *Endocrine (EN-do-krin) system*—producing the chemicals called hormones that help regulate most body activities and functions.
- *Musculoskeletal (MUS-que-lo-SKEL-et-l) system*—providing protection and support for the body and internal organs and permitting body movement.
- *Special senses*—providing sight, hearing, taste, smell, and the sensations of pain, cold, heat, and tactile responses (smoothness, roughness, softness, and the like).

In addition to the above, there is a system composed of the skin and related structures (hair, sweat glands), and a system to protect the body from disease-causing organisms.

1st RELATING STRUCTURES TO THE BODY

In this section, we will use a series of illustrations to show what you should be able to do as a First Responder considering the human body. Your problem is a complex one, requiring much thought and practice before you will be comfortable with the new knowledge to be gained in your training. As we stated earlier, your task is to know where structures are, in general, as you view the external body. On many of these illustrations, you will see a line representing the diaphragm. Being able to visualize the position of the diaphragm will greatly help you understand how the various organs and glands fit into the body.

Begin with Figure 2–5. Here we see the position of the heart in the chest cavity. As a quick point of reference, use your fingers to find a small,

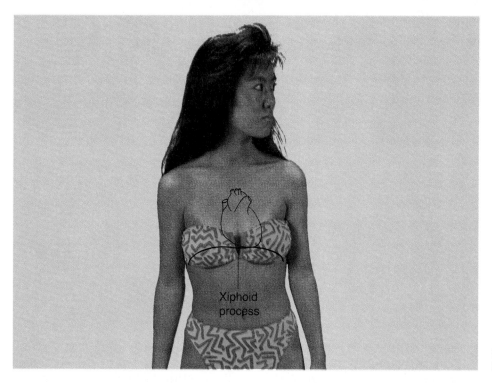

FIGURE 2–5.   Position of the heart.

hard spot just below your breastbone (sternum). This is the xiphoid (ZI-foyd) process, a major body landmark. You can find a point directly over the inferior (lower) border of the heart by measuring two finger-widths up from this point. Look at yourself in a mirror and find this point. Each time you look in the mirror during your training, try to visualize where your heart is located.

Figure 2–6 shows you the position of the lungs in the chest cavity. Notice that the lungs do not extend downward to the end of the rib cage. By studying Figure 2–6, you will have a good idea of the size, shape, and position of the lungs.

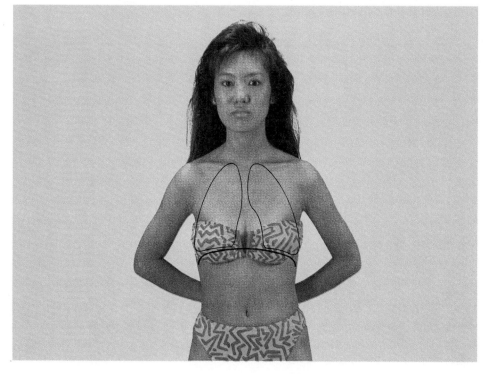

FIGURE 2–6.
Position of the lungs.

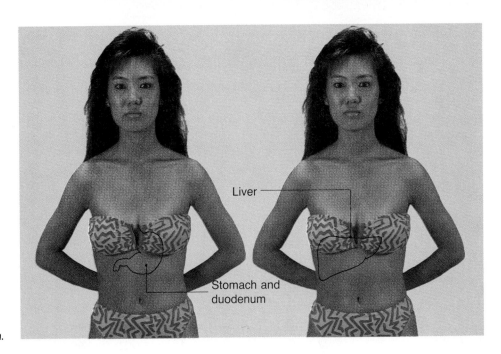

FIGURE 2–7. Position of the stomach, liver, and duodenum.

The two illustrations in Figure 2–7 show the position of the stomach, liver, and the first portion of the small intestine (called the duodenum: du-o-DE-num). Note how the lower ribs protect the stomach and liver. The level of the xiphoid process is where the esophagus enters the stomach, immediately after passing through the diaphragm. If this makes sense to you, then you are gaining a firm grasp of human anatomy. If it doesn't, then you need to set aside time to review the first part of this chapter.

The first portion of the small intestine is important in emergency medicine because it is held in a more rigid position than the rest of the small intestine. Forceful blows to the abdomen, often received in automobile accidents, may injure the first portion of the small intestine without causing any significant damage to the rest of the intestine.

Using Figure 2–8, you can quickly add the positions of three other structures based on what you have already learned. Think of the gallbladder as being behind the liver, the pancreas as behind the lower part of the stomach,

FIGURE 2–8. Position of the gallbladder, pancreas, and spleen.

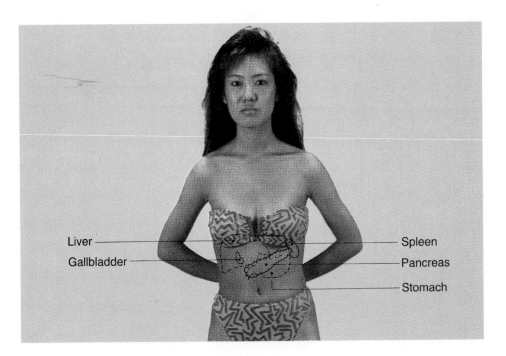

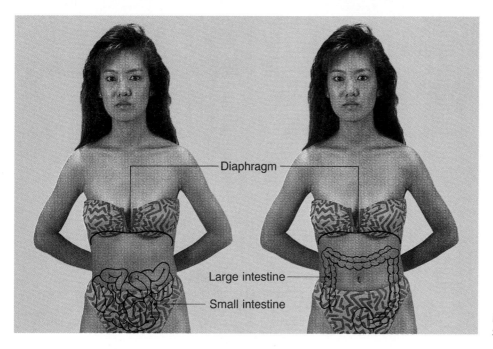

Diaphragm

Large intestine

Small intestine

FIGURE 2–9. Position of the small and large intestine.

and the spleen behind the left side of the stomach. These descriptions would not be good enough if you were a student of anatomy, but they are very useful to a First Responder in an emergency situation. Knowing these general locations will improve your chances of correctly assessing the severity of many injuries to the abdomen.

Figure 2–9 shows, on the left, the space occupied by the small intestine. As you can see, it fills most of the abdominal cavity. On the right you can see the space occupied by the large intestine. Do not try to memorize its shape, but note how it passes through each of the four abdominal quadrants as it "frames" the small intestine.

The kidneys and the urinary bladder are shown in Figure 2–10. Remember, the kidneys are behind the abdominal cavity and the bladder is in the pelvic cavity. Although they appear well protected, injuries to these structures are common in motor vehicle accidents. This is particularly true when occupants not wearing seat belts are thrown about the passenger

FIGURE 2–10.
The urinary system.

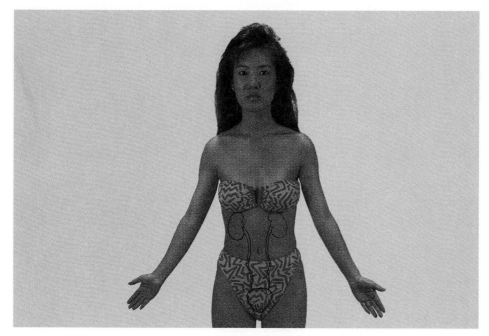

Major Body Organs

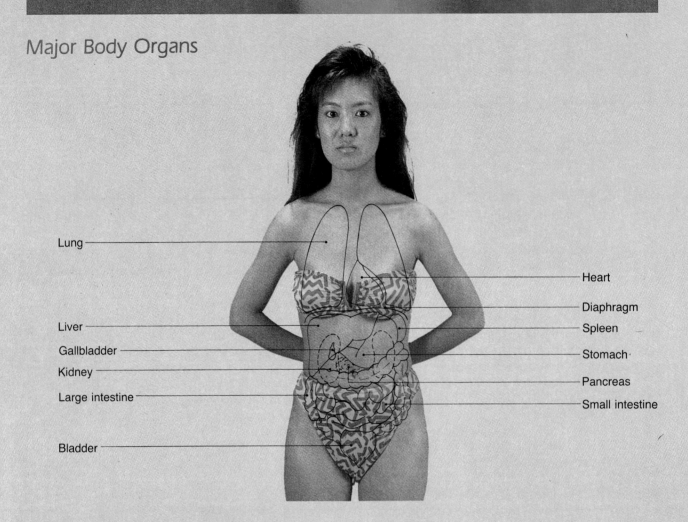

Lung
Liver
Gallbladder
Kidney
Large intestine
Bladder

Heart
Diaphragm
Spleen
Stomach
Pancreas
Small intestine

SOLID ORGANS

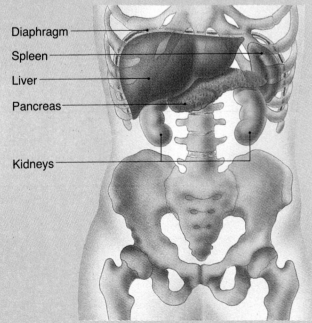

Diaphragm
Spleen
Liver
Pancreas
Kidneys

HOLLOW ORGANS

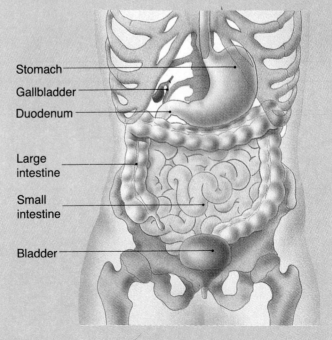

Stomach
Gallbladder
Duodenum
Large intestine
Small intestine
Bladder

compartment. Gunshot wounds, stab wounds, severe blows to the abdomen or back, and crushing injuries are other common sources of injury.

We have spent a good deal of time and effort on the illustrations dealing with the anterior cavities and their structures. Scansheet 2.1 sums up this material with an internal view, a view of the hollow organs, and a view of the solid organs. This shows you all that you have covered so far. Learning such drawings will not be of much help to you as a First Responder unless you spend the time to relate the positions of these organs to the body's exterior.

On occasion throughout this text we will look at the positions of other body structures. You will see the complexity of the neck, the regions of the spine, major nerve bundles, and many other anatomical structures.

SUMMARY

Before returning to the list of objectives on page 20, use your own body as a reference and:

1. Use the terms anterior, posterior, medial, and lateral.
2. Outline your own major body cavities. What do you find in each cavity?
3. Point to each of your abdominal quadrants. Can you name any of the organs found in each quadrant?
4. Look in a mirror. Where are your heart, lungs, xiphoid process, liver, stomach, gallbladder, pancreas, spleen, small intestine, and large intestine? Can you locate your bladder and kidneys?

Go back to the chapter objectives and be sure that you can meet every objective for this chapter. Then, through the rest of your training, continue to practice locating the positions of the body's organs and glands. Add new structures to your list as they appear in the text.

ANATOMY AND PHYSIOLOGY PLATES AND ATLAS OF INJURIES PHOTOGRAPHS

The anatomical plates included in this text are designed to help you learn the anatomy and physiology of the major body systems as you progress through your First Responder course. The plates are not grouped together to indicate that they should be learned all at once. You may wish to refer to them throughout your course as aids in learning the various body structures and systems as they are covered and needed in your training.

The injury photographs that follow show major types of body injuries.

Anatomy Plates

- Membranes, p. 32
- Special Senses, p. 33
- Skeleton, p. 34
- Muscles, p. 35
- The Heart, p. 36
- Blood Vessels, p. 37
- The Nervous System, pp. 38–39
- Respiration, p. 40
- Digestion, p. 41
- Excretion, p. 42
- Reproduction, p. 43

Atlas of Injuries, pp. 44–47

MEMBRANES

The Skin

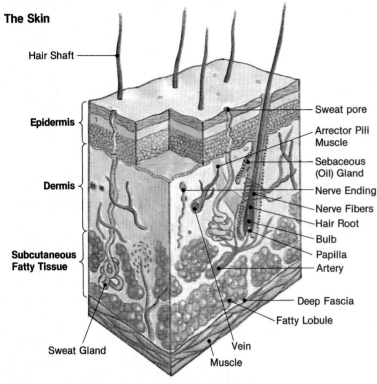

Hair Shaft

Epidermis

Dermis

Subcutaneous
Fatty Tissue

Sweat pore
Arrector Pili Muscle
Sebaceous (Oil) Gland
Nerve Ending
Nerve Fibers
Hair Root
Bulb
Papilla
Artery
Deep Fascia
Fatty Lobule

Sweat Gland

Vein
Muscle

The skin is the largest organ of the body. In the adult the skin covers about 3000 square inches (1.75 square meters) and weighs about 6 pounds. It is involved with protection, insulation, thermal regulation, excretion, and the production of vitamin D.

The Peritoneum

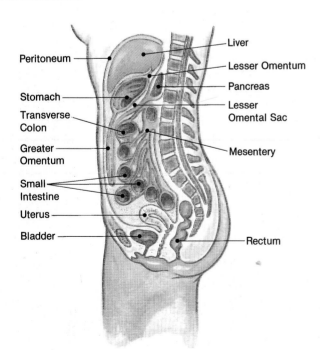

Peritoneum

Stomach

Transverse Colon

Greater Omentum

Small Intestine

Uterus

Bladder

Liver
Lesser Omentum
Pancreas
Lesser Omental Sac

Mesentery

Rectum

Membranes

Membranes cover or line body structures to provide protection from injury and infection. There are four major classes of membranes. Mucous membranes line those structures that open to the outside world (for example, the mouth, the airway, digestive tract, urinary tract, and vagina). Serous membranes line the closed body cavities and cover the outsides of organs. The cutaneous membrane is the skin. Synovial membranes line joints to reduce friction during movement.

A serous membrane that covers an organ is called a visceral layer. The term parietal layer is used for the part of the serous membrane that lines a cavity. The serous membrane in the thoracic cavity is called pleura (for example, the parietal pleura lines the chest cavity). In the abdominal cavity, it is called peritoneum (for example, the parietal peritoneum). A double layer of peritoneum is called mesentery. The membrane that lines the sac surrounding the heart is pericardium.

Synovial Joint

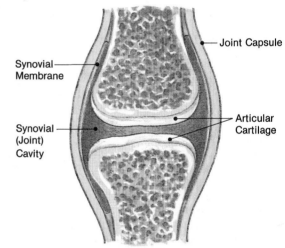

Synovial Membrane

Synovial (Joint) Cavity

Joint Capsule

Articular Cartilage

The Pleura

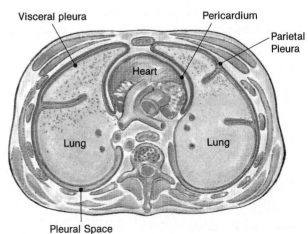

Visceral pleura

Pericardium

Parietal Pleura

Heart

Lung

Lung

Pleural Space

SPECIAL SENSES
The Eye and Ear

The Eye

The body has the sense of vision, hearing, balance and equilibrium, touch, pain, heat, cold, pressure, taste, and smell.

The eye can receive and focus light and then convert this energy into nerve impulses to be sent to the brain. The nerve impulses originate from the retina. Visual receptors in the retina called rods can work in low intensity light. They have no color function. The visual receptors called cones operate in high intensity light and do receive colors.

The ear's functions include hearing, static equilibrium (balance while standing still), and dynamic equilibrium (balance when moving). The outer and middle ear are responsible for sound gathering and its transmission. The inner ear has the nerve endings for hearing and equilibrium.

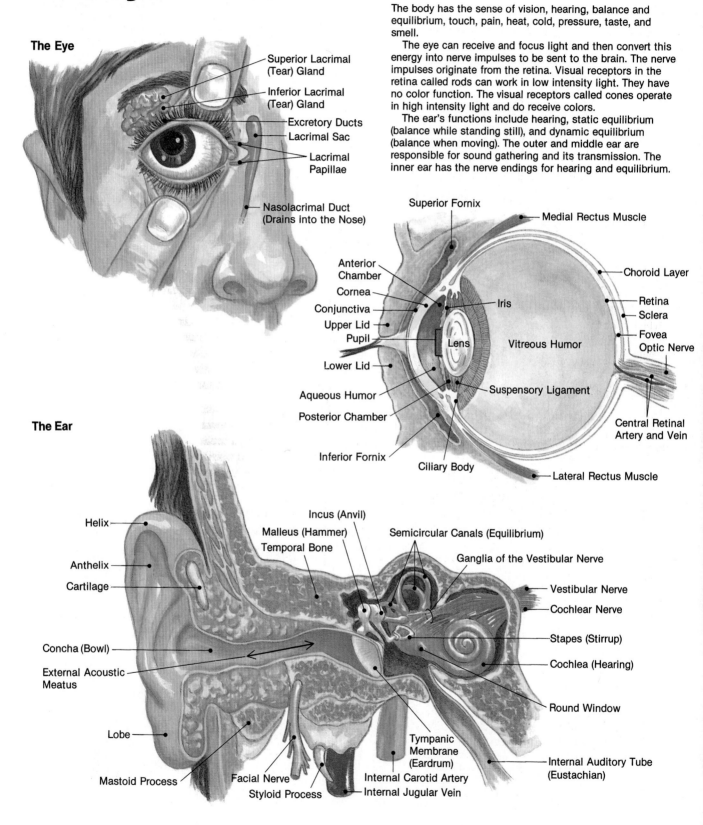

The Eye labels:
Superior Lacrimal (Tear) Gland
Inferior Lacrimal (Tear) Gland
Excretory Ducts
Lacrimal Sac
Lacrimal Papillae
Nasolacrimal Duct (Drains into the Nose)

Eye cross-section labels:
Superior Fornix
Medial Rectus Muscle
Anterior Chamber
Cornea
Conjunctiva
Upper Lid
Pupil
Lower Lid
Aqueous Humor
Posterior Chamber
Inferior Fornix
Ciliary Body
Iris
Lens
Vitreous Humor
Suspensory Ligament
Choroid Layer
Retina
Sclera
Fovea
Optic Nerve
Central Retinal Artery and Vein
Lateral Rectus Muscle

The Ear

The Ear labels:
Helix
Anthelix
Cartilage
Concha (Bowl)
External Acoustic Meatus
Lobe
Mastoid Process
Facial Nerve
Styloid Process
Incus (Anvil)
Malleus (Hammer)
Temporal Bone
Semicircular Canals (Equilibrium)
Ganglia of the Vestibular Nerve
Vestibular Nerve
Cochlear Nerve
Stapes (Stirrup)
Cochlea (Hearing)
Round Window
Internal Auditory Tube (Eustachian)
Tympanic Membrane (Eardrum)
Internal Carotid Artery
Internal Jugular Vein

SKELETON

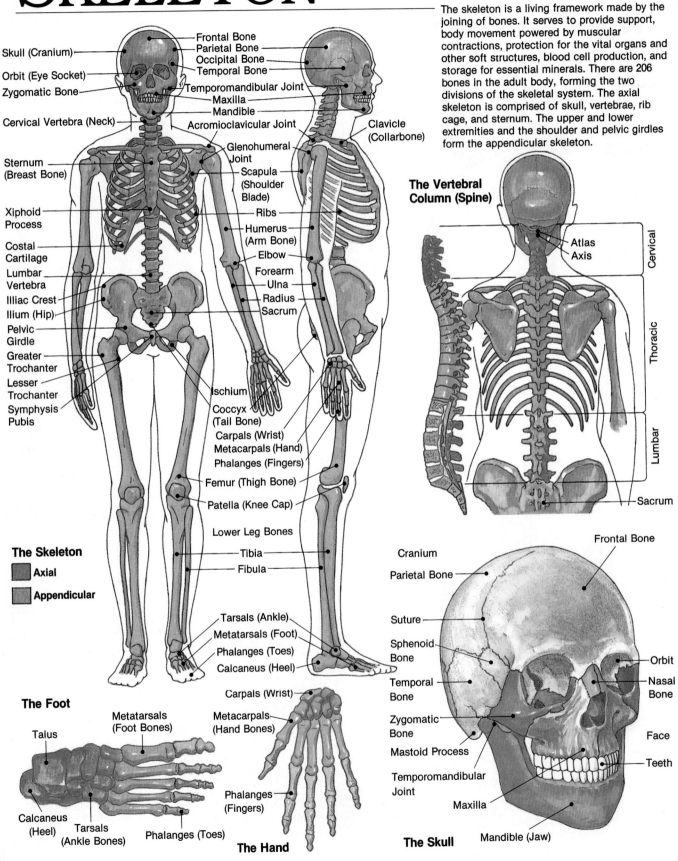

The skeleton is a living framework made by the joining of bones. It serves to provide support, body movement powered by muscular contractions, protection for the vital organs and other soft structures, blood cell production, and storage for essential minerals. There are 206 bones in the adult body, forming the two divisions of the skeletal system. The axial skeleton is comprised of skull, vertebrae, rib cage, and sternum. The upper and lower extremities and the shoulder and pelvic girdles form the appendicular skeleton.

Skull (Cranium)
Orbit (Eye Socket)
Zygomatic Bone
Cervical Vertebra (Neck)
Sternum (Breast Bone)
Xiphoid Process
Costal Cartilage
Lumbar Vertebra
Illiac Crest
Ilium (Hip)
Pelvic Girdle
Greater Trochanter
Lesser Trochanter
Symphysis Pubis

Frontal Bone
Parietal Bone
Occipital Bone
Temporal Bone
Temporomandibular Joint
Maxilla
Mandible
Acromioclavicular Joint
Glenohumeral Joint
Scapula (Shoulder Blade)
Ribs
Humerus (Arm Bone)
Elbow
Forearm
Ulna
Radius
Sacrum
Ischium
Coccyx (Tail Bone)
Carpals (Wrist)
Metacarpals (Hand)
Phalanges (Fingers)
Femur (Thigh Bone)
Patella (Knee Cap)
Lower Leg Bones
Tibia
Fibula
Tarsals (Ankle)
Metatarsals (Foot)
Phalanges (Toes)
Calcaneus (Heel)

Clavicle (Collarbone)

The Skeleton
- Axial
- Appendicular

The Vertebral Column (Spine)

Atlas
Axis
Cervical
Thoracic
Lumbar
Sacrum

The Foot
Talus
Metatarsals (Foot Bones)
Calcaneus (Heel)
Tarsals (Ankle Bones)
Phalanges (Toes)

The Hand
Carpals (Wrist)
Metacarpals (Hand Bones)
Phalanges (Fingers)

The Skull
Cranium
Parietal Bone
Suture
Sphenoid Bone
Temporal Bone
Zygomatic Bone
Mastoid Process
Temporomandibular Joint
Maxilla
Frontal Bone
Orbit
Nasal Bone
Face
Teeth
Mandible (Jaw)

MUSCLES
The Muscular System

The tissues of the muscular system comprise 40 to 50% of the body's weight. The skeletal muscles of the body are voluntary muscles, subject to conscious control. They exhibit the properties of excitability; that is, they will react to nerve stimulus. Once stimulated, skeleton muscles are quick to contract and can relax and very quickly be ready for another contraction. There are 501 separate skeletal muscles that provide contractions for movement, coordinated support for posture, and heat production. Muscles connect to bones by way of tendons.

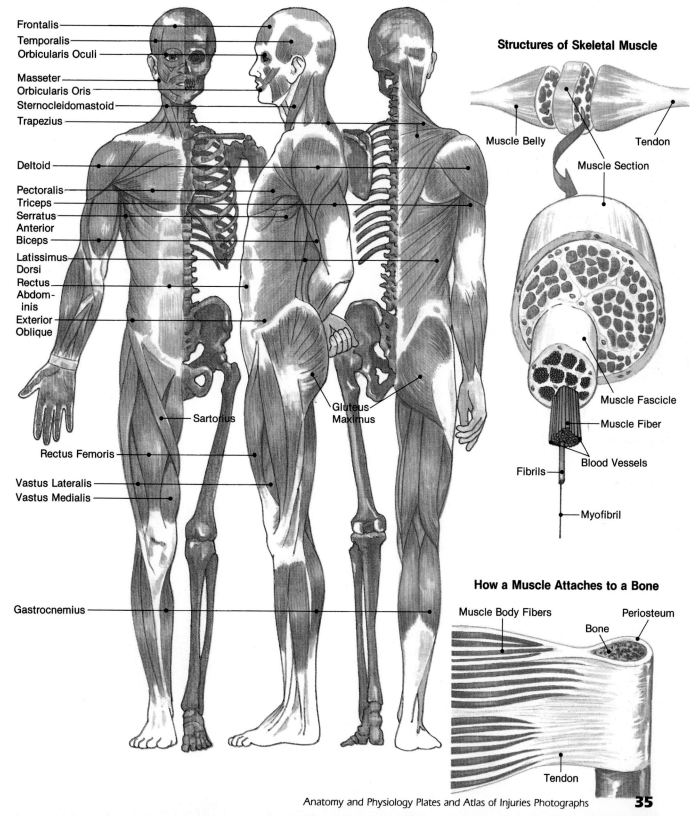

Frontalis
Temporalis
Orbicularis Oculi
Masseter
Orbicularis Oris
Sternocleidomastoid
Trapezius
Deltoid
Pectoralis
Triceps
Serratus Anterior
Biceps
Latissimus Dorsi
Rectus Abdominis
Exterior Oblique
Sartorius
Gluteus Maximus
Rectus Femoris
Vastus Lateralis
Vastus Medialis
Gastrocnemius

Structures of Skeletal Muscle

Muscle Belly
Tendon
Muscle Section
Muscle Fascicle
Muscle Fiber
Blood Vessels
Fibrils
Myofibril

How a Muscle Attaches to a Bone

Muscle Body Fibers
Bone
Periosteum
Tendon

THE HEART
The Cardiovascular System

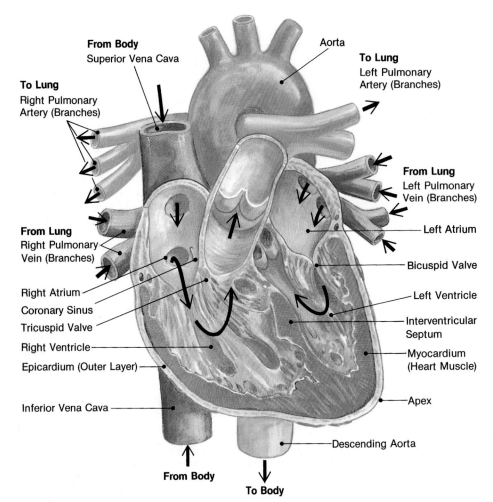

From Body
Superior Vena Cava

Aorta

To Lung
Left Pulmonary
Artery (Branches)

To Lung
Right Pulmonary
Artery (Branches)

From Lung
Left Pulmonary
Vein (Branches)

Left Atrium

From Lung
Right Pulmonary
Vein (Branches)

Bicuspid Valve

Right Atrium

Left Ventricle

Coronary Sinus

Tricuspid Valve

Interventricular
Septum

Right Ventricle

Epicardium (Outer Layer)

Myocardium
(Heart Muscle)

Inferior Vena Cava

Apex

Descending Aorta

From Body

To Body

The heart is a hollow, muscular organ that pumps 450 million pints of blood in the average lifetime. Its superior chambers, the atria, receive blood. Both atria fill and then contract at the same time. The inferior chambers are the ventricles. They pump blood out of the heart. Both ventricles fill and then contract at the same time. When the atria are relaxing, the ventricles are contracting.

The right side of the heart receives blood from the body and sends it to the lungs (pulmonic circulation). The heart's left side receives oxygenated blood from the lungs and sends it out to the body (systemic circulation).

The heartbeat originates at the sinoatrial node (pacemaker) and spreads across the atria to stimulate contraction. After a slight delay, the impulse is sent from the atrioventricular node, down the bundles of His, and out across the ventricles. This stimulates the ventricles to contract while the atria are relaxing.

The heart muscle (myocardium) receives its blood supply by way of the right and left coronary arteries. These vessels are the first branches of the aorta.

The Conduction System

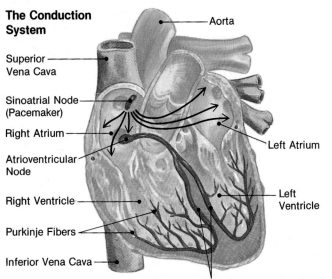

Aorta

Superior
Vena Cava

Sinoatrial Node
(Pacemaker)

Left Atrium

Right Atrium

Atrioventricular
Node

Right Ventricle

Left
Ventricle

Purkinje Fibers

Inferior Vena Cava

Right and Left Branches of the Bundle of His

The Coronary Arteries

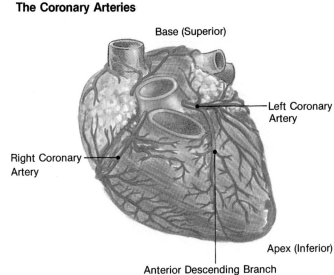

Base (Superior)

Left Coronary
Artery

Right Coronary
Artery

Apex (Inferior)

Anterior Descending Branch

BLOOD VESSELS
The Circulatory System

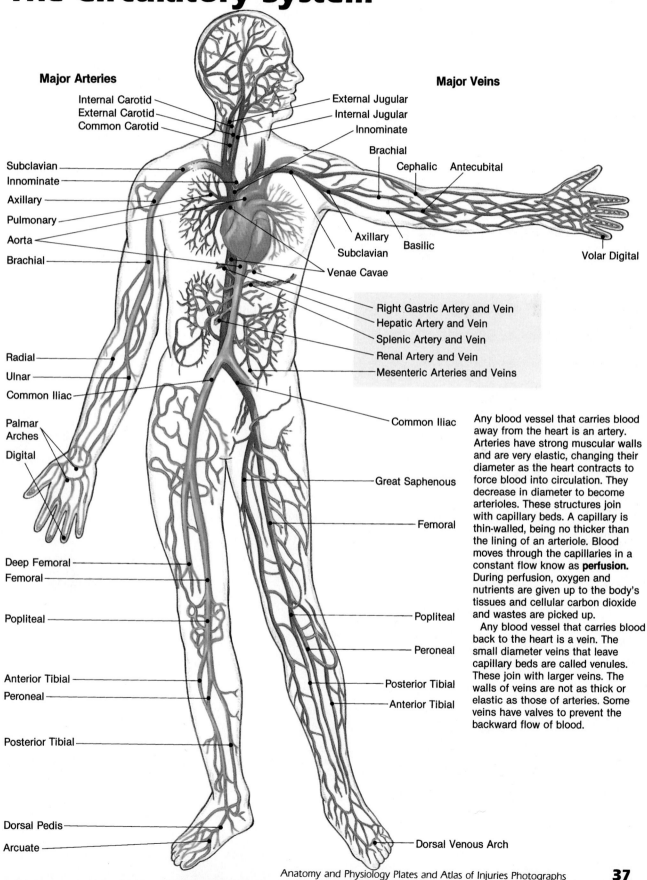

Major Arteries

- Internal Carotid
- External Carotid
- Common Carotid
- Subclavian
- Innominate
- Axillary
- Pulmonary
- Aorta
- Brachial
- Radial
- Ulnar
- Common Iliac
- Palmar Arches
- Digital
- Deep Femoral
- Femoral
- Popliteal
- Anterior Tibial
- Peroneal
- Posterior Tibial
- Dorsal Pedis
- Arcuate

Major Veins

- External Jugular
- Internal Jugular
- Innominate
- Brachial
- Cephalic
- Antecubital
- Axillary
- Basilic
- Subclavian
- Venae Cavae
- Volar Digital
- Common Iliac
- Great Saphenous
- Femoral
- Popliteal
- Peroneal
- Posterior Tibial
- Anterior Tibial
- Dorsal Venous Arch

Right Gastric Artery and Vein
Hepatic Artery and Vein
Splenic Artery and Vein
Renal Artery and Vein
Mesenteric Arteries and Veins

Any blood vessel that carries blood away from the heart is an artery. Arteries have strong muscular walls and are very elastic, changing their diameter as the heart contracts to force blood into circulation. They decrease in diameter to become arterioles. These structures join with capillary beds. A capillary is thin-walled, being no thicker than the lining of an arteriole. Blood moves through the capillaries in a constant flow know as **perfusion.** During perfusion, oxygen and nutrients are given up to the body's tissues and cellular carbon dioxide and wastes are picked up.

Any blood vessel that carries blood back to the heart is a vein. The small diameter veins that leave capillary beds are called venules. These join with larger veins. The walls of veins are not as thick or elastic as those of arteries. Some veins have valves to prevent the backward flow of blood.

NERVOUS SYSTEM

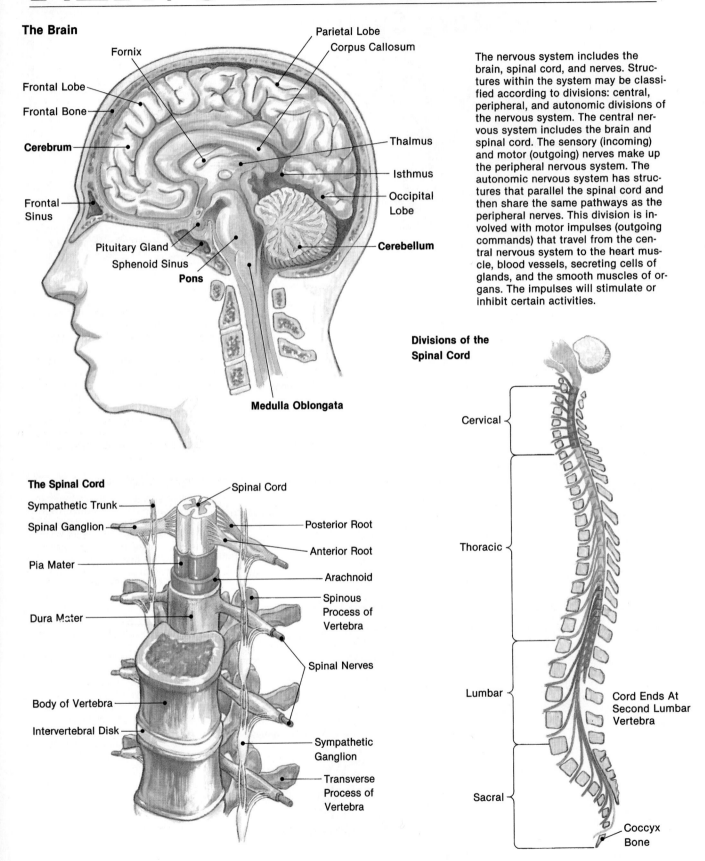

The Brain

Fornix
Parietal Lobe
Corpus Callosum
Frontal Lobe
Frontal Bone
Cerebrum
Thalmus
Isthmus
Occipital Lobe
Frontal Sinus
Pituitary Gland
Sphenoid Sinus
Pons
Cerebellum
Medulla Oblongata

The nervous system includes the brain, spinal cord, and nerves. Structures within the system may be classified according to divisions: central, peripheral, and autonomic divisions of the nervous system. The central nervous system includes the brain and spinal cord. The sensory (incoming) and motor (outgoing) nerves make up the peripheral nervous system. The autonomic nervous system has structures that parallel the spinal cord and then share the same pathways as the peripheral nerves. This division is involved with motor impulses (outgoing commands) that travel from the central nervous system to the heart muscle, blood vessels, secreting cells of glands, and the smooth muscles of organs. The impulses will stimulate or inhibit certain activities.

The Spinal Cord

Spinal Cord
Sympathetic Trunk
Spinal Ganglion
Posterior Root
Anterior Root
Pia Mater
Arachnoid
Spinous Process of Vertebra
Dura Mater
Spinal Nerves
Body of Vertebra
Intervertebral Disk
Sympathetic Ganglion
Transverse Process of Vertebra

Divisions of the Spinal Cord

Cervical
Thoracic
Lumbar
Cord Ends At Second Lumbar Vertebra
Sacral
Coccyx Bone

Nervous System Continued

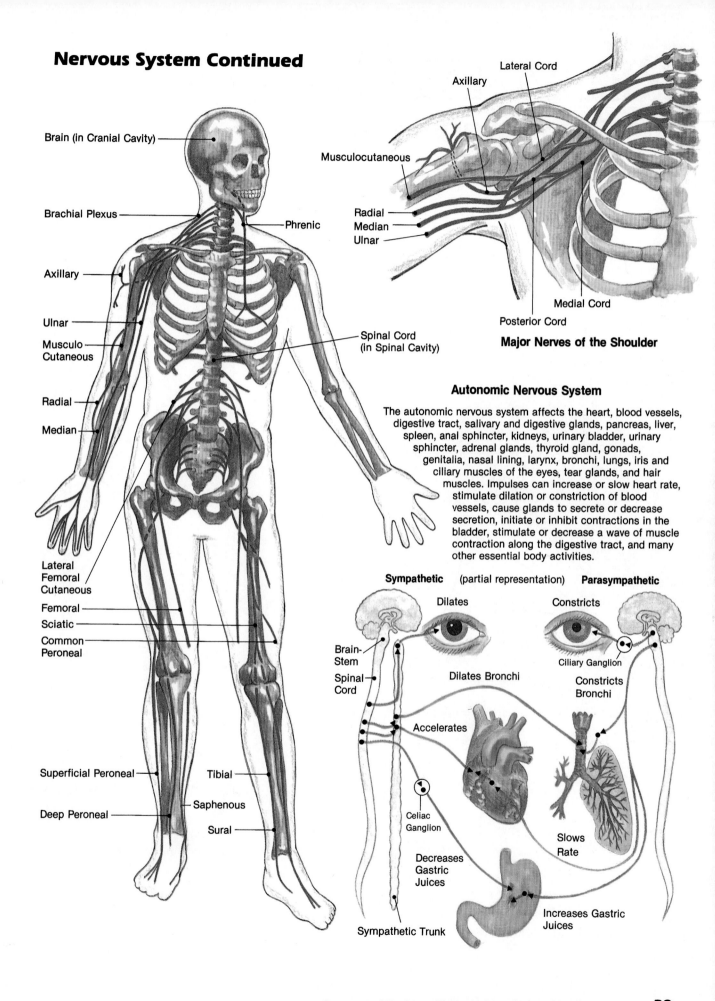

Brain (in Cranial Cavity)

Brachial Plexus

Phrenic

Axillary

Ulnar

Musculo Cutaneous

Radial

Median

Spinal Cord (in Spinal Cavity)

Lateral Femoral Cutaneous

Femoral

Sciatic

Common Peroneal

Superficial Peroneal

Deep Peroneal

Tibial

Saphenous

Sural

Major Nerves of the Shoulder

Lateral Cord

Axillary

Musculocutaneous

Radial
Median
Ulnar

Medial Cord

Posterior Cord

Autonomic Nervous System

The autonomic nervous system affects the heart, blood vessels, digestive tract, salivary and digestive glands, pancreas, liver, spleen, anal sphincter, kidneys, urinary bladder, urinary sphincter, adrenal glands, thyroid gland, gonads, genitalia, nasal lining, larynx, bronchi, lungs, iris and ciliary muscles of the eyes, tear glands, and hair muscles. Impulses can increase or slow heart rate, stimulate dilation or constriction of blood vessels, cause glands to secrete or decrease secretion, initiate or inhibit contractions in the bladder, stimulate or decrease a wave of muscle contraction along the digestive tract, and many other essential body activities.

Sympathetic   (partial representation)   Parasympathetic

Dilates

Constricts

Brain-Stem

Spinal Cord

Ciliary Ganglion

Dilates Bronchi

Constricts Bronchi

Accelerates

Celiac Ganglion

Slows Rate

Decreases Gastric Juices

Increases Gastric Juices

Sympathetic Trunk

RESPIRATION
The Respiratory System

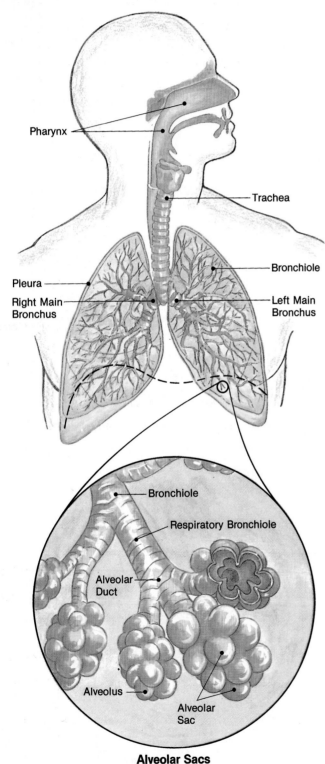

The airway consists of structures involved with the conduction and exchange of air. Conduction is the movement of air to and from the exchange levels of the lungs. Air enters through the nose (primary) and mouth (secondary) and travels down the pharynx to enter the larynx. After passing through the larynx, air enters the trachea. At its distal end, the trachea branches into the right and left primary bronchi. These bronchi branch into secondary bronchi, which then branch into the bronchioles. Some of the bronchioles end as closed tubes. Air movement in them helps the lungs expand. The rest of the bronchioles carry the air to the exchange levels of the lungs.

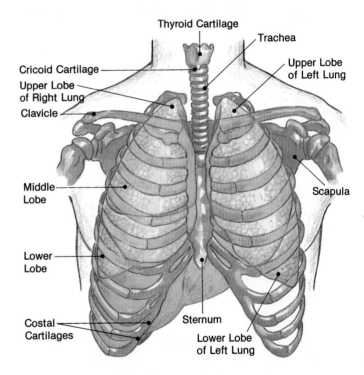

Alveolar Sacs

The respiratory bronchioles turn into alveolar ducts. These form alveolar sacs that are made up of the alveoli. Gas exchange takes place between the alveoli and the capillaries in the lungs.

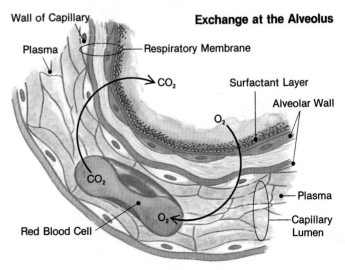

Exchange at the Alveolus

DIGESTION
The Digestive System

The digestive system includes the digestive tract and various supportive structures and accessory glands. The tract begins at the oral cavity with the teeth and tongue. The salivary glands release saliva into the mouth to moisten food for swallowing. The tract continues down the throat to the esophagus, through the cardiac sphincter, and into the stomach. Acid and digestive enzymes are added to the food to produce chyme. The chyme passes through the pyloric sphincter to enter the small intestine. Digestive enzymes from the pancreas and bile from the liver are added to the chyme. The process of digestion and absorption are completed in the small intestine. Wastes are carried through the ileoceccal valve into the large intestine. The wastes are moved to the rectum, from where they can be expelled through the anus.

Liver, Stomach, and Pancreas

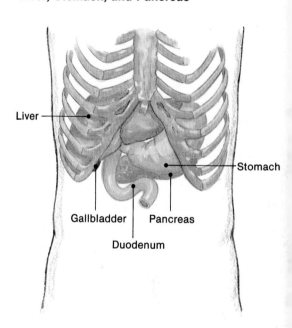

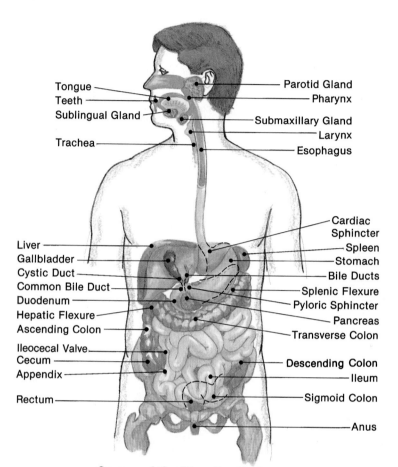

Tongue · Teeth · Sublingual Gland · Trachea · Parotid Gland · Pharynx · Submaxillary Gland · Larynx · Esophagus · Cardiac Sphincter · Spleen · Stomach · Bile Ducts · Splenic Flexure · Pyloric Sphincter · Pancreas · Transverse Colon · Liver · Gallbladder · Cystic Duct · Common Bile Duct · Duodenum · Hepatic Flexure · Ascending Colon · Ileocecal Valve · Cecum · Appendix · Rectum · Descending Colon · Ileum · Sigmoid Colon · Anus

Organs of the Digestive System

Large Intestine

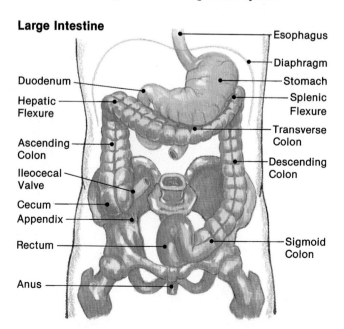

Duodenum · Hepatic Flexure · Ascending Colon · Ileocecal Valve · Cecum · Appendix · Rectum · Anus · Esophagus · Diaphragm · Stomach · Splenic Flexure · Transverse Colon · Descending Colon · Sigmoid Colon

Small Intestine

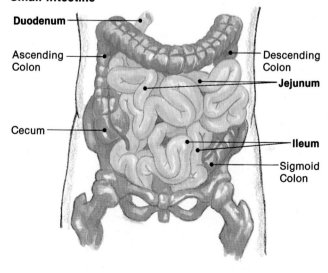

Duodenum · Ascending Colon · Cecum · Descending Colon · **Jejunum** · **Ileum** · Sigmoid Colon

EXCRETION
The Urinary System

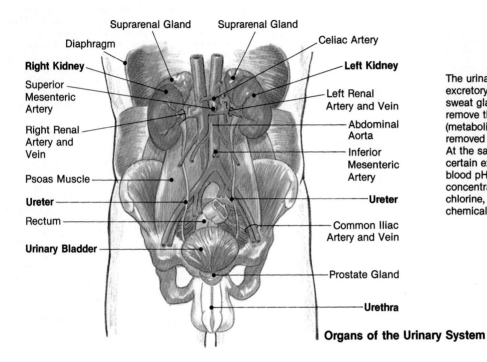

Suprarenal Gland
Diaphragm
Suprarenal Gland
Celiac Artery
Right Kidney
Left Kidney
Superior Mesenteric Artery
Left Renal Artery and Vein
Right Renal Artery and Vein
Abdominal Aorta
Inferior Mesenteric Artery
Psoas Muscle
Ureter
Ureter
Rectum
Common Iliac Artery and Vein
Urinary Bladder
Prostate Gland
Urethra

Organs of the Urinary System

The urinary system is part of the body's excretory structures (urinary system, lungs, sweat glands, and intestine). The kidneys remove the wastes of chemical activities (metabolism) in the body. These wastes are removed from the blood to produce urine. At the same time, the kidneys remove certain excess compounds, regulate the blood pH (acid-base balance), and the concentration of sodium, potassium, chlorine, glucose and other important chemicals.

The Nephron
Each kidney is made up of microscopic nephrons. Both wastes and needed chemicals are filtered from the blood. As these materials are passed through the nephron, the needed compounds (including water) are sent back into the blood. Wastes are collected as urine.

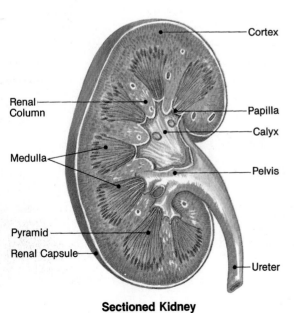

Cortex
Renal Column
Papilla
Calyx
Medulla
Pelvis
Pyramid
Renal Capsule
Ureter

Sectioned Kidney

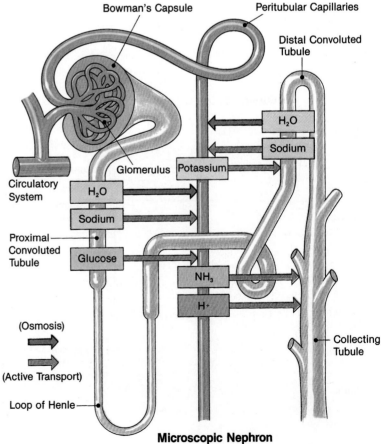

Bowman's Capsule
Peritubular Capillaries
Distal Convoluted Tubule
H_2O
Sodium
Glomerulus
Potassium
Circulatory System
H_2O
Sodium
Proximal Convoluted Tubule
Glucose
NH_3
H⁺
Collecting Tubule
(Osmosis)
(Active Transport)
Loop of Henle

Microscopic Nephron

REPRODUCTION
The Reproductive System

The reproductive system consists of the organs, glands, and supportive structures that are involved with human sexuality and procreation. In the male, spermatozoa and the hormone testosterone are produced in the testes. The female produces ova (eggs) and the hormones estrogen and progesterone in her ovaries. The union of ovum and sperm produce a single cell called a zygote. Through growth, cell division, and cellular differentiation (the formation of specialized cells) the new individual develops and matures.

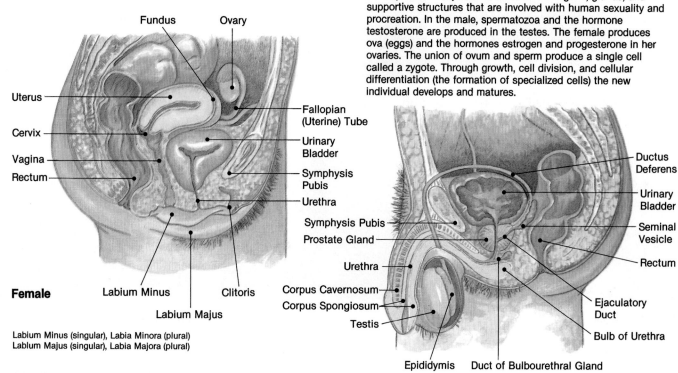

Female

Fundus
Ovary
Uterus
Cervix
Vagina
Rectum
Fallopian (Uterine) Tube
Urinary Bladder
Symphysis Pubis
Urethra
Labium Minus
Clitoris
Labium Majus

Labium Minus (singular), Labia Minora (plural)
Lablum Majus (singular), Labia Majora (plural)

Male

Ductus Deferens
Urinary Bladder
Seminal Vesicle
Rectum
Symphysis Pubis
Prostate Gland
Urethra
Corpus Cavernosum
Corpus Spongiosum
Testis
Ejaculatory Duct
Bulb of Urethra
Epididymis
Duct of Bulbourethral Gland

The Ovary

Suspensory Ligament of Ovary
End of Fallopian Tube
Released Ovum
Mature Follicle
Maturing Follicle
Primary Follicle (Ovum and Single Layer of Follicle Cells)
Ovarian Ligament
Ovum
Corpus Luteum (Produces Estrogen and Pregesterone)
Egg Nest
Corpus Albicans

The developing ovum and its supportive cells are called a follicle. Each month, follicle stimulating hormone (FSH) from the pituitary gland starts the growth of several follicles. Usually, only one will mature and release an ovum (ovulation). During its growth, the follicle produces estrogen. After ovulation, the remaining cells of the follicle form a specialized structure that produces both estrogen and progesterone.

The Breast

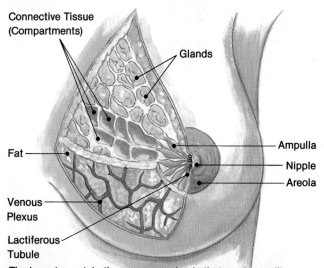

Connective Tissue (Compartments)
Glands
Fat
Ampulla
Nipple
Areola
Venous Plexus
Lactiferous Tubule

The breasts contain the mammary glands that produce milk (lactation). A mammary gland is a highly modified form of sweat gland. Estrogen stimulates the growth of the ducts, while progesterone stimulates the development of the secreting (milk-producing) cells. Lactic hormone from the pituitary stimulates milk production. Another pituitary hormone, oxytocin, stimulates the milk-producing cells to eject their milk into the ducts.

Atlas of Injuries

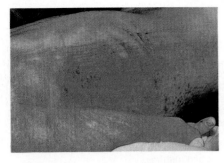

ABRASION (Gravel Roadway)

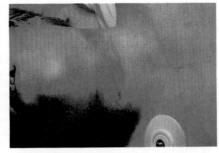

ABRASION (Rope or Cord)

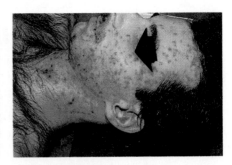

PITTED ABRASION

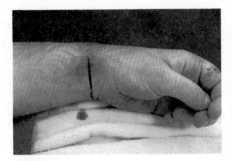

INCISION

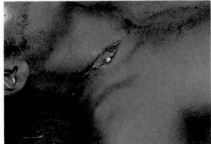

INCISION

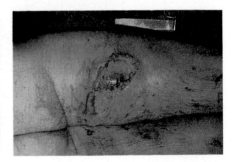

LACERATION (Jagged Margins)

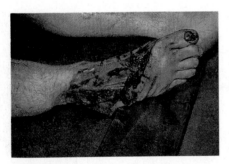

LACERATION (Tendons Still Intact)

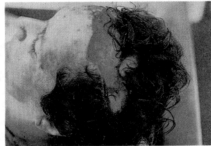

SCALP LACERATION (With Skin Separation)

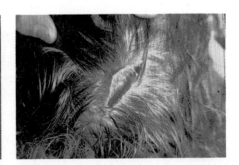

SCALP LACERATION (Minor)

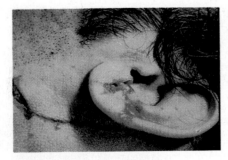

PUNCTURE WOUNDS (Stab Wounds)

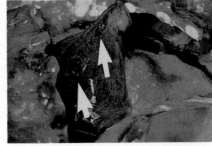

PUNCTURED LUNGS — FROM STAB WOUNDS (Autopsy)

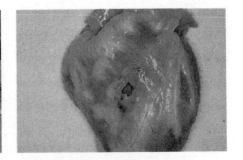

PERFORATED HEART (Bullet Wound)

ALL PHOTOGRAPHS ON THIS PAGE ARE FROM Dr. Lee J. Abbott. PO Box 1285, Laxahatchee, FL 33470

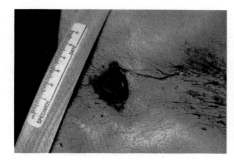

ENTRANCE WOUND (Bullet)

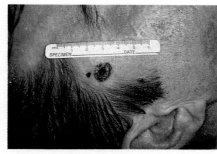

ENTRANCE WOUND (Bullet — Close Range)

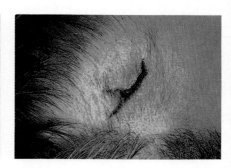

EXIT WOUND (Bullet)

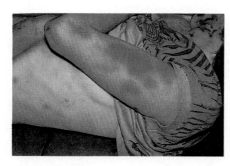

SHOTGUN WOUND

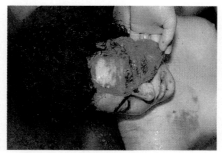

FACIAL AVULSION

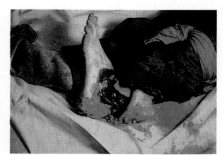

SKIN AVULSION (All Layers)

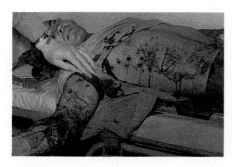

CONTUSIONS

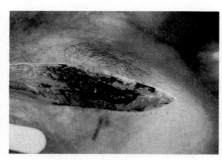

CONTUSION (Opened to Show Blood Accumulation)

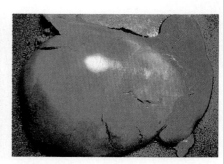

LACERATED LIVER (Abdominal Trauma)

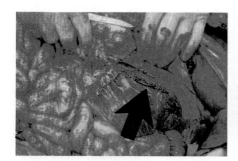

LACERATED SPLEEN

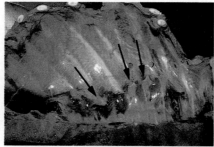

FRACTURED RIBS (Death due to Blood Loss from Lacerated Lungs)

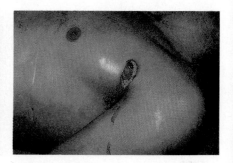

PERFORATED CHEST (Sucking Chest Wound)

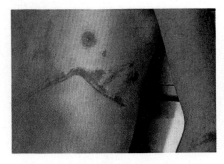

BLUNT TRAUMA TO CHEST

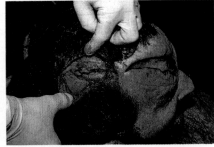

OPEN HEAD WOUND — SKULL FRACTURE

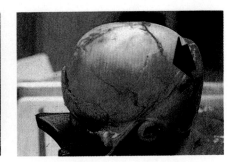

RADIATING SKULL FRACTURE (Blunt Trauma)

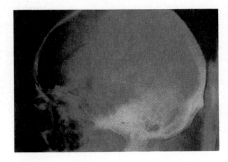

MULTIPLE SKULL FRACTURES (X-ray)

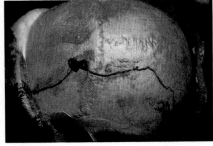

DEPRESSED SKULL FRACTURE (Force from Small Object)

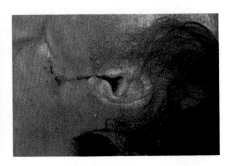

BLEEDING FROM EAR (Possible Skull Fracture)

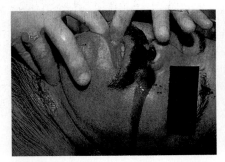

BLEEDING FROM NOSE (Possible Skull Fracture)

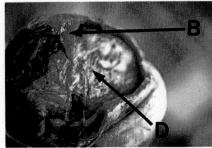

EPIDURAL HEMATOMA (D = Dura, B = Bone Fragment)

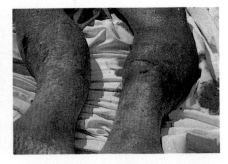

EXTENSIVE BILATERAL INJURY — LOWER EXTREMITIES (Impact with Car)

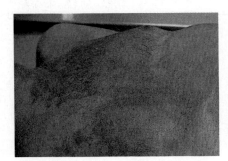

FIRST-DEGREE BURN

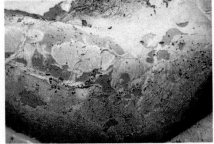

SECOND-DEGREE BURN

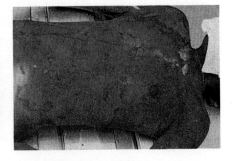

THIRD-DEGREE BURN

ALL PHOTOGRAPHS ON THIS PAGE ARE FROM Dr. Lee J. Abbott. PO Box 1285, Laxahatchee, FL 33470

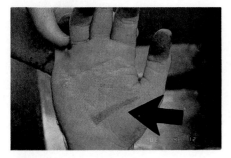

ELECTRICAL BURN
(Contact with Source) LJA

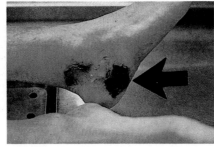

ELECTRICAL BURN (Exit)
LJA

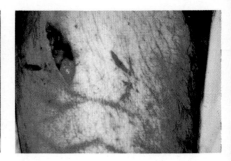

OPEN FRACTURE (Femur)
UT

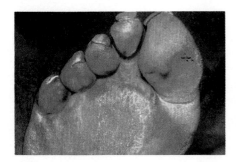

FROSTBITE

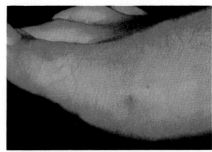

SNAKEBITE
UT

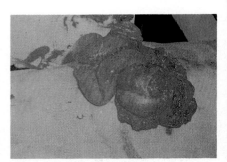

BOWEL EVISCERATION

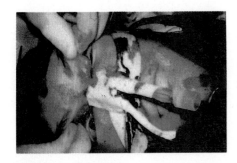

ORBITAL EDEMA

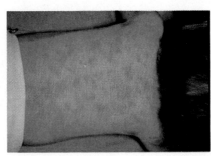

HIVES
AFIP Neg. No. 65-6982-4

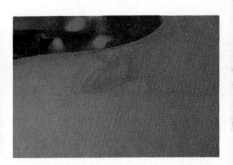

DOG BITE (Leg)
AFIP Neg. No. 62-12291

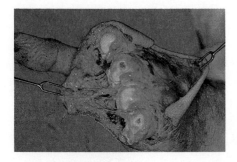

AMPUTATION (Fingers)
AFIP Neg. No. 75-20914

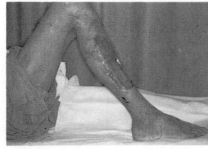

LACERATED LEG
AFIP Neg. No. 68-15269

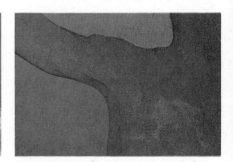

BURN (Hot Water)
AFIP Neg. No. 64-8320

LJA = Dr. Lee J. Abbott   AFIP = Armed Forces Institute of Pathology
UT = University of Tennessee, Memphis, Division of Forensic Pathology

ALL PHOTOGRAPHS ON THIS PAGE ARE FROM Dr. Lee J. Abbott. PO Box 1285, Laxahatchee, FL 33470

CHAPTER 3

Patient Assessment

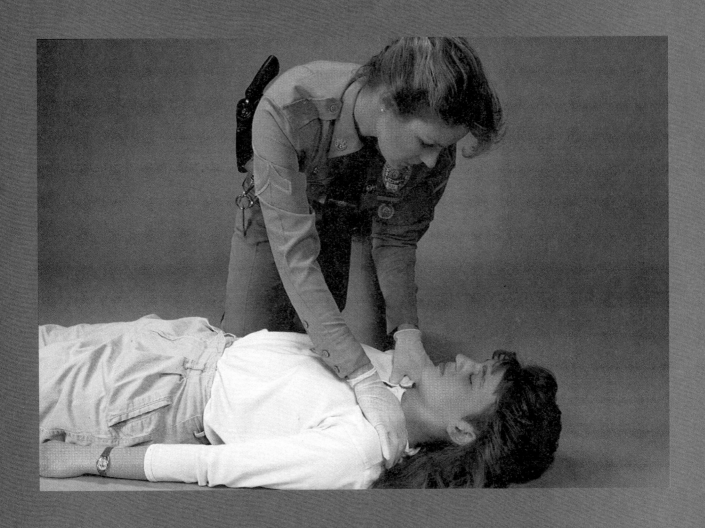

OBJECTIVES

By the end of this chapter, you should be able to:

1. List three major concerns to consider when you are gathering information. (p. 52)
2. State the three things you must say to a conscious patient upon your arrival at the scene. (p. 52)
3. List six quick sources of information. (p. 53)
4. Describe the personal protection to be worn by a First Responder during patient assessment. (p. 54)
5. Define primary survey, stating what it is, why it is done, when it is done, and what can be detected by using this procedure. (pp. 54–55)
6. Describe how to determine if a patient is responsive. (p. 55)
7. Describe how you ensure an open airway and how you check a patient for adequate breathing. (pp. 55, 58)
8. Describe how to take a carotid pulse. (p. 58)
9. Define secondary survey in terms of when it is done, why it is done, and what types of problems are searched for during this procedure. (pp. 59, 61)
10. Define interview and examination. (p. 61)
11. Define sign, vital signs, and symptom. (p. 61)
12. List some of the questions you should ask bystanders and patients. (pp. 61–63)
13. List in correct order the steps of the primary survey. (pp. 55, 58)
14. List in correct order the steps of the secondary survey. (p. 61)
15. Describe how to take vital signs and indicate what you are looking for in terms of rates, character, and what is considered normal. (pp. 65–71)
16. List in correct order the steps of the head-to-toe examination. (pp. 70–78)
17. State ten First Responder rules applying to the patient examination. (p. 80)

SKILLS

Upon completing this chapter and your class lectures and skills labs, you should be able to:

1. Determine a carotid (neck) pulse, a radial (wrist) pulse, a dorsalis pedis pulse, and a posterior tibial (ankle) pulse, noting both rate and character for the radial pulse.
2. Determine respiratory rate and character.
3. Determine relative skin temperature.
4. Determine blood pressure (optional).
5. Act out your arrival at an emergency scene. Show how you would safely gather information, do a primary survey, and do a secondary survey.

WARNING: Patient assessment procedures may bring you into direct contact with the patient's blood, body fluids, wastes, and mucous membranes. Be certain that you wear approved latex or vinyl gloves during assessment and care. Wear any other items of personal protection required for the emergency. Follow all Centers for Disease Control and local guidelines established to help prevent the spread of infectious diseases.

THE PRINCIPLES OF ASSESSMENT

Patient assessment—the gathering of information to determine the possible nature of the patient's illness or injury. It includes interviews and physical examinations.

Patients cannot receive appropriate care until their problems have been detected and understood by those trying to help them. The patient assessment is a procedure that helps determine the possible nature of most problems associated with illness or injury and provides direction in making decisions concerning the emergency care that must be rendered. It has been designed to allow you to gather information quickly from as many sources as possible.

The patient assessment is not a fixed system. This means that not all aspects of the assessment will apply to every patient and that the order of events may vary depending on the nature of the patient's problem. For most patients, the assessment should proceed as follows:

1. Ensure your own safety.
2. Make certain that the scene is safe for the patient.
3. Find out if the patient is responsive. Is he alert and what is the level of awareness (consciousness)?

The rest of the procedure changes slightly depending on the type of patient:

Conscious Patient—Medical Problem (No Injuries)

- Begin an interview. This should continue through the rest of the assessment and care.
- Determine vital signs (pulse, respirations, relative skin temperature, and, for some First Responders, blood pressure).
- Examine the patient as required regarding the complaints gathered during the interview.

Unconscious Patient—Medical Problem (No Injuries)

- Begin to interview any bystanders, but at the same time . . .
- Make certain that the patient has an open airway, is breathing, and has a pulse. Check for profuse bleeding. Provide care for any of these problems as they are found.
- Determine vital signs.
- Examine the patient for signs of the nature of the emergency.

Conscious Patient—Injuries

- Note anything that may indicate the cause of injury.
- Interview the patient while checking for adequate breathing and profuse bleeding.
- Determine vital signs if the patient appears to be unstable.
- Do a complete examination of the patient.
- Determine vital signs.

Unconscious Patient—Injuries

- Note anything that may indicate the cause of injury.
- Begin to question bystanders, but at the same time assess the patient for life-threatening problems. Does the patient have an open airway and adequate breathing? Does he have a pulse that indicates circulation? Is there serious bleeding? Care must be provided for any of these problems as they are found.
- Take vital signs if the patient appears to be unstable.
- Do a complete examination of the patient.
- Determine the patient's vital signs.

Sometimes the type of patient (injury or illness) is not so clearly defined. For example, a patient who is ill may fall and injure himself. Your interview of the patient and bystanders may alert you to this fact. Knowing this, you will have to conduct a complete physical examination. At other times, you might suspect that a medical problem may have caused the accident. Your interview will have to include questions to determine this.

OBTAINING INFORMATION

This chapter will not cover the problems that may be found at the scene of an accident or medical emergency. For now, don't worry about traffic, crowd control, fire, toxic gases, possible falling objects, and other dangers and difficulties. These things are important, but they will be discussed later in your training. For now, be concerned only about the patient's problems and how to gather information about them.

You must attempt to identify and correct any life-threatening problems. Keep this in mind throughout this chapter. It is foolish to be gathering statements from bystanders if the patient's heart is not beating (cardiac arrest). You would be a poor First Responder if you checked a patient's pulse and assumed that it would not change. Gathering information is a systematic process, but it is not always a straight step-by-step procedure. You may have to stop what you are doing and go back to a procedure completed only seconds after you arrived. No matter where you are in your information-gathering process, you must remember:

1st • Your primary concern is to identify and provide care for life-threatening problems.

• Your second concern is to identify any injuries or medical problems that are serious or could become serious, and provide care for these problems.

• Your third concern is to continue monitoring the patient in case her or his condition changes.

Arrival at the Scene

Again, at this point in your training, let us assume that the only problems at the scene will be injuries or medical emergencies. Start by identifying yourself to the patient and bystanders. Do this for the patient even when you believe that he or she is unconscious. You may find that a patient who at first appears to be unconscious is actually alert. If you are a uniformed law enforcement officer or firefighter, most bystanders and patients will respond to your uniform and let you take charge. Should you be out of uniform, or if you are an industrial or a public First Responder, then identification may prove to be critical in allowing you to go about your duties. State your name and then the following: "I am a First Responder. I have been trained to provide emergency care." True, most people do not know who or what a First Responder is, but this statement should allow you access to the patient and grant you the cooperation of bystanders.

Your next statement to the patient should be: "May I help you?" It is hard to understand, but many people in an emergency situation will say, "No." Usually, their fear is so great that they are confused. Simple conversation works best in gaining patient confidence.

If the patient is unconscious or unable to respond, then implied consent allows you to begin care at the First Responder level.

1st Upon arrival, you must:

1. State your name (and rank or classification).
2. Identify yourself as a trained First Responder. If necessary, explain what this means. Let the patient and bystanders know that you are with the emergency medical services system (do not say EMS System).
3. Ask the patient if you may help.

While you are doing this, remember to look for any life-threatening problems such as serious bleeding or the early indications of shock.

If you arrive at the scene and someone else has started to render care, identify yourself and let this person know that you are a First Responder. If the person's training is equal to or above your own, ask if you may assist. You should identify yourself to the patient and find out if he wishes you to help. Both actual and implied consent laws still apply.

Should you determine that you have more training than the person who has begun care, ask to take over responsibility for the patient. Do this with respect for the first provider. Take time to compliment him on what he has done and ask him to assist you. *Never* criticize or argue with the first provider. Unless you are a law enforcement officer or there are specific emergency care laws in your state, you cannot order the first person to stop so that you can provide care. In rare cases, you may have to supervise what is being done and take the necessary steps to protect the patient and to ensure proper care.

Quick Sources of Information

You are at the scene. Only a few seconds have passed as you identified yourself and asked if you could help. During this time period, there are other things you should be doing to gain information. Clues to the problem will come from:

- The scene itself.
- Patients, if they are conscious and able to respond.
- Any relatives or other bystanders.
- Any obvious mechanism of injury. What type of accident has occurred and how might it have injured the patient?
- Any noticeable deformities or obvious injuries.
- Any signs or characteristics of certain types of injuries or illnesses.

The above should be thought of in terms of being *quick* sources of information. Now is not the time to ask a lot of questions or look over the entire scene. What is to be gained must be accomplished in a matter of

FIGURE 3–1.
Some clues to the patient's problem can be gathered upon arrival at the scene.

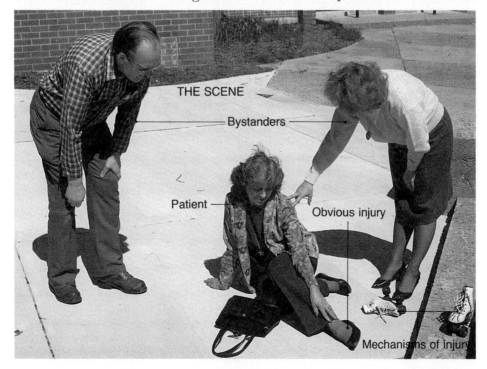

THE SCENE

Bystanders

Patient

Obvious injury

Mechanisms of injury

seconds as you move to the patient. All these things may be considered in depth, but not at this stage of the information-gathering procedure.

In a few seconds, you could gain valuable information such as:

The scene—Is it safe? Should the patient be moved? Is there more than one patient? Can you account for all the patients?

The patient—Is he alert, trying to tell you something or pointing to a part of his body?

Bystanders—Are they trying to tell you something? Listen, they might be saying, "He has a bad heart." "He fell off that ladder!" "We told him you couldn't mix pills and booze."

Mechanism of injury—Has something fallen on the patient? Was fire involved in the accident? Has the patient been injured by the steering column during an automobile accident?

Deformities or injuries—Does the patient's body appear to be lying in a strange position? Are there burns? Do you see any crushed limbs? Are there any wounds?

Signs—Is there blood around the patient? Has the patient vomited? Is the patient having convulsions?

Mechanism of injury—what forces caused the injury. The rescuer must consider the kind of force, its intensity and direction, and the area of the patient's body affected.

Remember that your personal safety comes first. Do not be so busy gathering information that you forget to look for dangers at the scene and control hazards according to your local protocols. Likewise, do not be so busy that you forget to put on any items that may be needed to protect yourself from infectious diseases (see pages 4 and 325). Patient assessment procedures may place you in direct contact with the patient's blood, body fluids, wastes, and mucous membranes.

As noted in Chapter 1, approved latex or vinyl gloves are recommended for all patient care procedures. This recommendation includes all assessment activities. Wearing gloves to avoid contact with disease-causing agents is part of the Centers for Disease Control (CDC) universal blood and body fluid precautions. These procedurs are referred to as *universal precautions.* Pocket face masks (page 92) and other special devices for the delivery of artificial respirations have been added to the list for all EMS personnal.

The CDC universal precautions include wearing gloves, masks, protective eyewear or face shields, and gowns or aprons. Most First Responders carry gloves. Protection for the eyes may be included as part of uniforms issued or other safety equipment. Masks, gowns, and aprons are seldom part of First Responder equipment and supplies, but this is changing. Follow your EMS System's guidelines for First Responders and wear what you have been issued for all recommended situations.

Other than gloves for all patient care procedures, how the rest of the universal precautions are used is a matter of special guidelines and common sense. Most patients would find it insulting if you "suited up" before approaching them. Some may not be very happy to see you wearing gloves. If the wearing of gloves causes any problems with patient, be certain to explain that the gloves help to protect the patient during care. If there is blood, body fluids, or wastes at an emergency scene, wear the necessary protective equipment.

THE PRIMARY SURVEY

NOTE: This section covers the major steps of the primary survey. The actions taken to care for problems that may be found during the survey will be covered in Chapters 4 through 8.

The primary survey is defined as a process carried out in order to detect life-threatening problems. As these problems are detected, life-saving measures are taken. Learning how to do a primary survey and then learning how to correct the problems found during this survey are the most important parts of your First Responder's training. You must begin the primary survey as soon as you reach the patient and initiate immediate life-saving procedures as required.

1st Three major life-threatening problems are considered during the primary survey. They are:

- **Respiration**—Is the airway open and is there adequate breathing?
- **Circulation**—Is there a pulse to indicate that the patient's heart is circulating blood?
- **Bleeding**—Is there serious bleeding, or did the patient lose a great quantity of blood before you arrived? Are there indications that the patient is developing shock?

These problems and the actions taken to correct them collectively are known as the ABCs of emergency care. This stands for:

A = airway (ensure an open airway)
B = breathe (maintain airway, rescue breathing)
C = circulate (chest compressions, control of bleeding)

1st As a First Responder, the procedures you should follow are:

1. See if the patient is responsive. A conscious patient indicates that there is breathing and circulation. The breathing may not be adequate and the need may exist for clearing the airway, but the patient is breathing. A conscious patient also indicates that the heart is circulating blood to the brain. Since all this could change rapidly, you must continuously monitor the patient's level of awareness.

   To check for responsiveness, gently shake the patient's shoulder and shout: "Are you okay?"

2. If the patient is unresponsive, it might be necessary to reposition the patient so that you can determine if he is breathing and has a pulse and to check for serious bleeding. You should try to make these assessments without moving the patient. This can be done in many cases, but you *must* reposition the patient if you cannot tell whether he is breathing and has a pulse, or if you suspect undetected serious bleeding.

   When the patient is an unconscious accident victim, you must assume that there are serious neck and spinal injuries. Moving this type of patient may cause serious injuries, but the risk may have to be taken to check for life-threatening problems. The medical patient who has not suffered an accident can be repositioned only if you are certain that an accident has not occurred. Several methods of repositioning and moving a patient will be covered in future chapters. For now, see the method described in Scansheet 3–1. This one-rescuer log roll is to be used only for basic life-support procedures when trained personnel are not on hand to assist the rescuer.

3. If the patient is unresponsive, check for breathing. This is a two-step procedure. First, ensure an open airway. Second, check for adequate breathing.

   - **Open airway**—For cases in which you do not suspect spinal injury, begin by positioning yourself at the patient's side. The patient should be lying on her or his back. (In automobile accidents, you may have to place the patient in a seated position.) Next, use the head-tilt, chin-life method as shown in Scansheet 3–2 to open the patient's airway. Procedures for patients with spinal injury will be covered in Chapter 4.
   - **Adequate breathing**—Look, listen, and feel for air exchange.

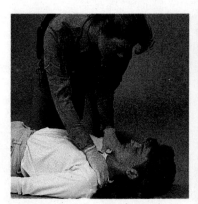

FIGURE 3–2.
Establish unresponsiveness.

■ SCAN 3-1.

Repositioning the Patient for Basic Life Support

WARNING:
THIS MANEUVER IS USED TO INITIATE BASIC CARDIAC LIFE SUPPORT WHEN YOU MUST ACT ALONE. FOR ALL OTHER REPOSITIONINGS, USE THE FOUR-RESCUER LOG ROLL.

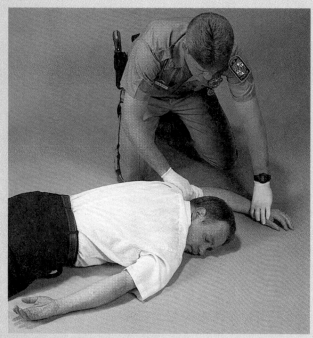

1 Straighten the legs and position the closest arm above the head.

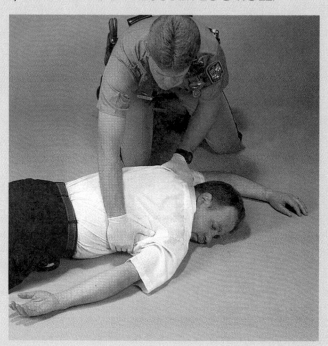

2 Cradle the head and neck, grasp under the distant armpit.

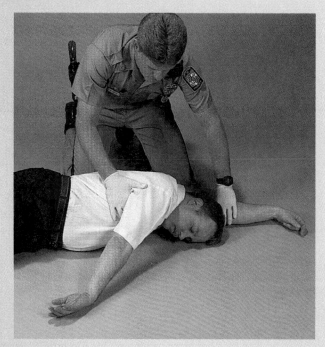

3 Move the patient as a unit onto his side.

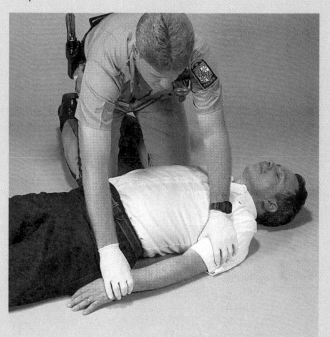

4 Move the patient onto his back and reposition the extended arm.

■ SCAN 3-2.

The Head-tilt, Chin-lift Maneuver

WARNING:
THIS PROCEDURE IS NOT RECOMMENDED IF THE PATIENT HAS POSSIBLE SPINAL INJURIES.

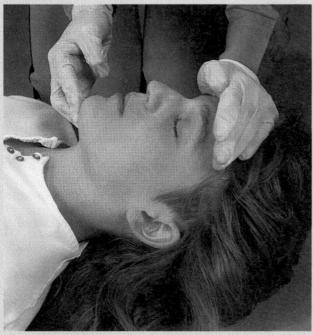

One hand is placed on the patient's forehead while the fingertips of the other hand are placed under the patient's chin.

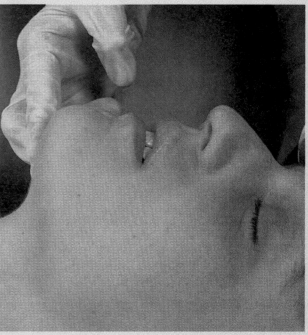

Keep the fingertips on the bony part of the chin. Do not compress the soft tissues that are under the lower jaw.

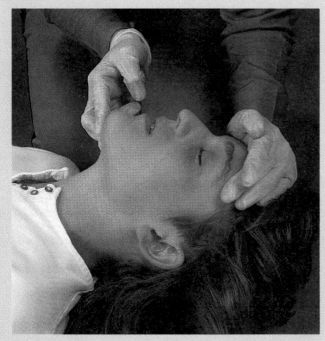

Most of the head-tilt is provided by the gentle pressure on the forehead. Lift the chin and bring it to a point where the lower teeth are almost touching the upper teeth. Do not allow the mouth to close.

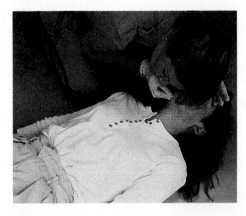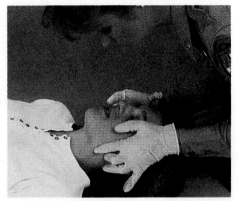

FIGURE 3–3.
LOOK, LISTEN, and FEEL for breathing.

Remaining in the same position, turn your head so that you can watch the patient's chest. Position your ear close to the patient's mouth and nose.

Look for chest movements associated with breathing. Note that males show chest movements in the region of the diaphragm, while females show more pronounced respiratory movements at the collarbones (clavicles).

Listen for the movement of air at the patient's mouth and nose.

Feel for air being exhaled through the patient's nose and mouth.
The determination of breathing should take only 3 to 5 seconds.

If the patient is breathing through an open airway, there will be a pulse. This means that you can go on to check for profuse bleeding. However, if there is airway obstruction or if the patient is not breathing, you **must take immediate action.** The procedures to follow are covered in the next chapter.

Carotid (kah-ROT-id) pulse— the pulse that can be felt on each side of the neck.

4. If the patient is not breathing, determine if there is a carotid (kah-ROT-id) pulse. For emergency situations, this pulse is considered to be more reliable than the wrist (radial) pulse. The procedures for taking a carotid pulse are as follows:

Begin by locating the patient's "Adam's apple." Place the tips of your index and middle fingers directly on the midline of this structure. Now, slide your fingertips to the side of the patient's neck closest to you. The palm side of your fingertips should be against the patient's neck. *Do not* slide your fingertips to the opposite side of the patient's neck. You may apply improper pressure and close the airway. Also, a sudden movement or convulsion by the patient may cause you to injure the patient, or you may apply too much pressure and stop circulation.

The pulse should be detected in the groove between the windpipe and the large muscle on the side of the neck. Very little pressure need be applied to feel the carotid pulse. Take 5 to 10 seconds to determine if the patient has a carotid pulse. You will need to practice this procedure in order to act swiftly and accurately during the survey.

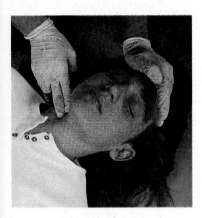

FIGURE 3–4.
Check for a carotid pulse.

Take no less than 5 but no more than 10 seconds to establish pulselessness.* The precise rate of the pulse is not important during the primary survey. You are simply trying to determine if heart action is circulating the blood. You should note if the pulse is very rapid or weak. This may be an indication of shock. If there is no pulse, begin CPR procedures (see Chapter 5). If there is a pulse, but still no respiration, artificial ventilation is required (see Chapter 4). Otherwise, concentrate on possible bleeding.

5. You must stop all bleeding that is life threatening. Any bleeding, if it continues will eventually prove to be life threatening. However, only

* For cases of hypothermia, take up to 1 minute to establish pulselessness (see page 344).

profuse bleeding is considered during the primary survey. Look for spurts of blood and free-flowing blood. Methods to control such bleeding will be covered in Chapter 7.

You may arrive to find a patient who has been bleeding slowly for a long time. There will be a significant amount of blood around the patient and he may have blood-soaked hair or clothing. You could find yourself thinking, "The rate of bleeding is slow. If this had just started, I wouldn't worry, but look at all the blood he's lost. I better do something now." In such cases, this slow bleeding will have to be considered life threatening. This is certainly the case if you know that there will be some delay before EMTs arrive on the scene.

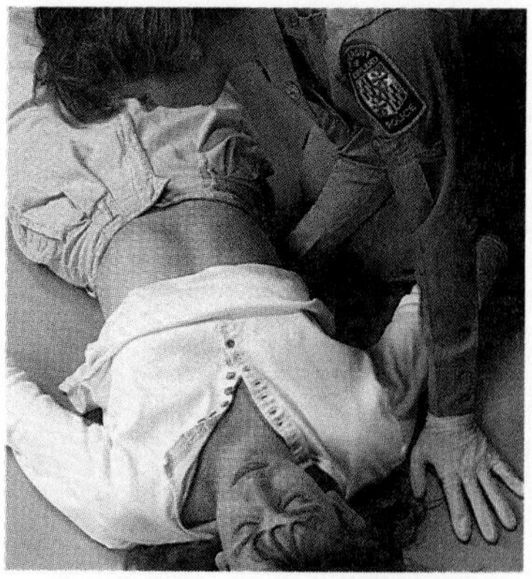

If the patient's airway is open, breathing is adequate, a carotid pulse can be found, and all profuse bleeding is under control, then you can continue to gather information by moving on to the secondary survey.

FIGURE 3–5.
Locate and control all profuse bleeding.

Special Considerations

You may be wondering about situations where there is more than one patient. For such cases, there is one firm rule:

Conduct all primary surveys and control all life-threatening problems before moving on to any secondary survey.

1st There is one special condition that you should consider at this time. What do you do if you see obvious profuse bleeding, where blood is spurting or flowing rapidly from a wound? Such bleeding would indicate heart action is still present. This requires a slight break in the primary survey procedures. As important as stopping bleeding is to saving the patient, respiration cannot be ignored. You will probably have to attempt to slow down the bleeding while you are looking for chest movements and other signs of breathing. You should do what you can to help control the bleeding, but you must place your emphasis on an open airway and adequate breathing.

Alerting Dispatch

There is a tendency for some people to want to call or have someone call the EMS System dispatcher as soon as they arrive at the emergency scene. It is best to wait until you know the type of emergency, how many patients there are, if any patients are unconscious, and if basic life-support measures have to be started. The time to have someone phone or radio dispatch is after you have checked for a carotid pulse. The information you can now give to dispatch may influence the type of response ordered. For example, if you have started CPR, dispatch may be able to send an advanced cardiac life-support unit to your location.

THE SECONDARY SURVEY

The main purpose of the secondary survey is to discover injuries or medical problems that could be a threat to the patient's survival if allowed to go untreated. The secondary survey is a very systematic way of gathering information and often helps to reassure the patient, family, and bystanders by indicating that there is concern for the patient and that something is being done.

Secondary survey—the patient assessment procedure that includes interviews, the head-to-toe survey, and the taking of vital signs.

■ SCAN 3-3.

Primary Survey

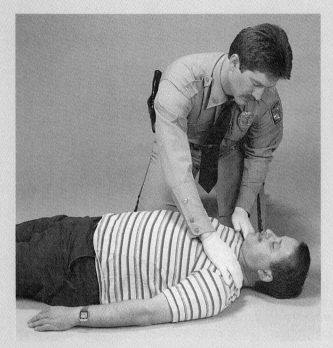

1 Responsiveness

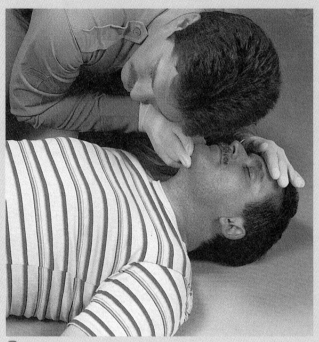

2 Open airway

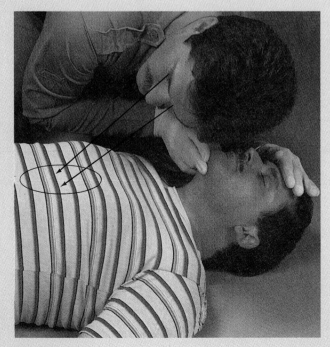

3 Breathing

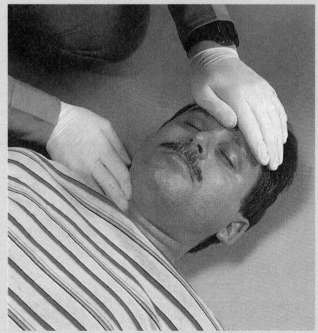

4 Circulation
- Pulse
- Profuse Bleeding

1st A special vocabulary goes with the secondary survey. Some of the more important terms include:

Interview—Gathering information by asking questions and listening. Whenever possible, the patient is your primary source of information. Relatives and bystanders will also be sources of information. This interview is sometimes called the subjective interview.

Examination—This is a head-to-toe survey of the patient, requiring you to use your senses in order to find injuries or indications of illness. This examination is sometimes called the objective examination.

Symptoms—What the patient tells you is wrong. Such things as chest pains, dizziness, and nausea are considered to be symptoms.

Signs—What you see, feel, hear, and smell when examining the patient.

Vital signs—Pulse, respirations, and relative skin temperature. In some First Responder courses, blood pressure is included in the required vital signs.

Symptom—what the patient tells about his or her injury or illness.

Sign—what you see, hear, feel, and smell in relation to the patient's illness or injury.

Vital signs—at the First Responder level, these include pulse, respiration, and relative skin temperature.

Before considering how these definitions apply to the secondary survey, remember that First Responders must be realistic. Asking a lot of questions while a patient wants you to look at a leg may only upset him. You should always acknowledge the patient's primary complaint and show some concern for the problem. This may lead to having to do two things at once during the secondary survey. The systematic approach to the survey is to be completed, but in a practical manner and in a way that does not upset the patient.

The Scene and the Patient

You will have to reconsider some of the things you did upon arrival at the scene. Since you were concerned with beginning a primary survey, you may have missed something. Now would be the time for you to:

- Look over the scene—Is it still safe? Do you see a mechanism for injury?
- Look over your patient—Are there obvious injuries or signs? Is the patient wearing a medical identification device you can read without moving him?

THE BYSTANDER INTERVIEW

If your patient is unresponsive or unable to converse with you for some other reason, you may have to depend on bystanders for information. Try to keep things flowing in an organized manner by asking specific questions. This will shorten the time required to gather needed information.

1st When interviewing bystanders, you should ask:

1. The patient's name. If the patient is a minor, you should ask if the parents are there or if they have been contacted.
2. What happened? You may be told that the patient fell off a ladder, appeared to faint, was hit on the head by a falling object, or any of hundreds of possible clues.
3. Did they see anything else? For example, was the patient holding his chest before he fell?
4. Did the patient complain of anything before this happened? Here is where you may learn of chest pains, nausea, worry about a funny odor where the patient was working, and other clues to the problem.
5. Did the patient have any known illness or problem? This may provide you with information about heart conditions, allergies, alcohol

problems, and other possibilities that could change conditions over the next few minutes.

6. Do they know if the patient was taking any medications? Try to use the words "medications" or "medicines." If you say "drugs" or some other term, bystanders may not answer, believing the question to be part of a criminal investigation.

Do not ask these questions as an isolated part of the secondary survey. You will have to be active, conducting the objective examination at the same time you are asking questions and listening to the answers. The patient may have moderate bleeding, an unnoticed injury, or some other problem that you cannot ignore while conducting the interview.

THE PATIENT INTERVIEW

If your patient is responsive and appears to be alert, do not direct your questions to bystanders. Being close to the patient and being concerned will help ease the fear that is a part of injury and illness. Ask questions clearly and at normal rate. Do not say such things as, "Everything will be okay," or "Take it easy, everything's fine." The patient knows differently and may have little confidence in you if you use such phrases.

1st When interviewing patients, you should ask;

1. Your patient's name. Simply state, "May I have your name?" This personal consideration is essential. You now have valuable information that must be learned quickly. Keep in mind that a conscious patient may not remain conscious. Once you have the patient's name, try to use it as often as possible during the rest of the interview. Do not be surprised to find that children will give only their first names until asked specifically for their last names.

2. Children's ages and how to contact their parents. As a First Responder, you will have little need for knowing more than the general age of an adult. The age of a child, though, may determine what type of care you must provide. Children expect to be asked their age. You would do well to ask adolescents for their age to be certain that you are dealing with a minor. Ask all minors how you can contact their parents. This question will sometimes upset children because it intensifies the fear they already have about being sick or hurt without their parents being there to help them. Be prepared to offer comfort and assure the child that someone will contact the parents.

3. What is wrong? No matter what the complaint, ask if there is any pain. If an extremity is involved, ask if there is numbness, burning, or a tingling sensation in the limb. This is a warning of possible nerve or spinal injury. As you learn more about various illnesses and injuries, you will see what additional questions can be asked to obtain a list of symptoms.

4. How did it happen? In cases of injury, knowing how someone has been injured will help direct you to problems that may not be noticeable to the patient. For patients you find lying down, always determine if they lay down, were knocked down, fell, or were thrown into that position. Do this even for those patients who have medical problems as their chief complaint. This information may indicate the possibility of spinal injuries or internal bleeding.

   In cases involving automobile accidents, word your questions with care. If you say, "What happened?" or "How were you hurt?", you will probably find yourself listening to a story of how the other driver was wrong. More specific questions such as, "Did you hit the dash (or windshield, steering wheel)?" "Were you thrown forward (or backward)?" "Were you thrown from the car?" will provide you with better information.

   How long they have felt this way? In cases of illness, you will need to know if this problem has occurred suddenly, or if it has been developing for the past few days or over a longer period of time.

5. Has this happened before or have they ever felt this way before? Asking if someone was ever hit by a truck before is not too practical. However, if the patient has fallen, it is important to know whether this is a recurring problem. If the patient complains of shortness of breath, dizziness, or chills, then you need to know if this is a first-time complaint. If a patient provides you with a symptom, find out if this problem has happened before.

6. About current medical problems. Are there any problems? Has the patient been feeling badly lately or been seeing a doctor?

7. If *any* medications are being taken.

8. If the patient has any allergies. Even a simple allergy can cause discomfort. If you know about a patient's allergy, then you may be able to help keep that substance away from the patient.

This list really does not offer that many new things for you to consider. It is not unusual for you to introduce yourself and to find out someone's name. If you saw the person was sick or in pain, you would ask what was wrong and how did it happen. Haven't you then asked, "Are you seeing a doctor?" and "Are you taking anything for the problem?" Asking about previous problems and allergies may not be part of your past experience. Certainly, you have asked children their ages and have asked about their parents.

There is a tendency to see that something is wrong and begin immediately to take care of the problem. This is correct for the primary survey, but it could be wrong during the secondary survey. For example, you note that the patient has a broken leg. Should you stop the interview to do something about this fracture? *Think!* You cannot stop a broken leg! True, as a First Responder you will know some courses of action to take with fractures, and you should do so at the proper time. What you can stop is bleeding, if you find it. What you can stop is additional injury to the spine and nervous system, if you think there are possible spinal injuries. What you may be able to do is slow down internal bleeding, if you suspect it may be occurring. To help the patient, you must know the possible problems. To be a First Responder, you *must* be able to conduct an interview.

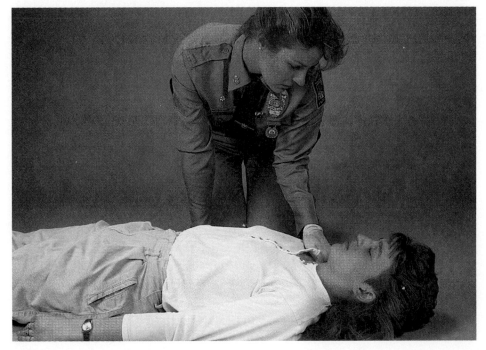

FIGURE 3–6.
Interviewing may continue through the secondary survey examination.

Can you be doing other things during the interview? Yes, providing you do not break contact with the patient and you do not do anything that may aggravate injuries, especially spinal injuries. Try to maintain contact with the patient. Eye-to-eye contact is best. If you look away while asking a question or while the patient is answering, then confidence and personal communication may be lost. When lost, they are replaced by fear.

You can touch the patient's forehead to note relative skin temperature. Not only are you gaining medical information but also you are communicating with the patient. In our culture, this is an indication of caring and attention. You also may begin to care for a problem that concerns the patient. For example, you might begin to stop minor bleeding on an arm while asking questions. Such actions may even improve communication with the patient. However, you must not be turning the patient's head or moving the arm until you are sure that spinal injuries are not part of the problem.

In situations where there is more than one patient, particularly when there are severe accident injuries, then this method of interviewing will have to be modified. This problem and the approaches to take will be covered later.

THE EXAMINATION

1st RULE 1: If anything about the patient's awareness or behavior does not seem right to you, consider that something is seriously wrong with the patient.

The objective examination should always begin with determining the patient's state of consciousness. If the patient is conscious, then you need to determine the level of alertness, responsiveness, rationality, confusion, and distress. All these factors must be considered and then reported when more highly trained personnel arrive at the scene.

1st RULE 2: Even patients who appear stable may worsen rapidly. You must be aware of all changes in a patient's condition.

Patients change condition as time passes. Sometimes this happens very quickly and other times this may take hours. Be on the alert for changing respiration, failing heart action, new profuse bleeding, and the onset of shock.

1st RULE 3: You must watch the patient's skin for color changes.

The body often indicates severe problems and injuries with changes in skin color. You need to note any odd colorations of the patient's skin and stay alert for color changes. The fingertips and lips are often the first areas that show any changes. Blacks and individuals with dark complexions may not show skin color changes as readily as people with lighter skin. For these patients, be aware of changes at the lips, tongue, nailbeds, whites of the eyes, and earlobes. Table 3–1 lists some of the skin coloration changes you might see and how they relate to specific medical problems. Do not try to memorize this table. Each of these changes will be considered at other points in this book.

1st RULE 4: You must observe the patient and note anything that looks wrong.

You do not want to contaminate wounds, aggravate fractures, or restart bleeding. Also, you do not wish to cause the patient any additional pain. Before you touch the patient, look carefully for obvious fractures, deformities, burns, wounds, swelling and puffiness, ulcers and blotches on the skin, and blood-soaked areas.

1st RULE 5: Unless you are certain that the patient has no spinal injuries (for example, a conscious patient with medical problem), *assume* the patient

TABLE 3–1. ASSESSMENT SIGN: SKIN COLOR

Observation	Possible Problem
Red	Heat stroke, high blood pressure, heart attack, diabetic coma
Pale, ashen	Shock, heart attack, bleeding, fright, reduced circulation, insulin shock
Blue	Airway problems, heart failure, lack of oxygen, lung disease, certain poisonings
Yellow	Liver disease
Black and blue	Seepage of blood under the skin surface

has spinal injuries. In emergency care, any unconscious injured patient is assumed to have spinal injuries.

We will cover spinal injuries in other chapters. For now, remember that you need to examine the patient without aggravating spinal injuries.

1st RULE 6: You must say that you are going to examine the patient and stress the importance of the examination.

When dealing with a conscious patient, tell him that you need to perform an examination. You must receive the alert patient's permission to conduct this examination. Assure the patient that you have noticed obvious injuries and have understood his complaints, but you must be certain that nothing else is wrong. Be honest with the patient and say that the examination may produce some pain and discomfort. Have the patient acknowledge or respond to what you are saying.

As you conduct the examination, let the patient know whenever you need to lift, rearrange, or remove *any* article of clothing. Always tell what you are going to do before you do it.

Vital Signs

1st For most First Responders the vital signs are pulse, respiration, and relative skin temperature. Many First Responders are also responsible for blood pressure determination (see Appendix 2). You might think that taking vital signs is not worth doing since you cannot give any medications. However, vital signs can provide you with important information on the patient's current condition. These signs also can alert you to problems that require immediate attention. When repeated, vital signs are good indicators of changes in the patient's condition.

As you go through your First Responder course, notice how certain combinations of vital signs point to possible illnesses and injuries. For example, cool, clammy skin, a rapid, weak pulse, and difficult breathing indicate possible shock. If the skin is hot and dry and the pulse is rapid and full, then heat stroke is a possibility.

In medicine, there are high-priority patients. These patients require a physician's attention immediately. A First Responder does not have the training or the facilities at hand to begin the care that a physician would. This does not mean that you cannot make a difference. You may be able to provide care that reduces the severity of shock. You may save a patient's life if you start basic life support should the patient stop breathing. The early indications of many high-priority situations are found by determining vital signs.

A continuous pulse rate below 50 beats per minute or above 100 beats per minute is considered serious. By keeping the patient at rest and providing care for shock, you may lessen the severity of this condition. Talking to the conscious patient, assuring that you will help and that more help is on the way, may prove to be significant. As the patient relaxes and stays aware, rapid pulse rates will often slow and low pulse rates will often stabilize. The changes may be slight, but these changes could be significant. Fear may not be the reason why the heart is beating too rapidly or too slowly, but fear will worsen the condition. Sometimes simple, reassuring conversation with the patient can change the pulse rate as much as 10 beats per minute. This could save a patient's life.

A respiratory rate above 28 breaths per minute or below 8 breaths per minute is considered to be a serious condition. Again, through keeping the patient at rest, caring for shock, and reassuring the conscious patient, you can make a difference.

These conditions are considered serious because they indicate very unstable situations that could be life threatening. The patient could worsen at any second and possibly go into respiratory arrest or cardiac arrest. Stay alert and constantly monitor the patient.

1st Pulse

Two factors, *rate* and *character*, must be determined when taking a patient's pulse. In terms of rate, you have to determine the number of beats per minute. This will provide you with the information necessary to decide if the patient's pulse rate is **normal, rapid,** or **slow.** Character considers the rhythm and force of the pulse. You will judge the pulse as being **regular** or **irregular** in regard to rhythm and **full** or **thready** (weak) in regard to force (strength).

Radial pulse—the wrist pulse. The site is in the lateral wrist.

During the secondary survey, a wrist pulse is measured. This is called a **radial pulse,** named for the radial artery found in the lateral portion of the forearm (remember the anatomical position) at the wrist. If for any reason you cannot measure the radial pulse, determine pulse rate and characteristics by using the carotid pulse. Should you have to move the patient's arm in order to measure a radial pulse, and you believe that the patient may have spinal injuries or injuries to the arm, use the other arm. If this is not possible, use the carotid pulse. If you find no pulse at the wrist, you must take a carotid pulse. *Do not* start CPR based upon the absence of a radial pulse.

1st To measure radial pulse rate, you should:

1. Use the three middle fingers of your hand. This approach enables you to stay fixed over the pulse site and judge the amount of pressure being applied. Do not use your thumb to measure pulse rate. The thumb has its own pulse, and you would be measuring your own pulse rate instead of the patient's.
2. Place your fingertips on the palm side of the patient's wrist, just above the crease between hand and wrist. Slide your fingers from this position toward the thumb side of the wrist (lateral side). Keeping the fingertip of the middle finger on the crease between wrist and hand will ensure you of placing the fingertip over the site of the radial pulse.
3. Apply moderate pressure to feel the pulse beats. If the pulse is weak, you may have to apply more pressure. Too much pressure can cause discomfort to the patient or problems with blood flow. By having three fingers in contact with the patient's wrist and hand, you should be able to judge how much pressure you are applying.
4. Once you can feel pulsations, make a quick judgment as to rate. Does this pulse feel normal, rapid, or slow? This is done in case something happens that prevents you from making a full assessment.
5. Count the number of beats for 30 seconds.
6. While counting, judge rhythm and force.
7. Multiply your count by 2 to determine the radial pulse rate in beats per minute.

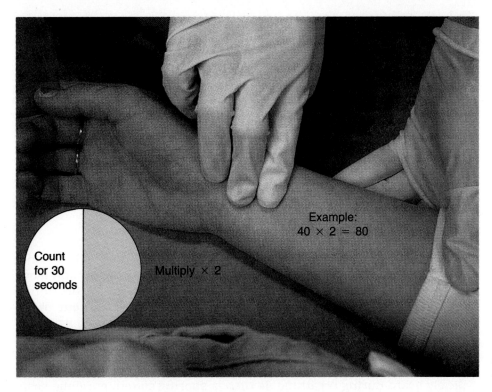

Count for 30 seconds

Multiply × 2

Example:
40 × 2 = 80

FIGURE 3–7.
Pulse rate and character are vital signs.

1st NOTE: If the patient's pulse feels irregular, count the beats for one full minute.

While you are determing the pulse rate, notice if the beats are regular, regardless of the rate of the pulse. A rapid, regular beat means something quite different from a rapid, irregular beat. At the same time, judge the force of the pulse. If it is strong, if you have the impression that a wave of blood is passing under your fingertips, then the pulse is full. If you feel a weak pulse, causing you to believe that the flow is "thin," then the pulse is thready. Before you finish counting the pulse beats to find rate, you should be able to say if the pulse is rapid or slow, regular or irregular, and full or thready.

Table 3–2 shows the relationship between pulse and certain emergency problems you might see as a First Responder. Do not try to memorize this table. These situations will be covered later.

The normal pulse rate for adults at rest is between 60 and 80 beats per minute. Any rate above 80 is rapid and any rate below 60 is slow. In emergency situations, it is not unusual for this rate to be maintained around 100 beats per minute. Consider a pulse above 100 beats per minute or below 50 beats per minute to be a serious situation. The exception is an athlete. Some well-conditioned individuals have a normal pulse rate at or below 50 beats per minute.

Newborn infants can have pulse rates around 150 to 180 beats per

TABLE 3–2. ASSESSMENT SIGN: PULSE

Observation	Possible Problem
Rapid, full	Internal bleeding (early stages), fear, heat stroke, overexertion, high blood pressure, fever
Rapid, thready	Shock, blood loss, heat exhaustion, diabetic coma, failing circulatory system
Slow, full	Stroke, skull fracture, brain injury
No pulse	Cardiac arrest

minute. Children up to 5 years old will show ranges from 65 to 160 beats per minute, depending on their age and size. Children from 5 to 12 will show ranges from 70 to 110 beats per minute, again depending on age and size of the child. Some children in this age group may have normal pulse rates as low as 60 or as high as 120 beats per minute. Use the 70 to 110 range as a guideline. Any child with a pulse rate below 60 is considered to be in serious condition. Adolescents typically have a pulse rate ranging from 55 to 105 beats per minute.

You will have to practice determining pulse rates. Practice on both males and females, adults and children. Try taking "at rest" pulse rates and also pulse rates after the individual has completed some mild exercise. This practice will help you in judging and measuring normal and rapid rates.

1st Respirations

The rate and character of respiration are both considered during the secondary survey. The respiratory rate is classified as **normal, rapid,** and **slow.** Character will include **rhythm, depth, sound,** and **ease** of the breathing.

A single respiration is the entire cycle of breathing in and out. While you are counting these cycles, note if the rhythm is regular or irregular. At the same time, decide if the depth of breathing is normal, shallow, or deep.

While measuring respiratory rate, listen for any sounds that are not typically heard during breathing. Is there a snoring sound, gurgling, gasping, or birdlike crowing sounds? Notice if the breathing is easy or whether it appears labored, difficult, or painful. If the patient is conscious, ask if he is having any problems or pain when he breathes.

Table 3–3 shows some of the problems that are associated with variations in respiration. Do not try to memorize this table. This information will be covered at other points in this text.

1st To measure respiratory rate and character, you should:

1. Remain in the same position you assumed for measuring pulse. Keep your fingers on the patient's wrist as if you are still monitoring pulse rate. Many individuals tend to vary their rate of respiration when they know someone is watching them breathe.
2. Watch the patient's chest movements and listen for sounds.
3. Count the number of breaths (one breath = one inspiration and one

TABLE 3–3. ASSESSMENT SIGN: BREATHING

Observation	Possible Problem
Rapid, shallow	Shock, heart problems, heat exhaustion, insulin shock, heart failure, pneumonia
Deep, gasping, labored	Airway obstruction, heart failure, heart attack, lung disease, chest injury, lung damage from heat, diabetic coma
Slowed breathing	Head injury, stroke, chest injury, certain drugs
Snoring	Stroke, fractured skull, drug or alcohol abuse, partial airway obstruction
Crowing	Airway obstruction, airway injury due to heat
Gurgling	Airway obstruction, lung disease, lung injury due to heat
Wheezing	Asthma, emphysema, airway obstruction, heart failure
Coughing blood	Chest wound, fractured rib, punctured lung, internal injuries

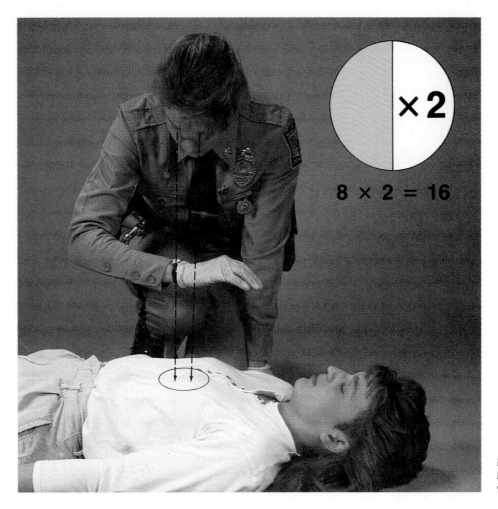

FIGURE 3–8.
Breathing rate and character are vital signs.

expiration) the patient takes in 30 seconds. Multiply this number by 2 to obtain breaths per minute.

4. While counting respirations, note rhythm, depth, sound, and ease of breathing.

If you have difficulty in establishing the respiratory rate, gently place your hand on the patient's chest, near the xiphoid process. This will allow you to feel each inspiration and expiration. Do not follow this procedure if there are obvious injuries to the chest or abdomen. Let the patient know you are going to touch his chest.

Normal respiratory rates for adults at rest fall into a range of 12 to 20 breaths per minute. Most people have 12 to 15 breaths per minute as their normal range. Older adults tend to breathe more slowly than young adults. Infants can have a range from 35 to 60 breaths per minute. For adults, a rate over 28 breaths per minute is serious. If the patient is a child from 1 to 5 years of age, a rate over 44 breaths per minute is serious. A rate over 36 breaths per minute is serious for children 5 to 12 years old.

1st Skin Temperature

Skin temperature is measured at the patient's forehead unless access to this area is not practical. Use the back of your hand to feel for **normal, hot, cool,** or **cold** skin temperature. At the same time, notice if the patient's skin is **dry, moist,** or **clammy.** Look for goose pimples often associated with chills.

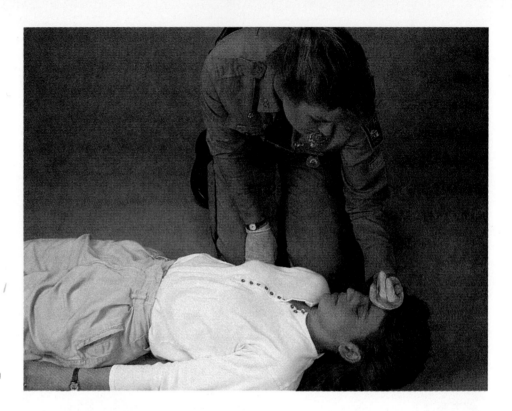

FIGURE 3–9.
Relative skin temperature is a vital sign.

Table 3–4 shows some of the problems associated with skin temperature. Do not try to memorize this table. These problems will be presented later in this text.

1st RULE 7: Take vital signs. This process will take a little over 1 minute. Information gained could save the patient's life.

TABLE 3–4. ASSESSMENT SIGN: SKIN TEMPERATURE

Observation	Possible Problem
Cool, moist	Shock, bleeding, loss of body heat, heat exhaustion
Cool, dry	Exposure to cold
Cool, clammy	Shock, heart attack, anxiety
Hot, dry	High fever, heat stroke
Hot, moist	Infection

Blood pressure

There is no doubt that the patient assessment is more reliable when the patient's blood pressure is taken and monitored. However, most First Responders do not carry a stethoscope and blood pressure cuff to measure this vital sign. If your EMS System has blood pressure determination as a required vital sign, see Appendix 2.

The Head-to-Toe Examination

This physical examination of the patient should take no more than 2 to 3 minutes. The entire survey need not be performed on every patient. This is true for minor accidents and obvious medical emergencies that do not

■ SCAN 3-4

VITAL SIGNS

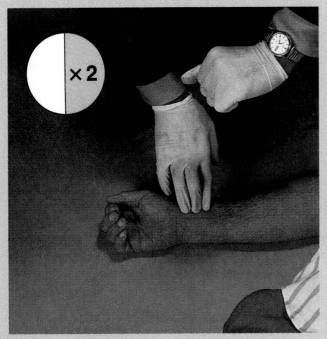

PULSE: Rate and character

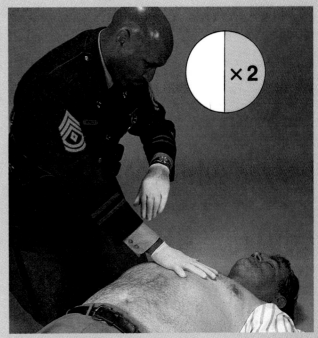

RESPIRATION: Rate and character

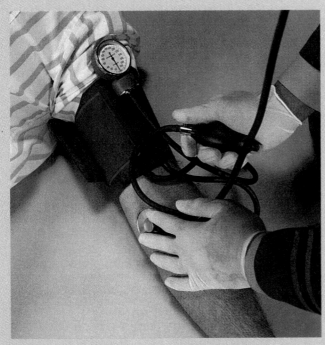

BLOOD PRESSURE: (Some First Responders)

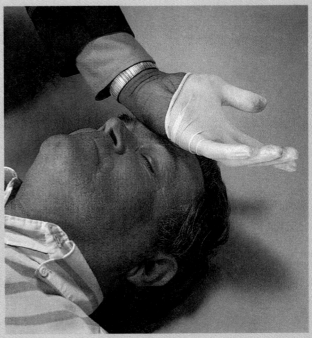

TEMPERATURE: (Relative skin)

involve injuries. Take a common sense approach. The total time of the secondary survey can be reduced if a second First Responder is present to take vital signs while you do the patient examination. During this examination, you must take great care not to move the patient. There could be neck and spinal injuries that have gone undetected by you and the patient.

The head-to-toe procedure may cause the patient some pain and discomfort. Therefore, you must know this procedure and each of its specific moves without any doubts. The more systematic you are in your approach and the more specific each of your moves is in the examination, the less pain and discomfort will be generated for the patient.

Again, take care not to contaminate wounds and aggravate injuries. *Do not* probe into wounds, fracture sites, and burns. If bleeding has obviously stopped, do not pull the clothing around the site, probe into the site, or pull on skin around the site. Your task is to find suspected injuries and medical problems and to provide care accordingly.

First Responders have little need to remove patient clothing during the head-to-toe examination. Readjust or remove only those articles of clothing that interfere with your ability to examine the patient. *Do not* try to pull clothing off the limbs of the patient. Such moves could greatly increase bleeding and injury. Most frequently, problems with clothing involve chest, back, and abdominal wounds. If you believe the patient has a wound in one of these areas, cut away, lift, slide, or unbutton the clothing so that you can examine the site of injury. Certain articles of clothing make the examination of the upper leg a difficult procedure. If there is suspected injury to the upper leg, clothing will have to be carefully cut away using scissors.

Penetrating wounds may have bleeding that will show or be felt on clothing. Internal injuries due to blunt object trauma often can be felt on examination or suspected because of the patient's reaction to your touch. An alert patient will direct you to many of these injuries. If the patient is not alert or is unconscious, you may have to remove or rearrange clothing to check the chest, abdomen, and back. If you believe that clothing has to be opened or removed, tell the patient what you are doing and why. Take great care to protect the modesty of the individual, and protect the individual from harsh weather conditions and low temperatures.

Some EMS Systems' standard operating procedures recommend having another woman present while a male First Responder examines a female patient. However, do not delay examining any patient. As a trained First Responder in an emergency situation, your intentions should be respected.

Some articles of clothing should be left in place. It is dangerous to remove gloves, particularly when they are tight fitting. Many times, if there is an open wound to the hand, the glove will help control the bleeding. When severe bleeding from the hand requires direct care of the wound site, a portion of the glove can be cut away so that you can control the bleeding. Take extra care if the bleeding is part of a crush injury to the hand.

The same rules apply to the removal of shoes and boots. Special practice is needed before you can properly deal with combat, work, and hiking boots. Ski boots require specialized training. (Contact a local ski patrol if applicable in your area.)

Technically, hairpieces and wigs are articles of clothing. When inspecting a patient's scalp, you may feel the netting of a hairpiece or see the border of the piece where it joins with the patient's natural hairline. *Do not* try to remove the hairpiece. Some have a permanent glue, while most are held by adhesive or tape. The removal of a wig may cause undesired movement of the patient's head and neck. Proper immobilization of the head and neck must be done by EMTs before a wig can safely be removed.

If the patient is wearing a hairpiece, make sure you notice any bleeding or deformity that can be felt through the netting. Also, do not judge a deformity in the netting to be a deformity of the patient's skull. *Do not* probe under a wig to inspect the scalp. To do so might cause additional injury to a head wound patient. It is best to leave the wig in place until EMTs can take over, unless life-threatening bleeding is coming from under the wig.

Begin the head-to-toe examination with another quick overview of the patient's body. Look for problems, listen for problems, feel for problems, and be aware of any strange odors that may indicate a problem.

1st RULE 8: Conduct a head-to-toe examination. Wear all the necessary items of personal protection. If *anything* looks, sounds, feels, smells, or "seems" wrong to you or to the patient, assume that there is something seriously wrong.

NOTE: The head-to-toe procedure is the traditional name for the objective patient examination. Actually, the neck should be examined first in an effort to improve the detection of possible spinal injuries. When the signs of these injuries are found, the head and neck can be stabilized to reduce the chances of causing additional injury (see Chapter 12). If the patient is unconscious, assume that there is spinal injury.

1st When conducting the head-to-toe examination, you should:

1. **Check the cervical spine for point tenderness and deformity.**

   That portion of the spinal column running through the neck is called the cervical (SER-ve-kal) spine. A painful response by the patient to gentle finger pressure is called point tenderness. Any point tenderness or deformity should be considered as an indication of possible spinal injury. **Where there is reason to believe a spinal injury has occurred, it is recommended that you stop the survey and immobilize the patient's head and neck.** Directions for doing so will be given later. After immobilizing the patient's head and neck, continue the head-to-toe examination.

   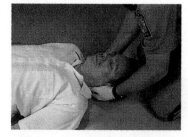

   FIGURE 3–10.
   Check the back of the neck for point tenderness. (Step 1)

   To check for *point tenderness* and *deformity* along the cervical spine, steady the patient's chin with one hand and check for midline point tenderness and deformities with your other hand. Be very careful and gentle during this procedure. Slide your fingertips in toward the patient's cervical midline at the region where head and neck meet. Keep the patient's head steady throughout the entire procedure. Warn the patient of possible pain.

   At this time, look for a medical alert identification device. Some people have such necklaces from the Medic Alert Foundation and other organizations. Be sure to note the information provided. *Do not* remove the necklace.

2. **Taking care not to aggravate neck or spinal injuries, check to see if the patient is a neck-breather.**

   This patient will have a surgical opening or a device in the front or side of the neck. Such patients will be covered in detail in Chapter 4.

   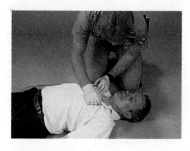

   FIGURE 3–11.
   Gently check the front of the neck for injuries and openings. (Step 2)

3. **Check the scalp for cuts and bruises.**

   Note: If you believe there is spinal injury, delay this procedure until the patient's head and neck can be immobilized. Take care not to move the patient's head. Run your fingers through the patient's hair, searching for blood. Gently feel for cuts, swelling, and any other indications of injury. *Do not* part the hair over possible injury sites to determine the nature of the wound and level of bleeding. Such action could restart bleeding. To examine the back of the head, gently slide your fingers under the back of the patient's neck and spread them upward to the back of the patient's head. Check your gloved fingers for blood.

   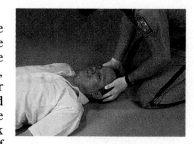

   FIGURE 3–12.
   Examine the scalp. (Step 3)

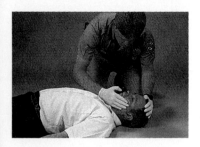

FIGURE 3–13.
After examining the scalp, check the skull and face. (Step 4)

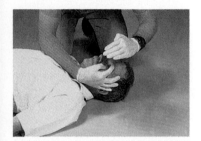

FIGURE 3–14.
Examine the eyelids, eyes, and pupils. (Step 5)

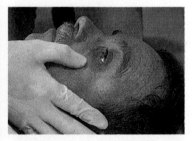

FIGURE 3–15.
Are the inner eyelids pale? (Step 6)

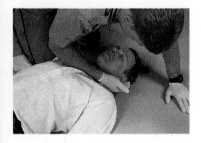

FIGURE 3–16.
Check the ears and nose for blood and clear fluids. (Step 7)

4. Check the skull for deformities and depressions and check the face.

While you are checking the scalp for cuts and bruises, note any depressions or bony projections that would indicate an injury to the skull. Check the facial bones for any signs of fracture (obvious breaks or crushing, swelling, heavy discoloration, or depressions of the bones).

5. Examine the patient's eyes.

Note any cuts, impaled objects, and any signs of chemical burns on the eyelids. (Chemical burns require immediate care.) Have the patient open his eyes or, in the case of the unresponsive patient, gently open his eyes by sliding back the upper eyelids. Look for cuts, foreign objects, impaled objects, and burns. Next, check the pupils for size, equality of size, and reaction to light. A pen light or other safe light source would be most helpful in this determination. Rate the pupils in terms of **dilated** or **constricted, equal** or **unequal,** and **bright** or **dull** (see Table 3–5). For our purposes, consider any variation listed in the table to be an indication of possible brain and spinal injury.

TABLE 3–5. ASSESSMENT SIGN: PUPILS

Observation	Possible Problem
Dilated, unresponsive	Unconsciousness, shock, cardiac arrest, bleeding, certain medications, head injury
Constricted, unresponsive	Central nervous system damage, certain medications
Unequal pupils	Stroke, head injury
Dull	Shock, coma

6. Look at the inner surface of the eyelids.

Are they pale? If so, this indicates the possibility of major blood loss to circulation. During the rest of the examination, be alert for external bleeding and indications of internal bleeding. A yellow color may indicate jaundice (possible liver injury or disease).

7. Inspect the ears and nose for blood, clear fluid, or bloody fluid.

A pen light or other source of light will be helpful. Blood in the nose may be the result of simple nasal tissue injury (a bloody nose). However, it could also mean a skull fracture. Blood in the ears or clear or bloody fluids in the ears or nose are strong indications of possible fractures in the skull bones.
WARNING: A conscious patient with clear fluids or blood in the nose and ears may refuse additional treatment and ask to leave. You must stress the importance of being examined by a physician. Make every effort to convince such patients to see a doctor.

Note also that parents may believe their child to be all right after an accident if there is no sign of severe injury. Tell them that fluids or blood in the nose or ears is a serious sign and that the child must be seen by a doctor.

8. Inspect the mouth for possible airway obstruction bleeding, and tissue damage.

When dealing with unconscious patients, you will have to open their mouths. Assume that the unconscious patient has neck and spinal injury. Follow the directions given in Chapter 4. For

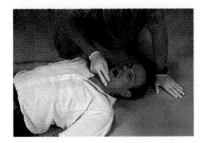

FIGURE 3–17.
Examine the mouth for
obstructions, bleeding, and
tissue damage. (Step 8)

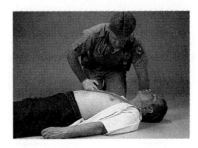

FIGURE 3–18.
Inspect the chest for wounds
and visible deformities. (Step 9)

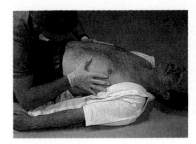

FIGURE 3–19.
Gently apply pressure to the
sides of the chest to check for
fractures. (Step 10)

all patients, look for broken teeth, dentures, bridges, and crowns
(caps). Check for chewing gum, food, vomitus, and foreign objects. If the patient is a child, take extra care in looking for toys,
balls, and other objects in the mouth or the back of the throat.
Should you find any objects, follow the directions given in Ch. 4.

While looking for airway obstruction, inspect the mouth for
blood. Move in close to the patient's mouth and note any odd
breath odors.

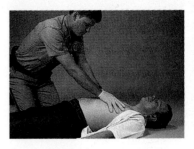

FIGURE 3–20.
Check for the equal expansion
of the chest. (Step 11)

9. **Inspect the chest for cuts, bruises, penetrations, and impaled
objects.**

If necessary, bare the chest and upper abdomen. *Do not* remove
any impaled objects. Follow your local protocols in regard to baring
the patient's chest. Usually, it is recommended to bare the chest
of an unconscious or injured patient.

10. **Examine the chest for possible fractures.**

After warning the patient of possible pain, gently apply pressure
to the sides of the chest with your hands. This process is called
compression. Pain indicates possible rib fractures.

11. **Check for equal expansion of the chest.**

Remain in the same position used to examine for chest fractures.
Feel for equal expansion of the chest. Look for chest movements
and note any section of the chest that appears to be floating or
moving in opposite directions to the rest of the chest. If you
cannot detect chest movements, bare the patient's chest and
look and feel for expansion. Provide female patients with as much
privacy as possible.

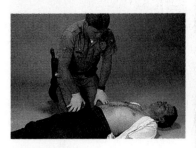

FIGURE 3–21.
Inspect the abdomen for
wounds and visible deformity.
(Step 12)

12. **Inspect the abdomen for cuts, bruises, penetrations, and impaled objects.**

13. **Feel the abdomen for tenderness.**

Prepare the patient for the possibility of pain. If the patient says
an area hurts, start away from this site. Gently press on the
abdomen with the palm side of your fingers, noting any rigid
areas, swollen areas, or reactions to pain. Many rescuers prefer
to do this by placing one hand on top of the other at the fingertips.
As you press, ask the patient, "Can you feel this?" and "Does
this hurt?" Note if the pain is **local** (confined to one spot) or
general (spread over a wide area). Be certain to check each abdominal quadrant and to relate any problems to specific quadrants.

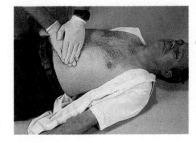

FIGURE 3–22.
Check for abdominal
tenderness. (Step 13)

14. **Feel the lower back for point tenderness and deformity.**

Take care not to move the patient. Check the area of the lower

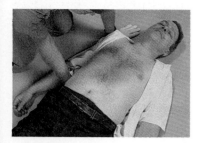

FIGURE 3–23.
Check the lower back for point tenderness. (Step 14)

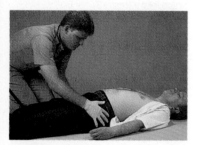

FIGURE 3–24.
Gently apply pressure to check for pelvic fractures. (Step 15)

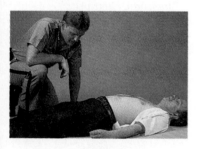

FIGURE 3–25.
Look for obvious injuries to the genital region. (Step 16)

back formed by the curve of the spine. **Gently** slide your gloved hands into position. Check your gloves for blood.

15. Feel the pelvis for injuries and possible fractures.

After checking the lower back, gently slide your hands from the small of the patient's back to the lateral "wings" of the pelvis. Warn the patient of possible pain and then lightly compress the pelvis toward the body's midline, noting any indications of pain or deformities.

16. Note any obvious injury to the genital region (groin).

Look for bleeding and impaled objects. *Do not* expose the area unless you believe there is an injury.

With male patients, check for priapism (PRI-a-pizm), the persistent erection of the penis caused by spinal injury. If there is any reason to suspect spinal injury and clothing prevents you from noting the presence of an erect penis, gently brush the genital region with the back of your hand. Priapism is an important indication of spinal injury and should be treated as a serious consideration during the head-to-toe examination.

17. Examine the legs and feet.

Examine each leg and foot individually. Always compare one limb to the other in terms of length, shape, and any apparent swellings or deformities. Do not move or lift the legs. Do not change the positions of the legs or feet from the position they were in at the beginning of the examination. Note any discolorations, bleeding, bone protrusions, and obvious fractures. If you think there is a fracture, warn the patient and then apply light fingertip pressure to the site. Note any point tenderness. **Do not touch possible fracture sites if the skin is broken.**

18. Check for a distal pulse.

The circulation of blood through the leg to the foot can be confirmed by feeling a distal pulse. In the majority of cases, the most useful pulse is the posterior tibial (TIB-e-al) pulse. This pulse can be felt behind the medial ankle as shown. If the patient is wearing boots, this pulse site might be obstructed. Removing the patient's boots may cause serious problems if there are spinal, leg, or foot injuries. Unless you must remove a boot to stop obvious bleeding, do *not* remove the boots of patients who have indications of crush injury to the leg or foot, objects impaled in the leg or foot, severe leg or foot fractures, or any indications or possibilities of spinal injury.

Another distal pulse, the dorsalis pedis (DOR-sal-is PEAD-is) pulse is located lateral to the large tendon of the big toe. This pulse can be of value in assessment because some patients do not have a posterior tibial pulse. Some EMS Systems do not

FIGURE 3–26.
Examine the legs and feet. DO NOT lift or move the legs or feet. (Step 17)

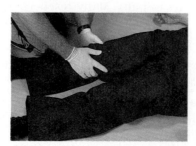

FIGURE 3–27.
When possible without risk to the patient, take a distal pulse. (Step 18)

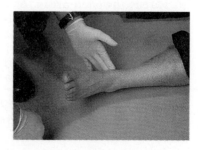

have First Responders use the dorsalis pedis pulse in the survey because they would have to unlace or remove the patient's shoe to feel this pulse.

REMEMBER: What you can do about the problem of circulation is minimal. Do not cause additional injury to the patient for the sake of taking a distal pulse. When possible, both legs must be checked for a distal pulse.

Some EMS Systems have the rescuer check for capillary refill at this point in the survey. See page 234 for more information.

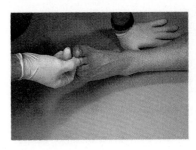

FIGURE 3–28.
Check for sensitivity in the toes of conscious patients. (Step 19)

19. **Check for nerve activity and possible paralysis to the legs and feet.**

This should not be performed on patients with possible fractures or dislocations of the lower limbs. Do not aggravate possible injuries by removing shoes. If you cannot rule out paralysis, assume the patient has spinal injury.

Begin by asking conscious patients to wave each foot by extending and then flexing it. Next, if the patient is responsive, touch a toe and ask the patient to tell you which toe you have touched. You may grasp a toe through the patient's shoe if you believe there are no injuries to the toes. Finally, have the patient gently press the sole of each foot against the palm of your hand. Consider all patients who fail these tests to have possible spinal injury. These tests must be done for both feet.

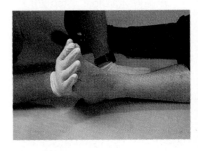

FIGURE 3–29.
Can the patient push his foot against the palm of your hand? (Step 19)

If the patient is not responsive, the above tests are useless. Most EMS Systems have guidelines calling for the unconscious patient to be treated as if neck and spinal injuries exist. As a First Responder, assume that all unconscious accident victims and all unconscious patients having an unwitnessed medical emergency have spinal injury.

Your EMS System may require you to perform special tests on the unconscious patient. Your instructor will tell you if this is the case for your locality. If so, you will have to hold the patient's leg at the ankle and pinch the most accessible area on the patient's leg. This is best done on the upper surface of the foot, near the ankle, if the patient's shoe allows access to this area. This procedure must be done on both feet. The patient, even though unconscious, should show a reflex action by pulling the leg away from the pain. Failure to do so must be considered the result of spinal injury.

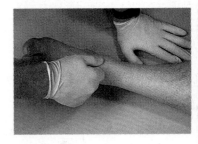

FIGURE 3–30.
If the patient is unconscious, pinch the most accessible area of the lower limbs. (Step 19)

Take great care in how you evaluate the results of this test. It is not very reliable under field conditions. If the patient merely moves his big toe, you may be confused by what you see. The downward movement of the toe is normal in the adult patient. An upward movement of only the toe may indicate possible injury to the brain. Again, you would do well to assume that the unconscious accident victim has neck and spinal injury.

20. **Examine the upper extremities from shoulders and collarbones (clavicles) to the fingertips.**

Each limb is examined separately. The procedures are like those for the lower extremities:

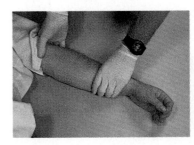

FIGURE 3–31.
Check the arms and hands for injuries. (Step 20)

- Note any cuts, bruises, impaled objects, bleeding, deformities, swellings, discolorations, protruding bones, or obvious fractures. Check for point tenderness at any suspected site of fracture. **Do not touch open fracture sites.**
- Confirm a radial pulse for both arms. Do not measure pulse rate. Simply confirm circulation. Your EMS System may have you check for capillary refill (see page 234).
- If alert, have the patient wave each hand, identify the finger you touch, and grip your hand. Remember, these tests must be done for both extremities.

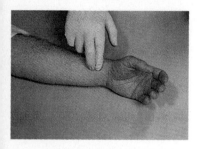

FIGURE 3–32.
Take a radial pulse. Remember, you did this for one arm when finding vital signs. (Step 20)

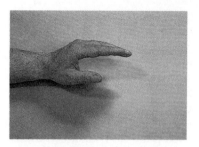

FIGURE 3–33.
Have the patient wave his hand. (Step 20)

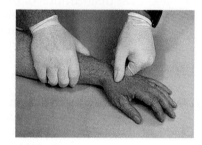

FIGURE 3–34.
Can the patient tell you which finger was touched? (Step 20)

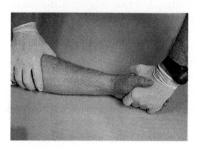

FIGURE 3–35.
Can the patient grasp your hand? (Step 20)

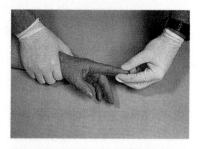

FIGURE 3–36.
If the patient is unconscious, pinch the hands. (Step 20)

- If the patient is not responsive, and your EMS System requires you to do so, pinch the patient's hand and look for reflex actions. Be certain to grasp the patient's arm as shown when pinching the hand. Remember, assume that the unconscious accident victim has neck and spinal injury.
- Look for a medical identification bracelet.

1st RULE 9: The failure of the patient to respond properly on any test for leg or arm nerve function *must* be considered a sign of spinal injury.

WARNING: Any awake and alert patient who cannot move his or her hands or arms may suddenly stop breathing. Constantly monitor the patient.

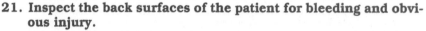

21. **Inspect the back surfaces of the patient for bleeding and obvious injury.**

Do not lift or roll the patient if there is any indication of skull, neck, or spinal injuries. It is best to consider any unconscious patient as having a neck injury. These injuries are difficult to detect and may be greatly aggravated if you lift or roll the patient.

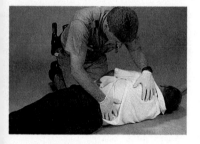

FIGURE 3–37.
If there are no injuries to the head, neck, spine, or extremities, inspect the back surfaces. (Step 21)

Upon completing the examination of the patient, you will have to consider all the signs found that could indicate an illness or injury. Certain combinations of signs can point to one specific problem. A finding as simple as pain in a certain body region could be significant. The lack of certain findings may also lead you to a conclusion. For example, if a patient has an obvious injury, but shows no reaction to pain, you will have to consider problems such as spinal injury, brain damage, shock, or drug abuse.

SECONDARY SURVEY

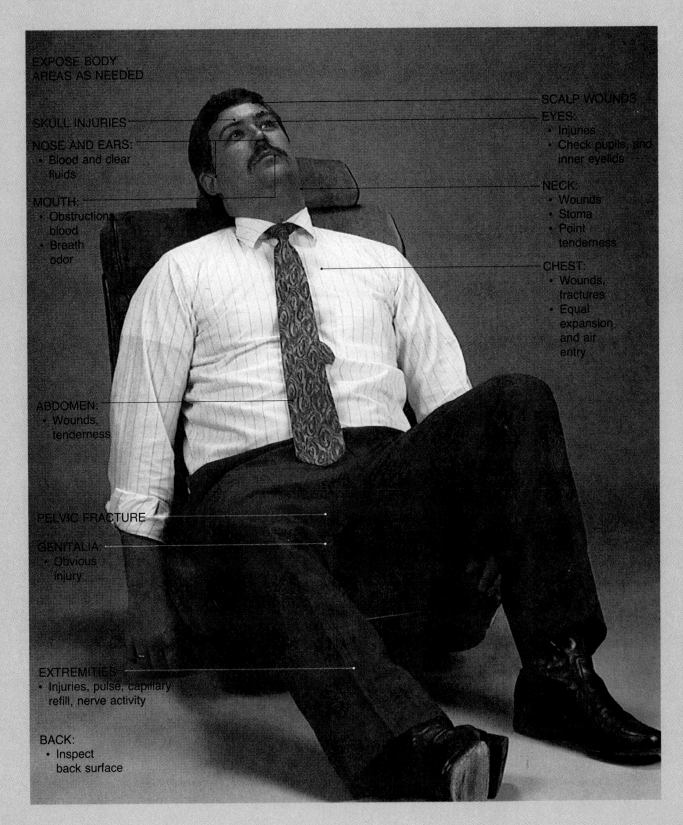

EXPOSE BODY
AREAS AS NEEDED

SKULL INJURIES

NOSE AND EARS:
• Blood and clear
fluids

MOUTH:
• Obstructions,
blood
• Breath
odor

ABDOMEN:
• Wounds,
tenderness

PELVIC FRACTURE

GENITALIA:
• Obvious
injury

EXTREMITIES:
• Injuries, pulse, capillary
refill, nerve activity

BACK:
• Inspect
back surface

SCALP WOUNDS

EYES:
• Injuries
• Check pupils, and
inner eyelids

NECK:
• Wounds
• Stoma
• Point
tenderness

CHEST:
• Wounds,
fractures
• Equal
expansion
and air
entry

As you learn to conduct the patient assessment, keep in mind the oldest emergency care rule:

1st RULE 10: *Do no harm.* Do only what you have been trained to do, avoiding additional injury and aggravating existing injuries and problems.

Later we will consider what you can do to help the patient based on the information gained in this head-to-toe survey. We will also consider how to help stabilize the patient and what to do if there is more than one patient.

TABLE 3–6. RULES FOR THE PATIENT EXAMINATION

For All Patient Examinations, the First Responder Must Follow These Rules:

Rule 1:	If anything about the patient's awareness or behavior does not seem "right," consider that something is seriously wrong.
Rule 2:	Patients who appear stable may worsen rapidly. You must be aware of all changes in a patient's condition.
Rule 3:	Watch the patient's skin for color changes.
Rule 4:	Look over the entire patient and note anything that appears to be wrong.
Rule 5:	Unless you are certain that the patient is free of spinal injury, assume he or she has spinal injury.
Rule 6:	Tell the patient you are going to examine him or her and stress the importance of the examination.
Rule 7:	Take vital signs.
Rule 8:	Conduct a head-to-toe examination. If anything looks, sounds, feels, smells, or "seems" wrong to you or the patient, assume that there is something seriously wrong with the patient.
Rule 9:	The failure of the patient to respond properly on any test for leg or arm nerve action must be considered to be a sign of spinal injury.
Rule 10:	*Do no harm.*

SUMMARY

The primary and secondary surveys are two of the most important things you will learn as a First Responder. Even though they may seem time consuming, they have to be done to allow you to find life-threatening problems and care for those problems as quickly as possible. Then, you must detect other problems that could become life threatening. Remember, it is impossible to provide quality First Responder care for a patient unless you have the information you need to tell you what that care should be.

Before going back to the chapter objectives, review the following:

Arrival—Gain information quickly from the scene, the patient, bystanders, mechanisms of injury, deformities or injuries, and signs.

Primary survey—Determine if the patient is responsive. Next, check for respiration, circulation, and profuse bleeding. Make certain that there is an open airway and adequate breathing. Confirm a carotid pulse. Stop all serious bleeding.

Secondary survey—Interview: Look over the scene, look over the patient, and look for medical identification devices. Now, gather information by asking questions and listening. The more organized you are in the interview, the better your chances of gaining needed information.

Secondary survey—Vital signs: As part of the examination phase of the secondary survey, take vital signs. Determine **pulse rate** and **pulse character.** Determine **respiratory rate** and the **character of respirations.** Determine relative **skin temperature.** Skin color should also be noted at this time, as well as the general condition of the skin. In some EMS Systems, blood pressure is measured.

Can you list all the characters of pulse and respiration that are considered when determining vital signs?

Secondary survey—Head-to-toe examination:

Determine level of consciousness

Neck—Examine the patient for possible injury and point tenderness of the **cervical spine.**

Neck—Recheck to see if the patient is a **neck breather.** Note obvious injuries and look for medical identification devices.

Head—Check **scalp** for cuts, bruises, swellings, and other signs of injury. Examine **skull** for deformities, depressions, and other signs of injury. Include the facial bones. Inspect the **eyelids** for injury and then do the same for the **eyes.** Determine **pupil** size, equality, and reactions to light. Note the color of the **inner surface** of the **eyelids.** Look for blood, clear fluids, or bloody fluids in the **nose** and **ears.** Examine the **mouth** for airway obstructions, blood, and any odd odors.

Chest—Examine the chest for cuts, bruises, penetrations, and impaled objects. Check for fractures. Look for equal expansion and note chest movements.

Abdomen—Examine the abdomen for cuts, bruises, penetrations, and impaled objects. Check for **local pain** and **general pain** as you examine the abdomen for tenderness.

Lower back—Feel for *point tenderness*, *deformity*, and other signs of injury.

Pelvis—Use **compression** to check for fractures and note any signs of injuries.

Genital region—Note any obvious injuries. Look for **priapism** when examining male patients.

Lower extremities—Examine for deformities, swellings, discolorations, bleeding, bone protrusions, and obvious fractures. Run point tenderness tests on suspected closed fracture sites.
Confirm a **distal pulse** for both legs. Do a capillary refill if required. Determine nerve activity.

Upper extremities—Examine for deformities, swellings, bleeding, discolorations, bone protrusions, and obvious fractures. Run point tenderness tests on all suspected closed fracture sites.
Confirm a **radial pulse** for both arms. Do a capillary refill if required. Determine nerve activity. Look for medical identification devices.

Back surfaces—Examine for obvious injuries.

Scansheets 3–4 and 3–5 will help you review the patient assessment.

CHAPTER 4

Breathing—
The Airway and
Pulmonary
Resuscitation

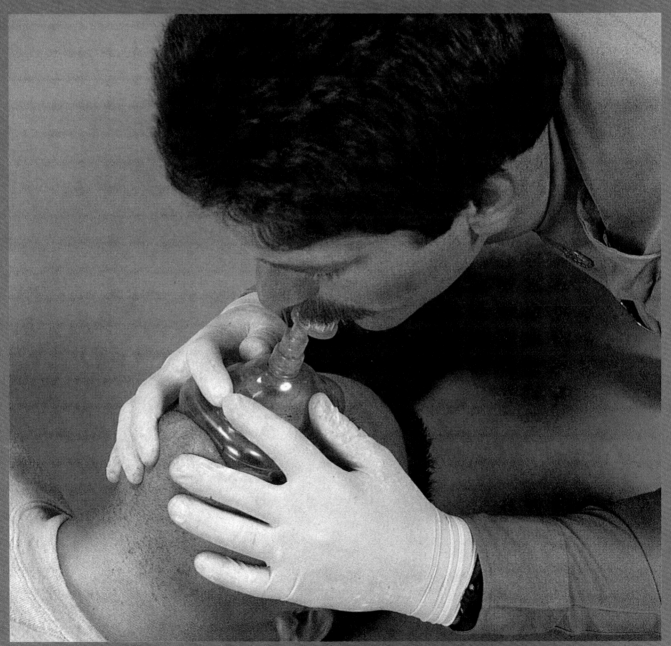

■ OBJECTIVES

By the end of this chapter, you should be able to:

1. State three reasons why we must breathe to stay alive. (p. 85)
2. Define clinical death and biological death, stating the approximate time in which brain cells will begin to die if they do not receive oxygen. (p. 86)
3. Name the major muscle used in breathing. (p. 87)
4. Relate, in a very general way, changes in volume and pressure in the lungs to the process of breathing. (pp. 87–88)
5. Label a drawing of respiratory anatomy, using everyday terms. (p. 89)
6. List the signs of adequate and inadequate breathing. (p. 89)
7. Describe, step by step, the head-tilt, chin-lift maneuver. (pp. 90–91)
8. Describe, step by step, the jaw-thrust maneuver, relating this maneuver to unconscious patients with possible neck and spinal injuries. (p. 91)
9. List the *seven steps* in the mouth-to-mask resuscitation technique and give the rate for delivering ventilations. (p. 93)
10. List the *nine steps* in the mouth-to-mouth resuscitation technique and give the rate of delivering ventilations. (p. 94)
11. Compare and contrast mouth-to-nose ventilation with mouth-to-mouth ventilation. (pp. 94–95)
12. List the *seven steps* in providing pulmonary resuscitation for an infant and for a small child, stating the rate for delivering ventilations. (p. 96)
13. State, in *four steps*, the special procedures used for the mouth-to-stoma technique. (p. 98)
14. Describe how to provide pulmonary resuscitation for the following patient: an automobile accident victim, still in the vehicle, who is unconscious with signs of possible neck and spinal injuries. (pp. 98–99)
15. State what *two* things a First Responder may do in relation to air in the patient's stomach (gastric distention) caused by artificial ventilation. (p. 99)
16. List *five* factors that may cause partial or complete airway obstruction. (p. 100)
17. List *three* signs of partial airway obstruction. (p. 100)
18. State when you should care for a partial airway obstruction as if it were a complete airway obstruction. (p. 100)
19. Describe *two* things you will commonly notice about a conscious patient with a complete airway obstruction. (p. 101)
20. Describe, step by step, the procedures for correcting airway obstructions, including:
    - back blows (infants only)
    - manual thrusts
      - abdominal thrusts
      - chest thrusts
    - finger sweeps (pp. 101–105)
21. State the sequence of combined procedures for correcting an airway obstruction when the patient is conscious. (pp. 106–107, 108)
22. State the sequence of combined procedures for correcting an airway obstruction when a conscious patient loses consciousness. (pp. 107, 109)
23. State the sequence of combined procedures for correcting an airway obstruction when the patient is unconscious. (pp. 107, 109)

WARNING: It is recommended that EMS personnel reduce the risk of contracting infectious diseases by using pocket face masks with one-way valves (see page 92) when ventilating patients. Latex or vinyl gloves should be worn during assessment and care (see page 4).

SKILLS

Upon completing this chapter and your class lectures and skills labs, you should be able to:

1. Determine if a patient is breathing adequately.
2. Apply the proper techniques and sequence of events for the relief of an upper airway obstruction, when given an adult and an infant manikin.
3. Properly demonstrate the head-tilt, chin-lift, and jaw-thrust maneuvers.
4. Correctly perform mouth-to-mask, mouth-to-mouth, and mouth-to-nose pulmonary resuscitation techniques on an adult manikin.
5. Correctly perform pulmonary resuscitation techniques on an infant manikin.
6. Correctly demonstrate the mouth-to-stoma technique.
7. Demonstrate the techniques used for patients with possible neck or spinal injuries.

BREATHING

Why We Breathe

Breathing is essential. If this basic process stops or if it becomes too inefficient, all other life processes will cease. Once breathing stops, the heart will soon stop beating. When this occurs, irreversible brain cell damage begins within 4 to 6 minutes. Within 10 minutes, the cells of the brain may start to die. In a very short period of time, cells making up the various organs and structures of the body begin to die. Death is not a reversible process. Once these cells die, they are no longer able to carry out their life functions and will never do so again. If enough cells die, the person dies.

The act of breathing is called **respiration.** During this process, oxygen is brought into the body and carbon dioxide is expelled. Oxygen is required by all body cells. This oxygen is used in chemical reactions to make compounds that store energy. All life processes require energy. The body uses energy to contract muscles, send nerve impulses, digest food, and build new tissues. When the body needs energy, it uses oxygen to help break down these storage compounds so they will release their stored energy. Energy cannot be properly stored, released, and used unless the cells receive oxygen.

In addition to supplying the cells with oxygen, breathing carries out the important function of removing carbon dioxide from our cells. As the body stores and uses energy, carbon dioxide is given off as a waste product. Carbon dioxide, if allowed to accumulate in the body's cells, soon becomes a deadly poison. Even if there is enough oxygen, an increase in carbon dioxide can cause dramatic events to take place. The individual will soon start panting, trying to rid the body of the excess carbon dioxide. Often, the person becomes restless or combative. Drowsiness will occur as the brain cells react to the excess carbon dioxide. Brain cells will start to malfunction, perhaps causing the individual to hallucinate (see things). Other brain functions, including those controlling respiration, will begin to fail. The individual will go into a coma and, unless something is done to reduce the level of carbon dioxide, the individual will die.

Along with bringing in oxygen and expelling carbon dioxide, the respiratory system plays a key role in keeping the blood from becoming too acidic or too alkaline (basic). If breathing is not adequate or if it fails completely, this balancing function stops. If our blood is too acidic or too basic, cells die. The brain is very sensitive to improper levels of acids and bases. Quickly, brain functions will cease, including those that control breathing.

Respiration—the act of breathing. The exchange of oxygen and carbon dioxide that takes place in the lungs.

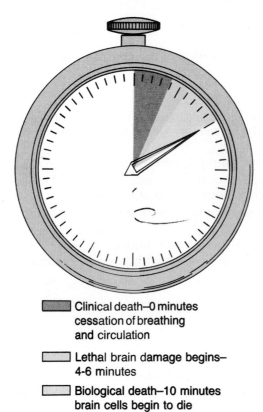

FIGURE 4–1.
Without oxygen, brain cells may begin to die within 10 minutes.

Clinical death–0 minutes cessation of breathing and circulation

Lethal brain damage begins– 4-6 minutes

Biological death–10 minutes brain cells begin to die

1st REMEMBER: Breathing allows the body to take in oxygen needed by the cells, to remove carbon dioxide that can poison cells, and to help control the acid–base balance of the blood.

1st As a First Responder, you need to know the difference between clinical death and biological death.

Clinical death—the moment that breathing and heart actions stop.

Biological death—when the brain cells die. This is usually within 10 minutes of respiratory arrest.

Clinical death—a patient is clinically dead the moment breathing stops and the heart stops beating.

Biological death—if a patient is not receiving oxygen, brain cells will usually be damaged in 4 to 6 minutes. Brain cell death may begin within 10 minutes. A patient is biologically dead when the brain cells die. Clinical death can be reversed; biological death is irreversible.

NOTE: The process of biological death may be delayed by cold temperatures, especially when related to cold-water drowning.

How We Breathe

Breathing is automatic. Even though you can control certain aspects of depth and rate, your control is short term and soon gives way to involuntary orders from the respiratory centers of the brain. If you try to hold your breath, these centers will urge you to breathe and then take over to force you to breathe. If you try to breathe slow, shallow breaths while running, these centers will automatically adjust the rate and depth of breathing to suit the needs of your body's cells. Asleep, or even unconscious, if there is no damage to these respiratory centers and the heart continues to circulate oxygenated blood to the brain, breathing will be an involuntary, automatic function. The needs of your cells, not your will, are the determining factors in the control of breathing.

The lungs are very elastic, always trying to expand. This expansion is

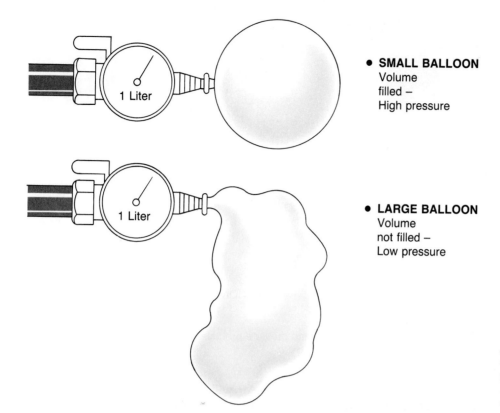

- **SMALL BALLOON**
  Volume
  filled –
  High pressure

- **LARGE BALLOON**
  Volume
  not filled –
  Low pressure

FIGURE 4–2.
An equal amount of air
delivered to each balloon will
not produce the same pressure.
If you increase the volume, you
decrease the pressure.

limited by the size of the chest cavity and the pressure within the cavity pushing back on the lungs. To inhale air (called an **inspiration**), the size of the chest cavity must increase and the pressure inside the cavity must be reduced. A simple law governs respiration: **as volume increases, pressure decreases.**

Inspiration—to inhale air. The process of breathing in.

If you take the air out of a small balloon and place this same amount of air into a larger balloon, the final pressure inside the large balloon will not be as great as it was in the smaller one. Why? The larger balloon has a greater volume to be filled. The air from the small balloon will produce less pressure inside the large one.

The volume of the chest cavity is increased by contracting muscles. This may sound a little backward because contractions usually make things get smaller. However, as you contract the muscles between your ribs, this action pulls the front of the ribs upward and forces them outward. This increases the volume of the chest cavity. When you contract your diaphragm, the major muscle of respiration, it flattens downward, increasing the space above it. The space above the diaphragm is the chest cavity (see Chapter 2). This means that the **volume** in the chest cavity **increases.** Each time the volume in the chest cavity increases, there is a **decrease** in the **pressure** within the cavity that pushes against the outside of the lungs.

1st The major muscle used in breathing is the **diaphragm.** When this muscle and the muscles between the ribs contract, the volume of the chest cavity increases and the pressure on the outside of the lungs decreases. See Figure 4–3, but do not try to memorize the various pressures cited in this figure. They have been shown so that you can see how the pressure decreases.

Diaphragm—the dome-shaped muscle that separates the chest and abdominal cavities. It is the major muscle used in breathing.

When the volume of the chest cavity increases and the pressure within the chest cavity decreases, the lungs will expand automatically. As the lungs expand, the volume inside each lung increases. This means that the pressure inside each lung will decrease. When the pressure inside the lungs becomes less than the pressure in the atmosphere, air will rush into the lungs, since air moves from high pressure to low pressure. (A punctured automobile

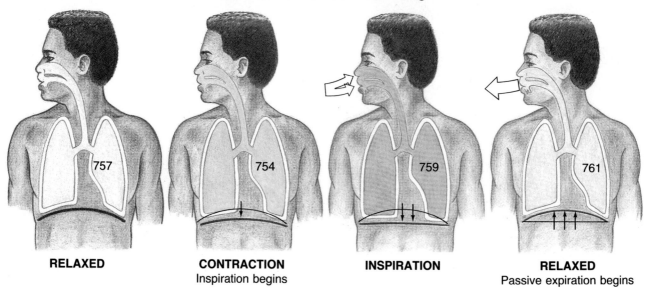

ATMOSPHERIC PRESSURE 760 mmHg

RELAXED	CONTRACTION	INSPIRATION	RELAXED
	Inspiration begins		Passive expiration begins

FIGURE 4–3. *Changes in volume and pressure produce inspirations and expirations (mm Hg = millimeters of mercury pressure).*

tire quickly demonstrates this fact.) Air will move into the lungs until the air pressure in the lungs equals the air pressure in the atmosphere.

1st When the lungs expand, the pressure inside the lungs becomes less than the pressure of the air in the atmosphere. Air moves from high pressure (atmosphere) to low pressure (lungs).

1st To exhale air **(expiration),** the process is reversed. The diaphragm and the muscles between the ribs relax, reducing the volume in the chest cavity. Pressure builds in the lungs until it becomes greater than the pressure in the atmosphere. This causes the air to flow from high pressure (lungs) to low pressure (atmosphere). Inspiration is an active process. You do work by contracting the diaphragm and the muscles between the ribs. Expiration is a passive process. No work has to be done for air to leave the lungs and return to the atmosphere.

Expiration—to exhale air. The passive process of breathing out.

Respiratory System Anatomy

1st You have already learned that there are respiratory centers in the brain. You have also learned that the diaphragm and the muscles between the ribs are the muscles of respiration. The other major structures of the respiratory system are the:

- Nose—the primary pathway through which air enters and leaves the system.
- Mouth—the secondary pathway through which air enters and leaves the system.
- Throat—the common passageway for air and food. This is also called the pharynx (FAR-inks).
- Voice box—the passageway for air found in the neck at the top of the windpipe. This region is also called the larynx (LAR-inks).
- Windpipe—the passageway for air flowing from the larynx. This is also called the trachea (TRAY-ke-ah).
- Bronchial tree—the tubes that branch out from the windpipe and take air to the exchange levels of the lungs.
- Lungs—the elastic organs containing microscopic air sacs (alveoli), where exchange of oxygen and carbon dioxide takes place with the blood.

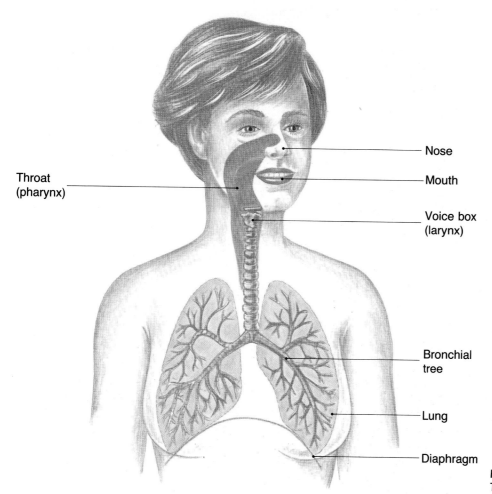

Throat (pharynx)

Nose

Mouth

Voice box (larynx)

Bronchial tree

Lung

Diaphragm

FIGURE 4–4.
The respiratory system.

ASSESSMENT SIGNS

1st Normal Breathing

- **Look** for the even rise and fall of the chest associated with breathing.
- **Listen** for air entering and leaving the nose or mouth. The sounds should be those typically heard in breathing (no gurgling, gasping, or other unusual (atypical) sounds).
- **Feel** for air moving into and out of the nose or mouth.
- **Observe** skin coloration. The skin should not be blue, gray, or ashen.
- **Note** that the rate and depth of breathing should be typical for the adult person when at rest (usually 12 to 15 breaths per minute).

1st Inadequate Breathing

- No chest movements or uneven chest movements.
- No air can be heard or felt at the nose or mouth.
- Breathing is noisy (see Chapter 3).
- The rate of breathing is too rapid or too slow. (Below 8 or above 30 breaths per minute could be critical for an adult.)
- Breathing is very shallow, or very deep and labored.
- The patient's skin is blue, gray, or ashen.

PULMONARY RESUSCITATION

Pulmonary resuscitation (PUL-mo-ner-e re-SUS-si-TAY-shun)—to provide breaths to a patient in an attempt to maintain artificially normal lung function.

Pulmonary (PUL-mo-ner-e) refers to the lungs. Resuscitation (re-SUS-si-TAY-shun) indicates any effort to revive or to restore normal function artificially. When you perform pulmonary resuscitation, you are providing artificial ventilations to the patient in an attempt to restore the normal function of the lungs: to put oxygen into the bloodstream and to remove carbon dioxide.

Since you will be delivering air to the patient's lungs that has already been in your lungs, there is often the feeling that you are not providing oxygen for the patient. The air you exhale still contains oxygen. In fact, it contains almost three times the amount of oxygen that is usually removed by the lungs during a normal inspiration. The atmosphere contains about 21% oxygen. The air being exhaled from your lungs into the patient contains almost 16% oxygen. This is more than enough oxygen to keep most patients biologically alive until they can receive supplemental oxygen and care at a hospital.

Opening the Airway

As part of the primary survey, make certain that the patient has an open airway and adequate breathing. The simple process of opening the airway will often relieve many problems of partial airway obstruction. This is particularly true for obstructions caused by the tongue. If a patient is conscious and is indicating a mechanical obstruction (for example, food in the airway), attempt to open the airway and go immediately to the procedures used for airway obstructions. Otherwise, as part of your primary survey, you should attempt to provide an open airway.

Repositioning the Head

WARNING: This procedure is not to be used on any patient who has possible injuries to the neck or spine.

1st For cases where the patient is conscious, simply repositioning the head may be enough to open the airway. If the patient's head is flexed forward, ask if the patient can hold his head in a normal position. Should the patient be lying down, be sure the head does not flex forward. If the patient is resting on several pillows or up against some object, reposition him so that the head is not flexed forward. Take care in positioning yourself so that the patient does not have to tilt his head forward to answer your questions.

NOTE: Patients under the influence of alcohol or drugs often have trouble with proper head positioning.

Head-tilt, Chin-lift Manueuver

WARNING: This procedure is not to be used on any patient with possible neck or spinal injuries.

This is the same procedure described in Chapter 3 for use during the primary survey (see Scansheet 3-2, page 57). During the head-tilt, chin-lift manuever, place one hand on the patient's forehead while placing the fingertips of the other hand under the chin, over its bony parts. Without compressing the tissues under the lower jaw, lift the patient's chin and move it to a point where the lower teeth are almost touching the upper teeth. *Do not* close the patient's mouth. You may find it necessary to use your thumb to pull back the patient's lower lip. While the lower jaw is being lifted, you should apply gentle pressure to the patient's forehead.

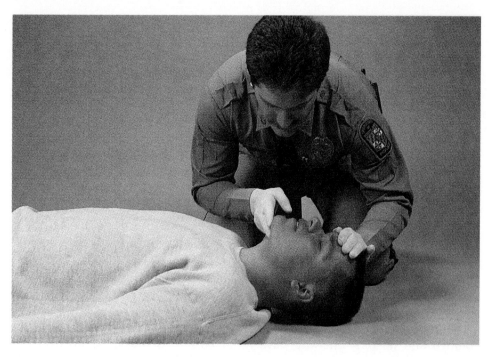

FIGURE 4–5. *If there are no spinal injuries, use the head-tilt, chin-lift maneuver to open the airway.*

Jaw-thrust Maneuver

NOTE: This is the only widely recommended procedure for patients with possible neck or spinal injuries.

1st Place the patient on his back and kneel at the top of head. Reach forward and carefully place one hand on each side of the chin, at the angles of the lower jaw. Push the jaw forward, applying most of the pressure with your index fingers. *Do not* tilt or rotate the patient's head.

FIGURE 4–6. *The jaw-thrust maneuver is used if there are possible neck or spinal injuries.*

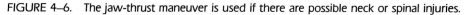

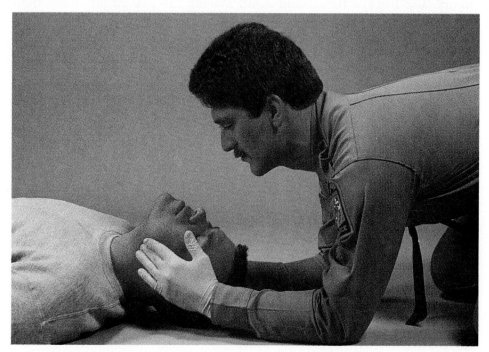

Rescue Breathing

The procedures for rescue breathing place the First Responder into direct contact with the patient's body fluids. In some cases, blood or vomitus may be present. As noted in Chapters 1 and 3, the rescuer should take all steps necessary to ensure protection from infectious diseases. The mouth-to-mask method is used to help prevent the transmission of infectious agents. It is the technique recommended for all First Responders. Your course may include the use of shields that are employed during rescue breathing to prevent direct contact. These shields should be those approved by your EMS System's medical advisors.

The mouth-to-mouth, mouth-to-nose, and mouth-to-mouth and nose methods presented here are done so for those readers who are taking certification in basic life support at the citizen level that allows for direct contact with the patient's mouth and nose.

Mouth-to-Mask Ventilation

This is the technique recommended for rescue personnel. It cuts down on the effort required to keep the patient's airway open and allows you to provide ventilations without having to make direct contact with the patient's mouth and nose. A one-way valve must be part of the mask so that the patient's saliva, mucus, vomitus, and blood do not reach the rescuer's mouth.

Pocket face mask—a device used to help provide mouth-to-mask ventilations. It has a chimney to allow the rescuer to provide breaths without touching the patient. A one-way valve is present in most models to prevent rescuer contact with the patient's blood and body fluids. Some masks have an inlet for supplemental oxygen.

The mask is made of soft materials that can be carried in your pocket. It is available with or without an oxygen inlet. Mouth-to-mask ventilations are provided through a chimney on the mask. If the mask has a second port for oxygen, you can simultaneously ventilate the patient with air from your own lungs and with additional oxygen from an oxygen source.

Another advantage of the pocket face mask is that it allows you to use both hands to maintain the proper head tilt and still hold the mask firmly in place. Keeping a good seal between the face mask and the patient's face is relatively easy with this device.

The pocket face mask can be used with or without an oropharyngeal airway in place (see p. 115). The patient's airway can be better maintained if an airway is in place.

WARNING: Extra care must be taken if there is any possibility of spinal injury. Use the jaw thrust and avoid moving the patient any more than necessary.

FIGURE 4–7. Pocket face masks. Note the chimney with one-way valve for mouth-to-mask ventilations.

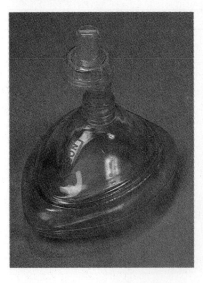
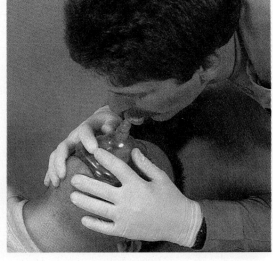

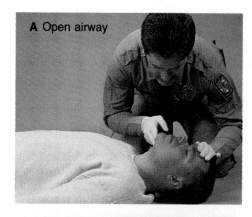

A Open airway

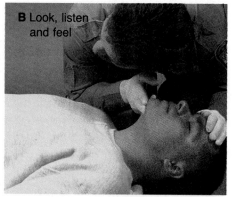

B Look, listen and feel

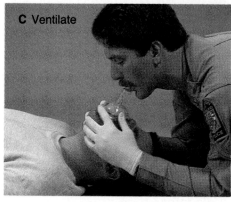

C Ventilate

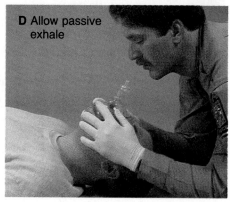

D Allow passive exhale

FIGURE 4–8.
Mouth-to-mask ventilation: (*A*) OPEN THE AIRWAY; (*B*) LOOK, LISTEN, and FEEL for air exchange; (*C*) VENTILATE, watching for the chest to rise; (*D*) ALLOW PASSIVE EXPIRATION, watching for the chest to fall.

1st To provide mouth-to-mask ventilations, you should:

1. Determine if the patient is unresponsive. If you are working alone, call out for help if the patient is unresponsive.
2. Properly position patient, then position yourself at the patient's head and open the patient's airway. If necessary, clear the patient's airway.
3. Maintain an open airway and determine if the patient is breathing and if the breathing is adequate.
   - **Look** for chest movements. Are they even and full?
   - **Listen** for air flowing into and out of the patient's mouth or nose. Note any unusual sounds (gurgling, crowing, snoring).
   - **Feel** for air exchange at the patient's mouth and nose.
   - **Note** anything that appears wrong, such as blue skin color. Take at least **3 TO 5 SECONDS** to determine if the patient is breathing.
4. Position the mask on the patient's face so that the apex (upper tip of the triangle) is over the bridge of the patient's nose and the base is between the lower lip and the projection of the chin.
5. *Firmly* hold the mask in place while maintaining the proper head tilt:
   - Place both thumbs at the dome of the mask, over the chin. Pressure can be applied along both sides of the mask.
   - Use the index, third, and fourth fingers of each hand to grasp the lower jaw on each side, between the angle of the jaw and the earlobe. The jaw is lifted forward.
6. Take a deep breath and exhale into the port of the mask chimney (1 to 1.5 sec). Watch for the patient's chest to rise.
7. Remove your mouth from the port and allow for a passive exhalation. Continue this cycle as you would for mouth-to-mouth ventilations, providing a breath every 5 seconds for the adult patient. If you are using a properly sized mask on a child, one breath every 4 seconds should be delivered. When providing ventilations for an infant, use the infant-size mask and deliver one breath every 3 seconds.

NOTE: Your EMS System medical advisors may allow you to use an infant-size mask for resuscitating infants. In some cases the advisors may approve the use of this mask for resuscitating neck breathers (see page 97). In the past, some guidelines have allowed adult masks to be inverted for use on children. Make certain that this procedure is approved by your state EMS medical advisors and that the mask you are using has been approved for this procedure by the manufacturer.

Mouth-to-Mouth Ventilation

This technique is a very efficient method of providing artificial ventilation (rescue breathing). It can be done by one person, without any special equipment. Keep in mind that it does expose the rescuer to the dangers of infectious diseases. For now, we will assume that the patient has no neck or spinal injuries. When performing mouth-to-mouth ventilation, you should:

1. Establish if the patient is unresponsive. When working alone, call out for help if the patient is unresponsive.
2. Properly position the patient; then open the patient's airway with the head-tilt, chin-lift or jaw-thrust maneuver.
3. While maintaining the proper head tilt, determine if the patient is breathing and if the breathing is adequate.
   - **Look** for chest movements. Are they even and full?
   - **Listen** for air flowing into and out of the patient's mouth or nose. Note any unusual sounds (gurgling, crowing, snoring).
   - **Feel** for air exchange at the patient's mouth and nose.
   - **Note** anything that appears wrong, such as blue skin color. Take at least **3 TO 5 SECONDS** to determine if the patient is breathing.
4. Keeping the patient in a position with maximum head tilt, pinch the nose closed with the thumb and forefinger of the hand you are using to hold the patient's forehead.
5. Open your mouth wide, taking a deep breath.
6. Place your open mouth around the mouth of the patient. Be certain to make a **tight seal** with your lips against the patient's face.
7. Ventilate the patient by exhaling slowly into the patient's airway until you see the chest rise and feel resistance to the flow of your breath. (Be certain that you do not have any objects, such as gum, in your mouth.) The ventilation should take 1 to 1.5 seconds. If this first attempt to provide a breath fails, reposition the patient's head and try again.
8. Break contact with the patient's mouth, allowing air to flow from the lungs. Quickly take in another deep breath and exhale this air into the patient's airway.
9. If the patient does not begin breathing again (spontaneous breathing), check for a carotid pulse to see if CPR must be started. Have someone alert dispatch after you check for a carotid pulse.
   If the patient has a pulse and is not breathing, you should continue with the following procedure, providing one ventilation every 5 seconds:
   - Take a deep breath.
   - Form a seal around the patient's mouth and exhale air into the patient's airway, taking 1 to 1.5 seconds per ventilation.
   - Break contact with the patient's mouth and release the pinch on the nose, allowing air to be released from the patient's lungs while you
   - Turn your head to watch the patient's chest fall and
   - Take a deep breath to begin the cycle again.

Between ventilations, the patient's lungs should passively deflate.

1st IMPORTANT: For the mouth-to-mouth technique, deliver breaths to the adult patient at **one breath every 5 seconds,** or at a rate of **TWELVE BREATHS PER MINUTE.** Every few minutes, stop and check for a carotid pulse. If there is no pulse, begin CPR. If the patient has a pulse, continue pulmonary resuscitation until the patient begins to breath unaided, until someone trained in mouth-to-mouth techniques can replace you, or until you are too exhausted to continue.

If you are following the correct procedures, and the patient's airway is not obstructed, you should be able to **feel** resistance to your ventilations as the patient's lungs expand, **see** the chest rise and fall, **hear** air leaving the patient's airway as the chest falls, and **feel** air leaving the patient's mouth as you allow the lungs to deflate. Stay alert to determine if the patient has begun to breathe unassisted.

The most common problems with the mouth-to-mouth technique are, in the following order:

- Failure to form a tight seal over the patient's mouth (often caused by pushing too hard in an effort to form a tight seal)
- Failure to pinch the nose completely closed
- Failure to establish an open airway because the patient's head is not tilted back far enough
- Failure to have the patient's mouth opened wide enough to receive ventilations
- Failure to deliver an adequate volume of air during a ventilation
- Providing breaths too quickly (take 1 to 1.5 seconds per breath)
- Failure to clear the upper airway of obstructions

WARNING: *Do not* practice mouth-to-mouth techniques on anyone. Such a warning may sound humorous; however, it is important to take this warning seriously. Practice on the manikins provided for your training.

Two additional related problems, forcing air into the patient's stomach and vomiting, will be covered later in this chapter.

Mouth-to-Nose Ventilation

Injuries to the mouth, complete obstruction of the airway through the oral cavity, and injuries to the lower jaw are examples of when mouth-to-mouth techniques will not work effectively. For such cases, you will have to employ the mouth-to-nose technique. Most of this procedure is the same as found in mouth-to-mouth usage. The head-tilt, chin-lift maneuver is still used. The first two ventilations are done. After this, breaths are delivered to the adult at a rate of **one breath every 5 seconds** to equal **TWELVE BREATHS PER MINUTE.** The differences in the mouth-to-nose procedure include:

- Keep one hand on the patient's forehead to tilt the patient's head back and use your other hand to lift the patient's lower jaw and close the mouth. The patient's nose is left open.
- After taking a deep breath, seal your mouth around the patient's nose.
- Ventilations are delivered through the patient's nose. Be certain that the patient's mouth is kept closed.
- When allowing the patient to exhale, break contact with the nose and slightly open the mouth. Keep your hand on the patient's forehead to keep the airway open.

NOTE: the jaw thrust can be used with the mouth-to-nose technique. When using this method, do not allow the lower lip to retract as you push with your thumbs. The patient's mouth should be sealed with your cheek.

Take a moment to compare and contrast the mouth-to-mouth technique and the mouth-to-nose technique. Note how they are the same except that you are using a different entry point to the patient's airway.

Special Patients

Until now, we have been considering adult patients without spinal injuries. As a First Responder, you may have to use artificial ventilation techniques on other types of patients, including infants and children, elderly patients, neck breathers, and accident victims (some with possible neck and spinal injuries).

Infants (Birth to 1 Year) and Children (1 to 8 Years)

1st When providing pulmonary resuscitation for an infant or child, you should:

1. Establish if the patient is unresponsive.
2. Lay both infants and children on a hard surface. However, when necessary, you may cradle infants in your arms.
3. Open the airway with the head-tilt, chin-lift technique and determine if the patient is breathing.

   CAUTION: Reduce the amount of head tilt to avoid closing the patient's airway, *but* be certain that the airway is adequate.
4. Properly position an approved face mask or other barrier approved by your EMS system. If you are using the mouth-to-mouth and nose technique, take a breath and cover both the *mouth* and *nose* of the infant or small child patient.
5. Use gentle but adequate breaths to ventilate infants and children. The volume of breath for either type of patient is determined by providing a ventilation until you *see the chest rise.*

   CAUTION: Stay alert for resistance to your breaths and for chest rise.
6. Uncover both the mouth and nose to allow the patient to exhale.
7. Ventilations are given at a rate of one breath every **3 seconds** for infants and one breath every **4 seconds** for children. Take 1 to 1.5 secons per breath.

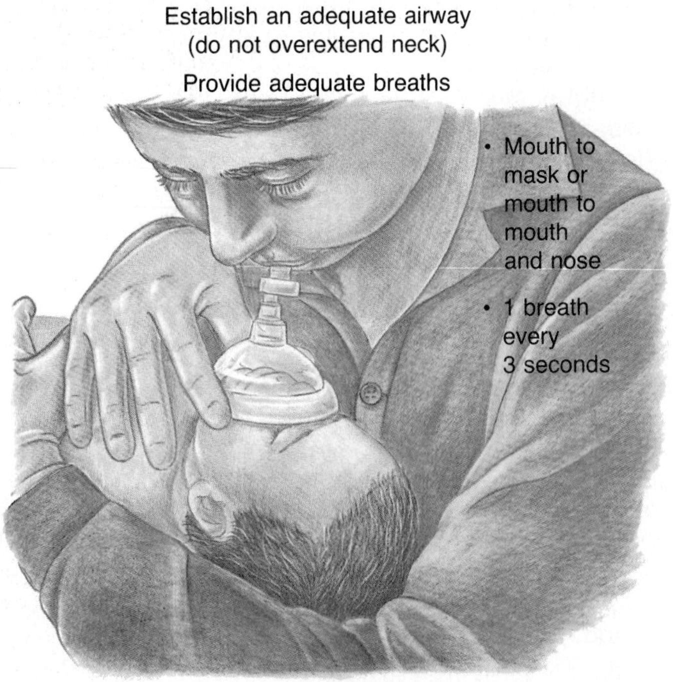

FIGURE 4–9.
Ventilating infants and small Children: Watch for chest rise.

Establish an adequate airway
(do not overextend neck)
Provide adequate breaths

• Mouth to mask or mouth to mouth and nose

• 1 breath every 3 seconds

Elderly Patients

You will find that elderly patients also require special care. First, the lungs may have lost some elasticity and the rib cage may be more rigid than in younger patients. Use the mouth-to-mask or the mouth-to-mouth procedures, but with great care. Stay alert and note resistance to your ventilations, and carefully note the rise and fall of the chest.

Second, realize that the elderly can have more brittle bones than do younger patients. If a fall has occurred, they are more likely to suffer injury to the spine. When such injuries are possible or when you are in doubt, the jaw-thrust maneuver is used in palce of the head-tilt, chin-lift maneuver.

You may have to use mouth-to-nose procedures for some elderly patients. This will happen with patients who have lost their teeth and have not been using dentures. These patients have receding chins that make the mouth-to-mouth seal impossible. The head-tilt, chin-lift technique works in most cases to open the airway.

Finally, as a First Responder you may be faced with bystanders who say such things as, "He's so old. Why make him suffer? Let him die in peace." It is not their right to make such decisions. You are charged with the responsibility to attempt to resuscitate all patients needing such care, unless direct orders have been given to you by a physician that no such measures should be taken (for example, terminally ill patient). What bystanders tell you may not be what the patient wants you to do.

Neck Breathers

Some people have undergone surgery that removes part or all of the voice box (larynx). Ater surgery, these individuals are called neck breathers or laryngectomees (LAR-in-JEK-to-me's). The upper airway is no longer complete, so air cannot travel from the throat to the windpipe. They must breathe through an opening in the neck.

1st The neck breather will have an opening called a **stoma** (STO-mah) in the front or side of the neck. Since air is no longer taken into the lungs

Stoma (STO-mah)—Any permanent opening that has been surgically made. The opening in the neck of a neck breather.

FIGURE 4–10. The neck breather's airway has been changed by surgery.

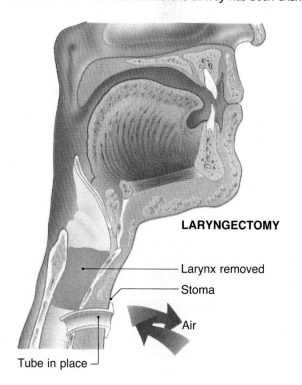

LARYNGECTOMY

— Larynx removed

— Stoma

Air

Tube in place ⌐

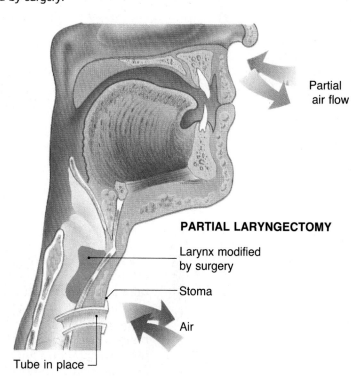

Partial air flow

PARTIAL LARYNGECTOMY

Larynx modified by surgery

Stoma

Air

Tube in place ⌐

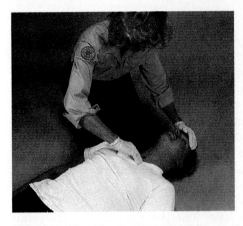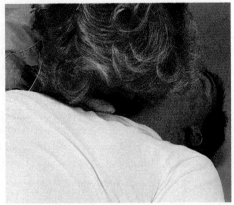

FIGURE 4–11. Mouth-to-stoma technique. If approved in your EMS System, use a pediatric-sized pocket face mask or other adjunct device.

by way of the nose and mouth, you will have to use the mask-to-stoma or mouth-to-stoma technique. When you attempt to open a patient's airway, always look to see if there is a neck opening or stoma. If so, and you must provide artificial ventilation, you should use the mask or shield recommended by your EMS System's medical advisors. Currently, there is no specific mask. Some advisors allow the use of a pediatric (infant's) mask. These masks are not commonly available to First Responders. Several shields sold to be used to protective barriers during rescue breathing may work for mouth-to-stoma ventilations; however, they have not been approved for such use by the AHA. Follow the recommendations of your EMS System's medical advisors. Remember, direct contact increases the risk of infection, but this problem is believed to be rare.

If you decide to use the mouth-to-stoma technique, then you should:

1. Keep the patient's head straight. *Do not* tilt the head.
2. Clean away any mucus or encrusted materials found on the neck opening or breathing tube. *Do not* remove the breathing tube.
3. Use the same procedures as in mouth-to-mouth resuscitation, except:
   - Do not pinch the patient's nose closed.
   - Place your mouth directly over the patient's stoma instead of the mouth or nose. Remember, this will increase your risk of exposure to infectious diseases since you will be in contact with the patient's mucus.

If the patient's chest does not rise, the patient may be a partial neck breather. This means that the patient takes in and expels some air through the mouth and nose. In such cases, you will have to pinch the nose closed and seal the mouth with the palm of your hand.

Accident Victims

The best results with pulmonary resuscitation can be achieved when the patient is lying down. This can be a problem when caring for automobile accident victims who are still in their vehicles. Be realistic. If you wait for other EMS personnel to arrive or if you take time to put on a rigid cervical collar and secure the patient to a spineboard, the patient will be biologically dead from lack of oxygen to the brain. If the patient is not breathing, **take immediate action**.

Without risking your own safety, reach the victim as quickly as possible. If the patient is lying down and not breathing, and you believe the mechanism of injury may have caused damage to the spine or neck, **use the jaw-thrust maneuver** and **mouth-to-mask,** or **mouth-to-nose** techniques. For the mouth-to-nose method you will have to seal the mouth with your cheek. If you try mouth-to-mouth techniques, you will have to seal the nose with your cheek. Many people find this maneuver difficult to perform. You should slightly tilt the head if, and only if, the airway will not open and you feel strong resistance to your efforts to ventilate the patient.

If the victim is seated and you do not suspect spinal or neck injuries, you can lay the patient flat on his back or, if this is not possible, cradle the patient with his neck on your upper arm. When cradling the patient, the head will tilt slightly and you can use the mouth-to-mask or mouth-to-mouth techniques. Should a patient in the front seat be positioned in a way that prevents easy access, go to the rear seat and deliver mouth-to-mask or mouth-to-mouth ventilations from this location.

The major problem occurs when you have a seated patient who is slumped forward or has been thrown backward. If there is a possibility of spinal or neck injury or an obvious broken neck, then all standard procedures may fail. Again, do not wait until you have help to place a rigid cervical collar and secure the patient to a spineboard. **Take immediate action!**

Make only one move with the patient. Rather than trying to reseat the patient, try to position him flat on the back. When by yourself, attempt to cradle the patient's head by wrapping one arm around the top of the head and holding the chin in your hand. Then slide the patient onto his back. If you have help, hold the patient's head and neck in line with the rest of the spinal column using both of your hands and forearms and work swiftly with your helpers to lay the patient flat. All this must be done very quickly, since the patient's brain cells may be near death.

Once again, be realistic. There is nothing you can do to fully protect the spine. The maneuvers mentioned here will not help in cases of severe neck injury. *But*, if you wait to begin resuscitation, you will surely have a dead accident victim. If you take immediate action, you still have a chance of having a live patient.

Air in the Stomach and Vomiting

1st One problem faced when performing pulmonary resuscitation on any patient is the possibility that some of the air from your lungs will be forced into the patient's stomach. This is called *gastric distention*. Assume that this is happening if the patient's abdomen starts to bulge while you are performing artificial ventilation. Do not worry about slight bulging; it is the case of very noticeable bulging that is of concern. The patient's diaphragm may be forced upward, causing ventilation to fail, or the patient may vomit. In cases of air in the stomach where you see a noticeable bulge, *reduce the force of your ventilations* and:

- Reposition the patient's head to provide a better airway, and
- Be prepared for vomiting, and turn the patient (not just the head) to one side if it occurs.

Do not reposition the head if you suspect spinal or neck injuries.

Do not push in on the stomach to release the air. Vomiting may block off the airway. Even more highly trained rescuers do not force air from the stomach unless they have suction equipment immediately available.

If the patient does vomit and you have turned him to one side, do not expect all the vomitus to simply flow out. You will probably have to use finger sweeps (see page 105) to clear the vomitus from the mouth. This is an unpleasant task, but remember, a person's life is at stake.

AIRWAY OBSTRUCTION

Causes of Airway Obstruction

1st Many factors can cause the airway to become partially or fully obstructed. These include:

- **Obstruction by the tongue**—the tongue falls back to block off the throat. This is a common problem, often occurring when the patient's head flexes forward, as in cases of unconsciousness, or when too large a pillow is placed under the head.
- **Obstruction by the epiglottis**—attempts made by the patient to force inspirations may create a negative pressure that can force the epiglottis (EP-i-GLOT-is) and perhaps the tongue to block off the airway. The epiglottis is a lidlike structure at the top of the larynx that prevents fluids, food, and foreign objects from entering the airway that passes through the larynx.
- **Foreign objects** (mechanical obstruction)—this can include pieces of food, ice, toys, dentures, vomitus, and liquids pooling in the back of the throat.
- **Tissue damage**—these accident-related tissue problems can be caused by punctures to the neck, crush wounds to the face, breathing hot air (as in fires), poisons, and severe injury due to a blow to the neck. Swelling of the throat and windpipe tissues presents major airway problems.
- **Diseases**—respiratory infections and certain chronic conditions (for example, asthma) can cause tissue swelling or muscle spasms that will obstruct the airway.

> **Epiglottis (EP-i-GLOT-is)**—a flap of cartilage and other tissues that is located above the voice box. It helps to close off the airway when a person swallows.

There is little that you can do if the obstruction is in the lower airway. Usually, this is the case when obstruction is due to respiratory disease. Likewise, foreign bodies in the lower airway cannot be cleared by ordinary First Responder-level procedures. Upper airway obstruction caused by foreign objects often can be relieved with a few simple procedures.

Signs of Partial Airway Obstruction

1st Partial airway obstruction is usually present if:

- The patient has unusual breathing sounds. Listen for:
  Snoring—probably caused by the tongue obstructing the back of the throat.
  Gurgling—probably caused by a foreign object in the windpipe or by blood in the airway.
  Crowing—probably caused by spasms of the voice box.
  Wheezing—may be due to swelling or spasms along the lower airway. However, wheezing often does not indicate any major problems of the airway.
- The patient is breathing, but has blue or blue-gray skin, lips, earlobes, fingernail beds, or tongue.
- The patient's breathing keeps changing from near normal to very labored.

1st If a conscious patient appears to have a partial airway obstruction, have the patient cough. A strong, forceful cough indicates that enough air is being exchanged. Encourage the patient to continue coughing in hope that any foreign materials will be dislodged and expelled.

1st In cases where the patient cannot cough or has a very weak cough, begin to care for the patient **as if there is a complete airway obstruction.** Do the same if the patient has poor air exchange or when good air exchange changes to poor air exchange.

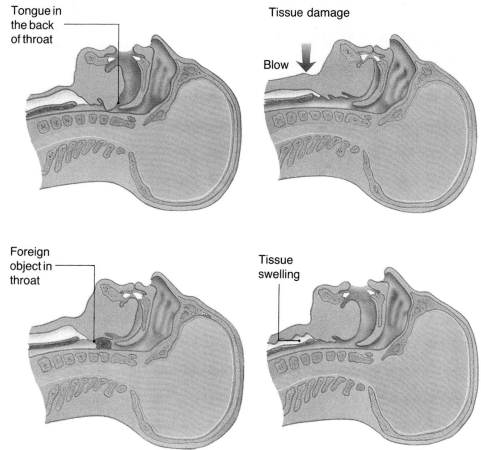

Tongue in the back of throat

Tissue damage

Blow

Foreign object in throat

Tissue swelling

FIGURE 4–12.   Four possible causes of airway obstruction.

Signs of Complete Airway Obstruction

1st The conscious patient will try to speak, but will not be able to do so. The patient will often grasp the neck and open the mouth widely in an effort to indicate inability to breathe. The unconscious patient will not have any of the typical chest movements or the other signs associated with good air exchange.

Correcting Upper Airway Obstruction—Foreign Body

In cases where a conscious patient is trying to tell you about an airway obstruction, move swiftly to clear the airway. When the patient is unable to communicate or is unconscious, quickly determine if there is an airway obstruction and take appropriate actions to clear the airway. Since so many cases of airway obstruction are caused by the tongue, always make certain that the airway is open. Once this has been done, move on to the recommended maneuvers to clear obstructions from the airway. We will look at each of these and the patterns that you should follow to correct airway obstructions.

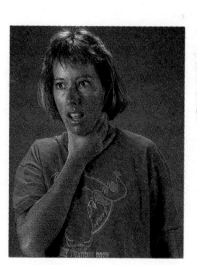

FIGURE 4–13.
The distress signal for choking.

Back Blows

1st If the patient is an *infant* with a complete airway obstruction, you should:

1. Cradle the patient, face down, on your forearm. Your hand must support the patient's jaw and chest. You can maintain better support of the patient if you are seated and rest your forearm on your thighs. The patient's head should be lower than the chest.

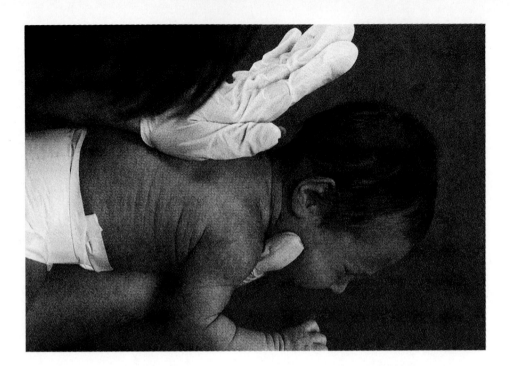

FIGURE 4–14.
Cradle the infant, face down, on your forearm.

2. Using the heel of your free hand, rapidly deliver *four sharp blows* to the midline of the patient's back, in the area between the shoulder blades.

NOTE: Do *not* place the infant or very small child into this head-down position if he has a partial airway obstruction and you observe that he is breathing adequately.

WARNING: The use of back blows is recommended for infants who have complete airway obstructions. Do not use this procedure on children and adults.

Manual Thrusts—Abdominal

Each abdominal thrust is applied in an effort to create a burst of air from the lungs that will dislodge the obstructing object.

WARNING: It is recommended that you do not use the full force of this procedure on your classmates when you are practicing this technique. It is best not to practice this procedure on anyone who has eaten a meal within 2 hours. *Do not* practice this procedure on anyone who has had any chest or abdominal surgery, heart problem, or hernia. *Do not* practice this procedure on anyone with abdominal or chest pains or who is pregnant.

NOTE: This procedure should not be used when the patient is pregnant. *Do not* use this procedure on infants and very small children.

1st If the patient with an airway obstruction is standing or sitting, you should:

1. Position yourself behind the patient.
2. Slide your arms under the patient's armpits, wrapping both of your arms around the waist.
3. Make a fist and place the thumb side of this fist against the midline of the patient's abdomen, just above the navel. Keep your fist below the patient's rib cage, taking extra caution to avoid the area just below the breastbone (sternum) at the level of the xiphoid process.
4. Grasp your fist with your free hand and apply pressure as an inward and upward thrust. This should press your fist into the patient's abdomen. Deliver **six to ten rapid inward and upward thrusts.**

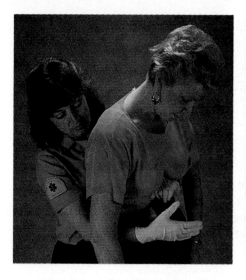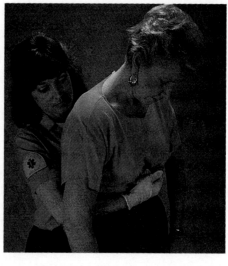

FIGURE 4–15. Correct positioning is essential when you deliver abdominal thrusts.

1st If the patient with an airway obstruction is lying down, you should:

1. Place the patient on his back.
2. Kneel and straddle the patient at the level of the hips.
3. Position the heel of one hand on the patient's abdomen at the midline, between the naval and the ribcage. Your fingers should point toward the patient's chest. Keep your hand below the patient's rib cage, avoiding the area just below the breastbone.
4. Place your free hand over the positioned hand and put your shoulders directly over the patient's abdomen.
5. Press your hands inward and toward the patient's diaphragm, as if you are trying to push toward the patient's upper back. Deliver **six to ten rapid abdominal thrusts.**

NOTE: If the patient is very large or if you are a small individual, you can deliver more effective thrusts if you straddle one leg of the patient. Depending on the position of the patient, it is often easier to straddle the entire patient, placing your knees at the level of the hips.

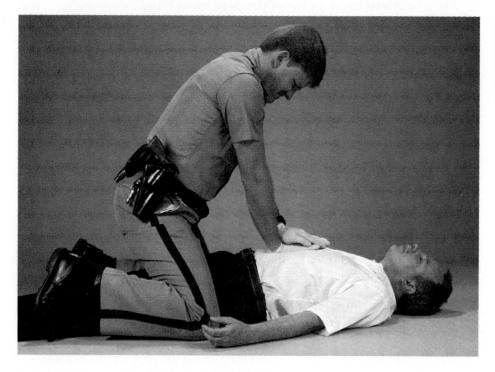

FIGURE 4–16. You can deliver abdominal thrusts to a patient who is lying down. Your shoulders must be directly over the patient's abdomen. Straddle the patient in order to deliver more effective thrusts.

Some danger exists if abdominal thrusts are used on infants or very small children who are still of infant size and weight range. Applying too much pressure can severely injure the patient. Improper application of the technique may break ribs, lacerate the liver, lungs, and heart, or internally damage the heart. The American Heart Association *does not* recommend abdominal thrusts for infants.

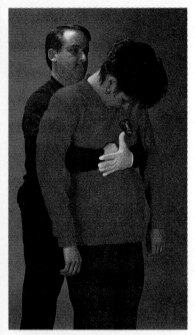

FIGURE 4–17. The chest thrust is used for pregnant patients.

Manual Thrusts—Chest

The technique of chest thrusts is used in place of abdominal thrusts when the patient is an infant, a very small child, or pregnant or in cases where the patient is so large that you cannot wrap your arms around the waist.

If you must employ the chest thrust technique for an adult patient who is standing or seated, you should:

1. Position yourself behind the patient and slide your arms under the armpits so that you can encircle the chest with your arms.
2. Form a fist with one of your hands and place the thumb side of this hand on the patient's breastbone. You should make contact with the region of the breastbone about two or three finger-widths above the lower tip of the breastbone.
3. Grasp your fist with your free hand and deliver **distinct thrusts** directly *backward* until the object is expelled or the patient loses consciousness. *Do not* exert this force in an upward or downward direction or off to one side.

1st If you must employ the chest thrust technique for an adult patient who is lying down, you should:

1. Kneel beside the patient's chest. Have both of your knees facing the patient (*note*: this is different from the position used for abdominal thrusts).
2. Place the heel of one hand on the midline of the breastbone, two to three finger-widths from the lower end of the breastbone. Lift and spread your fingers so that they will not apply pressure on the ribs.
3. Place your free hand on top of the positioned hand.
4. Lean forward until your shoulders are directly over the midline of the patient's chest.
5. Deliver **distinct thrusts** in a *downward* direction, applying enough force to compress the chest cavity. Continue until the object is expelled or the patient loses consciousness.

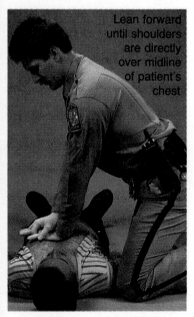

Lean forward until shoulders are directly over midline of patient's chest

FIGURE 4–18. The chest thrust can be given to a patient who is lying on his or her back.

NOTE: If the chest thrust must be done on a child (for example, abdominal injuries), use one hand to apply the compressions. While delivering the thrusts, kneel at the child's feet. You may place the child on a table and stand at his feet.

1st If you must employ the chest thrust technique for an infant, you should:

1. Cradle the infant, face down, on your forearm and deliver **four** back blows.
2. Sandwich the infant between your hands. Then turn the infant over to a face-up position on your thigh. Support the head throughout the entire process. When repositioned, the infant's head must be lower than the trunk.
3. Apply **four slow distinct** chest thrusts, using the tips of two or three fingers. Pressure should be exerted along the midline of the infant's breastbone, one finger-width below an imaginary line drawn directly between the nipples.

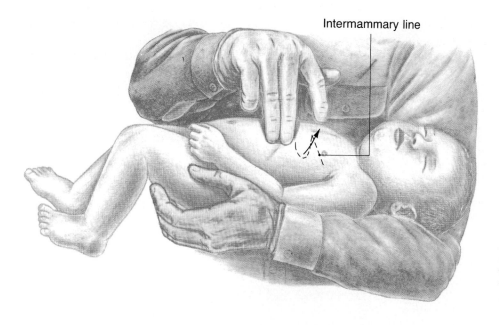

Intermammary line

FIGURE 4–19.
For infants, chest thrusts are to the midline of the sternum, one finger-width below the intermammary line.

Finger Sweeps

WARNING: Wear latex or vinyl gloves to avoid contact with the patient's blood and body fluids.

You can use your fingers to remove a foreign object from a patient's airway once the object is dislodged or partially dislodged. Take great care not to force the object back down the patient's throat. Be alert so that the patient does not bite your fingers. When you have to use finger sweeps to clear an object from the patient's airway, you should:

1. Place the patient on his back.
2. Use one hand to steady the patient's forehead, while you place the other hand's thumb against the patient's lower teeth and the index finger against the upper teeth.
3. Force open the patient's mouth by crossing your thumb and index finger. Once the mouth is open, hold the patient's lower jaw and tongue so the mouth cannot close. This is known as the tongue-jaw lift.
4. Release your grasp on the patient's forehead and use the forefinger of this free hand to sweep the patient's mouth, using your finger as a hook to capture any foreign materials. If you need to grasp an object, try to do so using your first and second fingers. You may have to turn the patient's head to one side in order to sweep an object from the mouth.

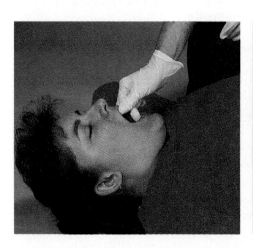
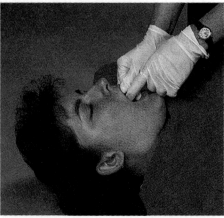

FIGURE 4–20. Open the patient's mouth using the crossed-fingers technique. Sweep foreign materials from the airway and mouth.

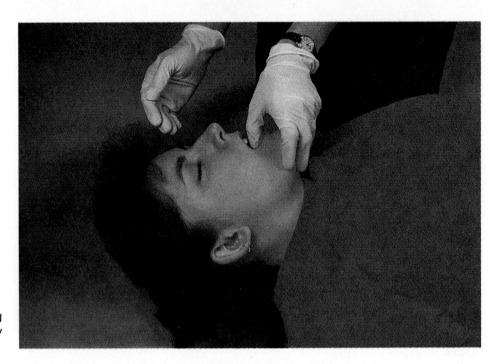

FIGURE 4–21.
The tongue-jaw lift can be used to open the mouth and airway of an unconscious patient.

WARNING: A conscious person has a gag reflex that may cause vomiting. The patient may vomit and inhale this vomitus into the lungs. The finger sweep technique should be used only on *unconscious* patients.

NOTE: *Do not* use "blind" finger sweeps and probes on infants and children. To do so might force objects into the airway. You *must* open the patient's mouth and look in to see an object before trying to grasp it with your fingers.

Correcting Airway Obstructions—Combined Procedures

The American Heart Association (AHA) has researched the proper techniques to be used in cases of partial and full airway obstruction. As part of their Basic Cardiac Life Support Program, the AHA has shown that a specific sequence of actions will provide the rescuer with the greatest chance of clearing the patient's airway. EMS Systems recognize the fine work done by the AHA and recommend the same combined procedure sequence.

Any procedure used to clear the airway is considered to be effective if, after it is applied, any of the following happens:

- The patient shows good air exchange or spontaneous breathing.
- The patient regains consciousness.
- Skin color improves.
- The foreign object is expelled from the mouth.
- The foreign object is expelled into the mouth where it is visible to the rescuer.

1st If the adult or child patient is *conscious*, you should:

1. Determine that there is **complete obstruction** or a partial obstruction that must be cared for the same as a complete one (poor air exchange).

Be certain to ask, "Are you choking," or "Can you speak?" Look, listen, and feel for the signs of complete obstruction or poor exchange. Quickly tell the patient you are going to help.

2. Give six to ten abdominal thrusts (or four chest thrusts if appropriate) in rapid succession. Should the patient's airway remain obstructed, you should . . .

3. Repeat the manual thrusts until the patient's airway is cleared or until the patient loses consciousness.

REMEMBER: Chest thrusts must be used if the patient is an infant, obese, or a pregnant woman.

1st If, during your attempts to clear the airway, the adult or child patient *loses consciousness*, you should:

1. Protect the patient from possible injury due to falling.
2. Have someone call the EMS System dispatcher.
3. Position the patient so that he is lying down on his back.
4. Use the tongue-jaw lift to open the mouth. Perform finger sweeps.
5. Attempt to open the patient's airway by the head-tilt, chin-lift maneuver.
6. Give **two adequate ventilations** as described in the section on mouth-to-mask ventilation. If your attempt to ventilate the patient fails, you should . . .
7. Perform six to ten abdominal thrusts in rapid succession. If this fails . . .
8. Check for foreign bodies in the mouth with the finger sweep method. You must be able to see the object in order to perform finger sweeps for the infant or small child. If you cannot find and remove the obstruction, you should . . .
9. Open the airway and repeat your attempt to ventilate the patient. If this fails . . .
10. Repeat the sequence of:
    a. Providing abdominal thrusts:
    b. Performing finger sweeps
    c. Attempting to ventilate

1st REMEMBER: You must continue these efforts until the obstruction is cleared. Even if you can do no more than partially dislodge the obstruction, you will then be able to keep the patient alive by mouth-to-mask ventilations.

1st If the adult or child patient is *unconscious* when you arrive at the scene, you should:

1. Use the method discussed in Chapter 3 to see if the patient is unresponsive. If you are working alone, call out for help.
2. Open the airway by the head-tilt, chin-lift or jaw-thrust procedure and determine if there is an obstruction, if the patient has poor air exchange or if the patient is not breathing.
3. Attempt to give the patient **two adequate ventilations.** If you are not successful, you should . . .
4. Reposition the patient's head and repeat your attempt to ventilate the patient. If this attempt fails, you should have someone alert the EMS dispatcher and . . .
5. Deliver six to ten abdominal thrusts and, if necessary, attempt finger sweeps to clear any foreign bodies from the airway. If these procedures fail, you should . . .
6. Attempt to ventilate and repeat the sequence of abdominal thrusts, finger sweeps, and attempt to ventilate until successful.

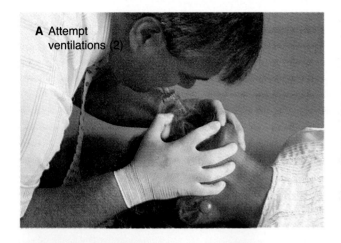

A Attempt ventilations (2)

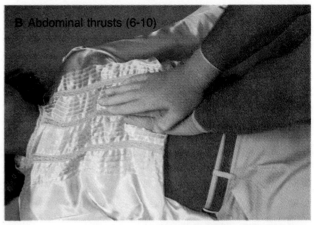

B Abdominal thrusts (6-10)

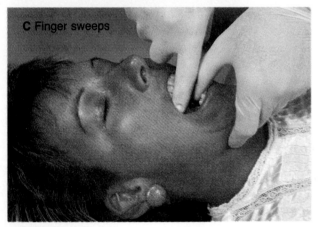

C Finger sweeps

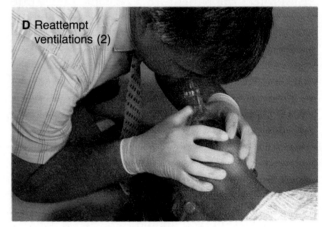

D Reattempt ventilations (2)

FIGURE 4–22.
The combined procedure for clearing the airway of an unconscious adult.

REMEMBER: Chest thrusts must be used for infants, obese patients, and pregnant women. You must be able to see the object before you attempt finger sweeps with infants.

1st You *must* continue this sequence of procedures until you clear the patient's airway or until you have dislodged the obstruction to the point where you can provide pulmonary resuscitation. If the patient's brain cells do not receive oxygen, lethal changes may begin within 4 to 6 minutes.

1st If the patient is a conscious infant who has an upper airway obstruction, you should:

1. Assess the breathing difficulties to make certain that the problem is due to an airway obstruction. When working alone, call out for help.
2. Provide full support for the infant's head. Use one hand and straddle the infant face down on your forearm. Use your thigh to support your forearm. Remember to keep the infant's head lower than his trunk.
3. Deliver **four back blows** in 3 to 5 seconds. If this fails . . .
4. Support the infant's head and sandwich him between your hands. Turn the infant over onto his back and keep the head lower than the trunk.
5. Deliver **four chest thrusts,** using the tips of two or three fingers. Make certain that you apply the compressions along the midline of the breastbone, with the index finger placed one finger-width below an imaginary line drawn directly between the nipples. The compressions are to be delivered more slowly than those that are applied during CPR (see Chapter 5).
6. Continue with the sequence of back blows and chest thrusts until the object is expelled or the infant loses consciousness.

1st If the infant loses consciousness while you are trying to clear the airway, you should:

1. Establish unresponsiveness. If you are working alone, call out for help.
2. Place the infant on his back and use the tongue-jaw lift and finger sweeps. Remember, you must see the object before applying the finger sweeps. Do **not** attempt "blind" finger sweeps.
3. Open the airway and attempt to ventilate. If this fails . . .
4. Deliver **four** back blows. If this fails . . .
5. Deliver **four** chest thrusts.
6. Use the tongue-jaw lift and look for and remove any visible foreign objects.
7. Reattempt to ventilate. If this fails . . .
8. Continue the sequence of back blows, chest thrusts, visible foreign object removal, and attempts to ventilate until you are successful.

1st If the infant is unconscious when you arrive, you should:

1. Establish unresponsiveness. When working alone, call out for help.
2. Position the infant on his back, remembering to support the head and neck.
3. Open the airway and establish breathlessness or poor ventilation (which must be cared for the same as a complete airway obstruction).
4. Attempt to ventilate using an approved mask-to-mouth technique or the mouth-to-mouth and nose technique. Should this fail . . .
5. Reposition the infant's head and reattempt to ventilate. If this fails . . .
6. Support the infant's head and straddle him face down on your forearm. Support your forearm with your thigh, keeping the infant's head lower than his trunk. Deliver **four back blows** in 3 to 5 seconds. Should this fail . . .
7. Sandwich the patient between your arms, and place him in a face-up position on your thigh. Deliver **four chest thrusts** in 3 to 5 seconds. If this fails . . .
8. Use the tongue-jaw lift and remove any visible foreign objects.
9. Open the airway and attempt to ventilate. Should this attempt fail . . .
10. Repeat the sequence of:
    - Four back blows
    - Four chest thrusts
    - Looking for and removing visible foreign objects and . . .
    - Attempts to ventilate until you are successful.

If the infant has developed respiratory arrest and you have cleared the airway enough to provide adequate ventilations, deliver two breaths and check for heart action to see if CPR *must* be started (see Chapter 5).

SUMMARY

There are several numbers that keep occurring when you study respiratory care. The number 2 is of great significance. When you begin artificial ventilation, you start with two adequate breaths.

The number 5 also should be of great importance to you. Artificial ventilations are delivered to the nonbreathing adult patient at a rate of one breath every 5 seconds. This rate can also be expressed as 12 breaths per minute

■ SCAN 4-1.

CLEARING THE AIRWAY-Unconscious Infant

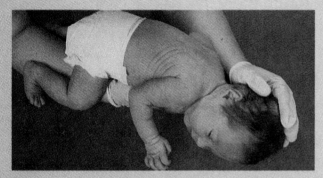

1 Establish unresponsiveness. Position the infant.

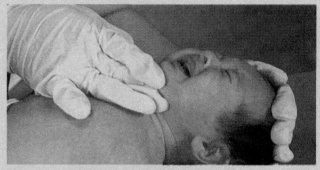

2 Open airway. Establish breathlessness.

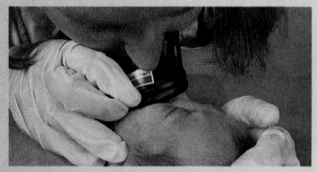

3 Attempt to ventilate. If this fails, reposition head and try again.

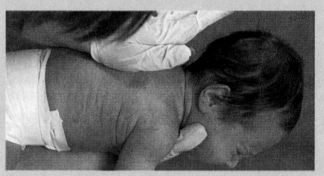

4 Deliver four back blows.

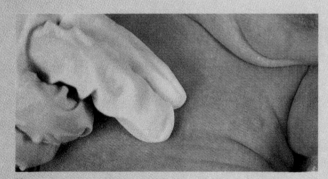

5 Deliver four chest thrusts.

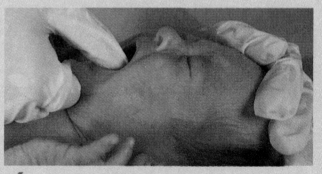

6 Remove visible objects.

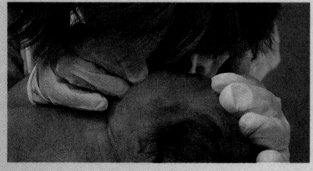

7 Reattempt to ventilate.

8 Repeat the sequence of:
- Back blows
- Chest thrusts
- Removing visible objects
- Reattempting ventilations

(60/5 = 12). The only variation here is in cases of children and infants, where the rate is one breath every 3 seconds for the infant and one breath very 4 seconds for the child.

When using abdominal thrusts to clear the airway, deliver six to ten abdominal thrusts in rapid succession. Chest thrusts, when appropriate, are delivered as four slow, distinct thrusts.

We breathe to bring in oxygen, remove carbon dioxide, and help regulate the acid–base balance of our blood. The major muscle of breathing, the diaphragm, and the muscles between our ribs contract to increase the volume of the chest cavity. This in turn decreases the pressure in the chest cavity, allowing the lungs to expand. As the lungs expand, the pressure inside decreases, allowing air to rush in from the atmosphere. When we exhale, just the opposite occurs. All this is an involuntary, automatic process, controlled mainly by the respiratory centers of the brain.

Clinical death occurs when an individual stops breathing and the heart stops beating. **Biological death** occurs when the brain cells start to die. Without oxygen, lethal changes take place in the brain cells within 4 to 6 minutes. Brain cell death may start within 10 minutes.

In addition to the respiratory centers in the brain, the diaphragm and the muscles between the ribs, the respiratory system includes the nose and mouth, the throat (pharynx), the voice box (larynx), the windpipe (trachea), the bronchial tree, and the lungs.

Look for chest movements, **listen** and **feel** for air exchange, and **note** anything that may indicate problems with breathing. Problems may be indicated in terms of rate and depth and by skin color changes.

Opening the airway is a primary procedure for First Responders. Simply repositioning the patient's head may solve breathing problems. The **head-tilt, chin-lift maneuver** is used to open the airway of patients without neck or spinal injuries. The **jaw-thrust maneuver** is used when there are possible neck or spinal injuries.

Mouth-to-mask ventilation is the recommended procedure for EMS personnel to use during rescue breathing. It requires the use of a pocket face mask with one-way valve. Follow your local guidelines.

Mouth-to-mouth ventilation is another form of pulmonary resuscitation. There are no shortcuts to this procedure. Learn all the steps provided in this chapter and how to use this procedure for the elderly, infants, and children. Learn the mouth-to-nose method as it applies to accident victims and the mouth-to-stoma method as it applies to neck breathers. Methods that do not use a mask or some other barrier increase the risk of infectious disease transmission.

Be alert for air forced into a patient's stomach. **Reposition the head,** adjust your ventilations, and be on guard for **vomiting.**

When considering accident victims, try to use the **jaw-thrust maneuver** to open the airway. Do what you can to protect the spine; however, if a patient not not breathing, **take immediate action!**

A variety of problems can cause partial or full airway obstruction. These include the tongue, epiglottis, foreign objects, tissue damage, and disease. In addition to the signs of inadequate breathing, **listen** for snoring, crowing, gurgling, and wheezing sounds. For cases of total obstruction, there will be no chest movements, no sounds of respiration, and no air exchange felt at the nose and mouth.

Encourage those patients with partial obstructions to cough. If they cannot cough, if their coughing is very weak, or if there is poor air exchange, **provide care as if there is a complete airway obstruction.**

Conscious patients with airway obstructions will often *grasp their necks* trying to communicate. Ask patients, *"Can you speak?"* or *"Can you cough?"* If they can, the obstruction is partial.

Correcting airway obstructions requires that you know the **combined procedures** of:

- Attempts to **ventilate**
- **Manual thrusts**
- **Finger sweeps**
- **Opening the airway** and reattempting **ventilations**

These various procedures are to be used in a specific pattern. Before you complete this chapter, make sure you know the combined procedures for conscious and unconscious adults and children (see Figure 4–22) and infants (see Scansheet 4–1).

CHAPTER 4-A

Aids to
Resuscitation—
Airways (Optional)

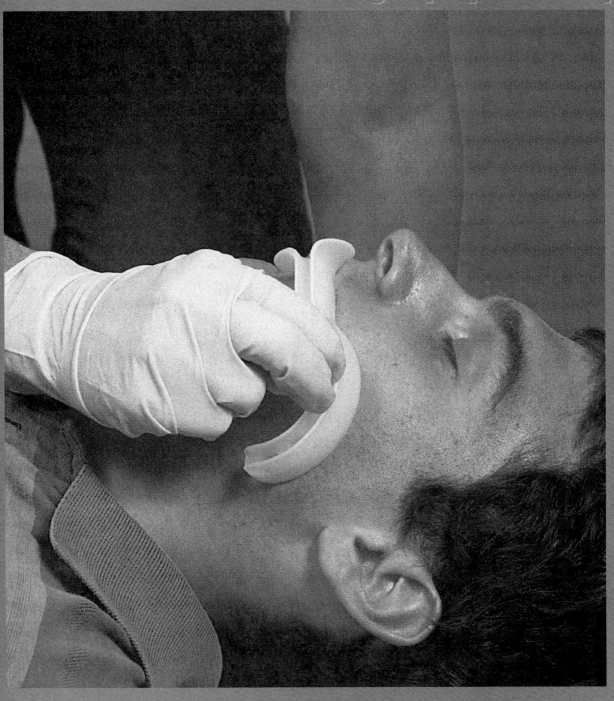

■ OBJECTIVES

By the end of this chapter, you should be able to:
1. Define and identify an oropharyngeal airway. (p. 115)
2. Describe how to insert an oropharyngeal airway. (pp. 116)
3. Describe how to provide artificial ventilations when using an oropharyngeal airway. (p. 118)

NOTE: There are many items of equipment and special techniques used in caring for patients with airway and breathing problems. *All* of this equipment and *all* these techniques require special *supervised* training.

Most areas do not require First Responders to know how to use special equipment and techniques in caring for breathing and circulation. This chapter is provided for those students requiring such skills. *Do not* try to learn from this chapter without your instructor's guidance and the opportunity to practice on manikins under your instructor's supervision. The pocket face mask with one-way valve is covered in Chapter 4, page 92. Students being trained in the use of the bag-valve-mask ventilator and oxygen therapy should refer to Appendix 3, Breathing Aids and Oxygen Therapy, p. 465.

SKILLS

Upon completing this chapter and your class lectures and skills labs, you should be able to:

1. Select and insert an oropharyngeal airway using a training manikin.
2. Demonstrate how to provide mouth-to-mask ventilation, using a manikin, an oropharyngeal airway, and a pocket face mask with one-way valve.

AIDS TO RESUSCITATION

Adjunct Equipment

The use of adjunct equipment can aid in providing effective respiratory and circulatory resuscitation. Most of the equipment is considered to be part of advanced life support, which is beyond the scope of First Responder training courses. Two pieces of adjunct equipment are commonly being taught for use in First Responder-level care. These devices are the oropharyngeal (o-ro-fah-RIN-je-al) airway and the pocket face mask (see page 92).

The major advantages of these two pieces of adjunct equipment are:

• They make it easier for the rescuer to maintain an open airway for the patient.
• They allow the rescuer to deliver more effective ventilations to the patient.
• They help reduce rescuer fatigue during resuscitation.

The major disadvantage of all adjunct equipment is the fact that its use can delay the beginning of resuscitation. *Never* delay the beginning of pulmonary resuscitation or cardiopulmonary resuscitation in order to locate, retrieve, or set up adjunct equipment.

Another disadvantage of some adjunct equipment is that it must be maintained and kept in working order. Unless cared for properly, adjunct devices can fail.

Oropharyngeal Airways

Once a patient's airway is opened, an oropharyngeal airway can be inserted to help keep the airway open. "Oro" refers to the mouth. "Pharyngeo" refers to the throat. An oropharyngeal airway is a device, usually made of plastic, that can be inserted into the patient's mouth and reach back into the throat. The oropharyngeal airway has a flange that fits against the patient's lips. The rest of the airway holds down the patient's tongue and curves back into the throat.

WARNING: Oropharyngeal airways are to be used only on **unconscious** patients who do not exhibit a gag reflex. These devices can induce vomiting in the conscious patient. The vomitus can be breathed back into the patient's lungs (aspirated). Also, airways can induce spasms along the airway of a conscious patient. If the patient is responsive, even if he is totally disoriented or confused, airways are not to be inserted. *The patient must be unconscious.*

Some EMS Systems allow First Responders to use oropharyngeal airways *only* for unconscious, nonbreathing patients. This is done to reduce the risk of vomiting. Since most First Responders do not have suction equipment, these EMS Systems consider it too risky to use the airway for unresponsive, breathing patients. They feel that the patient could regain consciousness, gag on the airway, and aspirate the vomitus before the rescuer has a chance to take action. *Follow your local guidelines.*

Rules for Using Airways

1. Open the patient's airway first. Insertion of an oropharyngeal airway does not replace this step.
2. Use only on unconscious patients. Any gagging by the patient indicates that the airway cannot be used.
3. Take great care not to push the patient's tongue back into the throat.
4. Constantly monitor the patient for gagging.
5. Remove the device immediately if the patient begins to gag. Continue to monitor the patient's airway and respiration.

Oropharyngeal (or-o-fah-RIN-je-al) airway—a curved airway that is inserted through the unconscious patient's mouth into the throat. It helps to maintain a clear airway (passage) for breathing or resuscitation.

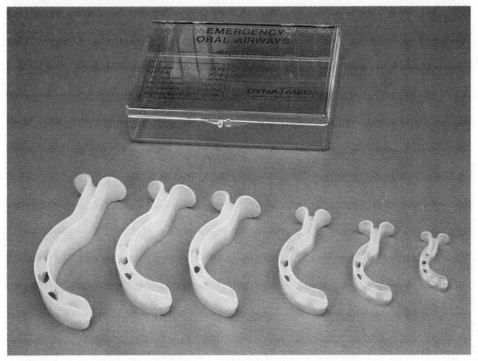

FIGURE 4A–1.
Various sizes of oropharyngeal airways.

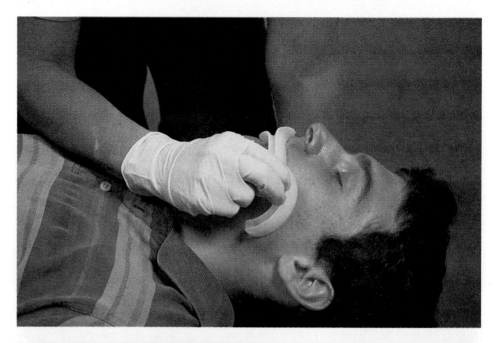

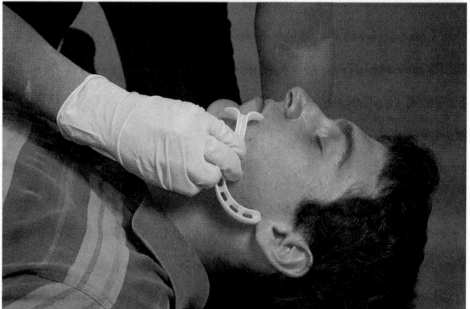

FIGURE 4A–2.
The airway is chosen and is checked for correct size.

Measuring the Airway

There are at least seven standardized sizes of oropharyngeal airways designed to fit infants, children, and adults. To use this device effectively, you must be able to select the correct size airway for the patient. An airway of proper size will extend from the center of the patient's mouth to the angle of the jaw bone (mandible). Before using an airway, hold the device against the patient's face and measure to see if it extends from the center of the mouth to the angle of the lower jaw. The airway also may be sized by holding it at the corner of the patient's mouth and seeing if it will extend to the tip of the ear lobe on the same side of the face. If the airway is not the correct size, *do not use* it on the patient.

Sometimes it is difficult to find the correct size oropharyngeal airway for a patient. If the airway is too long, it might cause the patient to vomit. In some cases, it might fall forward and push the tongue down the throat. If the device is too short, it could partially block the patient's airway. The device must be the correct size to be used.

Inserting the Airway

WARNING: Take special care if there is any possibility of spinal injuries. Open the airway by using the modified jaw-thrust technique. Avoid moving the patient any more than necessary.

To insert an oropharyngeal airway, you should:

1. Place the patient on his back, in the correct head-tilt position.
2. Cross your thumb and forefinger and then scissor open the patient's mouth at the corner.
3. Position the airway so that its tip is pointing toward the roof of the patient's mouth.
4. Insert the airway and slide it along the roof of the patient's mouth, past the uvula (the soft tissue hanging down at the back of mouth). Be certain not to push the tongue back into the throat.
5. Rotate the airway 180 degrees (one-half turn) until the tip is pointing down the patient's throat. Hold the tongue in place.

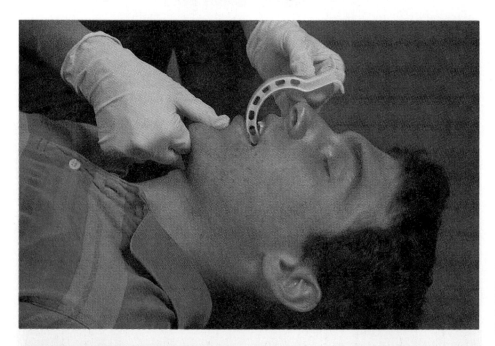

FIGURE 4A–3.
The airway is inserted with the tip pointing to the roof of the patient's mouth.

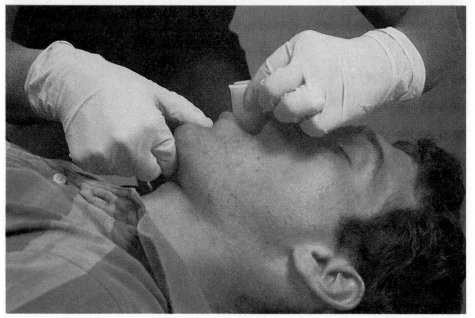

FIGURE 4A–4.
The airway is rotated into position.

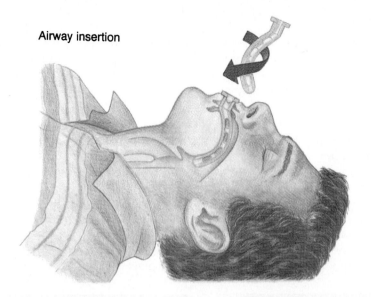

Airway insertion

FIGURE 4A–5.
Note that when the airway is properly positioned, the flange rests against the patient's lips.

6. Place the patient in a head-tilt position. Check to see that the flange of the airway is against the patient's lips. If the airway is too long or too short, remove it and replace with one of correct size.

7. Provide mouth-to-mask ventilations or deliver mouth-to-adjunct ventilations the same way you would provide mouth-to-mouth ventilations.

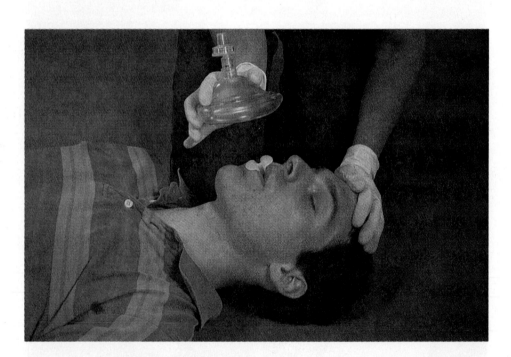

FIGURE 4A–6.
The patient is ready for ventilation.

WARNING: *Never* practice the use of airways on anyone. Manikins should be used for developing skills with airways.

CHAPTER 5

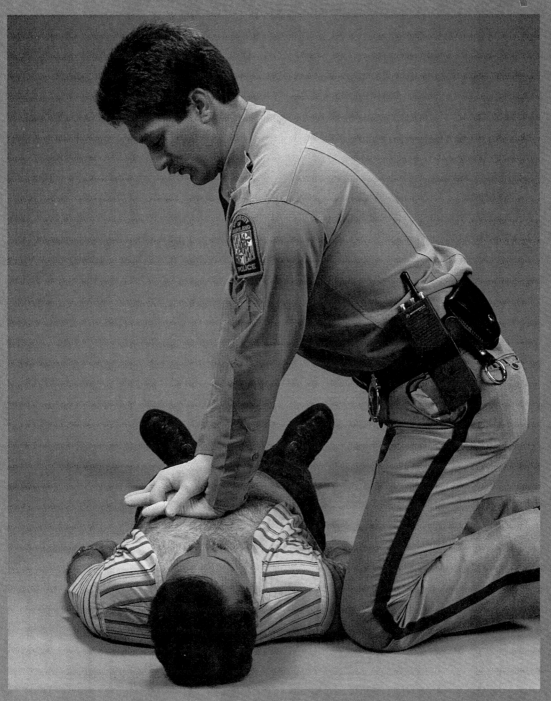

OBJECTIVES

By the end of this chapter, you should be able to:
1. Describe the relationship of heart, lung, and brain activity. (pp. 120–121)
2. List the signs of cardiac arrest. (pp. 121–122)
3. Define the ABCs of emergency care. (p. 122)
4. Explain how CPR keeps a patient alive. (pp. 122–123)
5. List the events that should occur during the primary survey that will lead to beginning CPR. (pp. 123–124)
6. Locate the CPR compression site on an adult, child, and infant. (pp. 124, 136)
7. Describe how to deliver external chest compressions and ventilations. (pp. 126–127, 136)
8. List the rates of compressions and ventilations used during CPR on adults, children, and infants. (pp. 129, 137)
9. State how you can determine that CPR is being performed correctly. (p. 129)
10. State why you should wait until you have checked for a carotid pulse before having someone call dispatch. (p. 124)
11. List, step by step, the procedures for performing CPR on adults, children, and infants. (pp. 130–137)
12. Describe the complications that can occur during CPR. (pp. 137–138)
13. State when you may stop CPR. (pp. 141–142)
14. Relate CPR techniques to the accident scene, electric shock, and drowning. (pp. 139–141)

WARNING: It is recommended that EMS personnel reduce the risk of infection by using pocket face masks with one-way valves (see page 92) when ventilating patients. Rescuers should wear latex or vinyl gloves to avoid contact with the patient's blood, body fluids, wastes, or mucous membranes.

SKILLS

Upon completing this chapter and your class lectures and skills labs, you should be able to:

1. Demonstrate how to evaluate a patient in order to detect cardiac arrest.
2. Perform one-rescuer CPR on an adult manikin.
3. Perform one-rescuer CPR on an infant manikin.

CIRCULATION

The circulatory system keeps blood moving in a constant, one-direction flow. At the center of this activity is the heart. As the heat beats, it performs as a pump. Blood from the body is taken into the heart and is then sent to the lungs. There the blood gives up excess carbon dioxide and picks up oxygen. This oxygen-rich blood is then sent back to the heart, where it is pumped out to the entire body. During the course of its circulation, the blood will take up nutrients from the small intestines, give up wastes to the kidneys, carry secretions from various glands to other areas of the body, and pick up carbon dioxide from the tissues.

1st There is a strong relationship among breathing, circulation, and certain brain activity. This relationship may be seen as follows:

- If breathing stops, the blood being pumped to the brain will not contain

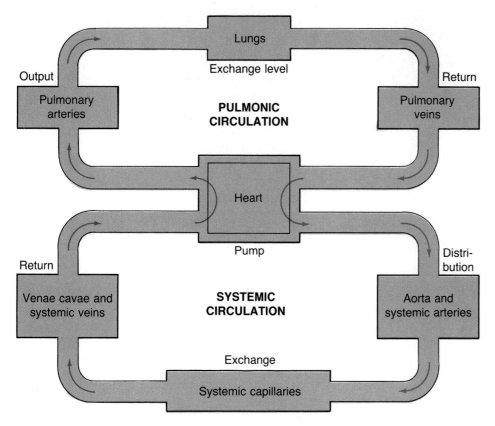

PULMONIC
CIRCULATION

Lungs
Exchange level

Output

Return

Pulmonary
arteries

Pulmonary
veins

Heart

Pump

Return

Distri-
bution

Venae cavae and
systemic veins

SYSTEMIC
CIRCULATION

Aorta and
systemic arteries

Exchange

Systemic capillaries

FIGURE 5–1.
The functions of the circulatory
system depend upon the heart
pumping the blood in a
constant, one-direction flow.

enough oxygen. Due to brain failure and a lack of oxygen for its own tissues, the heart will beat improperly and then stop beating altogether.

- When the heart stops beating, breathing stops almost instantly.

Cardiac Arrest

1st When the heart stops beating, a person is in cardiac arrest. The signs of cardiac arrest are:

- The patient is unresponsive.
- The patient is not breathing (respirations usually stop within 30 seconds of cardiac arrest).
- There is no carotid pulse.

Cardiac arrest—when the heart stops beating. Also, the sudden end of effective circulation related to highly irregular contractions of the lower chambers of the heart (ventricular fibrillation).

FIGURE 5–2.
The activities of the heart, lung, and brain are interdependent.

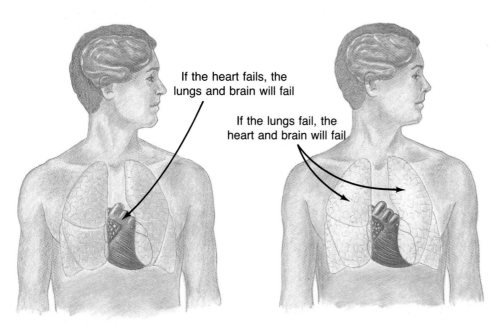

If the heart fails, the lungs and brain will fail

If the lungs fail, the heart and brain will fail

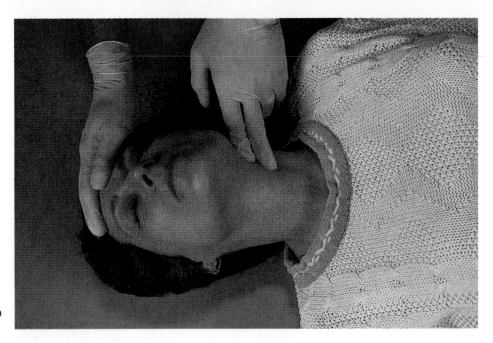

FIGURE 5–3.
The signs of cardiac arrest: unresponsive, no breathing, no pulse.

Note how the above are listed in the order in which they would be determined during the primary survey.

CPR—What It Is

Cardiopulmonary resuscitation (KAR-de-o-PUL-mo-ner-e re-SUS-ci-TA-shun), CPR—heart–lung resuscitation. A combined effort to maintain circulation and breathing artificially.

CPR is cardiopulmonary resuscitation. "Cardio" refers to the heart and "pulmonary" refers to the lungs. CPR is an emergency procedure applied when heart and lung actions have stopped.

1st Whenever you read about basic life support, you will see references made to the ABCs of emergency care. ABC stands for:

> A = Airway
> B = Breathing
> C = Circulation

1st In Chapter 4 you learned how to maintain an open airway and how to breathe for a patient in respiratory arrest. When applying CPR, you still are concerned with maintaining an open airway and breathing for the patient. In addition to these two procedures, you have to circulate blood to the lungs and the rest of the patient's body. Therefore, during CPR, you will have to perform procedures to:

- Maintain an open airway
- Breathe for the patient
- Force the patient's blood to circulate

CPR—How It Works

If clinical death and biological death were the same thing, CPR would not work (see Chapter 4). However, the delay that exists between the beginning of clinical death and the beginning of lethal changes in the brain allows you to employ the techniques of CPR to keep the patient from reaching biological death. The cutoff point is not 10 minutes in cardiac arrest. Many patients who have been in arrest for more than 10 minutes have been successfully resuscitated. This is particularly true in cases involving infants and children. In cold-water drownings, many people have survived after

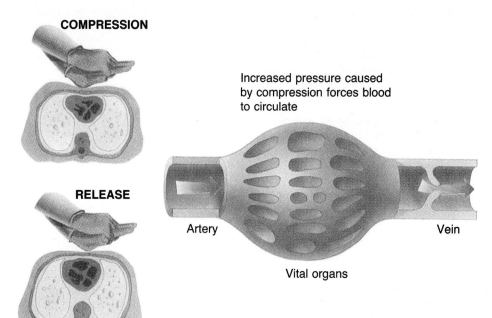

COMPRESSION

RELEASE

Increased pressure caused by compression forces blood to circulate

Artery

Vein

Vital organs

FIGURE 5–4.
During CPR, pressure in the chest cavity increases with compression. This forces blood into circulation.

20 minutes and some for periods much longer (for example, 45 minutes). This delay gives you time to apply CPR to prevent biological death.

NOTE: The above does not imply that starting CPR should ever be delayed. The patient's chances for survival increase if CPR is begun as soon as possible.

You already know that it is possible to provide breaths for a patient who is not breathing. This procedure will not benefit the patient unless the blood is circulating. In CPR, the rescuer causes the patient's blood to circulate by applying **external chest compressions.**

During the process of external chest compression, the patient's chest is compressed along its midline, at a point atop the breastbone (sternum). If the patient is lying face up on a rigid surface, this compression will cause pressure changes to take place in the chest cavity (thoracic cavity). The pressure increases and forces the blood to circulate. When the pressure is released, blood flows into the patient's veins and heart. One-way valves in the patient's heart and veins keep the blood moving in the proper direction.

1st When you provide CPR for a patient, your breaths provide oxygen to be taken up by the blood and your compressions cause this oxygenated blood to be ciruclated to the body's cells.

External chest compressions—measured compressions performed during CPR at a set rate over top of the CPR compression site. These compressions are applied to help create circulation of the blood.

THE TECHNIQUES OF CPR

We will begin our discussion of CPR by examining the various techniques used in the procedure as it is applied to the adult patient. Next, the complete procedure will be presented, step by step. Finally, we will cover CPR for infants and children.

When to Begin CPR

1st As a First Responder, always conduct a primary survey on each patient. The events leading to the beginning of CPR should be:

1. **Establishing unresponsiveness**—Is the patient responsive? Alert? Gently shake the patient on the shoulder and shout, *Are you okay?"*

Patients requiring immediate CPR will not be responsive. If the patient does not respond, you will have to have someone alert the EMS System dispatcher; however, this should wait until you have more information. You should ask someone at the scene to be prepared to phone dispatch, or if you are alone, you should *call out* for help.

2. **Position the patient**—Follow the procedures presented in Chapter 3, Scansheet 3-1.

3. **Establishing an open airway**—Use the head-tilt, chin-lift method or the jaw-thrust method. It is recommended that you check at this time to see if the patient is a neck-breather.

4. **Check for breathing**—Use the *look, listen, feel* method. This method requires checking for *3 to 5 seconds*. A patient who is breathing does not need immediate CPR. If the patient is not breathing, you should .. . .

5. **Deliver two adequate breaths**—Use the technique described in Chapter 4. If you note an airway obstruction, clear the patient's airway and provide two adequate breaths. If the airway is clear and he is not breathing on his own . . .

6. **Check for a carotid pulse**—Use the technique described in Chapter 3. You should take *5 to 10 seconds* to check for a pulse. If the patient is not breathing and there is no carotid pulse . . .

7. **Alert dispatch**—This must be done immediately. Make certain that the person tells the dispatcher that CPR has been started. If your EMS System has an advanced cardiac life-support (ACLS) unit available, it can be dispatched to the scene. If no such unit is available, the EMTs who respond will have oxygen and ventilation devices that will greatly improve the efficiency of CPR. *Do not delay CPR so that you can go and call the dispatcher.*

8. **Begin CPR.**

Locating the CPR Compression Site

External chest compressions are not effective unless they are delivered to a very specific site on the patient's chest. If you apply compressions to the wrong site, you will probably injure the patient or provide ineffective CPR and the patient will reach biological death.

1st After determining that the adult patient needs CPR, you should:

1. Begin by positioning yourself at the patient's side, with your knees pointed in toward his side.

2. Use the index and middle fingers of your hand closest to the patient's waist to locate the *lower margin* of the patient's rib cage. This should be done on the side of the patient's chest closest to your knees.

3. Run your fingers along the patient's rib cage until you find the *notch* where the ribs meet the breastbone. This will be found in the lower center of the patient's chest.

4. Keep your middle finger at the notch where the ribs connect to the breastbone. Your index finger should be positioned next to your middle finger, so that it rests over the lower end of the sternum.

5. The heel of your hand closest to the patient's head is placed over the middle of the breastbone, with the thumb side of the hand touching the index finger you used to locate the point where the ribs joined the breastbone.

At this point, the heel of your hand closest to the patient's head will be placed directly over the CPR compression site.

■ SCAN 5-1.

Locating the CPR Compression Site

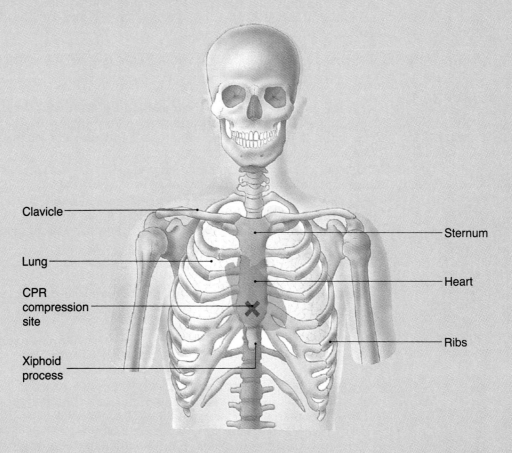

Clavicle

Lung

CPR
compression
site

Xiphoid
process

Sternum

Heart

Ribs

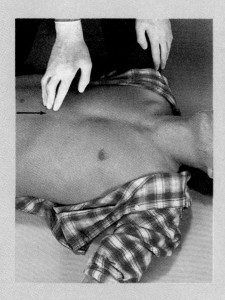

1 Use the index and middle fingers of the hand that is closest to the patient's feet to locate the lower border of the rib cage.

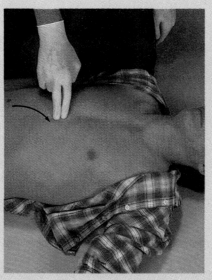

2 Move your fingers along the rib cage until you find the point where the ribs meet the breastbone. Keep your middle finger at the notch.

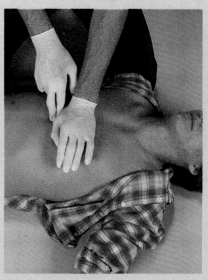

3 With your index finger over the lower end of the breastbone, move your other hand to the midline. Place its thumb side against the index finger of the lower hand.

External Chest Compressions

1st For external chest compressions to be effective, you must:

- Place the patient lying face up on a firm surface such as the ground or a floor. If the patient is in bed, move him to the floor or place a board under his back. *Do not* delay CPR in order to find a support or device.
- Make certain that you find the CPR compression site as described above. Remember, the heel of your hand closest to the patient's head is placed directly over this site (see above).

1st The correct procedure for providing external chest compressions includes:

1. With the patient properly positioned and the CPR compression site located, reposition the hand you used to locate the breastbone notch. This hand is now placed on top of the hand that is over the CPR compression site.
2. The heels of both hands should be parallel to one another, with the fingers of both hands pointing away from your body.
3. Your fingers can be extended or they may be interlaced, *but* your fingers **must be kept off the patient's chest.** Some people find it easier to deliver compressions if they grasp the wrist of the hand placed at the compression site (see Figure 5–6).
4. Straighten your elbows and lock them. *Do not* bend your elbows when delivering or releasing compression.
5. Position your shoulders directy over your hands so that you will deliver all compressions straight down onto the CPR compression site. Keep both of your knees on the ground.
6. Compressions must be delivered straight down. Apply enough force to the compression site of a typical adult so that you depress the breastbone 1½ to 2 inches. It is best if you move up and down at your waist.
7. After compression, fully release the pressure on the patient's chest. This allows the patient's heart to refill. *Do not* bend your elbows in order to release pressure. *Do not* lift your hands off the patient's chest. Lift up at your waist to return your shoulders to their original position. The release of pressure should take the same amount of time as the time required for compression (50% compression: 50% release).

FIGURE 5–5.
Positioning the hands at the CPR compression site.

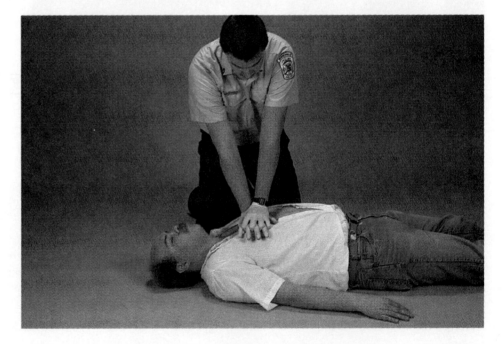

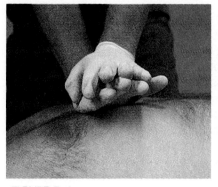
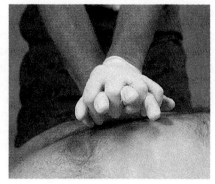
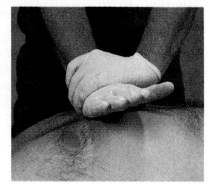

FIGURE 5–6.
Hand placement for
compressions.

WARNING: *Do not* practice CPR compressions on any person. This is an extreme emergency care procedure that may cause serious problems when applied to an individual with normal lung and heart actions. Practice only on the manikins provided for use in your course. Finding the landmarks for CPR (breastbone notch and compression site) may and should be practiced on people as well as the manikins.

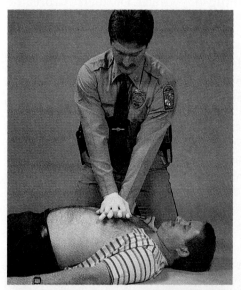
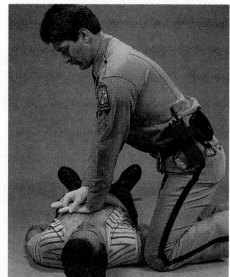
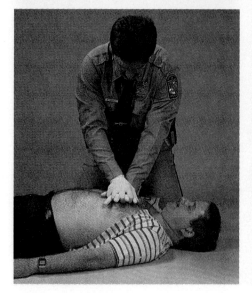
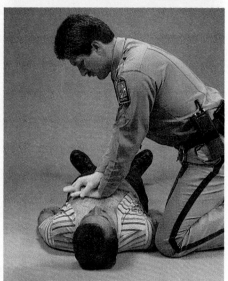

FIGURE 5–7.
The shoulders are placed
directly over the compression
site.

FIGURE 5–8.
Compressions
are delivered straight down.

Providing Breaths During CPR

Interposed ventilations—the breaths provided to the patient during CPR. They are delivered after a set number of external chest compressions.

Along with artificial circulation, you must provide artificial ventilation when performing CPR. The breaths that you supply to the patient have been traditionally called **interposed ventilations.** (Many CPR instructors prefer to use the term ventilation or rescue breathing.) They are provided between a set number of compressions, after a set number of compressions have been delivered. These breaths are provided to the patient, using the same basic technique employed in mouth-to-mask resuscitation (or the mouth-to-mouth, mouth-to-nose, or mouth-to-stoma technique). The patient's head must be placed in the correct head-tilt position by using the head-tilt, chin-lift, or jaw-thrust technique. Air should be delivered into the patient's lungs until you see the chest rise and feel resistance (usually a 1 to 1.5 second ventilation).

There are four special factors to consider when providing interposed ventilations during CPR:

- Deliver each breath in 1 to 1.5 seconds.
- Provide **two** breaths immediately after every **fifteen** compressions.
- *Do not* overventilate the patient. If you try to force too much air into the patient's lungs, you may cause gastric distention. Feel for resistance and watch the patient's chest rise.
- Establish a regular pattern of breathing for yourself. Do not try to breathe or hold your breath with each compression. To do so could lead to exhaustion.

The use of mouth-to-mask ventilations requires the rescuer to be at the patient's head to ensure a proper mask placement and seal. This is very difficult to do when moving to this position after delivering external chest compressions. Likewise, it is difficult to move from this head position to the patient's side in order to deliver compressions directly over the CPR compression site. Unless you are using a mask that is approved for use while positioned at the patient's side, you will have to place yourself at the top of the patient's head. This will take a lot of serious practice to develop the efficiency needed to provide effective CPR.

WARNING: *Do not* practice interposed ventilations on anyone. Use the manikins provided for your training.

FIGURE 5–9.
Deliver each breath in 1 to 1.5 seconds.

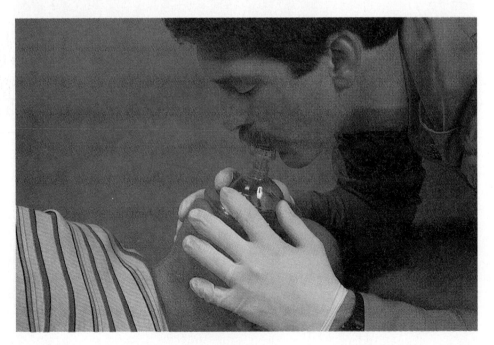

Rates of Compressions and Ventilations

1st The rate at which both compressions and ventilations are delivered is critical to providing effective CPR. CPR is very dependent on using the correct ratio of compressions and ventilations. As a First Responder, you must know the following:

- Compressions must be delivered at a rate of 80 to 100 per minute.
- Ventilations must be delivered at a ratio of 2 breaths every 15 compressions. These two breaths must be delivered at 1 ventilation every 1 to 1.5 seconds.
- CPR should never be interrupted for more than 7 seconds. If you must move the patient, 15 to 30 seconds is the maximum time to interrupt CPR.

In one-rescuer CPR, when compressions are delivered at a rate of 80 to 100 per minute, 80 to 100 compressions per minute are not actually delivered to the patient. The time taken up for ventilations will mean that about 60 compressions per minute are being delivered. To be certain that you are providing compressions at a rate of 80 to 100 per minute, use the following count as you deliver compressions:

State: "One-and, two-and, three-and, four-and, five-and . . ." until you reach fifteen compressions. Then, deliver two adequate ventilations, relocate the CPR compression site, and continue the next set of compressions.

Effective CPR

1st You can be certain that you are performing CPR correctly if:

- A person trained to take a carotid pulse can feel such a pulse each time you compress the patient's breastbone. *Do not* try to deliver compressions with one hand while you check for pulsations at the carotid artery.
- You see proper chest rise and fall associated with artificial ventilations.

If CPR is effective, you may notice the patient's skin color improves, but this is not always the case. Sometimes the patient may try to swallow, gasp, or move the arms and legs. This may not be that meaningful, but you should check for the return of breathing and a pulse when you observe these activities.

1st You should check for a carotid pulse after providing CPR for 1 minute. If the patient has a pulse, but is not breathing, stop CPR and provide pulmonary resuscitation. If there is no pulse, continue CPR and check for a carotid pulse every few minutes. The return of a heartbeat and spontaneous breathing are hoped for; however, in most cases you can provide effective CPR, but patients will not regain their own heartbeat and breathing. Most patients will require special medical procedures before they can ever regain heart and lung functions. CPR is used to keep patients biologically alive until these procedures can be provided.

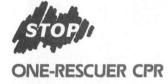

ONE-RESCUER CPR

Basic Procedures

CPR can be performed by one rescuer or by two rescuers. In this chapter, we will consider the techniques used by one rescuer providing CPR. It is essential for a First Responder to know how to perform both one-rescuer and two-rescuer CPR.

What follows is a step-by-step outline for performing one-rescuer CPR. The procedures covered here follow the recommendations of the AHA. Your instructor will inform you of any changes made by the AHA recently. Otherwise, learn the procedures exactly as they are presented. *Do not* try to develop your own method or look for apparent shortcuts. The extensive research done by the AHA has determined that the procedures presented here are the most efficient in saving the lives of patients in cardiac arrest.

1st 1. **Establish unresponsiveness**—A responsive patient does not need CPR. Gently shake the patient's shoulder and ask, "Are you okay?" If the patient is not responsive, call out for help.

1st 2. **Properly position the patient and yourself**—The patient should be placed flat, face up, on a hard surface. Position yourself beside the patient at chest level, with your knees pointing in toward the patient's chest. This is the position you assume when conducting a primary survey (Figure 5–12).

1st 3. **Establish an open airway**—Use the head-tilt, chin-lift method or the jaw-thrust method to ensure an open airway. At the same time, check to see if the patient is a neck-breather (has a stoma) (Figure 5–13).

1st 4. **Check for breathing**—*Look*, *listen*, and *feel* for air exchange. This should take about 3 to 5 seconds.

1st 5. **Provide two adequate breaths**—Use the procedures outlined for mouth-to-mask (or mouth-to-mouth, mouth-to-nose, or mouth-to-stoma) ventilation.

1st 6. If necessary, **clear the patient's airway**—Use the techniques of back blows (infants only), manual thrusts, finger sweeps, and ventilations as described in Chapter 4.

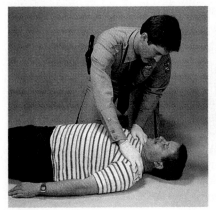

FIGURE 5–10.
Determine unresponsiveness.

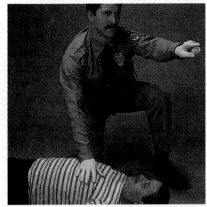

FIGURE 5–11. Call for help.

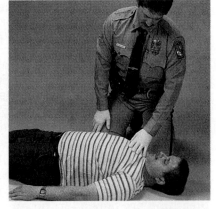

FIGURE 5–12. Properly position the patient and yourself.

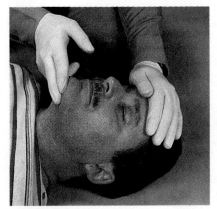

FIGURE 5–13.
Open the airway.

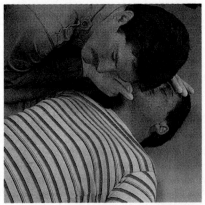

FIGURE 5–14.
Determine breathlessness.

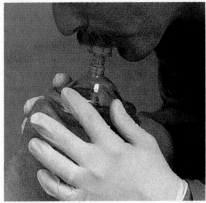

FIGURE 5–15.
Provide 2 breaths.

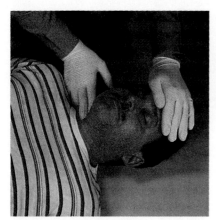
FIGURE 5–16.
Determine pulselessness.

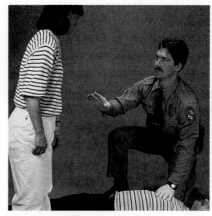
FIGURE 5–17.
Alert the EMS dispatcher.

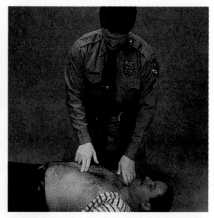
FIGURE 5–18.
Find the CPR compression site.

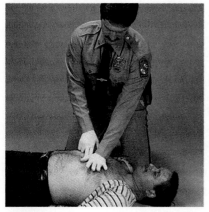
FIGURE 5–19.
Properly position your hands.

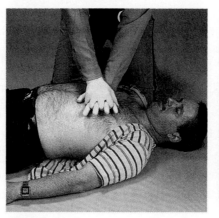
FIGURE 5–20.
Keep your fingers off of the patient's chest.

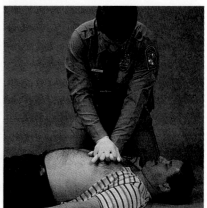
FIGURE 5–21.
Deliver 15 compressions.

REMEMBER: Artificial circulation will not be effective unless oxygen is reaching the exchange levels of the patient's lungs.

1st 7. **Establish cardiac arrest**—Check for circulation by feeling for a **carotid pulse.** This should take **5 to 10 seconds.** If the patient has a carotid pulse, but no respirations, provide one breath every 5 seconds. If the patient does not have a carotid pulse, you *must* make certain that someone alerts the EMS System dispatcher.

1st 8. **Find the CPR compression site**—Slide your index and middle fingers along the lower margin of the ribs until you locate the notch where the ribs join the breastbone (Figure 5–18).

1st 9. **Position your hands for delivering compressions**—Place your hand closest to the patient's head along the midline of the patient's chest. The heel of this hand should touch up against the index finger of the hand used to locate the compression site.

Next, move the hand used to locate the compression site. Place it on top of the hand positioned on the breastbone. The heels of both hands should now be parallel to one another, with your fingers pointing straight away from your body. The fingers may be interlocked or extended, or you may grasp the wrist of the hand placed at the compression site. Your fingers *must* be kept off of the patient's chest (Figure 5–20).

1st 10. **Deliver external chest compressions**—Keep your arms straight, elbows locked, and shoulders directly over the compression site. Bend at the waist when delivery compressions to utilize your upper body weight. **Remember:**

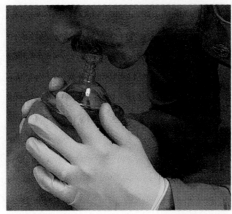

FIGURE 5–22.
Provide 2 breaths.

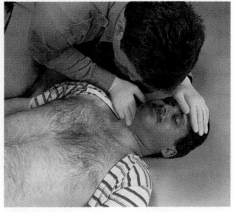

FIGURE 5–23.
Reassess the pulse.

A. Deliver compressions directly over the CPR compression site.
B. Compress the patient's breastbone 1½ to 2 inches.
C. Deliver compressions at a **rate of 80 to 100 per minute,** counting, "One-and, two-and, three-and . . . etc."
D. Release pressure completely to allow the heart to refill. Each release should take the amount of time as a compression. **REMEMBER:** *Do not* take your hands off the patient's chest.
E. **Deliver 15 compressions, then . . .**

1st 11. **Provide breaths**—Ventilations are provided at the **rate of 2 adequate breaths every 15 compressions.** Do this at a rate of one ventilation every 1 to 1.5 seconds. CPR compressions should not be interrupted for more than 7 seconds.

1st 12. **Continue CPR**—Deliver 15 compressions at the rate of 80 to 100 per minute, followed by two ventilations. Continue this cycle for one minute. This would be 4 sets of compressions and interposed ventilations.

1st 13. **Check for a carotid pulse**—After 1 minute of CPR, check for a carotid pulse (Figure 5–23). **Remember:** *Do not* interrupt CPR for more than 7 seconds in order to make this check. *If there is a pulse, stop CPR.* If the patient has a pulse, but is not breathing, provide breaths at the rate of one breath every 5 seconds. If there is no pulse, deliver 2 breaths and . . .

1st 14. **Continue CPR**—Check for a carotid pulse every few minutes. Provide CPR until another trained person can take over for you, the patient regains a pulse and breathing, or until you are too tired to continue.

CPR Techniques for Infants and Children

Many individuals highly trained in emergency medicine consider CPR for infants and children to be a major weakness in the EMS system. The members of the EMS System know how to perform CPR on infants and children; however, they have little practical experience due to the fact that few children need CPR away from a hospital setting. The vast majority of cases where CPR has been used for nonadult patients has been newborns in cardiac arrest. Such cases are rare. Anyone learning CPR needs to continually review and practice the techniques. Your review and practice *must* include CPR for infants and children.

1st Before learning the special techniques used on infants and children, consider the basic principles of CPR. These principles hold true for adult,

■ SCAN 5-2.

One Rescuer CPR

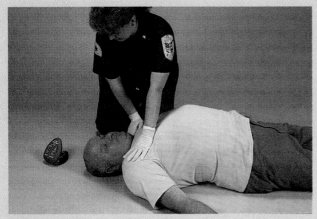

1 Establish unresponsiveness
Reposition

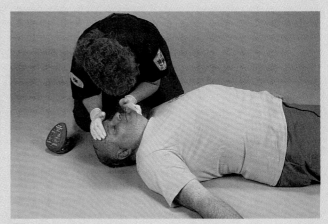

2 Open airway

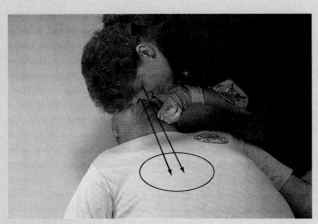

3 Look, listen and feel (3–5 seconds)

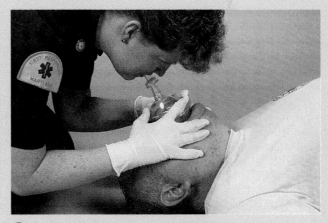

4 Ventilate twice (1–1.5 sec/ventilation)

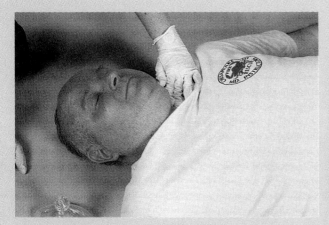

5 No pulse (5–10 sec.)

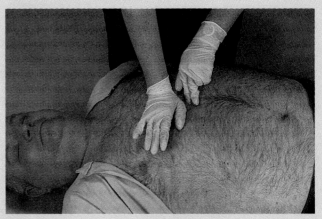

6 Locate compression site

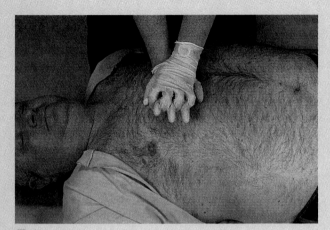

7 Position hands

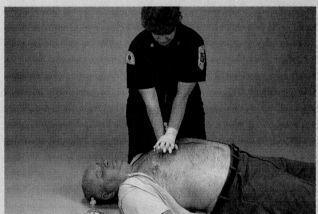

8 Begin compressions

Compressions delivered
at a rate of 80–100/minute
(15 per 9–11 seconds)

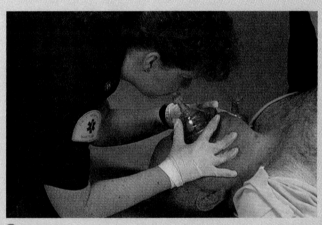

9 Ventilate twice

Provide 2 ventilations
every 15 compressions
(1–1.5 seconds/ventilations)

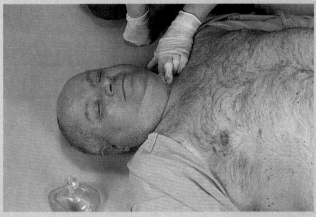

10 Recheck pulse after 4 cycles, then every few minutes

NOTE: When alone call out for help if patient is unresponsive. If off duty, have someone call dispatch after checking for pulselessness.

child, and infant. When providing CPR for an infant or a child, it will be necessary to:

1. Establish unresponsiveness
2. Call for help
3. Correctly position the patient
4. Open the airway
5. Establish breathlessness
6. Provide artificial ventilation, clearing airway obstructions when necessary
7. Establish the absence of a pulse
8. Have someone call dispatch
9. Provide chest compressions and ventilations

1st Infant or Child?

Since there are large infants, small children, and small adolescents, no hard and fast rule can be given. Instead, guidelines have been established for providing CPR. As a First Responder, you need to know:

- **Infant**—younger than 1 year of age
- **Child**—1 to 8 years of age

Anyone over the age of 8 years should be treated with adult techniques.

The size of the patient may lead you to make an error if you have to guess an age. Many infants and children are large for their age. Some adolescents are small enough to be mistaken for children. The above definitions are meant to be guidelines, not absolutes. The AHA has stated that "a slight error one way or the other is not critical."

Infant (AHA standard)—a person who is younger than one year of age.

Child (AHA standard)—a person who is 1 to 8 years of age.

Positioning the Patient

As with the adult patient, infants and children should be placed flat, face up, on a hard surface. Opening the airway of an infant or small child often lifts the back, preventing contact with the surface. When faced with such a situation, place one hand under the patient's back or have someone place a folded blanket or towel under the back to fill the void.

Opening the Airway

1st • **Infant**—use the head-tilt, chin-lift technique. A slight tilt is all that is needed, but be certain that the airway is *adequate.*

1st • **Child**—use the head-tilt, chin-lift method or the jaw thrust.
   Airway obstructions should be cared for as described in Chapter 4.

Establishing a Pulse

1st • **Infant**—*Do not* use the carotid or wrist pulse. You should use the brachial (BRAY-key-al) pulse that is found on the medial (inside) upper arm of the patient. You can find the brachial pulse by:

   1. Locating the point halfway between the patient's elbow and shoulder.
   2. Place your thumb on the lateral (outside) side of the patient's upper arm, at the midway point.
   3. Place the tips of your index and middle fingers at the midway point on the medial surface of the patient's upper arm.
   4. *Gently* press your index and middle fingers in toward the bone of the patient's upper arm in order to feel the brachial pulse.

Brachial (BRAY-key-al) pulse—the pulse found on the inside (medial) upper arm of the patient. It is used to evaluate circulation during the primary survey of an infant.

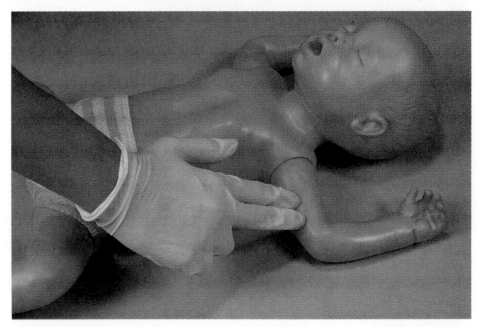

FIGURE 5–24.   For infants, determine circulation by feeling for a brachial pulse. The index and middle fingers are placed midway on the medial arm. The thumb should be placed on the lateral side of the arm during pulse determination.

1st • Child—determine circulation by finding a carotid pulse.

External Chest Compressions

1st • Infant—the size of the infant's chest and heart place the heart in a different position than what is found in the adult patient. Apply compressions to the breastbone, one finger-width below an imaginary line drawn directly between the nipples (see page 105). Deliver the compressions using the tips of two or three fingers. The breastbone of the infant should be depressed ½ to 1 inch.

1st • Child—use the heel of one hand to apply compressions to the breastbone, after finding the CPR compression site the same way as you would for an adult. The breastbone should be depressed 1 to 1½ inches.

FIGURE 5–25.   External chest compressions for infants and children. For infants, use tips of fingers and light pressure. For children, use heel of one hand only.

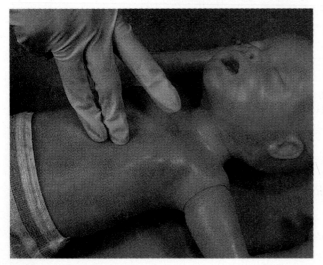

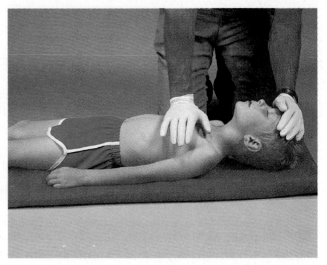

TABLE 5–1. CPR TECHNIQUES

Procedure	Adult	Child	Infant
Compressions			
• Method	2 hands	Heel of hand	2 to 3 fingers
• Depth	1½" to 2"	1" to 1½"	½" to 1"
• Rate	80 to 100/min	80 to 100/min	At least 100/min
Interposed ventilations			
• Method	Mouth-to-Mask	Mouth-to-Mask	Mouth-to-Mask
	Mouth-to-mouth	Mouth-to-mouth	Mouth-to-mouth
	Mouth-to-nose	Mouth-to-nose	and nose
Ratio			
Breaths:compressions	15:2	5:1	5:1
Count	1 and, 2 and, 3 and, 4 and, 5 . . . 15 and breathe, breathe	1 and 2 and 3 and 4 and 5 and breathe	1, 2, 3, 4, 5, breathe

Interposed Ventilations

1st • **Infant**—provide a gentle, but adequate breath of air to the infant's lungs using the mouth-to-mask (or mouth-to-mouth and nose) technique. Watch carefully for the rise and fall of the infant's chest.

1st • **Child**—provide a breath by way of the mouth-to-mask (or mouth-to-mouth or mouth-to-nose) technique. Watch carefully for the rise and fall of the child's chest.

CPR Rates

1st • **Infant**—deliver compressions at the rate of at least 100 per minute. Provide a breath after every fifth compression to give a ratio of 5:1.

1st • **Child**—deliver compressions at the rate of 80 to 100 per minute. Interpose a breath after every fifth compression to give a ratio of 5:1.

NOTE: To establish the correct rate for infants, count "One, two, three, four, five," and provide one breath. For children, you should count "One and two and three and four and five," and provide one breath.

PROBLEMS DURING CPR

CPR is not a simple process. Unless the proper procedures are carried out, it will not be effective and the patient will reach biological death. Ineffective CPR will result if:

- The patient is not placed upon a hard surface.
- The proper head-tilt is not performed.
- An improper seal is made over the patient's mouth, nose, mouth and nose, or stoma.
- The patient's nostrils are not pinched shut and the patient's mouth is not opened wide enough during mouth-to-mouth ventilation.
- The wrong compression site is selected or the hands are positioned improperly.
- Compressions are too shallow or upstrokes are too short.
- The wrong rates and ratios are used.
- CPR is stopped for more than 7 seconds.

Complications can occur during CPR. Some of these complications may arise from internal injuries, diseased organs, or weakened organs. As a

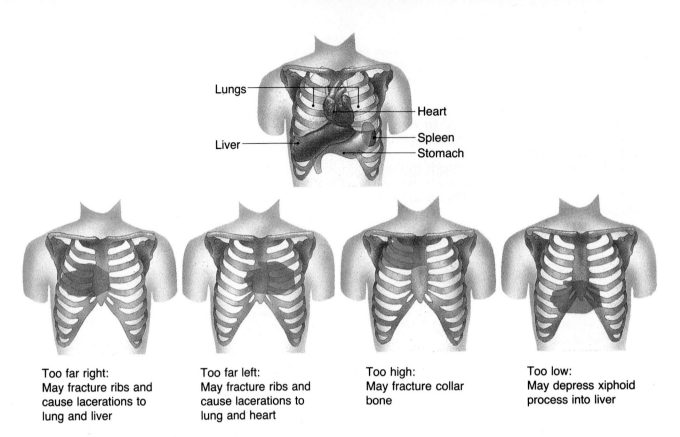

Too far right:
May fracture ribs and cause lacerations to lung and liver

Too far left:
May fracture ribs and cause lacerations to lung and heart

Too high:
May fracture collar bone

Too low:
May depress xiphoid process into liver

FIGURE 5–26.
Improper hand positioning can cause rib cage damage and injury to internal organs.

First Responder, there is nothing you can do when such complications arise. Regardless of the complication, you shoud still continue CPR.

1st Certain complications are associated with the improper positioning of the rescuer's hands during compressions. If your hands are too high on the patient's chest, you may fracture the collarbones. If your hands are too low, you may cut the patient's liver with the xiphoid process. Should you place your hands too far to the right, you may fracture the patient's ribs and possibly cut into the right lung. Placing your hands too far to the left might fracture the patient's ribs and cut into the left lung and the heart. Careful location of the CPR compression site and proper hand positioning will help you avoid these problems.

1st There are cases where ribs are fractured even during properly performed CPR. **Do not stop CPR** in such cases. Obviously, the patient would rather have a few fractured ribs than be allowed to die.

Another problem can occur if air is forced into the patient's stomach when providing ventilations. *Do not* try to force this air out of the stomach. To do so might cause the patient to vomit, blocking the airway. If the patient tries to breathe, vomitus could be aspirated (inhaled). If you try to provide breaths, you will force the vomitus into the lungs. Always look for the patient's chest to rise as you deliver ventilations. Adjust the size of your breaths accordingly. This will help reduce the amount of air that may be forced into the patient's stomach. Should air enter the stomach, reposition the head and adjust the size of your ventilations.

Should the patient vomit, **stop CPR.** Take time to clear the patient's airway as best you can by repositioning the patient for drainage and using finger sweeps. After clearing the airway, resume CPR.

SPECIAL CPR SITUATIONS

Moving the Patient

Usually, the only reason a First Responder has for moving a patient who is receiving CPR is because of immediate danger at the scene. Most of the time, the patient is moved after the EMTs have arrived and assumed responsibility for his or her care. The technique is shown in Scansheet 5–3, in case you have to assist the EMTs with the move. In the majority of moves, you probably will be asked to help lift and carry the patient. Since the EMTs will be using special devices and oxygen to assist with the ventilations, you probably will not be asked to ventilate the patient. Under certain circumstances, you may be asked to provide compressions. Note that this is a two-rescuer CPR procedure, with compressions delivered at the rate of 80 to 100 per minute, with a ventilation provided after every fifth upstroke.

The Accident Scene

Many factors can complicate CPR when dealing with the victim of an accident. Severe injuries to the patient's face may interfere with your attempts to provide ventilations. Crushing injuries to the patient's chest may lessen the effectiveness of external chest compressions. Head, neck, and spinal injuries may dictate special patient handling.

Your first priority at any accident scene is your own safety. *Do not* risk your own life. *Do not* place yourself in a position where someone else will have to rescue you. If you are a firefighter or law enforcement officer, you have been taught how to carry out your duties in hazardous situations. You also have been told the limits to the risks that you should take as part of your job. If you have no formal training for the accident scene, you must proceed with great caution. More will be said in Chapters 17–19 regarding what you may expect to find at the scene of an accident and what will be expected of you as a First Responder.

Many rescuers are a little hesitant to start CPR on certain patients. When they find obvious spinal injuries, they often wish to delay CPR until they can immobilize the patient's spine. If rescuers find a patient with a crushed chest, fear of causing internal injuries prevents them from providing external chest compressions. Patient injuries should not delay your start of CPR. True, it is possible that your actions may increase the severity of the patient's injuries. However, if you delay CPR, the patient will die.

Properly positioning the patient is a major problem at the accident scene. CPR is not effective if the patient is in a seated position. Nor is CPR likely to be effective if the patient is on a soft surface, such as a car seat. Patients *must* be moved to hard surfaces and placed on their backs. While doing so, take into account the possibility of neck and spinal injury.

When moving an adult, cradle the head in your forearm and apply a firm grip to the jaw. When moving an infant or a child, always use one hand to support the head and neck of the patient. Again, for CPR to be effective, the patient must be lying face up on a hard surface.

If you are by yourself or working with people who do not know CPR and have to move the patient once CPR has begun, then do so. True, it is best not to move the patient, but the dangers of the accident scene may force you to do so. Try not to interrupt CPR for more than 15 to 30 seconds during a move. The total move may have to be done in several stages.

If your patient has possible neck and spinal injuries, you must start CPR as soon as possible. **Do not delay CPR** in order to stabilize the neck and spine. Use the jaw-thrust method for ventilations in order to reduce the chances of causing greater injury to the patient.

Moving CPR

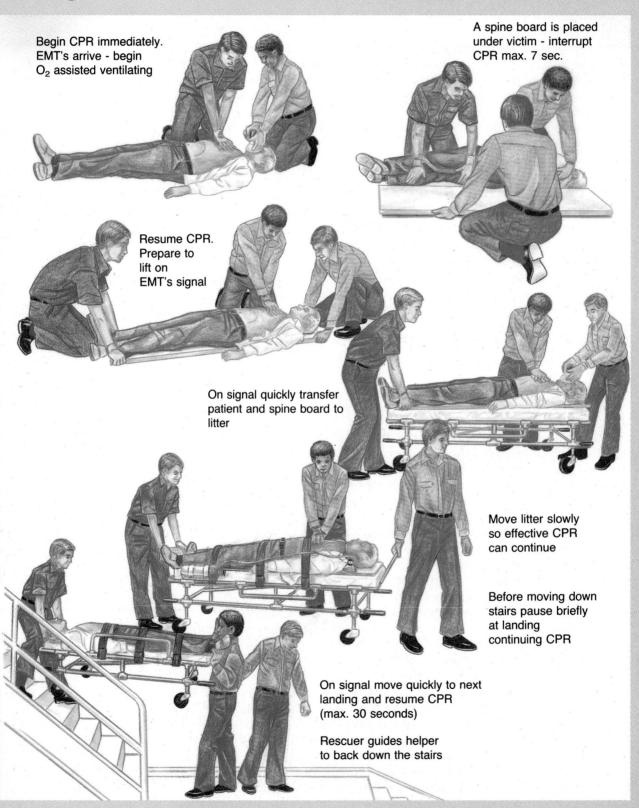

Begin CPR immediately. EMT's arrive - begin O$_2$ assisted ventilating

A spine board is placed under victim - interrupt CPR max. 7 sec.

Resume CPR. Prepare to lift on EMT's signal

On signal quickly transfer patient and spine board to litter

Move litter slowly so effective CPR can continue

Before moving down stairs pause briefly at landing continuing CPR

On signal move quickly to next landing and resume CPR (max. 30 seconds)

Rescuer guides helper to back down the stairs

Drowning

Rescuer safety and care procedures at the scene of a drowning or near drowning require special training in water rescue (see Chapter 20). In regard to CPR, you should begin as soon as possible. If you have been trained to do so, artificial ventilations should begin while the patient is still in the water. External chest compressions are not effective when the patient is in the water. Attempts to begin compressions while the patient is still in the water will only delay the removal of the patient from the water and the start of effective CPR.

NOTE: The American Red Cross is reevaluating the use of manual thrusts to expel water from the lungs of near-drowning victims. Follow your EMS System's guidelines.

Electric Shock

Some of the special problems of accident scenes involving electricity will be covered in Chapter 17. Your first priority is to avoid placing yourself in danger. Start artificial ventilations as soon as possible. CPR, when needed, is carried out the same way for the victim of electric shock as for any other patient in cardiac arrest.

CPR—RESPONSIBILITIES OF THE FIRST RESPONDER

As a First Responder, when dealing with cardiac arrest, your duty is to have someone alert dispatch and to **start CPR immediately.** Only a physician at the scene who has accepted responsibility for the patient may order you not to begin CPR. Bystanders and members of the patient's family may tell you that the patient would not want to be resuscitated. You are not to obey such requests. Even though the patient may have a terminal illness or may be very old, you are still to **provide CPR.** Without written directions confirmed by the patient's doctor or the EMS dispatcher, you have no way of knowing that this is what the patient would have you do.

The longer a patient has been in cardiac arrest before CPR is started, the less likely it is that CPR will be effective. However, there are documented cases of adults in cardiac arrest for over 10 minutes who have been resuscitated with no major brain damage. Children and infants usually can survive longer periods of time in cardiac arrest than can adults. Do not refuse to begin CPR simply because someone has been in cardiac arrest for 10 minutes. In most cases, if the patient has been in cardiac arrest for more than 10 minutes, CPR will probably not be effective. *However,* the moment the patient was seen to collapse and the moment of cardiac arrest are usually not the same. A patient may be unconscious with minimum lung and heart function for quite some time before actual cardiac arrest occurs. Set aside any doubts and **start CPR immediately.**

Cold-water drowning victims can be successfully resuscitated after long periods of cardiac arrest. There are documented cases of arrest that has lasted over 45 minutes before successful resuscitation (see Chapter 20). The same is true of people who have had their body temperatures lowered by cold (hypothermia). Resuscitation must be done for these individuals. The emergency department staff will continue resuscitation while they rewarm the patient's body. They will not declare biological death until the patient is rewarmed and all efforts to revive the patient have failed.

1st Once you have started, continue to provide CPR until:

- Spontaneous circulation begins; then provide artificial ventilations
- Spontaneous circulation and breathing begin

- An equally or more highly trained member of the EMS System or someone certified in CPR can take over for you
- You turn over the responsibility for the care of the patient to a physician
- You are exhausted and no longer able to continue

Many rescuers fear having to stop CPR when they are exhausted. You must be realistic about this problem. Should you reach such a point, realize that you have done all that you could to help the patient. It is not your fault that the EMS System could do no more for the patient. There will always be cases where a patient is too far away from the type of help required. CPR has its physical limitations on the performer. It also has its physical limitations on the patient. If, for example, you have provided CPR on a patient for 30 minutes to an hour, then realize that there is little hope for the patient at this point. This would be true even if a team of cardiac physicians arrived at the scene, bringing with them all the equipment modern medicine has to offer. You should not feel guilty if you cannot continue CPR.

If you wish to reduce the chances that you will have to stop CPR, then you should:

1. Keep yourself in good physical condition. Do exercises that will improve your heart and lung functions.
2. Become a CPR or basic cardiac life-support instructor. Help the AHA and American Red Cross in their efforts to train all citizens in basic cardiac life support. This will improve the chances of a bystander being able to assist you in providing CPR.
3. Support your local EMS System so that they may have the personnel and equipment needed to reach all victims in your area.
4. Practice what you have learned about CPR. Your instructor can tell you how you can review CPR, keep yourself up-to-date, and have access to manikins for practice.

Two factors, both possible to correct, could place you in a position where you will not be able to save a patient by using CPR. Rescuer hyperventilation is one such factor. Because of the irregular pattern of breathing established by performing CPR, you may start to breathe very deeply and very rapidly. This can prevent you from delivering ventilations and may even cause you to faint. Usually, someone in good physical shape will not hyperventilate during CPR. Many rescuers bring on hyperventilation by trying to breathe with each compression. During compressions, try to maintain a normal breathing rate. The practice with the manikins provided for your course will help you learn how to properly pace yourself.

If you are becoming exhausted and know that you will not be able to provide ventilations, look for help from bystanders. Even if they are not trained in CPR, you may be able to tell them what they should do to provide ventilations while you continue compressions. This is certainly better than stopping CPR.

The other factor that could lead to CPR being stopped is the inability to get help. In some cases, you may begin CPR knowing that only the best of luck will bring someone to the scene to help you. In most cases, bystanders or individuals near to the scene can go phone for help. (Remember that part of the procedures you have learned require you to call out for help.) As a First Responder, you should always have the EMS System dispatcher alerted so that other rescuers can respond to the scene.

If there is no one on hand to call dispatch, and there is little hope that someone will come along, you must try to call for EMS assistance. *Do not delay CPR* to phone for help. Provide CPR for 1 minute and then, if a phone is close by, quickly go and place the call.

SUMMARY

When someone stops breathing and the heart stops beating, **clinical death** results. Within 4 to 6 minutes, lethal changes take place in the brain. Within 10 minutes, **biological death** may occur when the brain cells start to die.

There is a strong relationship between breathing, circulation, and certain brain activity. When the heart stops beating, a patient is in **cardiac arrest** and will be unresponsive. The major signs of cardiac arrest are **no breathing** and **no carotid pulse.**

You should determine breathing by the **look, listen, and feel method.** Circulation is determined by feeling for a **carotid pulse.** If the patient is an infant (under 1 year of age), then feel for a **brachial pulse.**

If a patient is in cardiac arrest, you should take the **ABC** approach: **A** = Airway, **B** = Breathing and **C** = Circulation. After establishing that the patient is unresponsive, and after calling out for help, you should:

1. Correctly position the patient and open the airway. Take great care not to overextend the head tilt for infants.
2. Determine that the patient is not breathing.
3. Provide two adequate breaths (clear the airway if necessary).
4. Determine that there is no pulse.
5. Have someone phone the EMS dispatcher.
6. Find the CPR compression site:

   Adult—superior to the index finger of the hand used to locate the notch where the breastbone and ribs meet

   Child—along the midline of the breastbone, located in the same way that was done for an adult

   Infant—along the midline of the breastbone, one finger-width below an imaginary line drawn between the nipples
7. Correctly position your hands for compressions:

   Adult—The heel of your hand closest to the patient's head is placed on the CPR compression site. Your other hand is placed on top of this hand so that the heels of both hands are parallel and your fingers are pointing away from your body. Your fingers can be extended or interlaced. **Keep your fingers off the patient's chest.**

   Child—Deliver compressions with the **heel of one hand,** positioned over the child's CPR compression site.

   Infant—Deliver compressions with the **tips of two or three fingers,** positioned over the infant's CPR compression site.
8. Provide external chest compressions:

Adult—Depth	=	1½ to 2 inches
Rate	=	80 to 100/minute
Child—Depth	=	1 to 1½ inches
Rate	=	80 to 100/minute
Infant—Depth	=	½ to 1 inch
Rate	=	at least 100/minute

9. Provide ventilations:
   Adult—2 breaths every 15 compressions
   Child—1 breath every 5 compressions
   Infant—1 breath every 5 compressions

10. Check for a carotid pulse after 1 minute of CPR. Use the brachial pulse if the patient is an infant.

No pulse, no breathing—continue CPR, checking for a pulse every few minutes.

Pulse, but no breathing—stop compressions and provide artificial ventilations. Continue to monitor pulse every few minutes.

NOTE: The patient will not be breathing unless there is heart action.

You should not stop CPR for more than **7 seconds,** other than to move the patient because of danger at your location. If you have to move the patient, do not stop CPR for more than 15 to 30 seconds. Continue CPR until heart or heart and lung functions start, until you are relieved by an equally or more highly trained person, care for the patient is accepted by a physician, or until you can no longer continue due to exhaustion.

When a patient is in cardiac arrest, **start CPR immediately,** even if you may worsen existing injuries. Without CPR, the patient will quickly go from clinical death to biological death.

CHAPTER 6

Two-Rescuer CPR

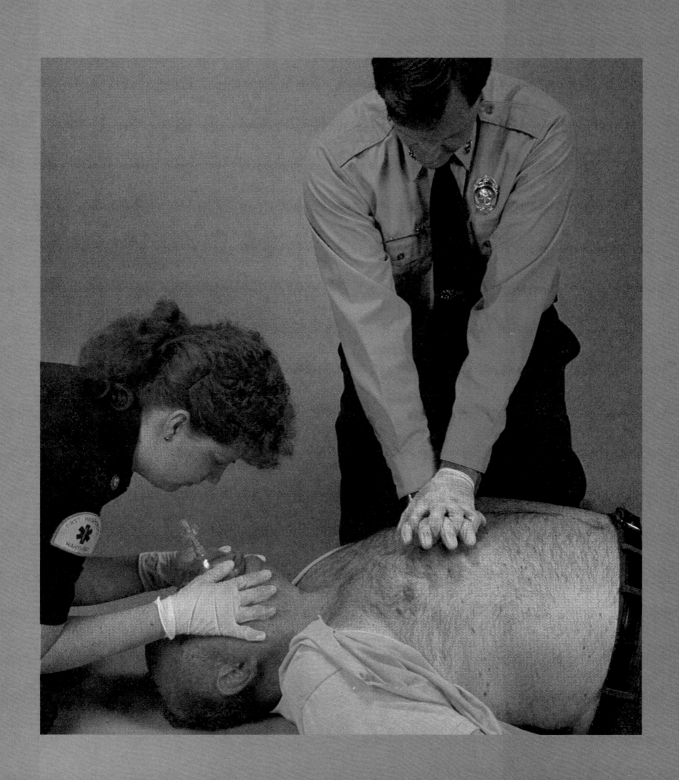

■ OBJECTIVES

By the end of this chapter, you should be able to:

1. State the advantages of two-rescuer CPR over one-rescuer CPR. (p. 146)
2. State the qualifications needed of volunteers wishing to help a First Responder in performing two-rescuer CPR. (p. 146)
3. Cite the rate of compressions and the rate of ventilations used when providing two-rescuer CPR. (p. 147)
4. List, step by step, the sequence of procedures for two-rescuer CPR. (pp. 147–149)
5. State how often you should check for a carotid pulse when providing two-rescuer CPR. (p. 149)
6. State how long compressions may be interrupted when checking for breathing and a carotid pulse. (p. 149)
7. List, step by step, the sequence of procedures for changing positions during two-rescuer CPR. (pp. 149–151)
8. State what you should do if you miss providing a ventilation to a patient during two-rescuer CPR. (p. 150)

SKILLS

Upon completing this chapter and your class lectures and skills labs, you should be able to:

1. Correctly perform two-rescuer CPR on an adult manikin, including at least two changes of position.
2. Repeat the skills demonstrated in two-rescuer CPR, but with a different partner.

INTRODUCTION

Two-rescuer cardiopulmonary resuscitation, if performed correctly, is a more efficient procedure than one-rescuer CPR. The patient receives more oxygen, chest compressions are not interrupted for as long, the rate of compressions allows for better filling of the heart, and the problem of rescuer fatigue is lessened.

1st When you are working with another member of the EMS System, there should be no major problems in the two of you performing CPR. You should both have the same training. However, as a First Responder, you will often have to care for patients without another member of the EMS System present. If a bystander has been trained by the American Heart Association or the American Red Cross to do two-rescuer CPR, then you can begin two-rescuer CPR. Make sure that the person wishing to help has been certified in two-rescuer CPR. Too many people have seen the procedure used on television and think they know the correct procedure without the benefit of training. Should you begin two-rescuer CPR and find that the volunteer is not able to perform correctly, *stop* the procedure and return to one-rescuer CPR. Since two-rescuer CPR has not been a part of the AHA citizen certification for a number of years, you may find that your helper is not up to date on CPR techniques. Also, it is unlikely that your helper will know how to use a pocket face mask. Quickly explain the risks of mouth-to-mouth ventilation.

1st CHANGING TO TWO-RESCUER CPR

NOTE: If someone arrives at the scene where you are performing CPR and dispatch has not been called, the first priority is to have that person call the dispatcher.

In many cases, one-rescuer CPR is initiated before a second trained rescuer arrives at the scene. To make a smooth transition from one-rescuer CPR to two-rescuer CPR, the following should be done when you arrive to help someone who is not a member of the EMS System:

1. The first rescuer is performing one-rescuer CPR. The second rescuer arrives and identifies himself or herself as a trained rescuer (or someone who is certified in CPR or basic life support).
2. The first rescuer, while continuing CPR, accepts the help.
3. The first rescuer continues one-rescuer CPR. The second rescuer must confirm that the patient is in cardiac arrest. He or she begins by checking for the pulse generated in the carotid artery each time the first rescuer provides a compression. Next, the second rescuer says, "Stop compressions." The first rescuer stops providing compressions. The second rescuer takes 5 seconds to simultaneously check for both respiration and pulse.
4. If there is no pulse, the second rescuer provides one interposed ventilation and says, "No pulse, continue CPR." If there is a pulse but no breathing, the second rescuer begins pulmonary resuscitation.
5. If CPR is continued, the first rescuer begins compressions at the rate of 80 to 100 per minute. The second rescuer will provide one ventilation at the rate of one breath every five compressions.

If you wish to join another member of the EMS System who is performing CPR, you should:

1. Ask to help.
2. Allow the first rescuer to complete a cycle of *15 compressions* and *2 ventilations.*
3. Take over as the compressor and allow the first rescuer to become the ventilator.

COMPRESSIONS AND VENTILATIONS

During two-rescuer CPR, the rate of compressions is five compressions every 3 to 4 seconds. Ventilations are delivered at *one every five compressions* to provide a rate of 12 per minute.

1st • *Compressions*: a rate of 80 to 100 per minute to actually deliver at least 60 per minute
1st • *Ventilations*: 12 per minute

The rescuer providing compressions will count out loud so that both rescuers will be able to establish and maintain the correct rates. The other rescuer will interpose a breath after every fifth compression using the mouth-to-mask technique, with the compressor pausing to allow for adequate ventilation. The count of 1 through 5 is repeated over and over again, as long as two-rescuer CPR is being provided for the patient.

CPR Procedure

1st Scansheet 6.1 outlines the complete sequence for two-rescuer CPR. Note that one rescuer will be called the ventilator and the other rescuer will be called the compressor. Both rescuers are shown on the same side of the

■ SCAN 6-1.

Two-rescuer CPR

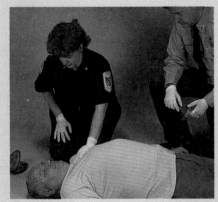

1 Determine unresponsiveness. Reposition patient.

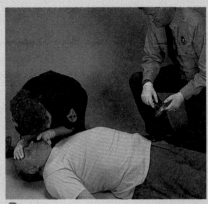

2 Open the airway and look, listen and feel for 3–5 seconds.

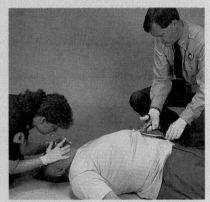

3 Ventilate twice (1–1.5 seconds per ventilation).

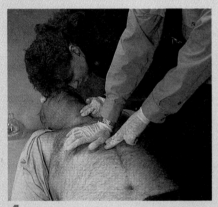

4 Determine pulselessness. Locate CPR compression site.

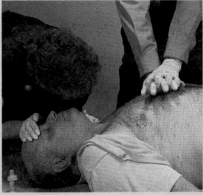

5 Say "No pulse." Begin compressions.

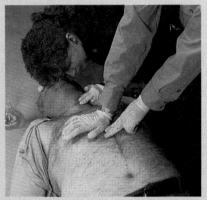

6 Check compression effectiveness. Deliver five compressions in 3–4 seconds. Rate = 80–100/minute.

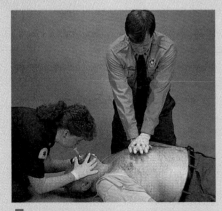

7 Ventilate once (1–1.5 seconds per ventilation). Stop for ventilation mouth to mask.

8 Continue with one ventilation every five compressions.

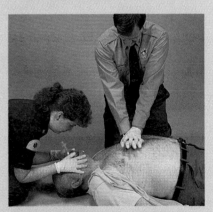

9 After ten cycles, reassess breathing and pulse. No pulse—ventilate and say "Continue CPR." Pulse—say, "Stop CPR."

NOTE: Assess for spontaneous breathing and pulse for 5 seconds at the end of the first minute, then every few minutes thereafter.

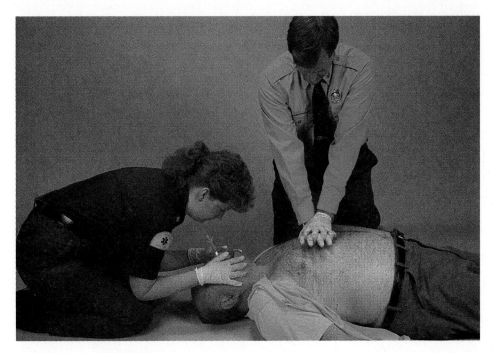

FIGURE 6–1. Positioning in two-rescuer CPR.

patient for teaching purposes. In actual two-rescuer CPR, the rescuers should place themselves on opposite sides of the patient. If a pocket face mask is being used, the ventilator may have to be positioned at the top of the patient's head.

The ventilator should frequently check for a pulse generated with each compression. If this pulse cannot be found, he or she should alert the compressor to check hand positioning and increase the force of compressions.

The ventilator constantly checks for spontaneous breathing. After 1 minute of two-rescuer CPR, the ventilator should stop CPR, take 5 seconds to simultaneously determine if there is breathing and a pulse, and then take appropriate action:

- Pulse, no breathing—provide pulmonary resuscitation.
- No pulse, no breathing—provide an interposed ventilation and say, "No pulse, continue CPR."
- Pulse and breathing—say, "Stop CPR." Both rescuers should monitor the patient.

If CPR is continued, the ventilator should check for spontaneous breathing and pulse every few minutes. This interruption should last for no more than 7 seconds.

Changing Positions

1st A change in position may be requested if either rescuer feels fatigued. Usually, it is the compressor who needs the break. In most cases, unless the ventilator finds that the compressor cannot generate a pulse during compression, the compressor should decide when a change in positions will take place. The ventilator is notified at the beginning of a compression cycle. The compressor will give a clear signal to change and complete a set of five compressions. At this point, the ventilator will provide one ventilation and the two rescuers will quickly change positions.

NOTE: Each rescuer must use his or her own pocket face mask with one-way valve.

It is best to do respiration and carotid pulse checks at the time of position change. The compressor, in moving into the ventilator position, can do both of these checks simultaneously for 5 seconds.

Problems

When two people begin to perform two-rescuer CPR, there are always some adjustments that must be made in terms of changing positions. Each person performs the change a little differently from the next person. For this reason, you should practice two-rescuer CPR with several different fellow students.

There is only 1 to 1.5 seconds for the ventilator to interpose a breath. Resistance from the patient's airway, fatigue, and many other factors can cause the ventilator to miss providing the breath to the patient. Whenever you miss a breath, do *not* wait another five compressions. Try to interpose this ventilation before the next set of compressions.

SUMMARY

In two-rescuer CPR:

- Compressions = 5 per 3 to 4 seconds
- Provide 1 ventilation every 5 compressions = 12 per minute
- The ventilator monitors the carotid pulse to check the effectiveness of the compressions.
- The compressor counts out loud the 1 to 5 cycles.
- The compressor signals the change of position.
- Check for breathing and carotid pulse every few minutes. This is best done by the new ventilator when changing positions.
- Do not interrupt CPR for more than 7 seconds.
- If you miss a breath, interpose a ventilation before the next set of compressions.

■ SCAN 6-2.

Changing Positions

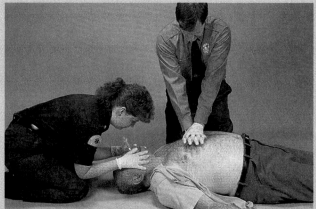

1 When fatigued, the compressor calls for the switch. Give a clear signal to change.

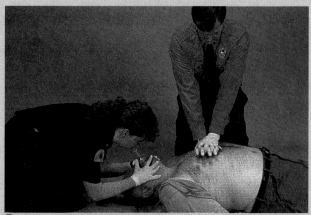

2 Compressor completes fifth compression. Ventilator provides one ventilation.

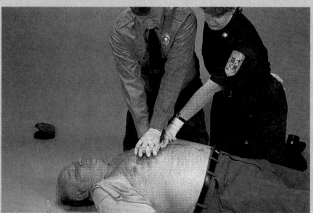

3 Ventilator moves to chest and begins to locate compression site. Compressor begins move to head.

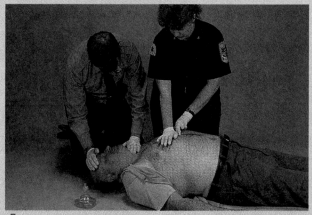

4 New compressor finds site. New ventilator checks carotid pulse (5 seconds).

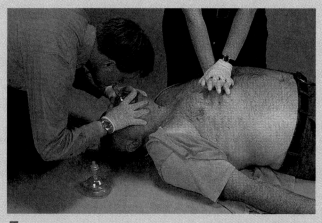

5 New ventilator says, "No pulse" and ventilates once (1–5 seconds).

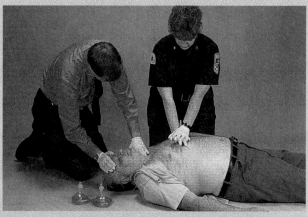

6 New compressor delivers five compressions (3–4 seconds) at a rate of 80–100 per minute. New ventilator assesses compressions.

■ SCAN 6-3.

CPR Summary

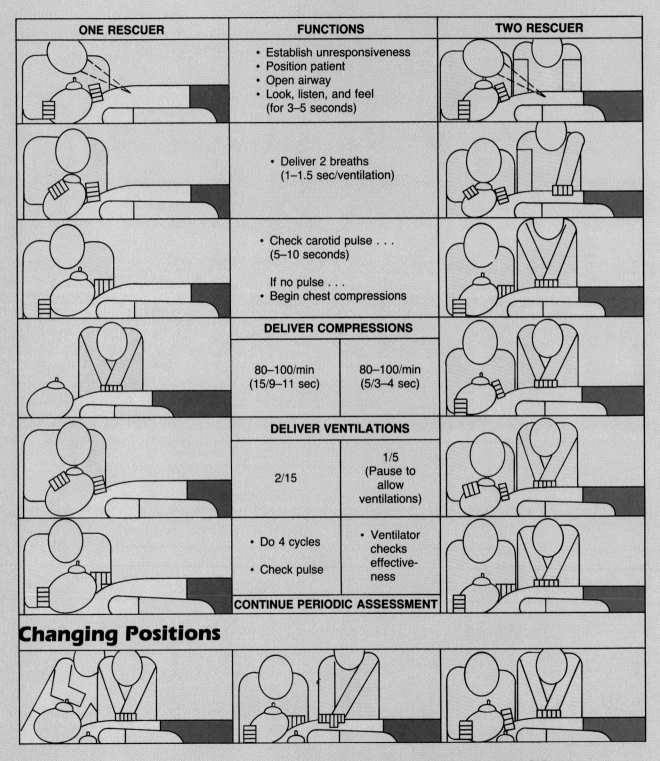

ONE RESCUER	FUNCTIONS		TWO RESCUER
	• Establish unresponsiveness • Position patient • Open airway • Look, listen, and feel (for 3–5 seconds)		
	• Deliver 2 breaths (1–1.5 sec/ventilation)		
	• Check carotid pulse . . . (5–10 seconds) If no pulse . . . • Begin chest compressions		
	DELIVER COMPRESSIONS		
	80–100/min (15/9–11 sec)	80–100/min (5/3–4 sec)	
	DELIVER VENTILATIONS		
	2/15	1/5 (Pause to allow ventilations)	
	• Do 4 cycles • Check pulse	• Ventilator checks effective-ness	
	CONTINUE PERIODIC ASSESSMENT		

Changing Positions

• Compressor: Signal to change; provide 5 compressions
• Ventilator: One ventilation

New ventilator checks pulse provides 1 ventilation

Continue CPR sequence

NOTE: Wear latex or vinyl gloves. Each rescuer should have his or her own pocket face mask with one-way valve.

CHAPTER 7

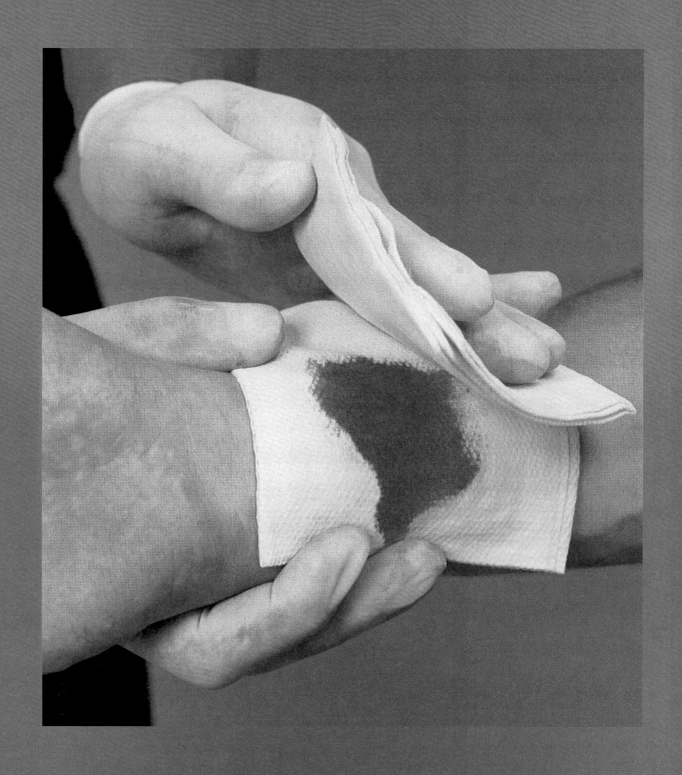

◼ OBJECTIVES

By the end of this chapter, you should be able to:

1. List the five major functions of blood. (p. 155)
2. List and define the three major types of blood vessels. (p. 156)
3. Define and describe arterial, venous, and capillary bleeding. (p. 156)
4. Classify bleeding as external or internal. (pp. 157–158, 167–169)
5. Relate profuse bleeding to First Responder actions during the primary survey. (pp. 157–158)
6. List the four methods used to control external bleeding, stating which method is most commonly used by First Responders. (p. 158)
7. Compare and contrast the methods used in direct pressure control of profuse bleeding to the methods used in direct pressure control of mild bleeding. (pp. 158–159)
8. Describe how to apply a pressure dressing. (p. 160)
9. Describe the use of elevation in controlling external bleeding, including the situations when elevation should not be used. (p. 161)
10. Define arterial pressure point and name the two major pressure point sites used by First Responders (pp. 161–162)
11. Describe, step by step, the pressure point procedures used to control bleeding from the arm. (p. 162)
12. Describe, step by step, the pressure point procedures used to control bleeding from the leg. (pp. 162–163)
13. State why tourniquets are used as a last resort, only after other methods to control bleeding have failed. (p. 164)
14. Describe, step by step, the procedures for applying a tourniquet, including all precautions for the procedure. (pp. 164–165)
15. List four factors that may cause difficulties when trying to detect internal bleeding. (pp. 166, 168)
16. List 10 conditions associated with internal bleeding. (p. 168)
17. Describe, step by step, First Responder procedures for controlling internal bleeding. (pp. 170–171)
18. Define shock. (p. 172)
19. List the symptoms and signs of shock. (p. 175)
20. Describe, step by step, the procedures used to care for shock. (pp. 176, 178)
21. Describe allergy shock (anaphylactic shock) in terms of what it is, how serious it is, what causes it, and what its signs are. (pp. 179–180)
22. Relate First Responder care for allergy shock to First Responder care for other types of shock. (p. 180)
23. Describe how to reduce a patient's chances of fainting. (p. 180)

SKILLS

Upon completing this chapter and your class lectures and skills labs, you should be able to demonstrate how to:

1. Control external bleeding by using direct pressure techniques, including the pressure dressing.
2. Control external bleeding by using direct pressure and elevation.
3. Control external bleeding by arterial pressure point techniques for bleeding from the arm and leg.
4. Correctly apply a tourniquet.
5. Survey for internal bleeding and apply the procedures needed to help control internal bleeding.

6. Survey for shock and allergy shock (anaphylactic shock) and utilize the procedures for caring for shock.
7. Carry out the procedure used to help prevent fainting.

REMEMBER: All care procedures should be done with rescuer safety being ensured. Avoid direct contact with the patient's blood, body fluids, and wastes.

THE BLOOD

The importance of blood has been stressed throughout your life. Blood carries oxygen to the body's cells and carries away carbon dioxide. It transports food to the cells and carries away certain waste products. The blood contains cells that destroy bacteria and cells that produce substances to help you resist infection (immunity). Compounds carried in the blood called hormones regulate most body activities. Without blood circulating through your body, you would quickly die.

1st The functions of blood are:

- **Respiration**—to carry oxygen and carbon dioxide.
- **Nutrition**—to carry food to the tissues.
- **Excretion**—to carry wastes from the tissues to the organs of excretion (kidneys, lungs, and skin).
- **Body regulation**—to carry hormones, water, salts, and other compounds needed to keep the body's functions in balance.
- **Defense**—to protect against disease-causing organisms.

Blood contains red blood cells, white blood cells, and elements involved in forming blood clots. All of these are carried by a watery, salty fluid called **plasma.**

The volume of blood in the typical adult's body is approximately 6 liters (about 12 pints). When bleeding occurs, the body not only loses blood cells and clotting elements, it also loses plasma and total blood volume. The loss of volume can be very significant since the volume of blood must be maintained at a certain level to have proper heart action, blood flow, and exchange between the blood and the body's cells. The body has more blood than is needed to produce minimum circulation. During bleeding, once this reserve is gone, the patient experiences circulatory system collapse, followed very quickly by death.

1st REMEMBER: The typical adult has 6 liters (12 pints) of blood. This volume must be maintained for proper circulatory function to take place.

TABLE 7–1 BLOOD VOLUMES AND SERIOUS BLOOD LOSS

Patient	Total Blood Volume	Lethal Blood Loss (rapid)
Adult male (154 pounds)	6.6 liters	2.2 liters
Adolescent (105 pounds)	3.3 liters	1.3 liters
Child (early to late childhood; depends on size)	1.5 to 2.0 liters	0.5 to 0.7 liters
Infant (newborn, normal weight range)	300+ milliliters	30 to 50 milliliters

Note: One liter equals about 2 pints. One milliliter is about the same as 20 drops from a medicine dropper.

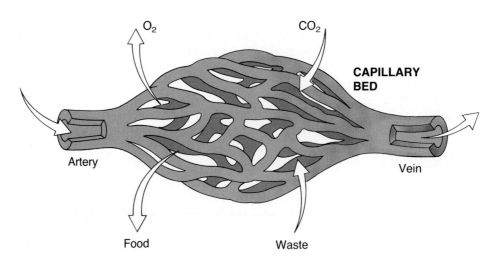

FIGURE 7–1. Blood vessels.

BLOOD VESSELS

Artery—any blood vessel that carries blood away from the heart.

Capillary—the microscopic blood vessels that connect arteries to veins. Where exchange takes place between the bloodstream and the body tissues.

Vein—any blood vessel that returns blood to the heart.

Perfusion—the constant flow of blood through the capillaries.

Blood is carried away from the heart in **arteries.** Exchange with the body's cells takes place through the thin walls of the **capillaries.** Blood is then returned to the heart by way of *veins.* The heart's beating action has the most influence on the arteries. Blood in the arteries is under greater pressure and travels faster than the blood in veins and capillaries. By the time blood reaches the capillaries, pressure and speed are greatly reduced and the beating action of the heart no longer causes pulsations. Blood moves through the capillaries in a constant flow called **perfusion.** (A reduction in blood volume can seriously affect perfusion.) Blood leaves the capillaries and is carried by veins leading to the heart. Both pressure and velocity in the veins are reduced in comparison to the arteries.

1st For now, you should know:

- Arteries—carry blood from the heart
- Capillaries—where exchange takes place
- Veins—return blood to the heart

TYPES OF BLEEDING

Bleeding can be **external** or **internal.** Both kinds of bleeding can be classified as to the type of blood vessel involved. Since a discussion of the vessels involved in internal bleeding is not very practical for First Responders, only external bleeding will be considered in relation to blood vessel type. Both kinds of bleeding will be presented in terms of assessment and care.

1st External bleeding may be classified by the First Responder as:

- Arterial Bleeding—Blood is flowing from an artery. The color of the blood is bright red. The flow from the wound is in spurts, often pulsating as the heart beats. Blood loss is rapid and extensive (profuse).
- Venous bleeding—Blood is flowing from a vein. The color of the blood is dark red, often so dark in color that it appears to be a deep maroon. The flow is steady, without the spurts seen in arterial bleeding. Venous bleeding can also be profuse.
- Capillary bleeding—Blood is oozing from a bed of capillaries. The color of the blood is red, usually less bright than arterial blood. The flow is slow, as seen in minor scrapes and shallow cuts to the skin.

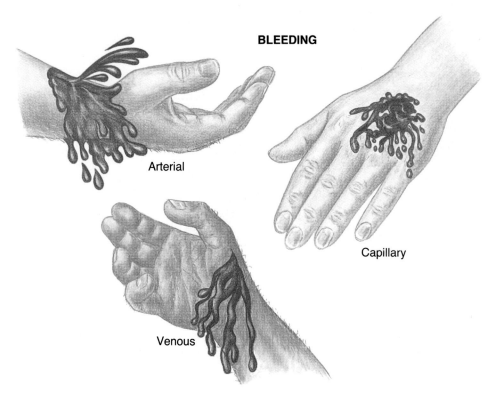

BLEEDING

Arterial

Capillary

Venous

FIGURE 7–2. Types of external bleeding.

EXTERNAL BLEEDING

Evaluating External Bleeding

Of the three types of external bleeding, arterial bleeding is the most serious. The loss of blood is quite rapid. The action of the heart and the pressure in the arteries prevent blood clot formation due to the rapid, pressurized flow. The thickness of artery walls creates problems in stopping the flow of blood. Sometimes the end of a completely severed artery will collapse and seal off the flow. More often, this collapse is not complete and the flow remains profuse. Since arteries are located deep within body structures, capillary and venous bleeding are seen more often than arterial bleeding.

Venous bleeding can range from very minor to very severe, leading to death within minutes. Some veins are located near the body surface. Many of these are large enough to be seen through the skin. Other veins are deep in the body and can be as large as arteries. Bleeding from a deep vein will produce rapid blood loss. Surface vein bleeding can be profuse, but the blood loss is not as rapid as that seen from arteries and deep veins because of the smaller vessel diameter. Veins have a tendency to collapse as soon as they are cut. This often reduces the severity of venous bleeding.

An additional problem is seen with venous bleeding that is usually not associated with arterial bleeding. Air bubbles may be sucked into open veins and carried to the heart. This situation can cause cardiac arrest. The greatest potential problem is with the large neck veins.

Most individuals experience little difficulty with capillary bleeding. The blood flow is slow and clotting is very likely to occur within 6 to 8 minutes. The larger the area of the wound, the more likely the chance of infection. Capillary bleeding requires care to stop blood flow and reduce contamination.

1st Finding and stopping profuse bleeding is part of the primary survey.

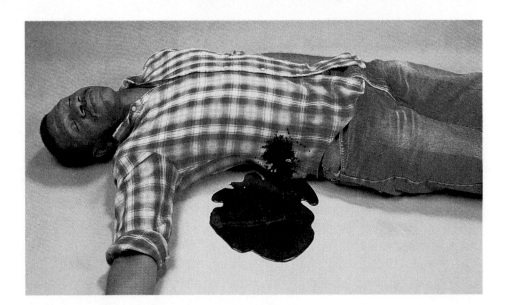

FIGURE 7–3. Estimating external blood loss; one-half liter (approximately 1 pint).

Arterial and large vein bleeding are given priority over small vein and capillary bleeding. If bleeding is deemed so severe as to be an immediate threat to life, control of the bleeding will have to begin while you are noting signs of breathing. Even though it may prove awkward, a First Responder can be faced with the task of stopping severe bleeding while, at the same time, evaluating airway and pulse.

Determining blood loss due to external bleeding requires some experience. The ability to make such a determination is of value to the First Responder in cases where slow bleeding has been occurring for a long time or in cases where both internal and external bleeding are present. A bleeding rate that normally could wait until after the secondary survey may be life-threatening because the patient has lost a large quantity of blood. To help yourself establish a feeling for blood volume lost, pour a pint of water on the floor next to a fellow student or a manikin. Try soaking an article of clothing with a pint of water and then note how much of the article is wet and how wet it feels.

Controlling External Bleeding

NOTE: In the following discussion, a dressing is the material placed over a wound and a bandage is the material that holds a dressing in place.
1st Four major procedures can be used by First Responders to control external bleeding:

1. Direct pressure
2. Elevation (used with direct pressure)
3. Pressure points
4. Applying a tourniquet

WARNING: Regardless of the method used to control bleeding, you *must* wear latex or vinyl gloves to avoid direct contact with the patient's blood.

Direct pressure—the quickest, most effective way to control most forms of external bleeding. Pressure is applied directly over the wound site.

1st *Direct Pressure*
Most cases of external bleeding can be controlled by applying direct pressure to the site of the wound. Ideally, a sterile dressing should be used. However, hunting in your pocket for a sterile dressing pack, going back to your

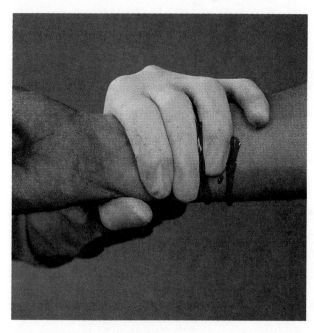

FIGURE 7–4. *In cases of profuse bleeding, do not waste time hunting for a dressing.*

car, going to a kit found in the next room, and other such activities are a waste of precious time. Always put on latex or vinyl gloves, but **do not let a patient bleed while you hunt for a dressing.**

In cases of profuse bleeding, as found during the primary survey, you should:

1. Not waste time hunting for a dressing.
2. Place your gloved hand directly over the wound and apply pressure.
3. Keep applying steady, firm pressure.
   In cases where the bleeding is mild or well controlled, you should:

1. Apply firm pressure using a sterile dressing or clean cloth. (You may have to use a clean handkerchief.)
2. Apply pressure until bleeding is controlled. In some cases, this may take 10 minutes, 30 minutes, or longer.
3. Hold the dressing in place with bandages only after you are certain that the bleeding is controlled.
4. *Never* remove or attempt to replace any dressing once it is in place. To do so may restart bleeding or cause additional injury to the wound site. If a dressing becomes soaked with blood, place another dressing directly over the blood-soaked one and hold both in place with firm pressure.

FIGURE 7–5. *Apply direct pressure with a dressing.*

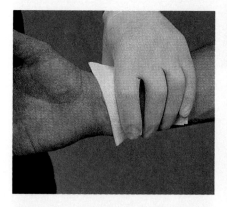
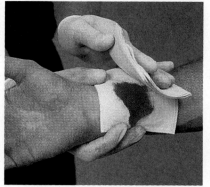
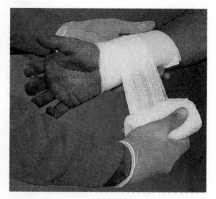

APPLY PRESSURE WITH DRESSING

APPLY ADDITIONAL DRESSING IF NECESSARY

BANDAGE WOUND

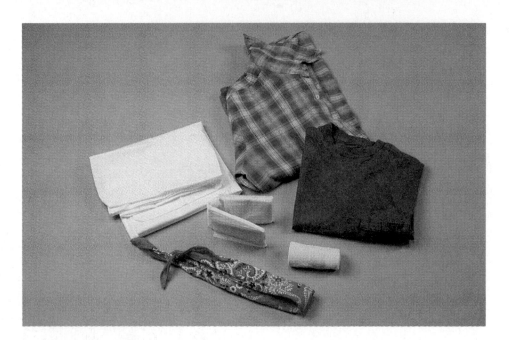

FIGURE 7–6. Dressings for use in emergencies.

A variety of dressings may be used in emergency situations. Some of these are shown in Figure 7–6. More will be said about dressings and bandages in Chapter 9.

Most bleeding can be controlled by a special form of direct pressure, the *pressure dressing*. To apply a pressure dressing, you need to:

1. Place several sterile gauze dressing pads directly on the wound and maintain pressure with your gloved hand.
2. Set a bulky dressing pad (multitrauma or universal dressing, sanitary napkin, or several handkerchiefs) over the gauze dressing pads. Continue to apply hand pressure.
3. Use self-adherent roller bandage to hold the entire dressing in place. It should be wrapped over the dressing and above and below the wound.
4. Wrap the bandage to produce enough pressure to control the bleeding.
5. Check for a distal pulse to be certain that the pressure has not restricted blood flow.

FIGURE 7–7. The pressure dressing. A bulky pad dressing is placed over the dressing pads. Roller bandage holds the dressings and is used to apply pressure.

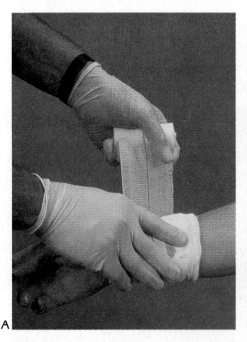

A

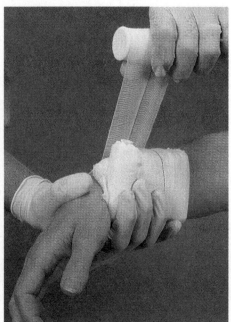

B

Once a pressure dressing is applied, it should not be removed. Should bleeding continue, you can add more pressure by using the palm of your gloved hand, apply more dressing pads, and continue the process of bandaging (do not remove the bandage to add more pads), or apply more bandage to increase the pressure. In very few cases (amputations and severe tearing injuries) will you have to create more bulk by adding additional dressings.

If you use your gloved hand or a dressing to apply direct pressure, you can apply a pressure dressing once the bleeding is controlled. If you are dealing with bleeding from an armpit, the abdominal wall, a large artery, or a deep vein, attempting to apply a pressure dressing may not be of any real use. Your best approach to such situations is to maintain pressure using your gloved hand and a dressing.

1st REMEMBER: Direct pressure is the quickest, most effective way to control bleeding.

1st Elevation

Elevation may be used in combination with direct pressure when dealing with bleeding from the arm or leg. The effects of gravity will help reduce blood pressure and slow the bleeding. This method should not be used if there are possible fractures to the extremities, objects are impaled in the extremities, or there is possible spinal injury. To use elevation, you should:

- Elevate the injured extremity. When practical, raise the extremity so that the wound is above the level of the heart. If the forearm is bleeding, you do not have to elevate the entire arm. Simply elevate the forearm.
- Continue to apply direct pressure to the site of bleeding as explained earlier in this chapter.

1st Pressure Points

Pressure points are sites where an artery, close to the body surface, lies directly over a bone. The flow of blood through such an artery can be inter-

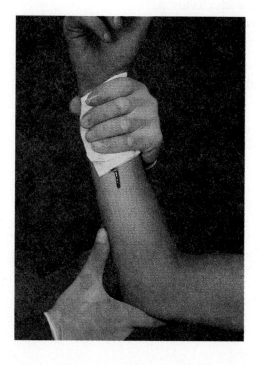

FIGURE 7–8. Combine elevation and direct pressure.

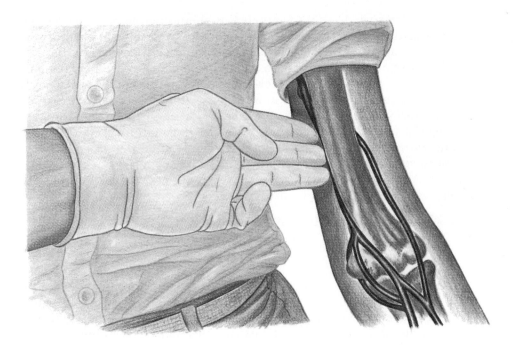

FIGURE 7–9. Using pressure points can stop profuse bleeding for an arm or leg.

rupted if pressure is applied to compress the artery. This procedure should be employed only after direct pressure or direct pressure with elevation has failed to control the bleeding.

There are 22 major pressure point sites used to control bleeding. They occur at 11 sites on each side of the body. Only the upper arm and thigh are commonly part of First Responder training. These pressure point sites are the:

Brachial (BRAY-ke-al) artery pressure point—the pressure point in the upper arm that can be used to help control serious external bleeding from the upper limb.

Femoral (FEM-o-ral) artery pressure point—the pressure point in the thigh that can be used to help control serious external bleeding from the lower limb.

- **1st** Upper arm—the brachial (BRAY-ke-al) artery pressure point for controlling bleeding from the arm.
- **1st** Thigh—the femoral (FEM-o-ral) pressure point for controlling bleeding from the leg.

1st For bleeding from the arm, you should:

1. Apply direct pressure.
2. If this fails, apply direct pressure with elevation.
3. Should this fail, extend the patient's arm, placing it at a right angle, lateral to the body. This angle will provide the best results, but may be reduced if a 90-degree extension is not possible. The palm of the patient's hand should be in the anatomical position.
4. Cradle the patient's upper arm in the palm of your gloved hand and position your fingers in the medial groove found below the biceps muscle. (See Figure 7–10).
5. Apply pressure to the brachial artery by pressing your fingers into this groove. Bleeding should stop and you should no longer be able to feel a radial (wrist) pulse.

1st For bleeding from the leg, you should:

1. Apply direct pressure.
2. If this fails, apply direct pressure with elevation.
3. Should this fail, locate the anterior, medial side of the leg where the thigh joins the lower trunk. The femoral artery has a pulse that can be felt at this location.
4. Use the heel of your gloved hand to apply pressure to this site. Keep your arm straight, using your body weight to help apply the pressure. The number of leg muscles, their size, and the fat content of the thigh

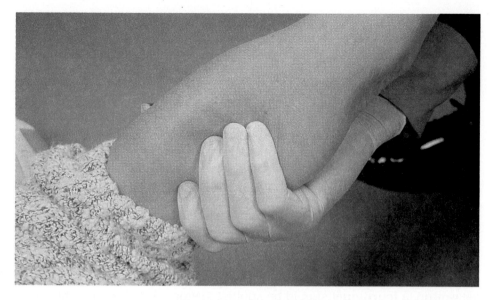

FIGURE 7–10. Apply pressure to the brachial artery pressure point to control bleeding from the arm.

will require you to exert much more pressure than you would use to compress the brachial artery in the arm.

5. Apply the necessary pressure to stop the bleeding.

1st Keep in mind that the upper arm and thigh pressure points are not to be used if there are possible fractures to the bone under the pressure point site. To do so could produce severe pain and could cause serious damage to the bone, soft tissues, nerves, and blood vessels in the area. You could cause more bleeding to take place rather than reduce the bleeding. If there are no possible fractures of the extremity and no indications of spinal injury, elevation and pressure point techniques can be combined to control bleeding.

1st REMEMBER: Pressure point techniques are to be used only after direct pressure or direct pressure and elevation have failed to control bleeding.

1st WARNING: Care must be exercised in the practice of pressure point techniques. As with most emergency care procedures, the application of pressure to compress an artery must be viewed as a drastic measure. A single compression of short duration will not harm a healthy adult. However,

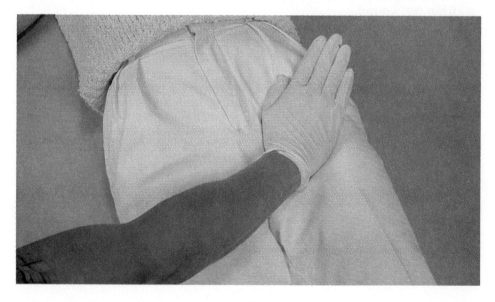

FIGURE 7–11. Apply pressure to femoral artery pressure point to control bleeding from the leg.

repeated practice on someone, applying pressure for more than a few seconds, and too much pressure applied to children can all cause problems. **Do not** attempt to practice or demonstrate this technique on children, infants, and adults with a history of heart problems, blood clot problems, or inflamed blood vessels.

1st Tourniquet

Tourniquet—the last resort used to control bleeding from an extremity. A band or belt is used to constrict blood vessels to help stop the flow of blood.

You must learn to consider the use of a tourniquet as one of the most extreme measures that can be applied by First Responders when providing emergency care. A tourniquet is a **last resort,** used only when the other methods of controlling life-threatening bleeding have failed. In most cases where you think that a tourniquet is to be used, a pressure dressing would be the better choice.

A partial amputation of the arm or leg may leave you with no other choice than to use a tourniquet. However, many total amputations do not have uncontrollable, profuse bleeding since the ends of the blood vessels tend to collapse. In cases where there is profuse bleeding from an arm or leg wound, a tourniquet should be applied to stop life-threatening bleeding after direct pressure, elevation, and pressure point techniques have failed. Be aware that the procedure could lead to the eventual loss of the arm or leg to which the tourniquet has been applied. If there is no other way to stop the bleeding and save the patient's life, then this is acceptable action.

1st REMEMBER: The use of a tourniquet is considered to be a last resort measure, used only to control life-threatening bleeding where other methods have failed.

1st WARNING: The application of a tourniquet is an extreme method of emergency care. *Do not* practice tightening a tourniquet on anyone!

1st If all other methods have failed and you must apply a tourniquet, note the following rules:

- Tourniquets are used only for wounds of the extremities. *Do not* apply a tourniquet on or below the elbow or on or below the knee.
- Once a tourniquet has been applied, it should not be loosened.

1st To apply a tourniquet, you should:

1. Locate the site for the tourniquet. This should be between the wound and the patient's heart, as close to the wound as possible without being on its edge. The most effective and safest location is about 2 inches from the wound.
2. A tourniquet pad should be placed on the site you have selected, over the artery. This pad can be a roll of dressing, a folded handkerchief, or a piece of cloth folded to about the same thickness as a folded handkerchief.
3. If you are using a manufactured tourniquet, carefully place it around the limb at the site. Pull the free end of the band through the friction catch or buckle and draw it tightly over the pad. You should tighten the tourniquet to the point where bleeding is stopped. *Do not* tighten it beyond this point. If you do not have a commercially manufactured tourniquet or you would have to leave the patient to retrieve one, use a flat belt, necktie, stocking, or long dressing material. *Do not* use any material that could cut into the patient's limb. Flat materials are best. The band should be at least ½ inch wide. Carefully slip the tourniquet around the patient's limb and tie a knot with the ends of the tourniquet. The knot should be over the pad. A device such as a long stick, wooden dowel, or metal rod should then be inserted into the knot (pens and pencils tend to break). Turn the device until bleeding has been stopped. *Do not* tighten the tourniquet beyond this point.

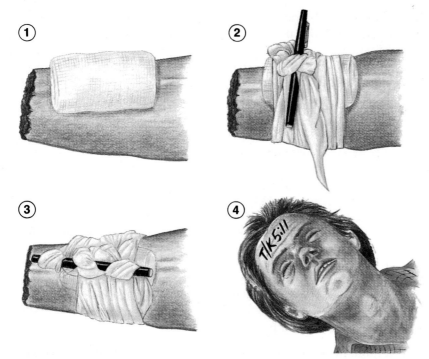

FIGURE 7–12. Apply a tourniquet as a last resort. 1. Apply pad. 2. Tighten tourniquet. 3. Fix in place. 4. Record time.

4. Once it is in place, **do not loosen the tourniquet.** To do so may cause great harm to the patient. The tightening device should be tied or taped in place.

5. Attach a note to the patient stating that a tourniquet has been applied and the time at which it was applied (for example, T/k—1:15 A.M.). If you do not have a tag, write the information, in ink, on the patient's forehead. If you do not have a pen, write the note in lipstick, crayon, or whatever is available at the scene. This note *must* be written so that the tourniquet does not go unnoticed and so that the hospital staff will know how long it has been in place.

6. Deliver care for shock (see page 176), but do not cover the tourniquet. This is an additional safeguard to prevent it from being missed by others who provide care for the patient.

NOTE: As a First Responder, you have the responsibility to advise the EMTs or other more highly trained personnel about the application of a tourniquet and the time it was applied.

Splinting

Splinting is not considered to be a primary First Responder-level method used to control bleeding. Some First Responders are trained to use air-inflatable splints. For long wounds on an arm or leg, the application of an air splint can help to control bleeding. This is actually a form of direct pressure. Using an inflatable splint requires special training in the application of the splint and knowing its limitations (see page 257). The air splint can be used even when there is no fracture to the bones of the limb. Combining the use of an air splint and elevation can work well on long, bleeding wounds. The splint also serves to immobilize the limb, helping to reduce the chances of patient movement restarting the bleeding. Since time is consumed by obtaining and applying air splints, this procedure is best done in cases of minor bleeding. The skilled rescuer can use air splints to control more serious bleeding if the splint is immediately at hand.

Special Cases of External Bleeding

Bleeding from the eye, ear, nose, mouth, and around impaled objects provides special cases that will be considered elsewhere in this book. For now, do not consider these sites while you are learning how to control bleeding.

There are situations where a deep cut will open a major artery or vein and then the cut will partially close. Such cuts do not always appear to be major and the bleeding from these cuts is often mild. Be alert for blood flow from wounds to change quickly from mild to profuse. If there is a wound to the arm and you cannot detect a wrist pulse, or if there is a wound to the leg and you cannot detect an ankle pulse, be prepared for profuse bleeding.

Do not let cuts to the chest and abdomen fool you. Some may appear minor, but they could be very deep and have produced internal injuries that are causing a great deal of internal bleeding. When you find an external wound, you must consider the possibility of internal injuries. **Do not open the wound to determine its depth.**

1st NOTE: You must have someone alert the EMS dispatcher for all patients with external bleeding except for the mildest cases (small areas of capillary bleeding) where there are no other signs of injury.
NOTE: Any patient who has suffered moderate to severe blood loss will benefit from receiving oxygen. If you are a First Responder who carries oxygen, administer 50% to 100% oxygen by mask, as needed.

INTERNAL BLEEDING

Significance of Internal Bleeding

Internal bleeding can range from minor importance to a major life-threatening problem. Most small, simple bruises are examples of minor internal bleeding. Such small blood loss is not of great significance. Of primary concern to First Responders are those cases of internal bleeding that produce a blood loss that could bring about shock, heart and lung failure, and eventual death. Some cases of internal bleeding are so severe that the patient dies in a matter of seconds. Other severe cases of internal bleeding take minutes to hours before death. First Responder-level care might keep these patients alive until the EMTs arrive.

Even when internal bleeding is not profuse, it does not take very long for serious reactions to occur in the body. The most important of these, shock, will be covered later in this chapter. The care you provide for internal bleeding and shock, even when the bleeding is not profuse, may save the patient's life.

Detecting Internal Bleeding

Internal bleeding can occur in many ways. It can be caused by wounds that are deep enough to sever major blood vessels or the vessels in organs, as in a deep wound to the chest or abdomen causing blood to flow freely into the body cavity. This type of wound is easier to imagine than one that severs a vessel in a muscle or bone, causing blood to flow freely in between the surrounding tissues.

Open wounds that have cut through major vessels to produce profuse internal bleeding may show only minor external bleeding. Many cases of

■ SCAN 7-1.

Methods of Controlling Bleeding

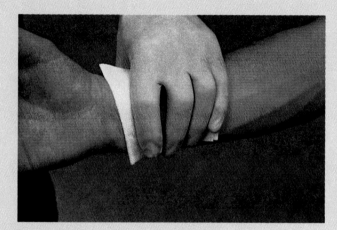

1 Direct pressure

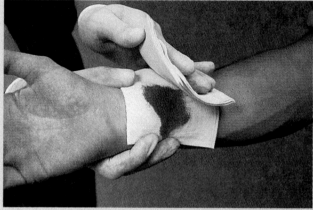

2 Pressure dressing

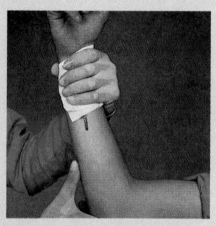

3 Direct pressure and elevation

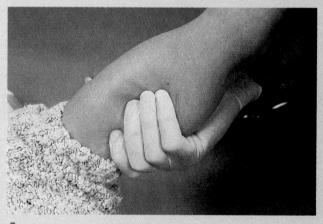

4 Pressure point: Arm

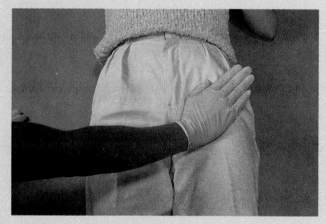

Pressure point: Leg

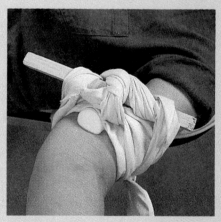

5 Tourniquet

internal bleeding occur even when there are no cuts in the skin or cavity walls. Internal organs and blood vessels may have been ruptured or crushed by a severe blow to the body that did not produce major external wounds. This is an example of blunt trauma, or injury caused by an object that was not sharp enough to penetrate the skin. The blunt instrument can be fairly large, such as the steering wheel of an automobile. Even though they do not tend to cause penetrating wounds, blunt instruments can deliver a great deal of force to the body, causing life-threatening internal bleeding.

Pay special attention to bruises on the neck, chest, and abdomen. Severe injury with internal bleeding may show no more than a bruise at first, to be followed by the rapid decline of the patient. Bruise detection can be particularly important in assessing possible internal bleeding when the patient is unconscious and thus unable to tell you of symptoms that would clearly indicate the problem.

To complicate your survey of the patient, there are cases where a blow to one side of the body may cause internal bleeding on the opposite side of the body cavity. In automobile accidents, blunt trauma to the lower right side of the rib cage can cause the spleen, on the left side of the body, to rupture and bleed freely, releasing about 1 liter (2 pints) or more of blood.

1st REMEMBER: Internal bleeding can be life-threatening. This may be hard to detect since it can occur in cases where bleeding from external wounds is minor, where external wounds are minor, away from the site of noticeable injury, or where there is no obvious external injury. Considering the mechanism of injury (falls, steering wheel injuries and the like) and conducting a proper secondary survey are of major importance in detecting internal bleeding.

1st Assume there is internal bleeding whenever you detect:

- Wounds that have penetrated the skull
- Blood or bloody fluids in the ears and/or nose
- The patient vomiting or coughing up blood (coffee-grounds or frothy red in appearance)
- Bruises on the neck
- Bruises on the chest, possible fractured ribs (possible cuts to the lungs and liver), and wounds that have penetrated the chest
- Bruises or penetrating wounds to the abdomen
- Hardness or spasms of the abdominal muscles
- Abdominal tenderness
- Bleeding from the rectum or vagina
- Fractures (with special emphasis on the pelvis and the long bones of the upper arm and thigh, and the ribs)

Notice how the items listed follow the secondary survey.

Assume there is internal bleeding if the patient has been injured and the symptoms and signs of shock are present. We will say more about shock later in this chapter, but for now you should know the basic symptoms and signs of shock used to detect possible internal bleeding.

1st Symptoms of shock associated with internal bleeding are:

- Patient feels weak.
- Patient is thirsty.
- Patient may feel cold.
- Patient feels anxious or restless.

1st The signs of shock associated with internal bleeding include:

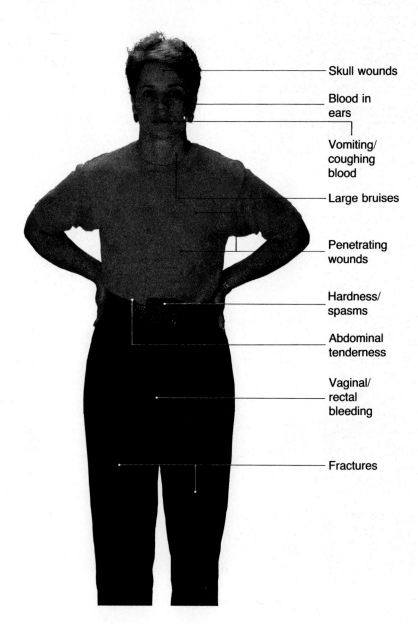

Skull wounds

Blood in ears

Vomiting/ coughing blood

Large bruises

Penetrating wounds

Hardness/ spasms

Abdominal tenderness

Vaginal/ rectal bleeding

Fractures

FIGURE 7–13. Any of the above indicates possible internal bleeding.

- Awareness—altered levels or unconsciousness
- Behavior—restlessness or combativeness
- Body—may be shaking and trembling (rare)
- Breathing—shallow and rapid
- Pulse—rapid and weak
- Skin—pale, cool and clammy (there may be profuse sweating)
- Eyes—pupils are dilated

Stop now and note how these signs fit into your survey of the patient during the physical examination.

NOTE: None of these symptoms and signs may be present in the early stages of internal bleeding. If the mechanism of injury is severe enough to make you think that there may be internal bleeding, assume that there is such bleeding and provide the necessary care.

1st You can detect internal bleeding by looking for injuries and mechanisms of injury that may cause internal bleeding, wounds, and the symptoms and signs of shock.

Some severe medical emergencies can produce internal bleeding. These will be covered in Chapters 13 and 15.

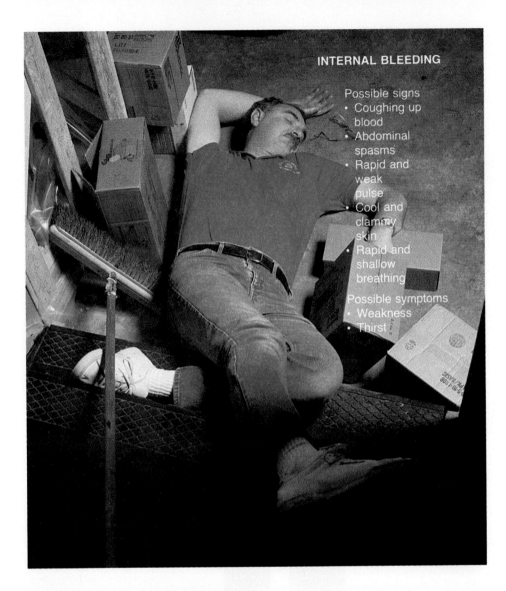

INTERNAL BLEEDING

Possible signs
• Coughing up blood
• Abdominal spasms
• Rapid and weak pulse
• Cool and clammy skin
• Rapid and shallow breathing

Possible symptoms
• Weakness
• Thirst

FIGURE 7–14. Internal bleeding.

Evaluating Internal Blood Loss

It is very difficult to determine the amount of blood lost in cases of internal bleeding. Special hospital procedures and tests are required. However, estimates can be made. Consider blood loss to be severe if there is penetration of the chest cavity over or immediately above the heart, if the spleen or liver may have been injured, or if the pelvis is fractured. Blood loss of at least 1 liter (2 pints) must be suspected if there is a major fracture in the upper arm or thigh bone. Where you find badly bruised skin, assume there is a 10% loss of total blood volume for each bruise the size of the patient's fist. For an adult, this is about a 1-pint loss. Such estimates will help you evaluate the chances of the patient going into shock, lung or heart failure, or cardiac arrest.

Controlling Internal Bleeding

1st The techniques for preventing or reducing the severity of shock will be covered later in this chapter. These techniques will help control internal bleeding. In general, the steps in the care for patients with suspected internal bleeding include:

1. Make certain that someone alerts the EMS dispatcher.
2. Maintain the airway and monitor breathing and pulse.

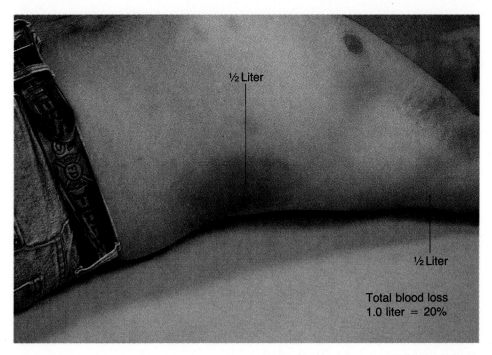

½ Liter

½ Liter

Total blood loss
1.0 liter = 20%

FIGURE 7–15. Estimating internal blood loss.

3. Care for shock, keeping the patient in the proper position and lying still.
4. Loosen restrictive clothing.
5. Be alert in case the patient starts to vomit.
6. *Do not* give the patient anything by mouth.
7. Apply pressure dressings if internal bleeding is in an extremity.
8. Report the possibility of internal bleeding as soon as more highly trained EMS personnel arrive at the scene.

NOTE: If you are a First Responder who carries oxygen, remember that any patient with possible internal bleeding will benefit from receiving 50% to 100% oxygen delivered by mask.

Internal bleeding in the abdominal cavity or the chest cavity is a life-

FIGURE 7–16. Certain types of injury may indicate serious internal bleeding.

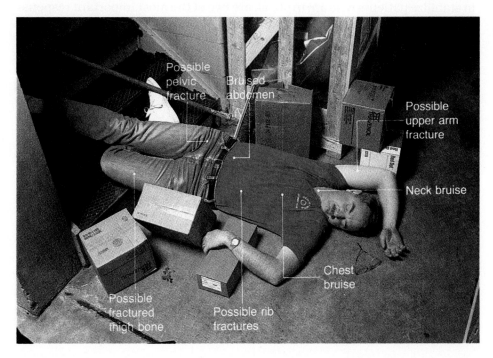

Possible pelvic fracture

Bruised abdomen

Possible upper arm fracture

Neck bruise

Chest bruise

Possible fractured thigh bone

Possible rib fractures

threatening situation requiring quick, safe transport to a hospital. Most areas in the country do not consider transport to be a First Responder's duty. Since EMTs and paramedics represent an extension of the hospital emergency department, directors of EMS believe it is better for patients if First Responders keep them at the scene. You must recognize that a patient unattended in the back seat of your car could go into cardiac arrest and die while you are trying to rush to the hospital. Improper transport also could aggravate spinal injuries, leading to the death of the patient.

Patients with internal bleeding need oxygen as part of their care. By transporting such patients to the hospital without oxygen, you may place them in greater risk than if you waited for EMS personnel to arrive with oxygen (and IV fluids).

Some localities may have special rules for First Responders in terms of patient transport (isolated areas with long EMT response time, and others). Follow the guidelines set for your locality.

Internal bleeding is very serious, often leading to death, even in cases where the bleeding begins once the patient is at the hospital. You may provide excellent First Responder care for a patient with internal bleeding, only to have him die on the scene. To be a good First Responder, accept the fact that there are limits to emergency care, at all levels. Some patients will die no matter what we do. The patient has a better chance to survive if you do as you have been trained.

SHOCK

Defining Shock

In emergency care there is the concept of the *"golden hour."* This is the first hour after serious injury or the sudden onset of certain illnesses. If shock can be prevented or if its severity can be reduced, the patient's chances for survival are greatly improved.

Any injury or illness must be rated as being more severe once the patient enters a state of shock. Keeping patients from going into shock and helping to stabilize patients who are in shock are two of the most important responsibilities of First Responders. If nothing is done for the patient who is in shock, death will almost always result.

Whenever the body is hurt, either by injury or illness, it reacts by trying to correct the effects of the damage. If the damage is severe, one reaction is shock. Shock indicates a problem with the circulatory system. The problem can be related to the:

- Heart—The heart must be pumping blood and doing so efficiently. If the heart fails to pump the required volume of blood or if it stops pumping altogether, shock will develop.
- Vessels—The circulatory system must be a closed system. If vessels are cut or burst open and enough blood is lost, shock will develop.
- Volume—There must be enough blood to fill the vessels. If there is loss of blood volume or if the vessels enlarge (dilate) to a size that no longer allows the system to be properly filled, shock will develop.

Shock—the reaction of the body to the failure of the circulatory system to provide enough blood to all the vital organs of the body. The failure of perfusion.

Basically, shock is the reaction of the body to the failure of the circulatory system to provide enough blood to all vital parts of the body. There must be enough blood being pumped efficiently to allow for a steady flow through the capillaries (perfusion) so that exchange can take place. Oxygen and carbon dioxide are exchanged, food and waste are exchanged, and fluid and salt balance must be maintained between the blood and the tissues. When perfusion cannot take place, shock develops.

The term "develops" means that shock occurs in a step-by-step process. This development can be rapid, or it can come about slowly. For most cases, you will have warning that the patient is going into shock. There is a saying used by EMS personnel: "Patients can go into shock a little at a time." This means that you will often have enough warning to prevent shock from occurring or to slow down the process, giving the patient a much better chance for survival.

Care for shock cannot be delayed. This is because the problem worsens with time. Think of shock as a reaction to a problem such as blood loss. This reaction causes more problems that, in turn, cause more problems.

FIGURE 7–17. The body's attempt to solve the circulatory problem may worsen the situation.

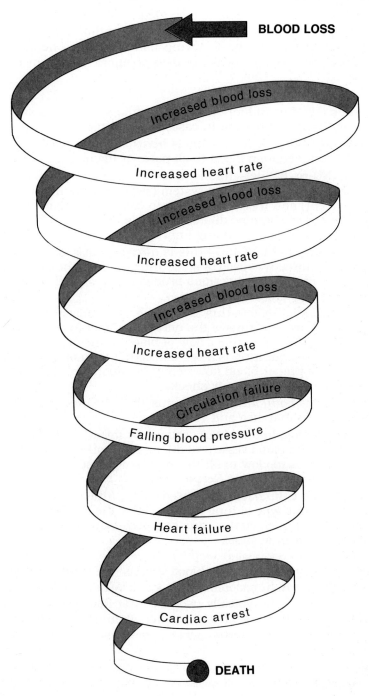

BLOOD LOSS

Increased blood loss

Increased heart rate

Increased blood loss

Increased heart rate

Increased blood loss

Increased heart rate

Circulation failure

Falling blood pressure

Heart failure

Cardiac arrest

DEATH

For example, if there is bleeding, the heart rate increases, attempting to circulate blood to all the vital parts of the body. By doing this, more blood is lost. The body's immediate answer to this problem is to try to circulate more blood by increasing the heart rate even further. The process of decline will continue until death occurs.

This process of decline must be stopped. The initial problem, such as bleeding, must be corrected, and any of the effects of shock must be treated. The procedures provided in First Responder-level care begin to correct problems and stop the decline.

1st REMEMBER: Shock occurs when there is a failure of the circulatory system to provide enough blood to all the vital parts of the body. Unless action is taken, shock can lead to death.

Types of Shock

Shock can be classified several ways because there is more than one cause of shock. *Do not* try to memorize the following list. It appears here so that you can see how many ways patients can develop shock. A patient in shock may have:

Bleeding shock, hemorrhagic (HEM-or-RIJ-ic) shock—the shock that develops due to the loss of blood or plasma.

- **Hemorrhagic shock** (HEM-or-RIJ-ic)—this is *bleeding shock*, caused by blood loss, or by the loss of plasma in cases of burn injury.
- **Cardiogenic shock** (KAR-di-o-JEN-ic)—this is *heart shock*, caused by the heart failing to pump enough blood to all parts of the body.
- **Neurogenic shock** (NU-ro-JEN-ic)—this is *nerve shock*, caused when something goes wrong with the nervous system (such as from an injury produced in an accident) and there is a failure to control the diameter of blood vessels. The vessels become dilated. There is not enough blood in the body to fill this new space, causing improper circulation.

Allergy shock, anaphylactic (AN-ah-fi-LAK-tik) shock—a severe allergic reaction in which a person goes into shock.

- **Anaphylactic shock** (AN-ah-fi-LAK-tik)—this is *allergy shock*, a life-threatening reaction of the body caused by something to which the patient is extremely allergic. This is such a serious problem that we will cover it as a special topic in this chapter.

Fainting, psychogenic (SI-ko-JEN-ic) shock—a self-correcting form of shock producing a temporary loss of consciousness when blood flow to the brain is reduced. Usually, this is due to the patient reacting to fear or stress; however, its cause may be more serious.

- **Psychogenic shock** (SI-ko-JEN-ic)—this is *fainting*. It usually occurs when some factor, such as fear, causes the nervous system to react and dilate the blood vessels. The proper flow of blood to the brain is interrupted. In most cases, fainting is a self-correcting form of shock, with the interruption of proper blood flow being a temporary condition. Fainting is not the same as neurogenic shock.
- **Metabolic shock**—this is *body fluid shock*, caused by the loss of body fluids as seen after severe diarrhea and vomiting.
- **Septic shock**—this is *bloodstream shock*, caused by infection. Poisons are released that cause the blood vessels to dilate. As in other cases of shock, the blood volume is too low to fill the circulatory system. This type of shock is seldom seen by First Responders.
- **Respiratory shock**—this is *lung shock*, caused by too little oxygen in the blood. It is due to some type of lung failure. Since the circulatory system is supplying blood to all vital organs and perfusion is taking place, this is not a true form of shock.

Whenever there is too little fluid in the blood vessels due to the loss of whole blood or plasma, the term *hypovolemic shock* can be used to describe the condition. This is not a term typically used by First Responders, but it is used by many EMTs and in many articles written about shock. Should you see or hear the term, remember that most people use it in place of hemorrhagic shock.

As a First Responder, you do not have to classify shock, with the exception of anaphylactic or allergy shock. For all cases other than anaphylactic or allergy shock, report that the patient has the symptoms and signs of shock and any factors you notice usually associated with shock (bleeding, loss of body fluids, and the like). If you cannot remember the term "anaphylactic shock," use the term "allergy shock." Other people in the EMS System will know what you mean and will ask you the questions needed to obtain information.

Symptoms and Signs of Shock

1st The symptoms of shock are:

- Weakness (this may be the most significant symptom)
- Nausea with possible vomiting
- Thirst
- Dizziness
- The patient indicates restlessness and fear. You may observe both of these conditions, thus considering them to be signs of shock. With some patients, such behavior may be the first indication of shock.

1st The signs of shock are:

- **Entire body survey:**
  1. Restlessness or combativeness
  2. Profuse external bleeding
  3. Vomiting or loss of body fluids
  4. Shaking and trembling (rare)
- **State of awareness**—the patient may become disoriented, confused, unresponsive, faint, or suddenly unconscious
- **Breathing**—shallow and rapid
- **Pulse**—rapid and weak
- **Skin**—pale, cool and clammy (may be profuse sweating)
- **Face**—pale, often with blue color (cyanosis) seen at the lips, tongue, and ear lobes
- **Eyes**—lackluster, pupils are dilated

The above list of symptoms and signs follows the order in which they may be detected during the initial patient survey. However, all the symptoms and signs of shock are not present at once, and they do not occur in the

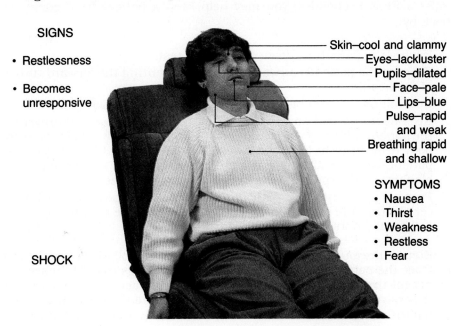

SIGNS

- Restlessness

- Becomes unresponsive

Skin–cool and clammy
Eyes–lackluster
Pupils–dilated
Face–pale
Lips–blue
Pulse–rapid and weak
Breathing rapid and shallow

SYMPTOMS
- Nausea
- Thirst
- Weakness
- Restless
- Fear

SHOCK

FIGURE 7–18. Symptoms and signs of shock.

order listed above. Since shock is a changing process, becoming worse with time, you should look for the following patterns:

1. *Increased pulse rate*—the body is trying to adjust to the loss of blood or inefficient circulation. This rate does not slow down in a few minutes as would be expected if it were due to the stress of an accident or the fear of needed help during a medical emergency.

2. *Increased breathing rate*—since circulation is not efficient, the demand for oxygen and the release of carbon dioxide are not being properly met. Breathing will not slow down as it usually does after experiencing stress.

3. *Restlessness or combativeness*—the patient is reacting to the body's attempt to adjust to the loss of proper circulatory function. The patient "feels" that something is wrong and may often look afraid. In some cases, this behavioral change may be the first sign of developing shock.

4. *Changes indicating possible shock*—skin, nail bed, and other color changes occur. The skin feels cool to the touch. Sweating will be profuse. Thirst, weakness, and nausea are noted.

5. *Rapid, weak pulse and labored, weakened respirations*—the body is failing in its attempt to adjust to the circulatory system failure.

6. *Changes in the state of awareness*—as adequate circulation to the brain continues to fail, the patient will become confused, disoriented, sleepy, or unconscious.

7. *Respiratory arrest*, then *cardiac arrest* can develop.

1st Provide care for all injured patients as if shock will develop. Do the same for all patients with problems involving the heart, breathing, abdominal distress, diabetes, drug abuse, poisoning, and abnormal childbirth. Carefully monitor all medical emergency patients for the early warnings of shock. If any are noticed, provide care as if the patient is developing shock. **NOTE:** Children and young adults may compensate for a loss of blood volume better than adults older than 35 years of age. This will delay the early indications of developing shock. However, once children and young adults begin to show the first signs of shock, its development may be rapid.

Preventing and Caring for Shock

1st Make certain that the dispatcher is alerted for cases involving shock or where shock may develop.

1st As a First Responder, you may help keep a patient from going into shock by:

1. Having the patient lie down and stay at rest.
2. Keeping the patient's airway open and preventing the forward tilting of the head.
3. Controlling external bleeding and splinting major fractures.
4. Keeping the patient warm with suitable covers. Take care not to overheat the patient. This will worsen the condition. You simply want to conserve body heat. Place at least one blanket under and one blanket over the patient, covering all body parts except the head. *Do not* try to place a blanket under a patient with possible spinal injuries.
5. Properly positioning the patient. Regardless of the position used, make certain that the patient has an open airway and be alert for vomiting. If there is no indication of spinal injuries, use one of the following positions:
   Elevate the lower extremities—This procedure is followed in most cases. Place the patient flat, face up, and elevate the legs 8 to 12 inches. *Do not* tilt the patient's body. *Do not* elevate any fractured limbs unless they have been properly splinted. *Do not* elevate the legs if there are fractures to the pelvis.

■ SCAN 7-2.

Developing Shock

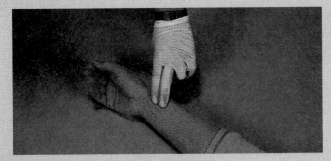

1 Increased pulse: 100+

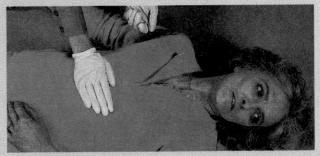

2 Increased breathing rate

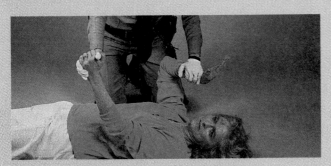

3 Restlessness or combativeness

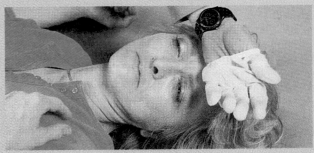

4 Skin changes and sweating

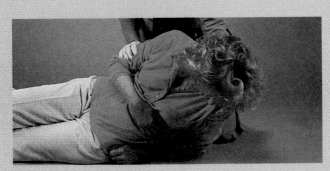

5 Thirst, weakness and nausea

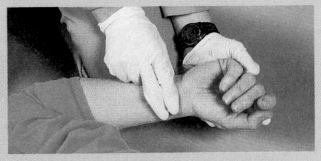

6 Rapid, weak pulse; labored, weak respirations

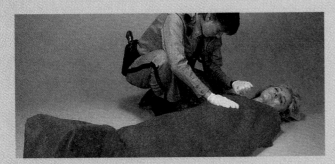

7 Loss of consciousness

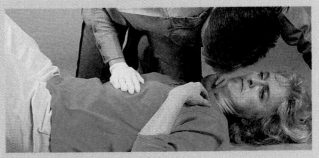

8 Clinical death may occur

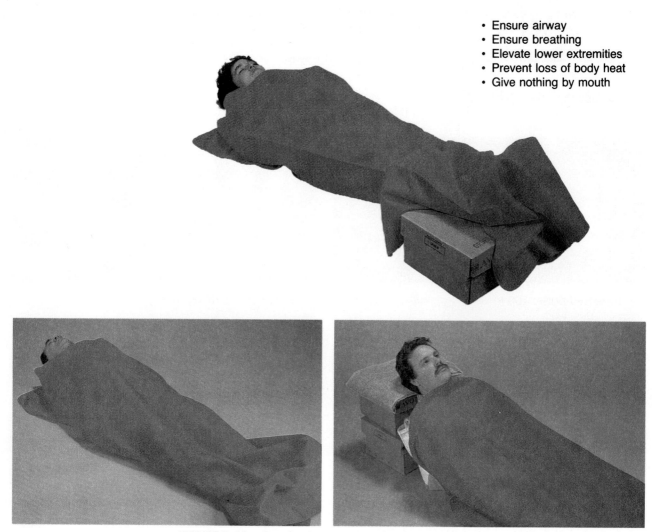

- Ensure airway
- Ensure breathing
- Elevate lower extremities
- Prevent loss of body heat
- Give nothing by mouth

FIGURE 7–19. Care for shock.

Lay the patient flat, face up—This is the supine position, used for patients with serious injuries to the extremities. If the patient is placed in this position, you must constantly be prepared for vomiting.
Slightly raise the head and shoulders—This position should be used *only* for conscious patients with no possible neck, spinal, chest, or abdominal injuries. This is done *only* for patients having difficulty breathing, but who have an open airway. A semiseated position can also be used for patients with a history of heart problems. It is not recommended for moderate to severe cases of bleeding shock. Be certain to keep the patient's head from tilting forward.
WARNING: Do not follow this procedure if there is a possibility of neck injury, if head injuries are severe, or if the patient is having any difficulty in maintaining an adequate airway.

6. Giving the patient nothing by mouth. Even if the patient expresses serious thirst, do not give any fluids or food.

7. Monitoring the patient's vital signs. This must be done no less than every 5 minutes. Stay alert for vomiting, give nothing to the patient by mouth, and provide emotional support to the conscious patient.

REMEMBER: Restlessness may be a sign of someone going into shock. The patient may want to assume a sitting position even when there are no problems with breathing. A patient has less chance of going into shock if kept lying down and at rest.

You will not be able to bring a patient out of shock, but you may be able to prevent shock or keep shock from worsening by following the above procedures. The care you provide may reverse the severity of certain aspects of shock and may help the patient avoid immediate danger.

NOTE: If you are trained to do so and if your state laws allow you to do so, oxygen can be very significant in helping shock patients. Provide the patient with 50% to 100% oxygen by mask.

Allergy Shock

Allergy shock is called anaphylactic shock. It sometimes occurs when people come into contact with a substance to which they are allergic. This is a true life-threatening emergency. There is no way of knowing if patients will stabilize, grow worse slowly or rapidly, or overcome the reaction on their own. Many patients in allergy shock decline rapidly. For some, death is a certain outcome unless special treatment is given quickly.

1st Many different things can cause anaphylactic shock, such as:

- Insect bites and stings, including bee stings
- Foods and spices
- Inhaled substances, including dust and pollens
- Chemicals, inhaled or when in contact with the skin
- Medications, injected or taken by mouth, including penicillin

1st The signs of allergy shock are:

- **Skin**—burning, itching, or "breaking out" (such as hives or some type of rash)
- **Breathing**—difficult and rapid, with possible chest pains and wheezing
- **Pulse**—rapid, very weak or not detected
- **Face**—the lips often turn blue (cyanosis), the face and tongue may swell
- **State of consciousness**—restlessness, often followed by fainting or unconsciousness

SIGNS OF ALLERGY SHOCK

- Restlessness
- Fainting, coma

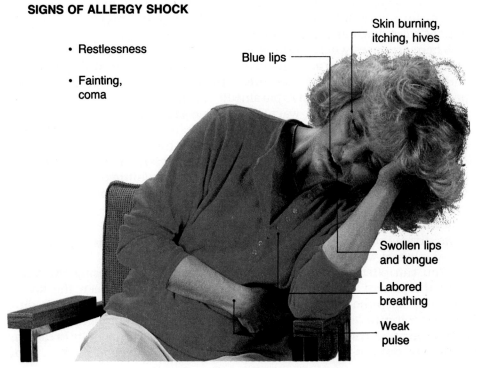

Skin burning, itching, hives

Blue lips

Swollen lips and tongue

Labored breathing

Weak pulse

FIGURE 7–20. Signs of allergy shock.

1st REMEMBER: When you interview patients, ask if they are allergic to anything and if they have been in contact with that substance. Look for a medical identification device that may indicate if there is an allergy problem. If you are in the patient's residence, look for a "Vial of Life" or similar type of sticker on the main entrance, the closest window to this main door, or the refrigerator door. This sticker indicates the presence of patient information and medications in a vial kept in the refrigerator.

To care for patients in allergy shock, follow the same procedures used for shock. Even though the danger to the patient may be immediate, do not attempt to transport the patient unless you are allowed to do so. Usually, it is better to wait for the EMTs to respond. In many cases, paramedics can respond to the scene and administer the medications required to stabilize the patient before transport.

Patients in anaphylactic shock need medications as soon as possible. In some states, certain First Responders are allowed to transport allergy shock patients immediately to a hospital. The EMS System dispatcher in the areas may decide that the EMT response time is too long and recommend that the First Responder provide transport. The First Responder may be allowed to transport allergy shock patients to a medical facility only if they have no injuries. Your instructor can tell you the policy for your own state or certain areas within your state. If you do transport allergy shock patients, be prepared for them to grow worse and be ready to provide pulmonary resuscitation or CPR.

1st REMEMBER: Anaphylactic shock is a true emergency.

Some people who are sensitive to bee stings or have other allergy problems carry medications to take in case of an emergency. These medications, usually epinephrine and/or antihistamines, can be administered by the patient. You may help the patient take medications. However, if the patient cannot do so or is unconscious, state laws will govern if you can administer the medication. Your instructor will inform you of local policies for the care of these patients.

Fainting

Fainting is usually a self-correcting form of mild shock. However, the patient may have been injured in a fall due to fainting. Be certain to examine the patient for injury. Even if there appear to be no other problems, keep the patient lying down and at rest for several minutes.

There are cases where fainting is caused by a sudden drop or elevation of blood pressure. If you are trained to do so and have the needed equipment, check the patient's blood pressure. Otherwise, have the patient's blood pressure checked by an EMT, paramedic, or nurse.

Fainting also can be a warning of some serious condition, including brain tumors, heart disease, undetected diabetes, and inner ear problems (do not cause the patient to faint again by telling him all these possibilities!). Always recommend that the person see a physician as soon as possible. In a polite but firm manner, tell anyone who has fainted not to drive or operate any machinery until after having been seen by a physician. Make certain that you have witnesses to this warning.

Your patient may have fainted due to fear, stress from problems, bad news, the sight of blood, or being in an accident. Be ready to provide emotional support when the patient is alert.

1st You can often prevent a person from fainting by lowering the head. Have the patient sit down and then lower the head between the knees. You *must* keep the patient from falling from this position. This procedure is *not* recommended for patients with fractures or possible spinal injuries. *Do not* carry out this procedure on anyone who is having difficulty breathing or on anyone with a known heart problem. For this type of patient, lying

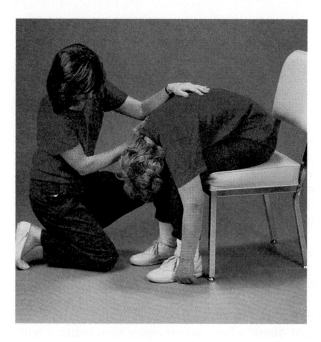

FIGURE 7–21. Try to prevent patient's fainting. Protect the patient from falling.

down with the feet slightly elevated and receiving emotional support will often prevent fainting.

SUMMARY

Bleeding can be **external** or **internal.** Both types of bleeding can range from minor to life-threatening.

Bleeding may be classified as:

- **Arterial**—profuse loss of bright red blood, spurting from an artery
- **Venous**—mild to profuse loss of dark red blood, flowing steadily from a vein
- **Capillary**—slow loss of red blood, flowing from a bed of capillaries, as seen in minor scrapes of the skin

The four major techniques for controlling external bleeding are:

1. **Direct pressure**—where your gloved hand, a sterile dressing or clean cloth, or a pressure dressing can be used to apply pressure directly to a wound to stop mild bleeding. *Never* remove a dressing once it is in place.
2. **Elevation**—usually used in combination with direct pressure to control bleeding from an extremity when there are no fractures to the limb or possible spinal injury.
3. **Pressure points**—using external hand pressure to compress an artery. This is most often performed on the brachial (upper arm) and femoral (thigh) arteries.
4. **Tourniquet**—a **last resort** procedure used to control bleeding from an extremity. The flat belt or band of a tourniquet is set over a pad placed close to the wound (about 2 inches), between the site of the wound and the patient's heart. The tourniquet belt is then tightened until bleeding stops. **Once the tourniquet is in place, do not loosen it.**

REMEMBER: Direct pressure is the first choice in controlling bleeding.

Internal bleeding can be very serious. Look for mechanisms of injury that may cause internal bleeding, look for wounds associated with internal bleeding, and examine the patient for the symptoms and signs of **shock.**

Care for internal bleeding is the **same as for shock.** In addition, pressure dressings can be applied for internal bleeding found in an extremity.

Shock is the body's reaction to the failure of the circulatory system to provide enough blood to all vital parts of the body. Unless the process is stopped, the patient will die.

The **symptoms of shock** may include weakness, nausea, thirst, dizziness, weakness, restlessness, and fear.

The **signs of shock** may include restlessness, combativeness, profuse external bleeding, vomiting or loss of body fluids, shaking and trembling (rare), altered states of awareness, shallow and rapid breathing, rapid and weak pulse, pale skin (with the face often turning blue), cool and clammy skin, lackluster eyes with dilated pupils.

REMEMBER: Look for a pattern of symptoms and signs to develop as shock progresses.

The **prevention** and **care** procedures for shock are the same. Keep the patient at rest, lying down and covered to stay warm. Maintain an adequate airway. Be sure that you have controlled external bleeding and have splinted major fractures. For most cases you should elevate the lower extremities.

Allergy shock (anaphylactic shock) is a **true life-threatening emergency.** This type of shock is brought about when people come into contact with a substance to which they are allergic (bee stings, insect bites, chemicals, foods, dusts, pollens, drugs).

The **signs of allergy shock** may include burning or itching skin, breaking out (hives), rapid and difficult breathing, a very weak pulse, swelling of the face, swelling of the tongue, blue coloration of the lips, and a sudden loss of consciousness.

The **care** for allergy shock is the same as for other cases of shock. The patient **must be transported to a hospital as soon as possible.** Follow the guidelines established for your state.

REMEMBER: Ask the patient about allergies during the interview. Be certain to look for a medical identification device.

Fainting is a mild form of self-correcting shock. Always look for injuries that may have been caused by falls due to fainting. Try to keep the patient at the scene until others arrive who can take readings of the patient's blood pressure as part of their assessment. **Discourage** patients who have fainted from driving a motor vehicle or operating machinery until they are examined by a physician. **Encourage** these patients to see a physician.

Fainting is often brought about by a reaction to stress or fear. Provide the patient with **emotional support**.

Fainting can often be **prevented** by placing the patient in a seated position and lowering the head between the knees. Stay alert in case the patient does faint. *Do not* follow this procedure for a patient who has fractures or possible spinal injuries. *Do not* follow this procedure for a patient who has difficulty breathing or known heart problems.

Considering the topics covered in this chapter, you should go back and review the **primary survey.** Remember, the purpose of the primary survey is to detect and control life-threatening problems. You should:

- See if the patient is responsive.
- Establish an airway as described in Chapter 4.
- If necessary, begin resuscitation techniques described in Chapter 4.
- Check for a carotid pulse, initiating CPR when needed as described in Chapters 5 and 6.
- Control all life-threatening bleeding by direct pressure, elevation, or pressure points.
- Use a tourniquet as a last resort for profuse bleeding from the extremities.
- If you are certain that there is severe internal bleeding, begin treating

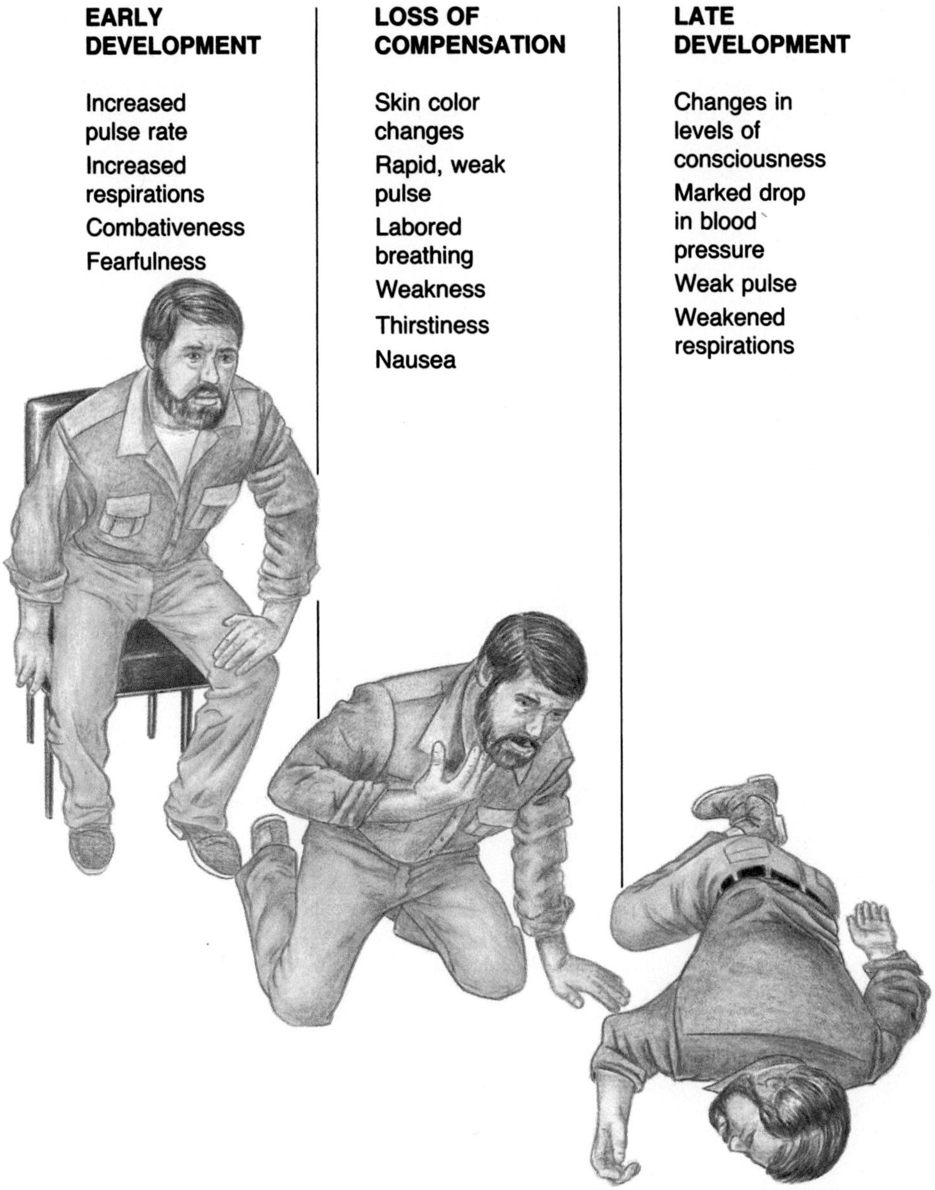

EARLY DEVELOPMENT	LOSS OF COMPENSATION	LATE DEVELOPMENT
Increased pulse rate	Skin color changes	Changes in levels of consciousness
Increased respirations	Rapid, weak pulse	Marked drop in blood pressure
Combativeness	Labored breathing	Weak pulse
Fearfulness	Weakness	Weakened respirations
	Thirstiness	
	Nausea	

FIGURE 7-22. The development of shock.

for shock. *Do not* elevate the limbs if there are indications of possible spinal injury.

You should relate the detection of **shock** to the **secondary patient survey.** What might you see that would indicate shock when you observe the entire patient? What will you find during the taking of vital signs (breathing, radial pulse, and skin temperature)? What should you notice about a patient's eyes if he or she is going into shock? What information is gained related to shock when you examine the head and face of a patient?

CHAPTER 8

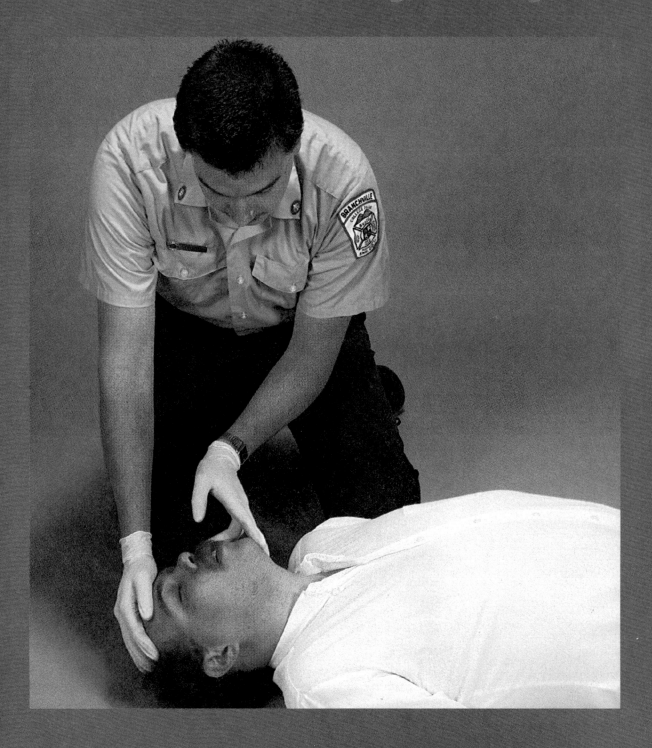

OBJECTIVES

By the end of this chapter, you should be able to:

1. List the steps of the primary survey, indicating why each step is performed.
2. State what may be detected during the primary survey and what can be done to:
   A. Open the airway
   B. Clear the airway
   C. Provide artificial ventilation
   D. Provide CPR
   E. Control profuse bleeding

SKILLS

Upon completing this chapter and your class lectures and skills labs, you should be able to:

1. Conduct a primary survey for a simulated emergency.
2. Provide all First Responder-level care for:
   A. Obstructed airway
   B. Respiratory arrest
   C. Cardiac arrest
   D. Profuse bleeding

THE PRIMARY SURVEY

Review of the Survey

This chapter lists the events of the primary survey. References are made to the techniques of care found in Chapters 4–7. Go through this list, noting any weaknesses you may have in terms of knowledge and skills. Page numbers are provided to allow you to stop and go back to specific chapter sections for review purposes.

1. Call for bystander help and put on any required items of personal protection.
2. Quickly look over the scene and the entire patient. Is the scene dangerous? Will you have to quickly move the patient? Are there any obvious mechanisms of injury? Are there obvious signs of possible spinal injury?
3. See if the patient is responsive. If not, call out for help.
4. Ensure an open airway by the head-tilt, chin-lift method (p. 90). If there are possible skull, neck, or spinal injuries, use the jaw-thrust method (p. 91).
5. Look, listen, and feel for breathing and indications of partial or complete airway obstruction (pp. 89, 100, and 101). Allow 3 to 5 seconds to determine if the patient is breathing. At this time, you can check to see if the patient is a neck-breather (has a stoma).
6. Airway obstruction:
   A. If the patient is conscious and has an airway obstruction, attempt to clear the airway by back blows (infants only) and manual thrusts (abdominal or chest, as appropriate). Continue until successful or until the patient loses consciousness (p. 107).
   B. If the patient becomes unconscious, perform finger sweeps and attempt to ventilate the patient. In cases where your ventilations are unsuccessful, use back blows (infants only), manual thrusts

(abdominal or chest, as appropriate), finger sweeps, and ventilations (p. 107).

C. If the patient is unconscious when you arrive, establish unresponsiveness, attempt to open the airway, and look, listen, and feel for adequate air exchange. When necessary, attempt to provide two adequate breaths (mouth-to-mask methods are suggested). Should your first attempt fail, reposition the patient's head and try to ventilate. If your efforts to ventilate fail, deliver back blows (infants only), manual thrusts (abdominal or chest, as appropriate), finger sweeps, and attempts to ventilate (p. 107).

REMEMBER: Do not use "blind" finger sweeps on infants and children.

7. When the unconscious patient is not breathing (in respiratory arrest) and there are no signs of obvious airway obstruction:
   A. Use the head-tilt, chin-lift or jaw-thrust maneuver to open the airway (p. 90). Do not hyperextend the head if the patient is an infant, but do ensure an adequate airway (p. 96).
   B. Attempt to provide two adequate breaths mouth-to-mask.
   C. Look, listen, and feel for breathing (3 to 5 seconds).
   D. If the patient is not breathing, feel for a carotid pulse (p. 58), or, in the case of an infant, a brachial pulse (p. 135). Take at least 5 seconds, but no more than 10 seconds, to check for the pulse.

8. Should the patient have a pulse, but is not breathing, have someone alert the EMS dispatcher indicating that the patient is not breathing. Provide pulmonary resuscitation.

   ADULT Ventilate using the mouth-to-mask (mouth-to-mouth, mouth-to-nose, or mouth-to-stoma) technique. Rate = 12 breaths per minute, or one breath every 5 seconds (p. 93).

   CHILD: Ventilate with small but adequate breaths utilizing the correct sized mask. At your own risk, you may opt to use the mouth-to-mouth method; or if the child is small, the mouth-to-mouth and nose technique. Rate = one breath every 4 seconds to provide 15 breaths per minute (p. 96).

   INFANT: Avoid excessive head tilt, but ensure an adequate airway. Ventilate with small but adequate breaths, delivered mouth-to-mask or mouth-to-mouth and nose (at your own risk). Rate = one breath every 3 seconds to provide 20 breaths per minute (p. 96).

   NOTE: It is rare to find a neck-breathing child or infant. However, you should be on the alert for a stoma with all patients.

9. If the patient is not breathing and does not have a pulse, have someone call the EMS System dispatcher. Have them alert the dispatcher to the fact that CPR has begun. Correctly position the patient and:

   ADULT: Provide CPR with a rate of 80 to 100 compressions per minute, at a rate of 15 compressions every 9 to 11 seconds. Compress the patient's breastbone 1½ to 2 inches. Interpose two adequate breaths every 15 compressions by the mouth-to-mask method (p. 128). Monitor for spontaneous breathing and check for a pulse after 1 minute of CPR. If there is no pulse, continue CPR. Check for a pulse every few minutes thereafter. If two-rescuer CPR is being used, deliver compressions at a rate of 80 to 100 compressions per minute, interposing one breath every 5 compressions (p. 152).

   CHILD: Provide CPR using one hand for compressions. Deliver compressions at a rate of 80 to 100 per minute (same for both one- and two-rescuer CPR), depressing the breastbone 1 to 1½ inches. Interpose one breath every 5 compressions (pp. 136–137).

   INFANT: Provide CPR using the tips of two or three fingers for compressions. Deliver compressions at a rate of at least 100 per minute, depressing the breastbone ½ to 1 inch. Interpose one ventilation every 5 compressions (pp. 136–137).

REMEMBER: Do *not* interrupt CPR for more than 7 seconds, unless you must move the patient or it is necessary to remove vomitus from the patient's airway. If you must move the patient, try not to interrupt CPR for more than 15 to 30 seconds. Continue CPR until heart action returns, breathing and heart action return, you are relieved by a trained person, a physician assumes the responsibility for care, or until you are too tired to continue (pp. 139, 141–142).

10. Control all profuse, life-threatening bleeding:
    A. Start with direct pressure (p. 158). When possible, apply a pressure dressing (p. 160).
    B. Use elevation when needed (p. 161).
    C. Next, try pressure points (p. 162).
    D. Use a tourniquet as a last resort (p. 164).
    E. Be prepared to care for shock (p. 176).

    There will be cases when bleeding is so profuse that it will be necessary to try to control the bleeding while checking for breathing and pulse. Since the cells of the brain may begin to suffer irreversible damage in 4 to 6 minutes when they are without oxygen, the priority of care is breathing, circulation, and bleeding. In severe cases, attempt to have bystanders help control bleeding while you provide resuscitation.

    The actions you take to keep the patient at rest and to control bleeding begin the care for shock. The complete care for shock requires you to perform elements of the secondary survey before wound care, splinting, and positioning of the patient are possible.

■ SCAN 8-1.

The Primary Survey and Basic Life Support

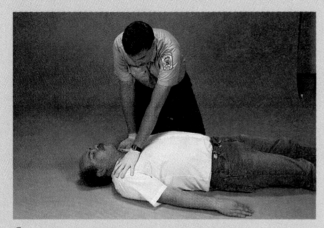

1. Establish unresponsiveness.

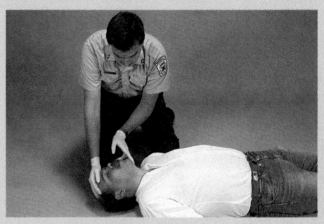

2. Open the airway.

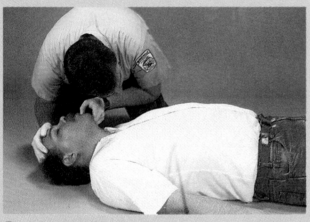

3. Look, listen, and feel.

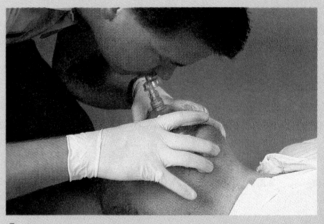

4. No breathing. Provide rescue breathing.

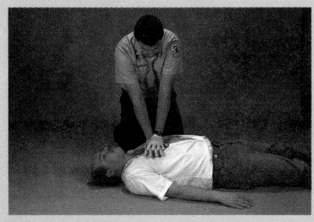

5. No pulse. Provide CPR.

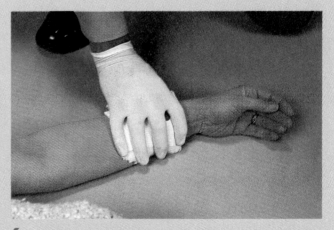

6. Control profuse bleeding. Provide care for shock.

This is a self-test. It has been designed for you to take on your own to evaluate your progress. After you have completed Chapters 1 to 8 and believe that you have met all the objectives listed for these chapters, take this test to see if you have any weaknesses in a specific area of study. Answers are listed at the end of the test. Page references are provided for each question so you can go back to the text to restudy any questions missed in the test.

If you wish to check your knowledge in more detail, note that the objectives listed at the beginning of each chapter can be read as questions and exercises. Go back to these objectives and see if you can list, describe, name, and so on, as directed in the objective statements.

Circle the letter of the best answer to each question.

1. A small child is injured, requiring First Responder emergency care. The child's parents cannot be contacted, but the child says that you can help. You can provide care because of (p. 14)

    A. The Medical   C. Informed consent
        Practices Act   D. Implied consent
    B. Actual consent

2. The anterior trunk of the body is composed of the abdomen, pelvis, and (p. 23)

    A. Cranial cavity   C. Spinal cavity
    B. Chest   D. Head and neck

3. The spleen is located in the (p. 25)

    A. Right lower   C. Right upper
        quadrant   quadrant
    B. Left lower quadrant   D. Left upper
                            quadrant

4. The order of the primary survey is level of responsiveness, then (p. 55)

    A. Respiration, pulse, bleeding
    B. Pulse, respiration, bleeding
    C. Bleeding, pulse, respiration
    D. Respiration, bleeding, pulse

5. For the average adult, the at-rest pulse rate is (p. 67)

    A. 50 to 70 beats/   C. 70 to 90 beats/
        minute   minute
    B. 60 to 80 beats/   D. 80 to 100 beats/
        minute   minute

6. During the primary survey of an adult patient, circulation is determined by taking a (p. 58)

    A. Pedal pulse   C. Carotid pulse
    B. Radial pulse   D. Apical pulse

7. Once respiratory arrest begins, lethal changes in the brain will usually start in (p. 85)

    A. 10 to 20 minutes   C. 30 to 60 minutes
    B. 4 to 6 minutes   D. 3 to 5 seconds

8. In dark-skinned people, blue coloration (cyanosis) due to a lack of oxygen is best observed on the (p. 64)

    A. Eyelids   C. Lips
    B. Palms of the hands   D. Abdomen

9. During a secondary survey of an injured person, you notice a white discoloration of the inner surface of a patient's eyelids. This usually indicates (p. 74)

    A. Loss of blood   C. Drug abuse
    B. Poisoning   D. Chemical burn

10. When an unconscious patient's head tilts forward, the airway often will be obstructed by the (p. 100)

    A. Voice box (larynx)   C. Throat (pharynx)
    B. Tongue   D. Tonsils

11. You find an unconscious patient and have called out for bystander help. Your next step is to (p. 93)

    A. Clear the mouth   C. Check for a pulse
    B. Ensure an open   D. Provide
        airway   ventilations

12. A First Responder is trying to correct a complete airway obstruction in an adult conscious patient. He should (p. 107)

    A. Attempt a finger sweep
    B. Try to reposition the patient's head
    C. Attempt to ventilate the patient
    D. Deliver 6 to 10 abdominal thrusts

13. You have failed in your efforts to clear a patient's airway of a total obstruction. The patient becomes unconscious. You try all the various techniques used to clear the airway and the patient still has the obstruction. You open the airway and attempt to ventilate. Which of the following is the correct sequence you should now follow? (p. 107)

    A. Ventilate, manual thrusts, finger sweeps
    B. Finger sweeps, ventilate, manual thrusts
    C. Manual thrusts, finger sweeps, ventilate
    D. Finger sweeps, manual thrusts, ventilate

14. In the mouth-to-mask resuscitation of an adult patient, you should provide a breath every (p. 93)

    A. 2 seconds   C. 5 seconds
    B. 4 seconds   D. 10 seconds

15. In the pulmonary resuscitation of an infant, breaths are provided every (p. 96)

    A. Second
    B. 2 seconds
    C. 3 seconds
    D. 4 seconds

16. When providing mouth-to-mask resuscitation for a patient with spinal injury, you should use the (p. 92)

    A. Neck lift, head tilt
    B. Jaw thrust
    C. Chin lift, head tilt
    D. None of the above

17. Which of the following comes first in CPR? (p. 123)

    A. Ensure an open airway
    B. Call dispatch
    C. Establish unresponsiveness
    D. Establish breathing

18. During the CPR of an adult, the breastbone (sternum) should be compressed (p. 126)

    A. 1½ to 2 inches
    B. 3 inches
    C. ½ to 3 inches
    D. 1 inch

19. The compression rate for one-rescuer CPR is (p. 129)

    A. 80 to 100 per minute
    B. 60 to 80 per minute
    C. 30 per minute
    D. 15 per minute

20. The rate of ventilations (breaths provided) during one-rescuer CPR is (p. 129)

    A. 1 every 5 compressions
    B. 1 every 15 compressions
    C. 2 every 5 compressions
    D. 2 every 15 compressions

21. The compression rate for two-rescuer CPR is (p. 147)

    A. 80 to 100 per minute
    B. 60 per minute
    C. 30 to 60 per minute
    D. 10 per minute

22. The rate of interpose ventilations (breaths provided) during two-rescuer CPR is (p. 147)

    A. 1 every 5 compressions
    B. 1 every 15 compressions
    C. 2 every 5 compressions
    D. 2 every 15 compressions

23. To establish a pulse in an infant, you should use the (p. 135)

    A. Apical pulse site
    B. Brachial pulse site
    C. Carotid pulse site
    D. Pedal pulse site

24. During CPR in infants, compressions are delivered with (p. 136)

    A. The heel of one hand
    B. Both hands
    C. One finger
    D. Two or three fingertips

25. The CPR compression site in the adult is (p. 124)

    A. Directly between the nipples
    B. The width of one hand below the collarbone
    C. Two finger widths above the sternal notch
    D. Three finger widths below the left nipple

26. During the emergency care for bleeding, your best line of defense against infectious diseases is to (p. 158)

    A. Wear latex or vinyl gloves
    B. Apply a bulky dressing
    C. Apply an occlusive dressing
    D. Wear a gauze mask

27. The best method to control bleeding is (p. 158)

    A. Tourniquet
    B. Direct pressure
    C. Pressure point
    D. Applying a dressing

28. To care for internal bleeding in the abdomen, First Responders should (pp. 170–171)

    A. Apply pressure dressings
    B. Apply hand pressure over the possible site
    C. Provide care for shock
    D. Apply constricting bands (cravats)

29. As patients develop shock, the pupils are usually (p. 175)

    A. Unequal
    B. Dilated
    C. Constricted
    D. Normal

30. A patient going into shock has difficulty breathing, a weak pulse, swollen face, and itching skin. This is probably (p. 179)

    A. Allergy shock (anaphylactic shock)
    B. Bleeding shock (hemorrhagic shock)
    C. Heart shock (cardiogenic shock)
    D. Nerve shock (neurogenic shock)

31. Below is a list of procedures carried out during the patient examination phase of the secondary survey. These procedures are not in the correct order. A set of blanks, listed 1 through 20, has been provided. Place the letter of a procedure in the blank that corresponds with the procedure's correct order in the secondary survey. (pp. 73–80)

    ___ 1   A. Inspect chest for penetration
    ___ 2   B. Feel pelvis for fractures
    ___ 3   C. Inspect scalp for wounds
    ___ 4   D. Check each arm for injury and paralysis
    ___ 5   E. Inspect the back surfaces
    ___ 6   F. Inspect pupils for equality and reaction
    ___ 7   G. Inspect mouth for blood
    ___ 8   H. Inspect genital region for obvious injury
    ___ 9   I. Inspect chest for fractures
    ___ 10 J. Check lower back for point tenderness
    ___ 11 K. Inspect ears and nose for blood or clear fluids
    ___ 12 L. Check each leg for injury and paralysis
    ___ 13 M. Inspect chest for equal expansion
    ___ 14 N. Inspect abdomen for penetration
    ___ 15 O. Inspect mouth for potential airway obstructions
    ___ 16 P. Inspect inner surfaces of eyelids
    ___ 17 Q. Feel abdomen for tenderness

(continued)

___ 18   R.   Feel cervical spine for point tenderness
___ 19   S.   Sniff for odd breath odor
___ 20   T.   Reinspect anterior neck for stoma

ANSWERS

Each of the following is worth 3 points:

1. D	11. B	21. A
2. B	12. D	22. A
3. D	13. C	23. B
4. A	14. C	24. D
5. B	15. C	25. C
6. C	16. B	26. A
7. B	17. C	27. B
8. C	18. A	28. C
9. A	19. A	29. B
10. B	20. D	30. A

Each response in question 31 is worth ½ point, or a total of 10 points for the entire question.

1. R	8. S	15. J
2. C	9. T	16. B
3. F	10. A	17. H
4. P	11. I	18. L
5. K	12. M	19. D
6. O	13. N	20. E
7. G	14. Q	

Start with 100 points. For questions 1 through 30, subtract 3 points for each wrong answer. In question 31, subtract ½ point for each wrong answer. You should try for a perfect score. If you scored between 80 and 100, you are doing well, but you should go back and check anything you missed. A score from 70 to 79 is good, but shows that you are having many problems and require more study. Anything below 70 means that you are having trouble, and you should see your instructor for additional help or hints for studying.

CHAPTER 9

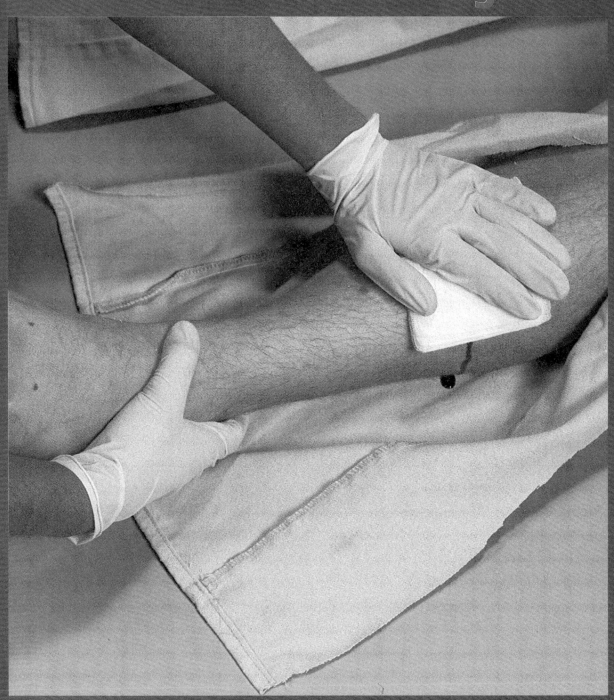

By the end of this chapter, you should be able to:

1. Define closed wound and open wound. (p. 196)
2. Classify open wounds by using the definitions for scratches and scrapes (abrasions), smooth and jagged cuts (incisions and lacerations), penetrating and perforating punctures, avulsions, amputations, and crush injuries. (pp. 196–198)
3. Cite the basic procedures used in caring for a closed wound. (pp. 199–200)
4. Cite the basic procedures used in caring for open wounds. (p. 200)
5. List the six steps used in caring for wounds with impaled objects. (p. 201)
6. Cite the basic procedures used in caring for avulsions, amputations, and crush injuries. (p. 202)
7. Define dressing, bulky dressing, occlusive dressing, and bandage. (pp. 203–204)
8. State the four basic rules applying to the dressing of wounds. (p. 205)
9. State the five basic rules applying to bandaging. (p. 205)
10. Cite the procedures of caring for cuts, burns, and foreign objects in the eye. (pp. 209–211)
11. List the special care for an eye injury with an impaled object. (pp. 211–212)
12. Describe the basic care for injuries to the ear. (p. 212)
13. Describe the basic care for nosebleeds and other nonfracture injuries to the nose. (p. 213)
14. Describe the basic care for injuries to the mouth. (pp. 213, 215)
15. List at least five signs of neck injury. (p. 215)
16. State the procedures for controlling arterial bleeding and venous bleeding from the neck. (pp. 215–217)
17. List at least seven signs of abdominal injury. (p. 217)
18. State the procedures used when caring for abdominal injuries. (p. 218)
19. Describe the basic care for injuries to the genitalia. (pp. 218–219)

SKILLS

Upon completing this chapter and your class lectures and skills lab, you should be able to:

1. Determine types of soft tissue injuries.
2. Control bleeding and apply the proper dressing and bandage for a given injury to the scalp, face, eye, ear, nose, mouth, neck, abdomen, pelvis, and genitalia.
3. Demonstrate the special care procedures for:
   - Impaled object in the eye
   - Severe bleeding from a neck vein
   - Severe bleeding from a neck artery
   - Impaled object in the cheek
   - Saving avulsed body parts
   - Amputations

RECOGNIZING INJURIES

As we grow from child to adult, we learn about injuries. Scratches, cuts, and bruises are learned in early childhood. Burns and fractures are recognized as injuries by the time we are in school. The idea of amputations and crush injuries are at least known, if not witnessed, before we enter our teens. Our own experiences and those of the people around us lead to our general understanding of injuries.

This prior knowlege will be useful to you. To be a First Responder, you will have to refine this knowledge, learning how to recognize and provide care for various injuries. However, you should not forget your basic understanding of injuries. Most of your patients will, at best, have the same level of understanding that you had when you started this course. Remembering this will help you with patient interviews and in providing explanations and reassurance. Also, recalling what you knew about injuries as you went through childhood will help when dealing with children who have suffered injuries.

So far, we have considered bleeding as a sign of injury. In this chapter and Chapters 10 through 12, you will learn to look for deformities, swellings, tenderness, breaks in the skin, and other signs of injury. Except for cases of spinal injury and certain types of internal injury, most adults can look at someone and often tell if there is an injury. Your training will build upon this ability so that you will not miss detectable injuries. This is why so much attention was paid to patient assessment and the secondary survey. As you progress through this course, you will be trained to determine the extent of injury and what specific emergency care procedures to use for given injuries.

In this chapter, we are concerned with injuries to soft tissues and to the internal organs of the body. Since you have just finished a study of life-threatening problems and basic life support, you might think that the injuries in this chapter are the next most serious problems faced by First Responders. With few exceptions, they are not. Look at the priorities of care on page 424 in Chapter 19. Some of these injuries are very serious, but many are not of a life-threatening nature. The more serious injuries are cared for first.

All this does not mean that the First Responder-level care for soft tissue and internal organ injuries is not important. Often, if left untreated, these injuries will lead to shock. In some cases, bleeding that has stopped will start again unless care is provided for the patient's soft tissue injuries.

Soft tissues—the tissues of the body that make up the skin, muscles, nerves, blood vessels, fatty tissues, and the cells that line and cover organs and glands. Bones, cartilage, and teeth are hard tissues.

FIGURE 9–1. Soft tissues.

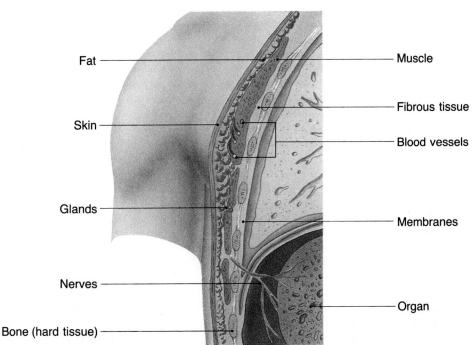

Fat — — Muscle

— Fibrous tissue

Skin — — Blood vessels

Glands — — Membranes

Nerves —

— Organ

Bone (hard tissue) —

The risk of infection is greatly reduced through proper soft tissue injury care. In addition to these considerations, there is the emotional well-being of the patient and the bystanders. The care provided at the First Responder level is usually understood by the patient and others at the scene. It is a comfort to them to see that something is being done.

Types of Injuries

When considering soft tissue injuries, a general classification can be used:

Closed wound—an internal soft tissue injury in which the skin is not broken.

1st Closed Wounds

A closed wound is an internal injury. The skin is not broken. As noted in the study of bleeding, internal injuries are usually caused by the impact of a blunt object. Bleeding can range from minor to major, while the extent of injury can range from a simple bruise to the rupturing of internal organs.

Bruises—simple closed wounds in which blood flows between soft tissues, causing a discoloration. A *contusion* (kun-TU-zhun).

BRUISES. The vast majority of closed wounds detected during First Responder care are bruises (contusions). There is always some internal bleeding associated with a bruise. Since the skin is not broken, the blood flows between tissues, causing a discoloration ranging from a brownish-yellow to black and blue. Keep in mind that large bruises can mean serious blood loss and that there may be fractures or extensive tissue damage under the site of the bruise.

Open wound—an injury to the body in which the skin or its outer layers are opened.

1st Open Wounds

The skin is damaged in cases of open wounds. The extent of injury can range from a single scrape to a tearing or cutting open of the skin. A simple scraping of the skin may produce no bleeding, while the more severe open wounds can have minor to life-threatening bleeding associated with the injury. Open wounds may be classifed as:

Scratches and scrapes—the simplest forms of open wounds that damage the skin surface but do not break all the layers of skin. Collectively, these injuries are called *abrasions* (ab-RAY-shuns).

SCRATCHES AND SCRAPES. Wounds such as skinned elbows and knees, "mat burns," "rug burns," and thorn scratches are minor open wounds known as abrasions (ab-RAY-shuns). Although scratches and scrapes may be painful, tissue injury is usually not serious since the skin is not fully penetrated and the force causing the injury does not crush or rupture underlying structures. There may be no detectable bleeding, or only minor capillary bleeding. Wound contamination tends to be the most serious problem faced when caring for abrasions to the skin.

FIGURE 9–2. Bruises are the most common form of closed wounds.

FIGURE 9–3. Scratches and scrapes (abrasions) are the least serious form of all open wound.

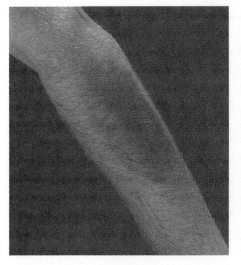

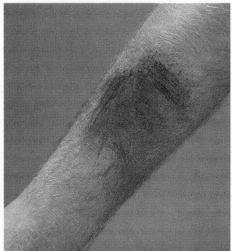

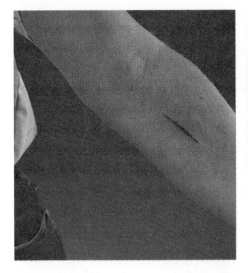

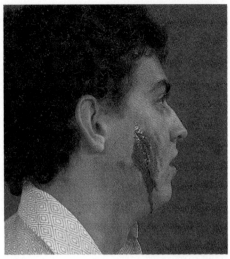

FIGURE 9–4. The edges of a smooth cut (incision) are straight.

FIGURE 9–5. Tissues along the edges of a jagged cut (laceration) will be torn and rough.

CUTS. In cases of cuts, the skin is fully penetrated, with injury also occurring to tissues lying under the skin. Cuts may be classified as **smooth** or **jagged:**

- Smooth cuts are called **incisions.** They are produced by very sharp objects, such as razor blades, knives, and broken glass. The edges of a smooth cut appear straight, with no apparent tears or jagged areas. Deep incisions can cause severe tissue damage and life-threatening bleeding.
- Jagged cuts are called **lacerations.** Tissue along the edge of the wound will be torn and a rough edge is produced. Sometimes jagged cuts can be produced from the impact of a blunt object. Usually, they occur when the skin is cut by an object that does not have a very sharp edge.

Cuts—soft tissue injuries in which all the layers of skin are opened and the tissues immediately below the skin are damaged. Smooth cuts are *incisions* and jagged cuts are *lacerations.*

PUNCTURES. Objects such as knives, nails, and ice picks can produce puncture wounds. An object puncturing the body will tear through the skin and usually proceed in a straight line, damaging all the tissues in its path. A puncture wound may be a **penetrating wound,** ranging from shallow to deep. Another type of puncture wound is a **perforating wound.** This injury, often seen with gunshot wounds, has an entrance and an exit wound, as the object passes through the body.

Punctures—an open wound that tears through the skin and damages tissues in a straight line. If there is an entrance and an exit wound, the puncture is called a *perforating* wound. If there is only an entrance wound, the puncture is called a *penetrating* wound.

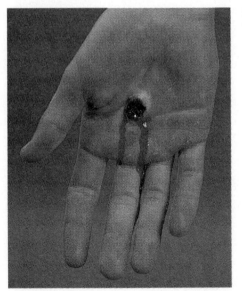

FIGURE 9–6. A penetrating puncture wound.

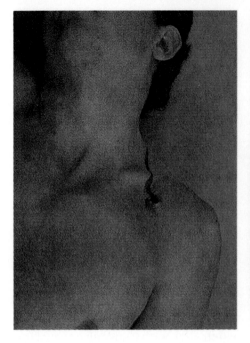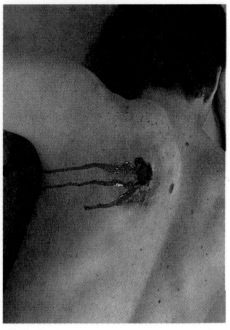

FIGURE 9–7. Puncture wounds can be perforating, having both an entrance wound and an exit wound. Often, the exit wound is the more serious of the two.

Avulsions (a-VUL-shuns)—a soft tissue injury in which flaps of skin are torn loose or torn off.

Amputations—soft tissue injuries that involve the cutting or tearing off of a limb or one of its parts. Often, hard tissues are also injured.

Crush injuries—soft tissue injuries produced by crushing forces. Soft tissues and internal organs are crushed and hard tissues are usually damaged.

AVULSIONS (a-VUL-shuns). These wounds most frequently involve the tearing loose or the tearing off of large flaps of skin. A torn ear, an eyeball removed from its socket, and the loss of a tooth are also examples of avulsions.

AMPUTATIONS. These wounds involve the cutting or tearing off of the fingers, toes, hands, feet, arms, or legs. Since amputation can be done as a surgical procedure, the injury is often called a traumatic (tra-MAT-ik) amputation.

CRUSH INJURIES. Most of the time, when people see an accident in which a body part has been crushed, their first thoughts are in terms of fractures. Soft tissues and internal organs are also crushed, often rupturing. Both external and internal bleeding can be profuse.

FIGURE 9–8. Avulsions are open wounds.   FIGURE 9–9. Amputation.

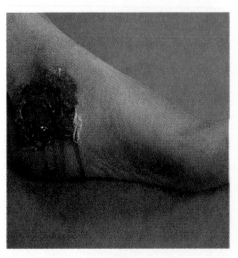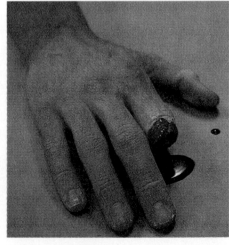

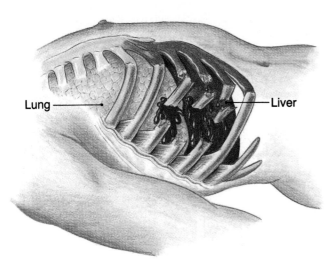

FIGURE 9–10. Soft tissues and internal organs are damaged in crush injuries.

BASIC EMERGENCY CARE

NOTE: Providing care for soft tissue injuries may place you in contact with blood and body fluids. Wear latex or vinyl gloves.

Closed Wounds

The most frequently seen closed wound is the bruise. Generally, bruises do not require emergency care in the field. However, bruises are a warning sign of possible internal injuries and related bleeding. Look for large bruises or large areas of the body covered with bruises. Remember that a deep bruise the size of the patient's fist equals a serious blood loss of about 10%. Be certain to look for swellings and deformities that may indicate fractures. Note if the patient's abdomen is rigid, if the patient is coughing up blood, or if there is blood in the mouth, nose, or ears.

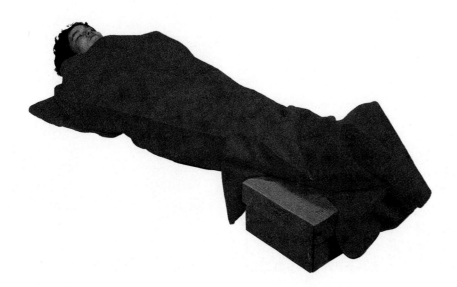

FIGURE 9–11. Always assume that there is serious internal bleeding when caring for closed wounds.

Later in this chapter we will consider some specific cases of internal injuries to soft tissues and body organs. For now, one general rule applies to the care given to patients with closed wounds:

1st Care for closed wounds as if there is internal bleeding, providing care for shock (see Chapter 7).

Open Wounds

1st In general, to care for open wounds you should:

1. **Expose the wound**—clothing over and around an open wound must be cut away. Avoid aggravating the patient's injuries. *Do not* try to remove clothing by pulling the items over the patient's head or limbs. Simply lift aside or cut the clothing away from the site of injury.

2. **Clear the wound surface**—remove foreign matter from the surface of the wound. If you have a sterile gauze pad, use this to clear the wound. This method will reduce the chances of contamination from your gloved fingers and will protect your fingertips. *Do not* try to clean the wound or pick out any particles or debris. If bleeding from the wound is controlled, take care not to restart or increase the flow of blood.

3. **Control bleeding**—start with direct pressure or direct pressure and elevation. If the bleeding continues, try pressure point control. A tourniquet should be used as a last resort for life-threatening bleeding from a limb.

4. **Prevent further contamination**—use a sterile dressing, clean cloth, or clean handkerchief to cover the wound. After the bleeding has been controlled, bandage the dressing in place.

5. **Keep the patient lying still**—any patient activity increases circulation. Keep the patient lying down, using a blanket or other form of covering to provide protection from the elements.

6. **Reassure the patient**—this will reduce patient movement and may help to lower the patient's blood pressure toward a normal level.

7. **Care for shock**—this applies to all but the simplest of wounds. *Do not* elevate a limb if there is the possibility of a fracture.

FIGURE 9–12. 1. Expose the wound. 2. Unless bleeding is profuse, clear the wound surface. 3. Apply direct pressure to control bleeding and prevent further contamination. 4. Keep the patient lying down, provide care for shock, and reassure the patient.

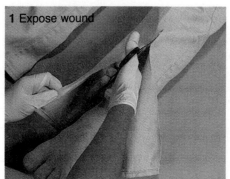

1 Expose wound

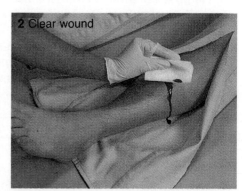

2 Clear wound

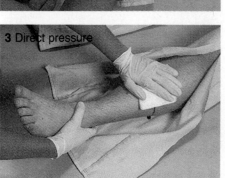

3 Direct pressure

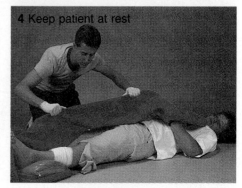

4 Keep patient at rest

REMEMBER: *Do not* remove a dressing once it is in place.

NOTE: If you have to control serious bleeding from an extremity, or the wound on the limb is a long cut, immobilize the limb with a splint (see Chapters 10 and 11) after dressing the wound. If you carry an air-inflated splint as part of your First Responder equipment, use this splint to help control the bleeding.

Puncture Wounds

1st When dealing with any puncture wound, assume that there is extensive internal injury and internal bleeding. Always look for an exit wound, realizing that exit wounds can be more serious than entrance wounds. Care for entrance and exit wounds as you would any open wound in soft tissue.

1st If the puncture wound contains an impaled object (such as a shard of glass, a knife blade, or a piece of wood, metal, or plastic), do the following:

1. **Do not remove the impaled object.**
2. Expose the wound, without disturbing the impaled object. *Do not* lift clothing over the object.
3. Control bleeding by direct hand pressure (wear gloves). **Caution:** Take special care not to cut your hand on the impaled object. Spread your fingers around the object and apply pressure to the wound site. *Do not* put any pressure on the object or the tissues that are up against the edge of a sharp impaled object.
4. Attempt to stabilize the impaled object by using bulky dressings. Several layers of dressings, cloths, or handkerchiefs placed on the sides of the object will help stabilize it. An alternate approach is to cut a hole in the center of a bulky dressing, making the cut slightly larger than the impaled object. *Gently* pass the dressing over the object. Bandaging these dressings in place will improve stability.
5. Keep the patient at rest and reassured.
6. Care for shock. *Do not* elevate a limb if the object is impaled in it, the abdomen, or the pelvis.

NOTE: The above procedures do not apply to objects impaled in the eye or in the cheeks. The correct procedures for these two cases will be covered later in this chapter.

Adhesive tape often does not stick to the skin around an impaled object wound site. Blood and sweat on the skin, even when the surface is cleared, may cause the tape to slip. Cravats (cloth ties) can be used to tie the dressings in place. These cravats should be made from folded cloth. Once folded, the cravats should be at least 4 inches wide. If the object is impaled in the chest or abdomen, a thin splint or coat hanger can be used to push the cravats under the natural void in the patient's back so that the cravat can be tied around the patient's trunk.

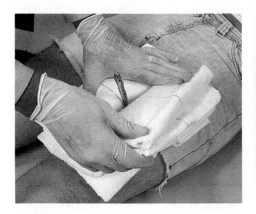 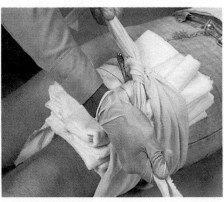

FIGURE 9–13. A. Expose the wound and control bleeding. B. Stabilize the impaled object.

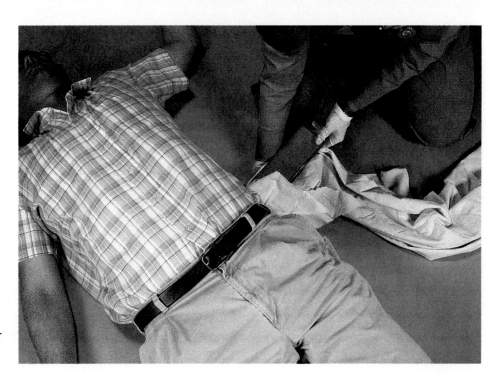

FIGURE 9–14. A flat splint or coat hanger can be used to position the cravat.

Avulsions

1st If flaps of skin have been torn loose, but not off, you should:

1. Clear the surface of the wound.
2. Gently fold the skin back to its normal position.
3. Control bleeding and care as you would for any open wound, using bulky pressure dressings.

1st If skin or another body part is torn from the body, you should:

1. Care for the wound with bulky pressure dressings.
2. Save and preserve the avulsed part. This is best done by placing the avulsed part into a plastic bag or wrapping the part in plastic wrap or sterile dressing. If possible, keep the part cool (not cold, avoid freezing). *Do not* place the avulsed part in water or in direct contact with ice.

Amputations

1st In most cases, bleeding can be controlled by direct pressure applied with a dressing held firmly over the stump. Pressure point techniques should be tried along with direct pressure if the bleeding continues. Should this fail, then apply a tourniquet. If possible, wrap or bag the amputated part in plastic and keep it cool.

Protruding Organs

1st A deep open wound to the abdomen may cause organs to protrude through the wound opening. In such cases:

- *Do not* try to replace the organ(s).
- Place a plastic covering over the exposed organs. If possible, apply a thick pad dressing over top of this covering to help conserve heat.
- Provide care for shock, and do not give the patient anything by mouth.

DRESSING AND BANDAGING

Many people, when first studying emergency care procedures, are worried about learning all the special procedures used in "bandaging" wounds. Actually, in First Responder care, there are few "special" techniques for you to learn. If the patient will benefit from a special procedure, this procedure will be presented. Otherwise, if you follow the basic principles of dressing and bandaging wounds, you will provide effective care for the patient. **1st** To begin, you should know the following definitions:

- **Dressing**—any material used to cover a wound that will help control bleeding and help prevent additional contamination.
- **Bandage**—any material used to hold a dressing in place.

Types of Dressings

Whenever possible, dressings should be sterile. This means that they have been processed so that all germs, and the spores that can grow into active germs are killed. Dressings are also aseptic, meaning that all dirt and foreign debris have been removed. Commercially prepared dressings are aseptic and are usually sterile. Typically, they are gauze pads, individually wrapped. They come in a variety of sizes, with the most common size being 4 inches square. They are referred to according to size, such as 2 by 2's and 4 by 4's.

Throughout this text, you will find reference to **bulky dressings** and multitrauma dressings. These are thick dressings, often large enough to allow for the complete covering of large wounds. They are used to help control very serious bleeding and to stabilize impaled objects. Sanitary napkins can be used in place of these dressings. They are available individually wrapped. While sanitary napkins are not sterile, they are very clean on

Dressing—any material used to cover a wound that will help control bleeding and reduce contamination.

Bandage—any material that is used to hold a dressing in place.

Bulky dressing—a thick single dressing or a buildup of thin dressings used to help control profuse bleeding, stabilize impaled objects, or cover large open wounds.

FIGURE 9–15. Dressings cover wounds, while bandages hold dressings in place.

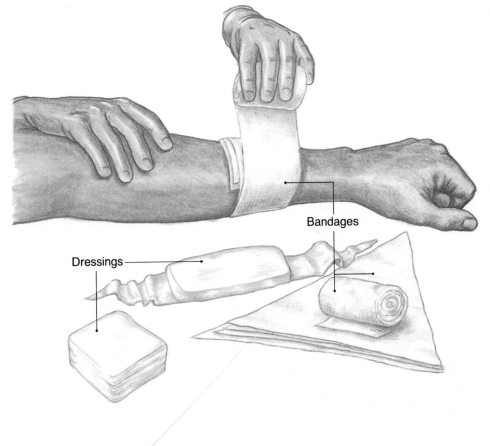

Bandages

Dressings

their surfaces (avoid applying any adhesive surface directly to the wound). Bulky dressings can be formed simply by applying many layers of simple gauze dressings.

Occlusive dressing—a dressing used to create an airtight seal or to close an open wound of a body cavity. Usually, it is made of plastic.

Another type of special dressing is the **occlusive dressing.** This is used when it is necessary to close an open wound that penetrates a body cavity. Commercially prepared occlusive dressing pads are available. If these are not on hand, you can use folded plastic wrap or a plastic bag to help seal off a penetrating wound to the chest or abdomen.*

1st Often, a First Responder will not have any dressing materials at the scene of an emergency. In such cases, you will have to use clean handkerchiefs, towels, sheets, and other similar materials. The patient's wound has already been contaminated. Your task is to avoid further contamination by using the cleanest material available. The hospital has special wound-cleansing procedures and antibiotics to care for wound contamination and infection. In the field you must be concerned with controlling bleeding and reducing contamination. When you improvise to make a dressing, it will not be sterile, but it can be used to help provide proper care for the patient.

Bandaging Materials

1st Dressings are more effective if they are held in place. Usually, this is done by taping or tying. The adhesive bandage has a sticky backing that will adhere to the patient's skin. If no such bandaging material is on hand, tie a dressing in place by using gauze roller bandage, a handkerchief, strips of cloth, or any other material that will not cut into the patient's skin. *Do not* use elastic bandages that are often used for strains and sprains to the joints. This type of bandage may restrict circulation and will apply undesired pressure to the injured tissues.

The use of self-adherent, form-fitting, gauze roller bandage eliminates the need for highly specialized bandaging techniques. Most of these techniques were developed for use with ordinary gauze roller bandage. The self-adherent roller bandage does not have an adhesive backing, yet clings to itself, making the task of wrapping the bandage around the dressing easier, quicker, and more efficient.

Have the students give examples of what items at the emergency scene may be used for dressings and bandages.

* Some EMS Systems allow aluminum foil to be used instead of plastic. There are reports that this foil can cut internal organs.

FIGURE 9–16. The application of self-adherent roller bandage.

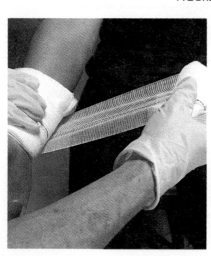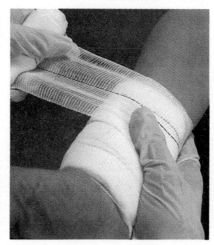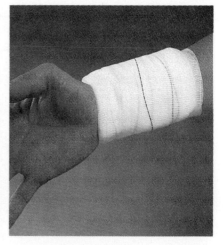

Rules for Dressing and Bandaging

1st The following rules apply to dressing wounds:

1. **Control bleeding**—it does little good to apply a dressing and bandage it in place if the dressing does not help to control bleeding. Continue to apply dressing material and pressure as needed to control bleeding.
2. **Use sterile or clean materials**—avoid touching the dressing in the area that will come into contact with the wound.
3. **Cover the entire wound**—the dressing should cover the entire surface of the wound and, if possible, the immediate area surrounding the wound.
4. **Do not remove dressings**—once a dressing is applied to a wound, it must remain in place. Add new dressings on top of blood-soaked dressings.

When a dressing is removed from a wound, there may be a restart of bleeding or an increase in the rate of bleeding. Because of this, a dressing should remain in place once it is applied to a wound. Removal should be done in the emergency department. There is an exception to this rule in some EMS Systems (do only what you have been trained to do). If a bulky dressing becomes blood-soaked, you may have to remove it so that direct pressure can be reestablished or a new bulky pad or dressing can be applied.

You may prevent an increase in bleeding rate or damage to wound tissue if you apply simple gauze dressing pads to the wound site before applying a bulky dressing. This will improve the chances of removing the bulky dressing without directly disturbing the wound.

1st The following rules apply to bandaging:

1. **Do not bandage too tightly**—hold the dressing snugly in place, but *do not restrict blood supply to* the affected area.
2. **Do not bandage too loosely**—the dressing must not be allowed to move on top of the wound or slip from the wound.
3. **Do not leave loose ends**—keep in mind that the patient will have to be moved. Loose ends of tape, dressing, or cloth might get caught on objects when the patient is being moved.
4. **Do not cover fingers and toes**—dressing materials and bandages should not cover the tips of the patient's fingers or toes unless the digits are injured. These areas must be exposed so that you can watch for color changes indicating a change in circulation or that the bandage is too tight. Blue skin, pale skin, and complaints of numbness, pain, and tingling sensations all indicate that the bandage may be too tight.
5. **Bandage from the bottom of a limb to the top** (distal to proximal)— the bandage should be wrapped around the limb starting at its far (distal) end and working toward its origin or near (proximal) end. Taking such action will reduce the chances of restricting circulation and wrapping too tightly.

Two additional rules for bandaging must be considered when the wound is on a limb:

1. Avoid applying the bandage to a small area. This can produce enough pressure to restrict circulation. Instead, wrap a large area of the limb, making certain to maintain uniform pressure as you wrap the bandage.
2. Do not bend a joint if it is bandaged. Sometimes it is necessary to apply the bandage across a joint. Once the bandage is in place, movement of the joint may restrict circulation or cause the bandage and dressing to loosen.

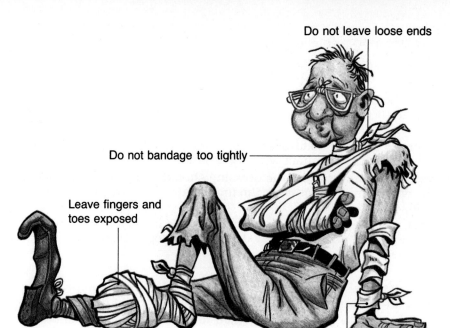

Do not leave loose ends

Do not bandage too tightly

Leave fingers and
toes exposed

Do not bandage loosely

FIGURE 9–17. The rules of
bandaging.

SPECIFIC INJURIES

In this section we will be concerned with specific injuries to soft tissues and to the internal organs of the abdomen and pelvis. Injuries to bony tissue will be considered in Chapters 10 through 12. Chest injuries will be covered in Chapter 12.

The Scalp and Face

Injuries to the scalp and face can be difficult to treat because of the numerous blood vessels found in both regions. Many of these vessels are close to the surface of the skin, producing profuse bleeding even from minor wounds. Additional problems arise if the bones of the skull are involved, the airway is obstructed, and neck injuries occur.

Injuries to the scalp and face require an extra effort on the part of the First Responder to provide emotional support for patients. These injuries tend to be very painful, produce bleeding that frightens many patients, and are in a body region where everyone worries about scars and deformities. Talk to patients in a calm, professional manner. Always let them know what you are going to do before you do it. Make certain that they know additional help is on the way.

1st The procedures for the care of soft tissue injuries covered earlier in this chapter apply to the care you should provide for injuries to the soft tissues of the scalp and face. However, there are three exceptions:

Exception 1: *Do Not* attempt to clear the surface of a scalp wound. This will often cause additional bleeding and may cause great harm if there are fractures to the skull.

Exception 2: *DO NOT* apply finger pressure to the wound if there is any chance of skull fracture.

Exception 3: *DO* remove impaled objects from the cheek if the object has penetrated the cheek wall and may become an airway obstruction.

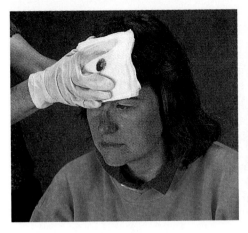
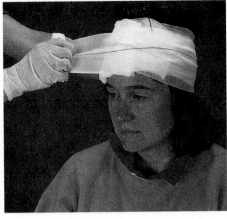

FIGURE 9–18. Providing care for scalp wounds: control bleeding with a sterile or clean dressing and then bandage dressing in place.

1st Care of Scalp Wounds

1. Do not clear the wound.
2. Control bleeding with a dressing held in place with controlled pressure. Avoid exerting any finger pressure if there are signs of a fractured skull or the injury site feels "spongy."
3. Adhesive bandages will not work well. Roller bandage or gauze can be wrapped around the patient's head to hold dressings in place once bleeding has been controlled. If there is any indication of neck or spinal injuries, *do not* attempt to wrap the patient's head. *Do not* wrap the bandage around the patient's lower jaw or neck.
4. If there are no signs of skull fracture, or injuries to the spine, neck, or chest, you may position the patient so that the head and shoulders are elevated.

An optional approach to holding a dressing in place over a scalp wound is to use a commercially prepared triangular bandage or one made from gauze or some other cloth. The steps for this procedure are shown in Figure 9–19.

FIGURE 9–19. Fold the bandage several times to make a two-inch hem along its base. B. Have the folded edge face out when you position the bandage on the patient's forehead, just above the eyes. Make certain that the point of the bandage hangs down behind the patient's head. C. Draw the ends of the bandage behind patient's head and tie them over the point of the bandage. D. Next, pull the ends to the front of the patient's head and tie them together. E. Finally, bring the point of the bandage down and tuck it into the crossed folds.

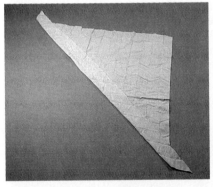

A

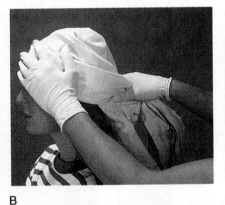

B

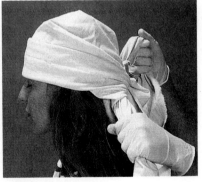

C

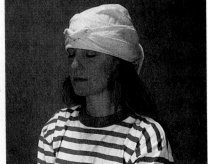

D

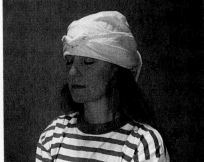

E

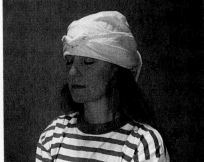

Care of Facial Wounds

The first concern when caring for facial injuries is to make certain that the patient's airway is open and breathing is adequate. Even though bleeding appears to be the only problem, check the airway and establish the presence of a carotid pulse. Continue to watch the patient to be sure that the airway remains open.

1st When caring for patients with facial injuries, you should:

1. Correct breathing problems, taking care to note and properly care for neck and spinal injuries.
2. Control bleeding by direct pressure, taking care not to press too hard since many facial fractures are not obvious.
3. Apply a dressing and bandage.

1st If you find the patient has an object impaled in the cheek that has passed through the cheek wall and is sticking into the mouth, you may have to remove the object from the cheek. This should be done if the object is loose and may fall into the airway. To remove an impaled object from the cheek, you should:

1. Look into the mouth and probe to see if the object has passed through the cheek wall.
2. If you find penetration, *pull* or safely *push* the object out of the cheek wall, back in the direction that the object entered the cheek. If the object has not penetrated the cheek wall, or if you cannot easily remove the object, stabilize it with dressings applied to the outer surface of the cheek.
3. In all cases, except for neck and spinal injuries, turn the patient so that blood will drain from the mouth. If there are neck or spinal injuries, *do not* turn the patient. Use dressing material packed against the inside wound to control the flow of blood.
4. If you removed an impaled object, pack the inside of the patient's mouth with dressing material. Place the material between the wound and the patient's teeth, leaving some of the dressing outside the mouth so that it can be held to prevent swallowing. Watch closely to be sure this material does not work its way loose and into the airway. Do not assume that the patient's swallow reflex will prevent this material from becoming a major obstruction.
5. Dress and bandage the outside of the wound.

FIGURE 9–20. Care of soft tissue injuries to the face.

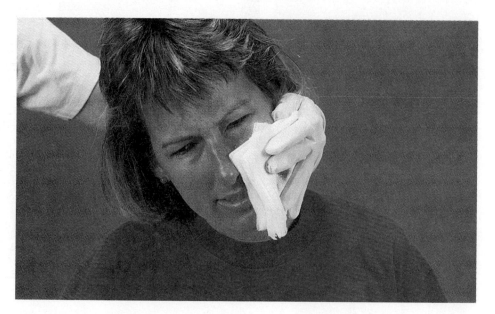

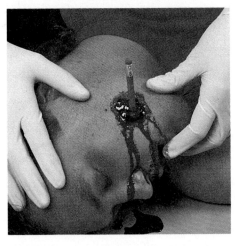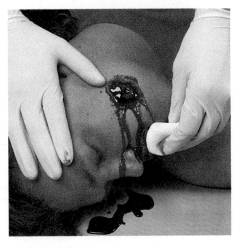

FIGURE 9–21. Removing an impaled object from the cheek.

Eye Injuries

Two rules of soft tissue injury care apply when caring for an eye injury. *Do not* remove any impaled objects and do not try to put the eye back into its socket. When caring for a cut eyeball, there is one major exception to the procedures listed for soft tissue injury care:

1st Exception

Do not apply direct pressure on a cut eyeball. There are jellylike fluids inside the eyeball that cannot be replaced. A loose bulky dressing will help the formation of blood clots to control the bleeding.

Problems resulting from foreign objects in the eyes are common occurrences. These problems can range from minor irritations to permanent injury caused by sharp objects. If the patient's own tears do not wash away the foreign object(s), use running water to remove them. **Do not apply the wash if there are impaled objects in the eye or cuts in the eye.**

Apply the flow at the corner of the eye socket closest to the patient's nose. You may have to help the patient hold open the eyelids. As you pour the water into the eyes, direct the patient to look from side to side and up and down. Before completing the wash, have the patient blink several times. When possible, continue the wash for 20 minutes or for the time recommended by your EMS System's medical advisor.

FIGURE 9–22. Foreign objects can be washed from the eye.

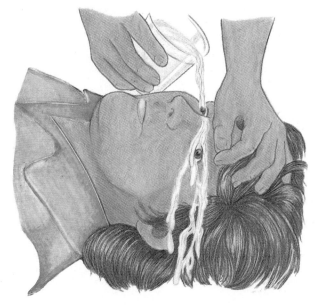

1st It is critical that you:

- *Do not* remove impaled objects (including what may appear to be small pieces of glass impaled in the globe of the eye).
- *Do not* probe into the eye socket.
- Reduce the patient's eye movements. If there are sharp objects in the patient's eye, do not direct the patient to move the eyes during the wash, even though they will have some natural movement. After the wash, keep the patient's eyes shut. Cover both eyes, bandaging the materials in place.

NOTE: After debris is washed from the eye, the patient must be examined by someone with more advanced training. A physician or qualified eye care specialist should see the patient.

Whenever you are caring for a patient with eye injuries, you will have to cover both eyes. In most cases, only one eye will actually be injured. However, when one eye moves, the other eye will also move (sympathetic movement). If you cover the injured eye and leave the uninjured eye uncovered, the uninjured eye will continue to react to activities and movement. Each time the uninjured eye moves, so will the injured eye. Having both of the patient's eyes covered reduces eye movements.

Obviously, a patient with both eyes covered will not be able to see, causing fear and uncertainty. Tell the patient why you are covering the uninjured eye. Keep close to the patient or have someone else stay close. Try to maintain contact with the patient through conversation and touch. If a friend or loved one of the patient also has been injured, reassure the patient that care is being provided for others.

If the patient is unconscious, it is best to keep someone with him or her at all times. This person can reassure the patient if consciousness returns and can help prevent the patient from reaching for his covered eyes. Should the unconscious patient have to be left unattended, you may tie the hands at the waist to prevent the grabbing of the eyes should consciousness be regained. Even though this may produce a fearful moment for the patient, it is better than the additional injury that could take place. Any procedure that requires the tying of the patient's hands must be approved by your EMS System.

1st Always remember to close the eyelids of unconscious patients. Since unconscious people do not blink, moisture is quickly lost from the eye surface, damaging the eye. If you notice that the patient is wearing contact lenses, be sure to point this out to the EMTs who take over the care of the patient.

Burns to the eye must always be considered serious, requiring special in-hospital care. The actions taken by a First Responder can often make the difference as to whether or not the patient's sight can be saved. As a First Responder, you may have to care for burns to the eyes caused by heat, light, or chemicals.

- **1st Heat burns**—most often, only the eyelids will be burned. *Do not* try to inspect the eyes if there are signs of heat burn to the eyelids. With the patient's eyelids closed, cover the eyes with loose, moist dressings. If you have no means to moisten the dressings, then apply loose, dry dressings. *Do not* apply any burn ointment to the eyelids.
- **Light burns**—"snow blindness" and "welder's blindness" are two examples of light burns. Close the patient's eyelids and apply dark patches over both eyes. If you do not have dark patches, then use thick dressings or dressings followed with a layer of an opaque material such as dark plastic.
- **Chemical burns**—many chemicals cause rapid, severe damage to the

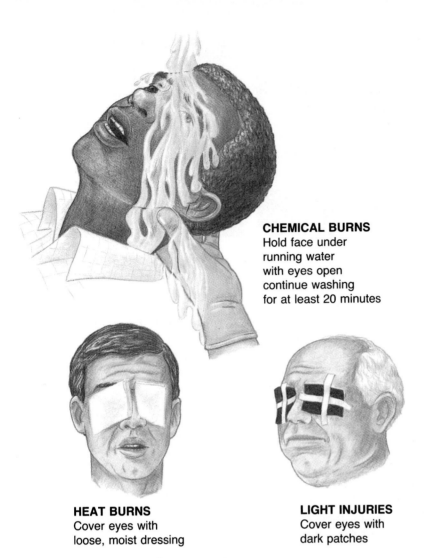

CHEMICAL BURNS
Hold face under
running water
with eyes open
continue washing
for at least 20 minutes

HEAT BURNS
Cover eyes with
loose, moist dressing

LIGHT INJURIES
Cover eyes with
dark patches

FIGURE 9–23.   Basic care for burns to the eyes.

eyes. Flush the eyes with water. Do not delay care by trying to locate sterile water. Use any source of clean drinking water. If possible, continue the washing flow for at least **20 minutes.** After washing the patient's eyes, close the eyelids and apply loose, moist dressings.

1st If you find an object impaled in the globe of a patient's eye, you should:

1. Use several layers of dressing or small rolls of gauze to make thick pads to be placed on the sides of the object. If you have only enough material for one thick pad, cut a hole, equal to the size of the eye opening, in the center of this pad. Set the pad over the patient's eye, allowing the impaled object to stick out through the opening cut into the pad.
2. Fit a disposable cardboard drinking cup (do *not* use Styrofoam) or paper cone over the impaled object. This will serve as a protective shield. Rest the cup or cone onto the thick dressing pad, but do not allow this protective shield to come into contact with the impaled object.
3. Hold the pad and protective shield in place with self-adherent roller bandage or with a wrapping of gauze or other cloth material.
4. Use dressing material to cover the uninjured eye and bandage this dressing in place. This will reduce eye movements.
5. Provide care for shock.
6. Provide emotional support to the patient.

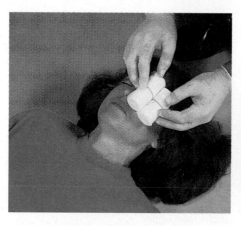 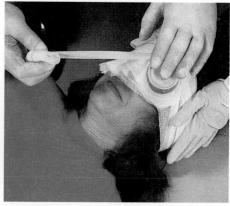

FIGURE 9–24. Caring for a patient who has an object impaled in the globe of the eye.

Wrapping a paper cup or cone with gauze is very tricky and cannot be done easily unless you practice. Ideally, you should wrap around the cup and then continue around the patient's head and wrap around the cup again. This procedure is repeated until the cup is stable. *Do not* wrap the gauze over the top of the cup. *Take great care* not to push the cup down onto the impaled object or pull the cup out of place.

1st If the eye is pulled out of the socket (avulsed eye), the care provided is the same as for an object impaled in the eye.

External Ear Injuries

- Cuts—apply dressing and bandage in place.
- Tears—apply bulky dressings, beginning with several layers behind the torn tissue.
- Avulsions—use bulky dressings, bandaged into place. Save the avulsed part in a plastic bag or plastic wrap. Keep the part dry and cool. If no plastic is available, then wrap in dressing material. Be certain to label the bag, wrap, or dressing.

Internal Ear Injuries

NOTE: Any bleeding from the ear must be considered a sign of serious head injury. Bloody or clear fluids draining from the ear may indicate the presence of cerebrospinal fluid (see Chapter 3) associated with severe head injury. For such cases, assume there is serious injury and provide the necessary care. More will be said about head injuries in Chapter 12.

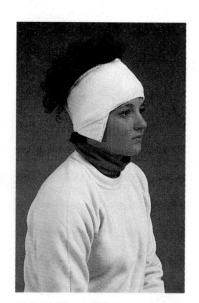

FIGURE 9–25. When caring for injuries to the external ear, apply a dressing and bandage in place.

- Bleeding from the Ears—*Do not* pack the external ear canal. To do so may cause increased internal injury. Apply external dressings and hold these in place with bandages. Report this bleeding to the EMTs.
- Foreign Objects in the Ear—*Do not* attempt to remove the objects. Apply external dressings if necessary and provide emotional support to the patient.
- Bloody or Clear Fluids Draining from the Ears—*Do not* pack the external ear canal. Apply a loose, external dressing. This dressing should be sterile, but any clean dressing will do if a sterile dressing is not available (see Chapter 12).
- "Clogged" or "Stopped up" Ear—damage to the ear drum, fluids in the middle ear, and objects in the ear canal all can cause the patient to complain of "clogged" or "stopped up" ears. *Do not* probe into the ears. Many of these problems will go away without care or quickly after hospital care. As a First Responder, your main duty in such cases is to prevent the patient from hitting the side of the head in an effort to clear the ears. These blows may cause severe internal ear damage.

Nose Injuries

1st For now, we will assume that there are no skull fractures or spinal injuries. When dealing with any nasal injuries, you will have two duties:

1. Maintain an open airway
2. Stop bleeding

You may be called upon to care for:

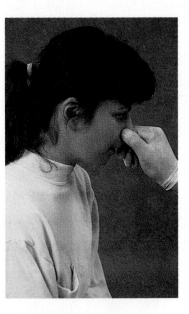

- **1st** Nosebleeds—maintain an open airway. Have the patient assume a seated position, leaning slightly forward. This position will help prevent blood and mucus from obstructing the airway or draining down the throat and causing nausea and vomiting. Next, have the patient pinch the nostrils. Bleeding is usually controlled when the nostrils are pinched shut. If the patient cannot pinch them shut, you will have to do so. However, if other patients are in need of your help, do not delay their care while you sit pinching someone's nose. Have a bystander put on gloves and pinch the patient's nose and inform you of any problems as you continue to care for the other patients. *Do not* pack the patient's nostrils.

FIGURE 9–26. Caring for nosebleeds. Remember to position the patient for proper drainage.

- Nosebleeds (unconscious patients)—if patients are unresponsive or injured in such a way that they cannot be placed into a seated position, lay them back with the head slightly elevated or place them on one side with the head turned to provide drainage from the nose and mouth. Attempt to control bleeding by pinching the nostrils shut.

REMEMBER: A First Responder must apply knowledge to make decisions. You must judge the severity of bleeding in cases of nosebleeds. Most are minor, requiring very little attention. However, nosebleeds can be serious, with profuse bleeding. You will have to care for them accordingly.

- Fluids Draining from the Nose—*Do not* pack the nose. Bloody or clear fluids may indicate skull fractures (see Chapter 12).
- Foreign Objects in the Nose—*Do not* remove objects or probe into the nose. *Do not* allow the patient to blow his nose if he is bleeding from the nostrils or has recently controlled a nosebleed.
- Avulsions—apply a pressure dressing to the site. Save the avulsed part in plastic or a sterile or clean dressing. Keep the part cool.

NOTE: Nasal fractures will be covered in Chapter 12.

1st Injury to the Mouth

As with all injuries that occur along the pathway of respiration, your first concern will be to ensure an open airway. If there are no suspected skull, neck, or spinal injuries, position the patient in a seated position with the head tilted slightly forward to allow for drainage. If the patient cannot be placed in a seated position, position him or her on one side with the head turned slightly downward to provide some drainage for blood and other fluids.

- Cut Lips—use a rolled or folded dressing. Place this dressing between the patient's lip and gum. Take great care that the patient does not swallow this dressing.
- Avulsed Lips—apply a pressure bandage to the site of injury and save the avulsed part in plastic or a sterile or clean dressing. Keep the avulsed part cool.
- Cuts to the Internal Cheek—*Do not* pack the mouth with dressings.

■ SCAN 9–1.

Soft Tissue Injury Care: The Head

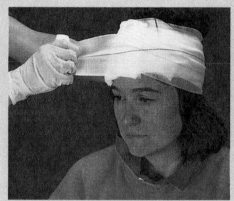

Scalp

Control bleeding.

Dress.

Wrap with roller bandage.

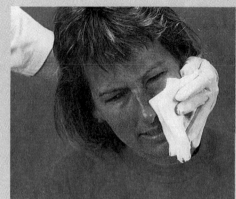

Facial

Ensure airway.

Control bleeding.

Dress and wrap with roller bandage.

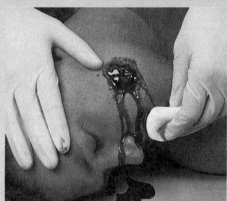

Cheek

Ensure airway.

Remove impaled objects.

Control bleeding.

Dress and bandage (external).

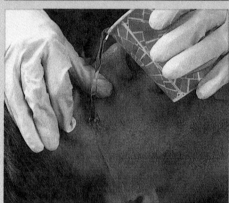

Debris In Eye

If eye is not cut, wash objects from surface.

Eye Burns

Wash chemical burns.

Loosely dress heat burns.

Dark patches for light burns.

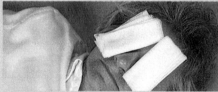

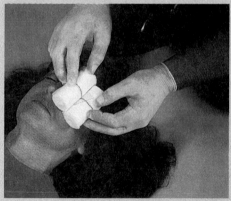

Impaled Object: Eye

Stabilize object. Apply rigid protection.

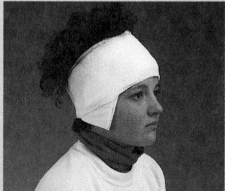

Ear Wound

Do not pack canal.

Dress and bandage.

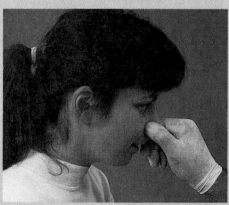

Nose Bleed

Pinch nostrils shut.

Any dressing positioned between the patient's cheek and gum will have to be held in place by a gloved hand. Always leave 3 to 4 inches of dressing material outside the patient's mouth. This will allow for quick removal. This is necessary to prevent the patient from swallowing the dressing. If possible, position the patient's head to allow drainage.

NOTE: Injuries to the bones of the skull and face and avulsed teeth will be covered in Chapter 12.

1st Neck Wounds

Blunt and sharp injuries can occur to the neck (fractures will be covered in Chapter 12). As a first Responder, be aware of the following signs that indicate neck wounds:

- Difficulty with speaking, loss of voice
- Airway obstruction when the mouth and nose are clear and no object can be dislodged from the airway. This is often due to swollen tissues.
- Obvious swelling or bruising of the neck
- Tracheal deviation (windpipe pushed off to one side)
- Depressions in the neck
- Obvious cuts or puncture wounds

1st For all profuse bleeding from blood vessels in the neck, make certain that someone alerts dispatch, informing them of the problem and the need for immediate EMS transport. Cut or severed arteries in the neck require the following procedure:

1. *Immediately* apply direct pressure over the wound using the palm of your gloved hand.
2. Try controlling the bleeding with a pressure dressing, taking care not to close the airway and not to apply pressure to both sides of the neck.
3. Once the bleeding is controlled, place the patient on the left side. If possible, lay the patient on a surface that can be slanted (table, long bench, plywood) so that the entire body can be tilted into a head-down position. The slant should be no more than 15 degrees. This will help trap any air bubbles that may have entered the bloodstream.
4. Provide care for shock.

FIGURE 9–27. When possible, place the patient on the left side with the body slanted into a head-down position.

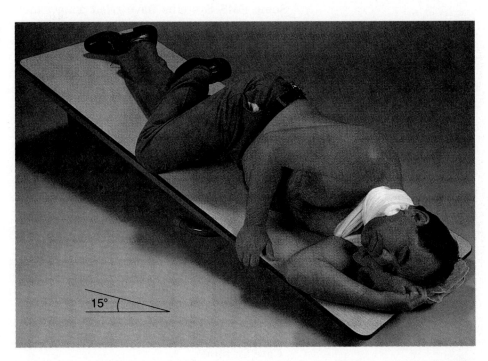

15°

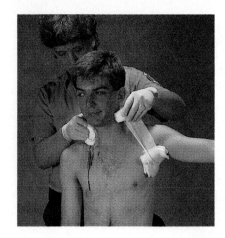 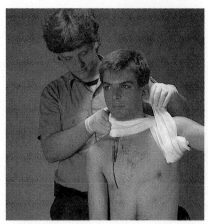 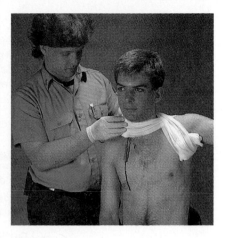

FIGURE 9–28.   Use an occlusive dressing to help control bleeding from the neck.

WARNING: *Do not* attempt to reposition the patient if there are indications of spinal injury (very likely), if the bleeding was very difficult to control (usually the case), or if you had difficulty carrying out the dressing and bandaging procedures (true for most rescuers).

1st Bleeding from large cut or severed neck veins usually cannot be controlled by pressure dressings. For such emergencies, you should:

1. *Immediately* apply direct pressure to the wound using the palm of your gloved hand.
2. Apply an occlusive dressing of plastic wrap.
3. Use tape to seal this dressing on all sides. When completed, the dressing must be airtight.
4. Position the patient on the left side, with the body slanted as described above (see WARNING). There is a greater chance of air entering the blood when a large vein is opened.
5. Provide care for shock.

If you do not have the materials to make an occlusive dressing, use any sterile or clean dressing material and attempt to control bleeding by direct pressure.

Some EMS Systems have tried a new method for controlling profuse bleeding from the blood vessels in the neck. Their success indicates that other EMS Systems may be adopting this method. Your instructor will tell you if this technique is approved for use in your state.

The newer method uses the same procedure for both arterial and venous bleeding. If the patient is bleeding from the neck, you should:

1. *Immediately* apply direct pressure over the wound using the palm of your gloved hand.
2. Place a plastic occlusive dressing over the wound and continue to apply pressure using the palm of your hand. *Do not* use a single layer of plastic wrap. It is too thin and may be sucked into the wound. Ideally, the occlusive dressing should extend 1 inch beyond the wound on all sides.

*Another roll can be placed between the wound and the trachea to help reduce pressure on the trachea.

3. Place a roll of gauze dressing or dressing materials over the occlusive dressing and continue to apply pressure.*
4. While maintaining pressure, secure the entire dressing with a figure-eight wrap of self-adherent roller bandage (see Figure 9–29). This eliminates the problem of trying to make adhesive tape stick to a bloody surface.
5. Place the patient on the left side, with the body slightly slanted in a head-down position.
6. Care for shock.

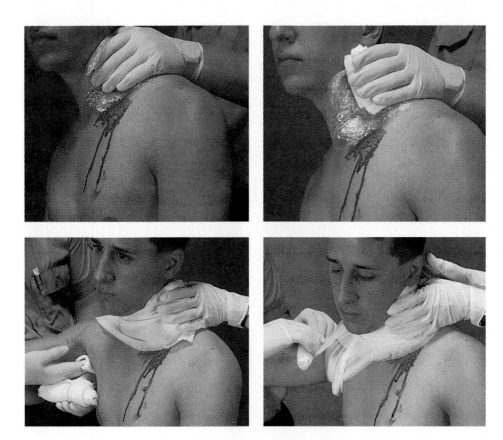

FIGURE 9–29. Securing the dressing in cases involving profuse bleeding from the neck.

All these methods take a great deal of practice and review if they are to be done correctly in the field.

Should your attempts to control the bleeding fail, a last-resort method would be to place your gloved finger or fingers into the wound and attempt to compress the vessel or pinch shut the ends. This a very difficult procedure that has little chance for success. If the vessel has been severed, the ends may have shifted or rolled away from the wound opening, making success even less likely. Again, this is a last resort to be used only when standard First Responder-level care procedures have failed to control life-threatening profuse bleeding.

Abdominal Injuries

In Chapter 2, we studied the positions of the various body organs. Before continuing with this section of Chapter 9, study Figures 9–30 and 9–31 to review the locations of the major hollow and solid organs of the abdomen and pelvis.

Internal bleeding can be severe when an internal organ ruptures. In addition, hollow organs can rupture and drain their contents into the abdominal and pelvic cavities, producing a very serious and painful reaction. As a First Responder, you should be aware of the following signs that indicate injury to the abdominopelvic organs:

- Any deep cut or puncture wound to the abdomen, pelvis, or lower back
- Indications of blunt trauma to the abdomen or pelvis
- Pain or cramps in the abdominopelvic region
- The patient is protecting the abdomen (guarded abdomen)
- The patient is trying to lie still with legs drawn up
- Rapid, shallow breathing and a rapid pulse
- Rigid and/or tender abdomen

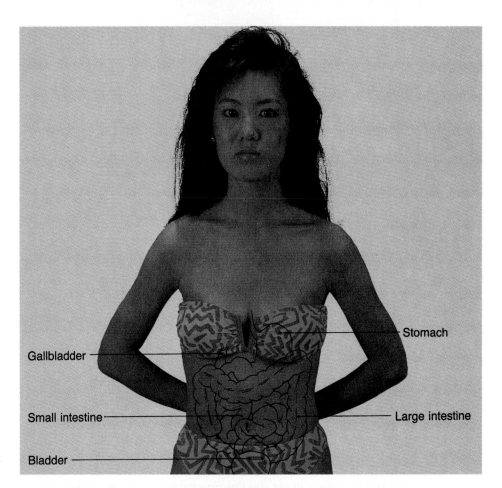

FIGURE 9–30. The hollow organs of the abdominopelvic cavity.

Gallbladder

Small intestine

Bladder

Stomach

Large intestine

FIGURE 9–31. The solid organs of the abdominopelvic cavity.

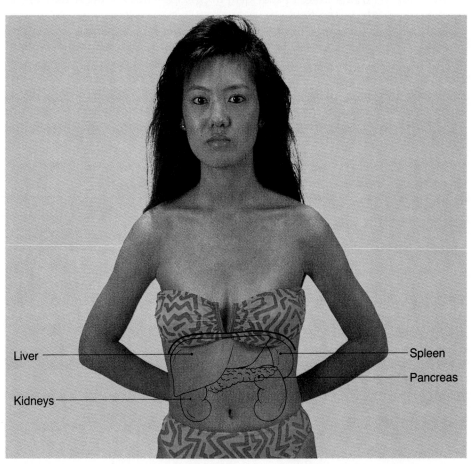

Liver

Kidneys

Spleen

Pancreas

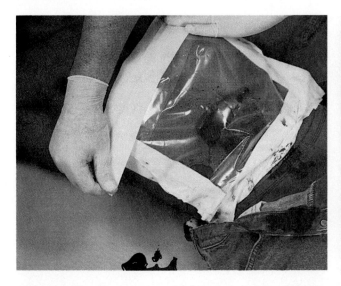
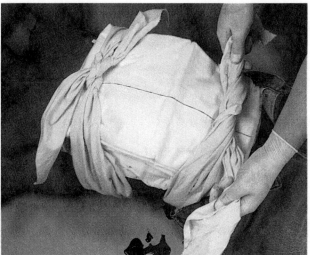

FIGURE 9–32. For open wounds in the abdomen, apply an occlusive dressing and cover to prevent heat loss.

Care for *all* possible abdominal and pelvic injuries by:

1. Dressing all open wounds.
2. Laying the patient back, with the legs flexed. Do not flex the legs if there are any signs of injury to the pelvic bones or lower limbs.
3. Caring for shock (see Chapter 7), constantly monitoring vital signs.
4. Being alert for vomiting.
5. Being certain that you *do not* touch any exposed internal organs. Cover them with an occlusive dressing, such as plastic wrap. Maintain warmth to the organ by placing dressings or a towel over the occlusive dressing. (NOTE: Some EMS Systems provide sterile materials to allow the First Responder to apply a moist sterile dressing in place of the occlusive dressing.)
6. Being certain that you *do not* remove any impaled objects. Stabilize the object with bulky dressings.

NOTE: Many patients with abdominal pain find some relief by hugging a bulky, soft object against the abdomen. A pillow works quite well for this purpose.

Injury to the Genitalia

1st Because of their location, the external reproductive organs are not a common site of injury. The pelvis and the thighs usually prevent injury to these organs, which are known as the external genitalia. When injury does occur, two types of soft tissue injury are commonly seen:

Genitalia (jen-i-TA-le-ah)—the external reproductive organs.

- Blunt Trauma Injury—such injury is very painful, but little can be done by the First Responder. An ice pack, if available, will help reduce the pain.
- Cuts—bleeding should be controlled by direct pressure. A sterile dressing or a sanitary napkin should be used. If either of these is not available, then use any clean, bulky dressing. Once bleeding is controlled, the dressing can be held in place with a large triangular bandage, applied in the same manner as a diaper.

Other soft tissue injury care procedures also apply when treating injuries to the genitalia:

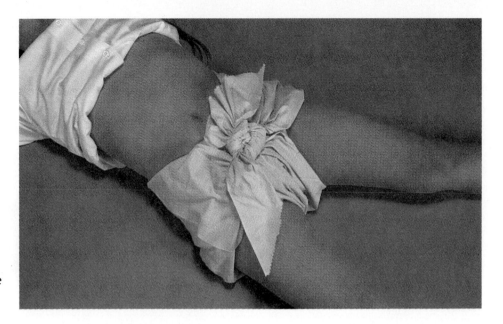

FIGURE 9–33. Dressings applied to the genitalia can be secured with a triangular bandage.

- Do *not* remove impaled objects.
- *Save* avulsed parts, wrapping them in plastic, sterile dressings, or any clean dressing.

First Responders are a part of the professional health care team. As such, you must carry out your role in a manner that will reduce embarrassment for the patient. Tell the patient what you are going to do. Tell the patient why you must examine and care for the genitalia. Protect the patient from the sight of onlookers by having them leave the scene. If this is not possible, have them turn their backs to the patient. Then, provide care without any hesitation. Conduct all procedures in the same manner as you would in caring for an injury to any other part of the body. This is essential if you are to provide proper **total patient care.**

SUMMARY

Closed wounds and **open wounds** cause soft tissue damage. Internal body organs may also be involved. **Bruises** (contusions) are the most common form of closed wound, while **scratches** and **scrapes** (abrasions) and **cuts** (lacerations and incisions) are the most common forms of open wounds.

Puncture wounds are open wounds, classified as **penetrating or perforating.** Perforating wounds have both an entrance wound and an exit wound.

Avulsions occur when skin or a body part (tip of the nose, fleshy part of a fingertip, external ear, tooth, lip, and so on) is torn loose or off the body. The cutting or tearing off of fingers, toes, hands, feet, arms, or legs is called an **amputation.**

Crush injuries can have open wounds with severe soft tissue damage. Both internal and external bleeding are problems seen with such injuries.

Always care for closed wounds as if there is **internal bleeding.**

When providing care for open wounds, take adequate measures to ensure personal safety and begin by **exposing the wound.** After **clearing the wound surface,** you should **control bleeding.**

In cases of open wounds, your first priority after the airway and circulation is to control bleeding. Once this is done, continued control of bleeding and wound contamination is achieved by **dressing the wound.**

Whenever you are dealing with an open wound, it is necessary to keep the patient **lying still.** Care for **shock.** Remember to care for the entire patient. Provide **emotional support** by reassuring the patient.

If you are caring for a patient with a puncture wound, assume that there are extensive internal injuries and bleeding. Remember to look for **exit wounds.**

Do not remove impaled objects. Control bleeding and stabilize the impaled object. If the object is in the cheek wall and has passed though into the mouth, causing a possible airway obstruction, then you should remove the object back in the direction of its entry.

Partially avulsed skin can be folded back to its normal position. If skin is torn loose, preserve the part in plastic wrap or a plastic bag. **Do not** try to replace an avulsed eye. **Do not** try to replace any protruding organs. In cases of avulsion, control bleeding, cover with a dressing (sterile, if available), and be prepared to care for shock.

When confronted with an amputation, attempt to control bleeding with direct pressure applied to a dressing held firmly over the stump. If necessary, use pressure point techniques to help control the bleeding. Your last resort is a tourniquet.

Dressings cover wounds and **bandages** hold dressings in place. Dressings can be single-layered or built up into bulky dressings. **Occlusive dressings** are used when an **airtight** seal is required.

The procedures for dressing a wound require you to **control bleeding,** to use sterile or clean materials, and to cover the entire wound. Remember, *do not* remove any dressing once it is in place.

The procedures for bandaging require you to secure the bandage so that it is not too loose or too tight and to be sure that there are no loose ends. Remember, *do not* cover the patient's fingertips and toes. Bandage limbs from distal to proximal (bottom to top).

Specific care procedures require you to remember certain rules and exceptions. For example:

Scalp wounds—*Do not* try to clean the surface of the scalp and *do not* apply finger pressure if there is any chance of a skull fracture. Control bleeding with a dressing, held in place with roller bandage.

Facial wounds—Maintain an open airway, control bleeding, and dress and bandage the wounds. Remember, you can remove impaled objects from the cheeks, if the object has passed through the cheek wall into the mouth. If there are no skull, neck, or spinal injuries, reposition the patient for proper drainage from the mouth.

Eye wounds—You need to remember:

- *Do not* apply direct pressure to a cut eyeball.
- *Do not* remove impaled objects. Remember to cover with dressing pads and a rigid shield (for example, a paper cup).
- *Do not* replace an extruded eyeball (pulled from its socket).
- *Do not* open the eyes of a patient with burns to the eyelids.
- Wash foreign objects from the eye.
- Care for chemical burns by washing the patient's eyes.
- Keep the patient's eyelids closed.
- Always cover both of the patient's eyes.

Ear wounds—*Do not* probe into the external ear canal and *do not* pack the external ear canal. For cuts and bleeding from the ear, apply a dressing and bandage. Save avulsed parts in plastic.

Nose injuries—Maintain an open airway. *Do not* pack the nostrils.

Bleeding from the nostrils is best controlled by pinching them shut. Avulsed parts are best saved in plastic, sterile dressings, or clean dressings.

Injury to the mouth—Maintain an open airway and allow for drainage. *Do not* pack the mouth with dressing material. Use dressing material and direct pressure to control bleeding—but hold the dressing in place.

Neck wounds—Always look for signs of neck wounds. Provide care for arterial bleeding with pressure dressings. Care for venous bleeding with an occlusive dressing. You may apply other dressing material over top of the occlusive dressing.

Abdominal injuries—Look for the signs of abdominal injury, including a rigid abdomen. Care for shock and be alert for vomiting. If there are no injuries to the pelvic bones or lower limbs, flex the patient's legs to help reduce pain.

Injuries to the genitalia—Conduct your examination and provide care in the strictest professional manner. Control bleeding by direct pressure applied with a dressing. Save avulsed parts in plastic or dressings (sterile, if available).

REMEMBER: Always ensure personal safety. Wear latex or vinyl gloves approved by your EMS System.

Examples of General Dressing and Bandaging

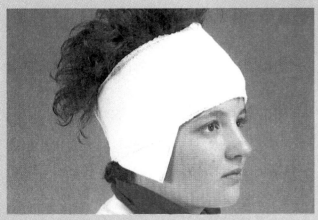

Forehead (No Skull Injury) or Ear. Place dressing and secure with self-adherent roller bandage.

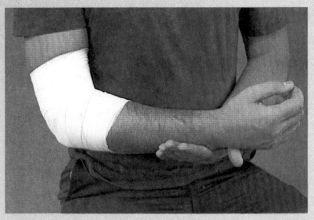

Elbow or Knee. Place dressing and secure with cravat or roller bandage. Apply roller bandage in figure 8 pattern.

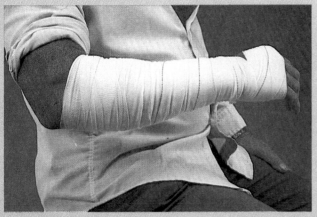

Forearm or Leg. Place dressing and secure with roller bandage, distal to proximal. Better protection is offered if palm or sole is wrapped.

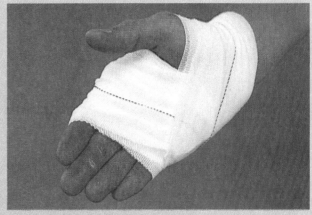

Hand. Place dressing, wrap with cravat, and secure at wrist. Use same pattern for roller bandage.

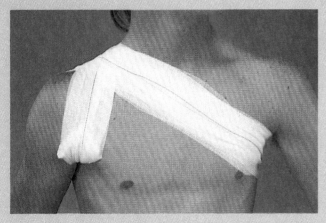

Shoulder. Place dressing and secure with figure 8 of cravat or roller dressing. Pad under knot if cravat is used.

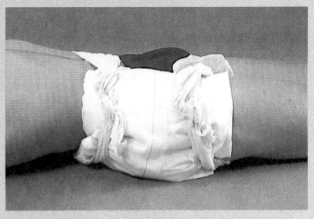

Hip. Place bandage and large dressing to cover hip. Secure with first cravat around waist and second cravat around thigh on injured side.

CHAPTER10

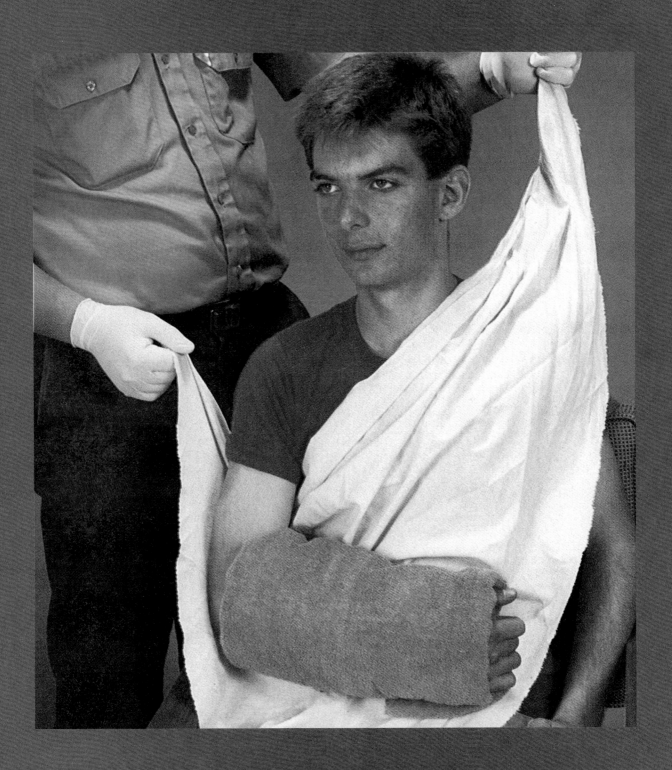

■ OBJECTIVES

By the end of this chapter, you should be able to:

1. List the functions of the skeletal system. (pp. 227–228)
2. Locate and name, using common terms, the major bones of the extremities. (pp. 228–230)
3. Define open fracture and closed fracture. (p. 231)
4. Define angulated fracture. (p. 231)
5. Define dislocation, sprain, and strain. (p. 232)
6. State the initial First Responder care provided for given injuries of the upper and lower extremities. (pp. 235–247)

NOTE: Many First Responders do not carry splints, nor do they have the training to use many of the commercial splints available for the initial care of fractures. Most of the time, splinting will be done by EMTs when they arrive at the scene. Their job could be made more difficult if improper splinting is done before they arrive.

This chapter provides you with the basic information needed to detect injuries to the extremities and to provide care without using rigid splints. The basics of rigid splinting will be covered in Chapter 11.

SKILLS

Upon completing this chapter, your class lectures, and skills labs, you should be able to:

1. Identify injuries to the extremities based on symptoms and signs.
2. Provide initial First Responder care for simulated injuries to the extremities.

INTRODUCTION

There is a problem that occurs when individuals begin to study injuries to the bones and joints of the body. With a little study, students soon learn the names and locations of bones, how to classify and detect injuries, and how to provide care for these injuries. However, while they are learning this new information, they often forget what they have been taught about soft tissues. Unfortunately, this carries over into the field, with some First Responders becoming so concerned about detecting and caring for fractures that they no longer notice other injuries.

Since the main thrust of this chapter is injury to the bones and joints of the extremities, we should reconsider other structures before they lose their importance. Figure 10–1 shows the major blood vessels and a few of the major nerves found in the arms and legs. Note, too, the large amount of muscle and other soft tissues. You need not remember every structure shown here, but you *must* remember how complicated the human body is in terms of soft tissue anatomy. Keep in mind that, in cases of fractures, the damage to soft tissues may present greater problems for the health care team.

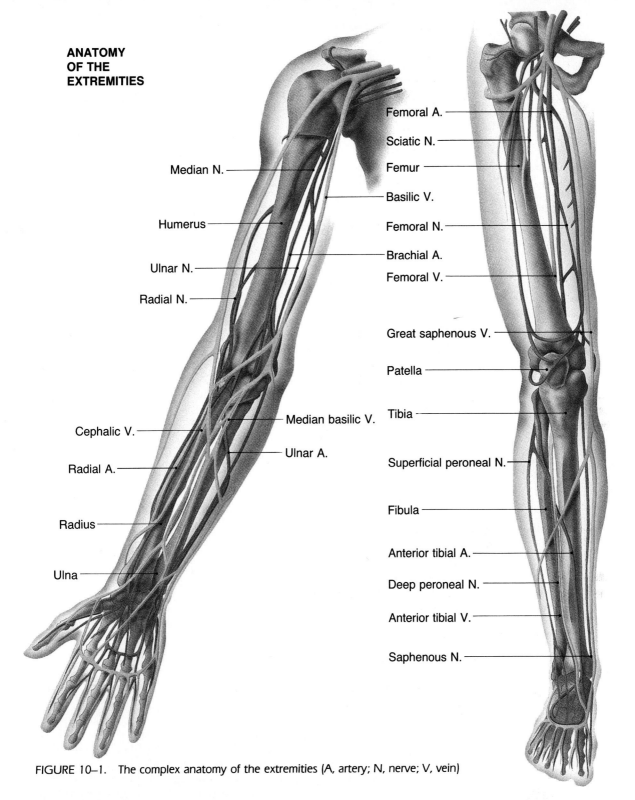

Median N.

Humerus

Ulnar N.

Radial N.

Cephalic V.

Radial A.

Radius

Ulna

Median basilic V.

Ulnar A.

Femoral A.

Sciatic N.

Femur

Basilic V.

Femoral N.

Brachial A.

Femoral V.

Great saphenous V.

Patella

Tibia

Superficial peroneal N.

Fibula

Anterior tibial A.

Deep peroneal N.

Anterior tibial V.

Saphenous N.

FIGURE 10–1.   The complex anatomy of the extremities (A, artery; N, nerve; V, vein)

THE SKELETAL SYSTEM

Functions of the Skeletal System

The skeletal system is made up of all the bones and joints in the body. At first, this may seem to be a simple system, but remember, bones are alive. If you think that bones are mineral deposits, requiring less care than the body's soft tissues, you may provide improper care.

1st The skeletal system has four major functions. The bones **support,** acting as a framework to give form to the body and to provide a rigid structure

Skeletal system—all the bones and joints of the body. The system is involved with support, movement, protection, and blood cell production.

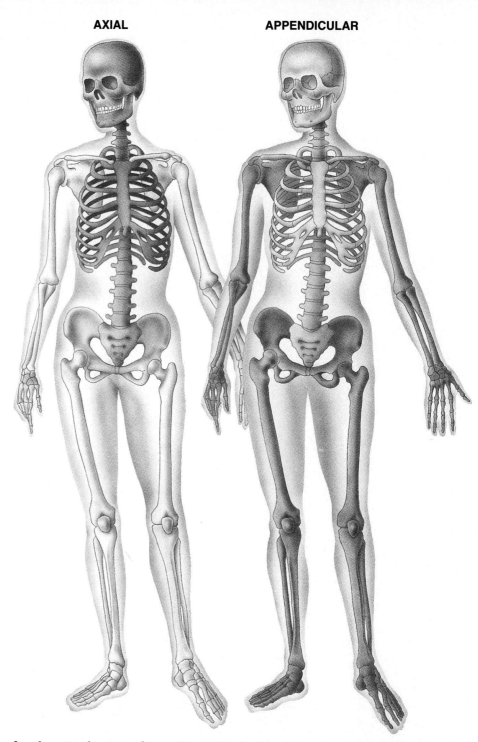

AXIAL   **APPENDICULAR**

FIGURE 10–2. The major divisions of the skeletal system.

for the attachment of muscles and other body parts. Acting with muscles, bones and the joints they form allow for body **movement.** Many of the bones in the body provide **protection** for the vital organs. The skull protects the brain and the backbone protects the spinal cord. The ribs protect the heart, lungs, liver, stomach, and spleen. The urinary bladder and internal reproductive organs are protected by the pelvis. In addition, some bones have cells involved in **blood cell production.**

Main Parts of the Skeletal System

1st There are two major divisions of the skeletal system:

- Axial (Ak-si-al) skeleton: all the bones forming the upright axis of the body, including the skull, backbones, breastbone, and ribs.
- Appendicular (Ap-en-DIK-u-ler) skeleton: all the bones forming the upper

Axial (AK-si-al) skeleton—the bones and joints that form the upright axis of the body. It includes the skull, spine, breastbone, and ribs.

Appendicular (ap-en-DIK-u-ler) skeleton—the bones and joints that form the upper and lower extremities.

and lower extremities, including collarbones, shoulder blades, arm bones, wrist bones, hand bones, and the bones of the hip, legs, ankles, and feet.

In this chapter, we will consider the structures that make up the appendicular skeleton. The axial skeleton will be covered in Chapter 12.

The Upper Extremities

First Responders are not required to learn the medical names for each bone in the body. Common names are used in First Responder training, so that you will spend more time learning how to recognize injuries and how to provide proper care. Medical names for bones will be provided only for reference. The following is a list of the bones of the upper extremities. The number of bones forming various structures has been provided.

Common Names	Medical Names
Shoulder girdle	Pectoral (PEK-tor-al) girdle
Collarbone (1/side)	Clavicle (KLAV-i-kul)
Shoulder blade (1/side)	Scapula (SKAP-u-lah)
Upper arm bone (1/arm, from shoulder to elbow)	Humerus (HU-mer-us)
Forearm bones (2/arm, from elbow to wrist: 1 medial, 1 lateral)	Ulna (UL-nah)—medial Radius (RAY-de-us)—lateral
Wrist bones (8/wrist)	Carpals (KAR-pals)
Hand bones (palm bones, 5/palm)	Metacarpals (meta-KAR-pals)
Finger bones (14/hand)	Phalanges (fah-LAN-jez)

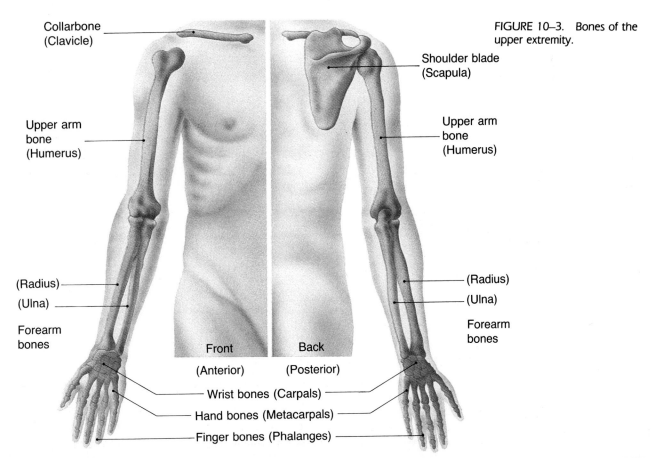

Collarbone (Clavicle)

Shoulder blade (Scapula)

Upper arm bone (Humerus)

Upper arm bone (Humerus)

Upper arm bone (Humerus)

(Radius)

(Ulna)

(Radius)

(Ulna)

Forearm bones

Forearm bones

Front
(Anterior)

Back
(Posterior)

Wrist bones (Carpals)

Hand bones (Metacarpals)

Finger bones (Phalanges)

FIGURE 10–3. Bones of the upper extremity.

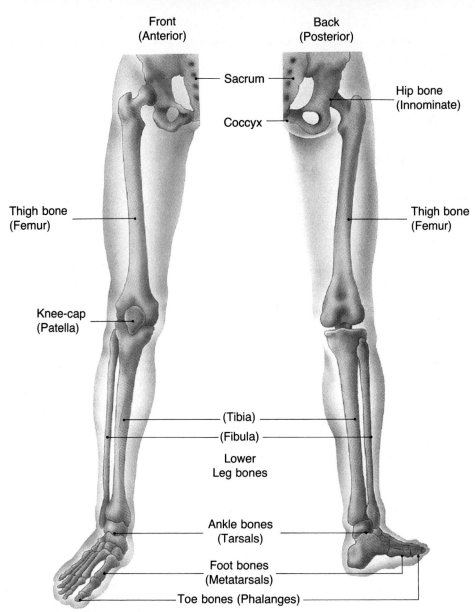

Front
(Anterior)

Back
(Posterior)

Sacrum

Coccyx

Hip bone
(Innominate)

Thigh bone
(Femur)

Thigh bone
(Femur)

Knee-cap
(Patella)

(Tibia)

(Fibula)

Lower
Leg bones

Ankle bones
(Tarsals)

Foot bones
(Metatarsals)

Toe bones (Phalanges)

FIGURE 10–4. Bones of the lower extremity.

The Lower Extremities

The lower extremities are made up of the pelvis and both legs, down to and including the toes. The following is a list of all the bones in the lower extremities. The medical names are given for reference. You need to remember only the common names. The number of bones forming various structures has been provided.

Common Names	Medical Names
Pelvic girdle (pelvis and hips)	Os coxae (os KOK-se)
Thigh bone (1/leg)	Femur (FE-mur)
Kneecap (1/leg)	Patella (pah-TEL-lah)
Lower leg bones (shin bones, 2/leg: 1 medial, 1 lateral)	Tibia (TIB-e-ah)—medial
	Fibula (FIB-yo-lah)—lateral
Ankle bones (7/foot)	Tarsals (TAR-sals)
Foot bones (5/foot)	Metatarsals (meta-TAR-sals)
Toe bones (14 to 15/foot, some people have two bones in the little toe, others may have three)	Phalanges (fah-LAN-jez)

NOTE: In First Responder care, the term "hip" means the upper end of the thigh bone (femur).

It should be noted that the term "arm" when used by itself means the upper arm only. The term "leg" is used to refer to the lower leg only. In First Responder training and care, such a distinction is not necessary. Most people use the term "arm" to refer to both upper arm and forearm. Likewise, they use the term "leg" to mean both the thigh and lower leg.

INJURIES TO BONES AND JOINTS

Types of Injuries

1st Anytime a bone is broken, including chips, cracks, splintering, and complete breaks, a **fracture** has occurred. There are two basic types of fractures. A **closed fracture** occurs when a bone is broken, but soft tissue damage does not extend from the fracture site out through the skin. The ends or pieces of bone have not been forced outward to rip open the skin. In some cases, soft tissue damage can be great and internal bleeding can be profuse, even though there are few external signs of injury. An **open fracture** occurs when a bone is broken and soft tissues are damaged from the fracture site, up through the skin. The ends or pieces of bone tear through the skin. This type of injury also can be produced by a penetrating wound that opens the skin and causes a fracture (for example, gunshot wounds).

1st Angulated fracture describes a fracture that causes a bone or a joint to take on an unnatural shape. For example, the straight upper arm bone may be bent or twisted somewhere between the shoulder and the elbow. Due to fractures, the joint at the knee may bend forward. Angulated fractures can be mild or severe. They may occur with both open and closed fractures.

Bone fractures can be caused in a variety of ways. Most cases of fractures seen by First Responders will be caused by direct violence (force), occurring when the bone is broken at the point of contact with an object. Indirect violence also will fracture bones. This happens when forces are carried from the point of impact to the bone. For example, someone may fall, land on a hand, and break an arm. Twisting forces, as seen in sports injuries, can cause bones to break. Aging and disease also can cause bone fractures. With age, the bones become weak and brittle, making them easier to fracture. The bones of individuals with certain diseases, such as bone cancer, may fracture due to even the mildest of forces.

Since possible fractures may be hard to detect, you should always consider if the accident is of the type known to cause broken bones. The mechanism of injury is very important. Look for indications of falls, the patient

Fracture—any break, crack, chip, split, or crumbling of a bone.

Closed fracture—a broken bone with no associated opening of the skin.

Open fracture—a broken bone with an associated opening of the skin. The cause of the opening may be from bone ends or fragments tearing out through the skin or a penetrating injury that has damaged a bone.

Angulated fracture—a fracture that causes a bone or joint to take on an unnatural shape or bend.

FIGURE 10–5. Basic types of fractures.

FIGURE 10–6. Angulated fractures.

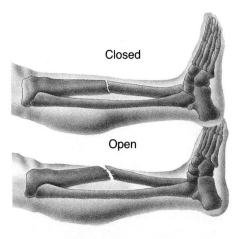

Closed

Open

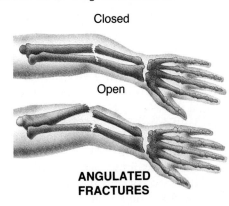

Closed

Open

ANGULATED FRACTURES

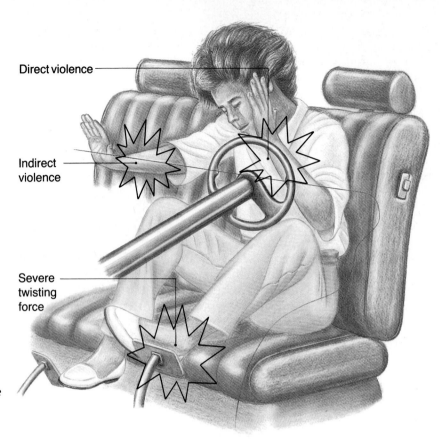

Direct violence

Indirect violence

Severe twisting force

FIGURE 10–7. Bones may be broken in a variety of ways.

Dislocation—the pulling or pushing of a bone end partially or completely free of a joint.

Sprain—a partially torn ligament.

Strain—the overstretching or mild tearing of a muscle.

being thrown against or struck by objects, and indications of body parts being caught and twisted.

1st Whereas most injuries to the bones are fractures, most serious injuries to joints are **dislocations.** One end of a bone making up a joint is pulled or pushed out of place. Soft tissue damage can be very serious in cases of dislocation. Sometimes the dislocation of a bone will cause it or an adjoining bone to fracture.

1st Ligaments connect bone to bone, helping to form joints. When ligaments are partially torn, **sprains** occur. These are different from **strains,** where muscles are stretched or where mild tearing of the muscle takes place.

1st NOTE: First Responders should consider all injured extremities to have serious fractures until proven otherwise. Dislocations, sprains, and some strains are difficult, if not impossible, to distinguish from fractures. In many cases, the exact nature of the injury cannot be determined until a physician examines x-rays of the patient.

Symptoms and Signs of Injury to Bones and Joints

1st The symptoms and signs of a fracture can include:

- Deformity—a part of a limb appears different in size or shape than the same part on the opposite side of the patient's body. (Always compare both arms to one another and do the same for both legs.) If a bone appears to have an unusual angle, consider this deformity to be a sign of possible fracture. Feel gently along the patient's limbs, noting any lumps, fragments, or ends of fractured bones.
- Swelling and discoloration—these begin shortly after injury. The discoloration is usually a reddening of the skin. Typical black and blue bruises will not occur until several hours after a bone is fractured.
- Tenderness and pain—tissues directly over the fracture will be very tender. The patient often experiences severe and constant pain at the

TABLE 10–1. FRACTURES: EXAMPLES OF MECHANISMS OF INJURY

Structure	Mechanism
Upper Extremities	
Shoulder	
• *Collarbone*	Fall on lateral shoulder, direct blow, blow to upper back and posterior shoulder, downward blow striking the bone
• *Shoulder blade*	Direct blow, severe downward blow to the shoulder (for example, falling objects), fall on the lateral shoulder
• *Proximal arm bone*	Direct blow to the lateral arm (falls or striking vehicle compartment wall in crash)
Arm bone (shaft)	Direct blow from striking an object (motor vehicle accidents), direct blow from a fall, fall on the elbow, fall on the hand of an outstretched arm
Elbow	
• *Distal arm bone*	Direct blow to flexed elbow, indirect force of landing on outstretched arm, forceful hyperextension of elbow
• *Proximal forearm bones*	Direct blow to elbow, indirect force from fall on outstretched arm, elbow dislocation
Forearm bones	
• *Shaft*	Direct blow (often to forearm while raised to protect face), compression occurring from a fall (usually to children)
• *Distal forearm*	Fall on hand, forced flexion or extension of hand
Wrist	Forced flexion or hyperextension, direct blow, indirect force from falling on an outstretched hand, crush injury, force of thumb being driven back into its joint with the wrist
Hand	Direct blows (falls), objects striking the distal fingers, falling objects striking the hand, forced flexion or hyperextension of fingers, twisting force to the fingers, impact to the fist
Lower Extremities	
Pelvis	Fall (landing on the buttocks), fall (more common with elderly), forceful direct blow, crush injury, strenuous activity (young patients)
Hip	Direct blow to knees (for example, striking dashboard), direct blow (for example, vehicle strikes pedestrian's hip), posterior dislocation
Thigh bone	
• *Femoral head*	Direct blow, anterior dislocation
• *Proximal shaft*	Fall on hip, fall on hip with twisting forces
• *Shaft*	Severe blow to thigh, severe blow to knees
Knee	
• *Distal thigh bone*	Direct blow (usually motor vehicle accidents or falls), hyperextension or severe twist of the knee
• *Proximal lower leg*	Direct force from a fall, transfer of force from falling and landing on the feet, object strikes leg (for example, vehicle strikes pedestrian)
• *Kneecap*	Direct blow (for example, falls, knee strikes dashboard), severe muscle contractions (for example, from the force of a fall)
Lower leg bones	Direct blow, twisting forces, blow to the side of the knee
Ankle	Twisting forces, crush injury, falls (landing on the feet)
Foot	Heel strikes ground during fall, forced extreme flexion or hyperextension of foot, severe ankle twist, direct blow to the toes (falling object or kicking an object)

injury site. Gently touch the area along the line of a bone to determine if there is a possible fracture and the exact location of the injury. This should not be done if the injury is an open fracture or there is obvious deformity.

• Loss of use—the patient will be unable to move a limb or part of a limb. Sometimes movement is possible but it produces intense pain. If the patient can move an arm, but not the fingers, or if a patient can move a leg, but not the toes, a fracture may have caused severe damage to nerves and blood vessels.

- Numbness or tingling sensations—this may indicate damage to nerves or blood vessesls caused by bone ends or fragments.
- Loss of distal pulse—bone ends or fragments may have compressed or severed an artery.
- Slow capillary refill—capillary refilling takes longer than 2 seconds (see below).
- Grating—when the patient moves, the ends of the fractured bone rub together to produce a sound. *Do not* ask a patient to move in order to confirm this sound or to reproduce a sound reported by the patient or bystanders.
- Sound of breaking—this is told to you by the patient or bystanders. Consider this enough information to assume a fracture has occurred.
- Exposed bone—the fragments or ends of fractured bone may be visible where they break through the skin in cases of open fractures.

A capillary refill test can be performed to indicate the rate at which blood will refill an area in a nailbed after pressure has forced blood out of a portion of its capillary beds. You can use your finger and thumb to apply pressure over a nailbed on the injured limb and then quickly release this pressure. This pressure should be applied to an uninjured finger. The nailbed will turn white (blanches) for a moment and then regain its normal color as blood refills the capillaries.

If capillary refill does not occur within 2 seconds, you must assume that there is impaired circulation. The reliability of this test is very poor if the patient has been exposed to a cold environment.

Dislocation typically produces deformity of the joint involved. Swelling at the joint is a common sign. In most cases, there will be constant pain with additional pain upon movement. The patient may lose use of the joint or may complain of a locked or "frozen" joint. If the patient's only sign of extremity injury is deformity at a joint, it is more likely a dislocation than a fracture. However, as a First Responder, you should still consider the possiblity of a fracture.

Sprains may be present if there is swelling or discoloration, and the patient complains of pain on movement. The only sign of strain will be pain, usually associated with movement. If swelling occurs, the injury is more likely to be a fracture, dislocation, or sprain.

As a First Responder, you should treat a suspected sprain as if it were a fracture. If you think the patient has a strain, you should keep the patient at rest, not moving any part of the body and provide the same care you

FIGURE 10–8. Typical signs of fracture.

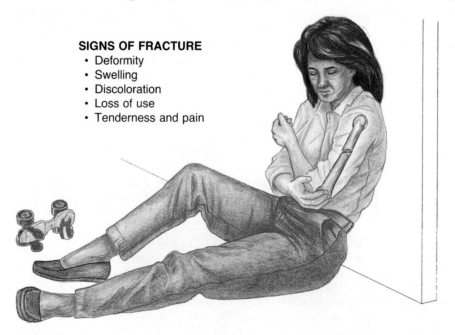

SIGNS OF FRACTURE
- Deformity
- Swelling
- Discoloration
- Loss of use
- Tenderness and pain

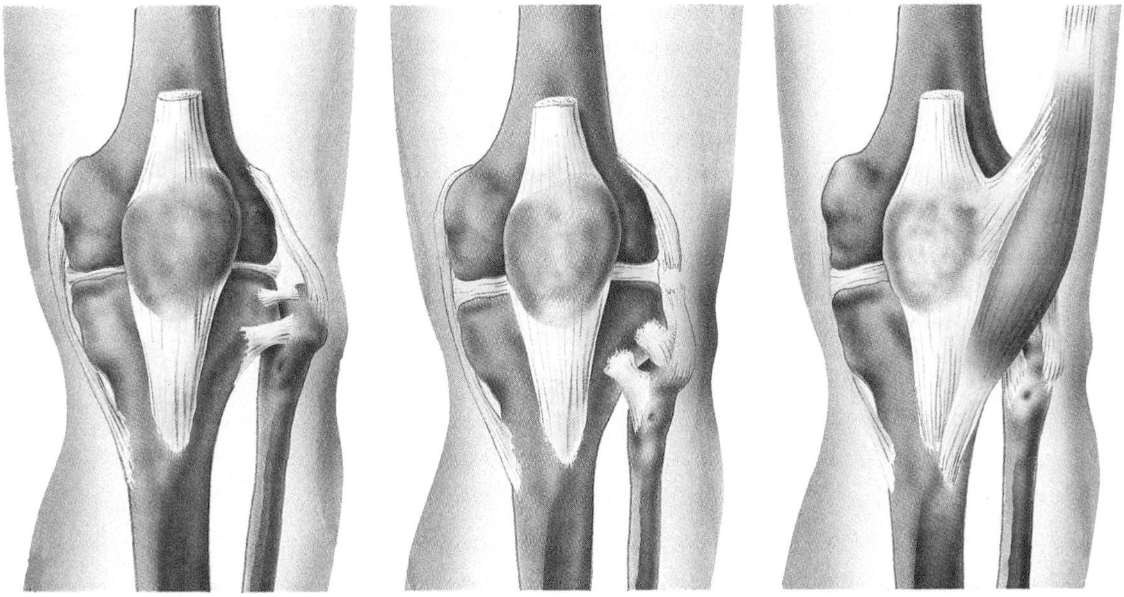

TYPE	DISLOCATION Joint deformity	SPRAIN Ligament torn	STRAIN Muscle over- stretched

INJURY			

SIGNS	• Deformity • Joint swelling • Constant pain • Increased pain on movement • Loss of movement • "Frozen joint"	• Swelling • Discoloration • Pain on movement	• Pain

FIGURE 10–9. Musculoskeletal injuries other than fractures.

would for a fracture. Even though a strain may appear obvious, you cannot rule out a fracture. The diagnosis must be done by a physician.

1st Care for all possible strains and sprains as if they were fractures.

INJURIES TO THE UPPER EXTREMITIES

WARNING: When providing care for possible fractures, always wear latex or vinyl gloves.

NOTE: Make certain that dispatch is alerted for all cases involving possible fractures and dislocations.

Total Patient Care

Too often, those arriving at the scene of an accident wish to begin care procedures with the treating of fractures. This is not the proper course of action for a First Responder. Remember to conduct a primary survey and a secondary survey, with an interview. You must detect and correct life-threatening problems as quickly as possible. Respiration, circulation, and bleeding are more important considerations than fractures. Detecting neck and spinal injuries is more important than starting care of fractures of the extremities. Caring for open chest wounds and open abdominal wounds should be done before you care for fractures. Shock and serious burns should be cared for before considering fractures, even if the fractures are major.

There is an order of care for various fractures. First priority is given to possible fractures of the spine. Next come possible fractures to the skull, pelvis, thigh, rib cage (when sections of ribs are broken loose), and any fracture where there is no distal pulse (as detected during the secondary survey). Possible fractures to the arm, lower leg, and individual ribs are considered last. The bleeding associated with pelvic and thigh fractures is often severe. The sooner care begins for these sites, the better the chances are for preventing serious shock.

1st Immobilizing fractured bones is usually the first thing that comes to mind when caring for an injured extremity. However, you may have to control bleeding, applying a pressure dressing, or dress an open wound before you can provide care for the fracture. Open fractures must be detected so you can apply any needed dressings.

Clothing should be cut away, folded back, or lifted off to expose the injury site. (*Do not* remove clothing by pulling it over an injured arm or leg.) This must be done so that you can clearly see the site of injury. Any serious bleeding must be controlled. An assessment of the injury should be made. All open wounds must be dressed and bandaged.

Emotional support is important when caring for a patient with suspected fractures. You may need to remind the patient that fractures can be set at the hospital and that bones with fractures will heal. Let the patient know that new techniques reduce the time spent wearing a cast or having the injured part immobilized. Emotional support will help keep the patient at rest and may help lower blood pressure, pulse rate, and breathing rate.

Injuries to the Shoulder Girdle

Fractures and dislocations of the shoulder girdle may be detected by looking for the typical symptoms and signs of bone and joint injuries. A common sign for fractures to the shoulder blade and collarbone is a condition known as "knocked down" shoulder or "dropped" shoulder. The patient's shoulder, on the injured side, will appear to droop. The patient usually holds the arm up against the side of the chest. This also may be seen in cases of shoulder dislocation.

Fractures and dislocation of the shoulder joint often produce what is known as anterior dislocation. The end of the upper arm bone that forms the shoulder joint can be felt in front of the shoulder.

1st In providing care for patients with shoulder injuries, you should:

1. Care for life-threatening problems and other injuries that have priority over fractures.
2. Check for a radial pulse and capillary refill on the injured side. If there is no pulse, the patient will need EMT transport as soon as possible. Note the time that you observed the absence of the distal pulse or slow capillary refill.
3. Check for nerve function by testing for feeling in, and movement of, the fingers on the injured side. If there is no nerve function, the patient will need EMT transport as soon as possible.
4. Apply a sling and swathe. If there are signs of anterior dislocation, place a pillow between the patient's arm and chest on the injured side before applying the sling and swathe (see Scansheet 10–1). Use a rolled blanket, rolled towel, or other form of padding in place of a pillow.
5. Reassess the wrist pulse and nailbed capillary refill. If the pulse is absent or capillary refill has been slowed, the arm on the injured side may have to be repositioned or the sling and swathe may have to be reapplied. In such cases, it is best to phone or radio the emergency department physician for directions before repositioning the limb.

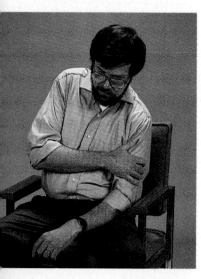

FIGURE 10–10. "Knocked down" shoulder indicates a fracture to the collarbone or shoulder blade.

On occasion, a dislocated shoulder will correct (reduce) itself. If you observe this, or are told this has happened by the patient, still proceed to take a radial pulse and check for nerve function. Even if both are good, apply a sling and swathe. This patient still has to see a physician. Arrange

The Extremities—Select Mechanisms of Injury

MECHANISM OF INJURY—
The force that produced the injury, its intensity and direction, and the area of the body that is affected.

DIRECT FORCE—
Any bone or joint can be injured by the direct force produced in a fall, striking an object, or being struck by an object.

DOWNWARD BLOW –
Clavicule
and
Scapula

LATERAL BLOW –
Clavicule
Scapula
and
Humerus

FORCED FLEXION
OR
HYPEREXTENSION –
Elbow
Wrist
Fingers
Femur
Knee
Foot

TWISTING FORCE –
Hip
Femur
Knee
Leg bones
Ankle
Shoulder
Elbow
Forearm
Wrist

INDIRECT
FORCE –
Pelvis
Hip
Knee
Leg bones
Shoulder
Humerus
Elbow
Forearm bones

LATERAL BLOW –
Knee
Hip
Femur
(Very forceful)

for transport, making certain to tell the EMTs that the dislocation apparently corrected itself and the time at which it took place.

The Sling and Swathe

A sling is a triangular bandage used to support the shoulder and arm. Once the patient's arm is placed in a sling, a swathe can be used to hold the arm against the side of the chest.

A sling and swathe can be used to immobilize an upper extremity. In addition to restricting the movement of the extremity, a sling and swathe support the arm on the injured side. When used alone, the sling and swathe can be applied for injuries to the shoulder girdle. If a pad is placed between the patient's arm and chest, the sling and swathe can be used for anterior dislocations of the shoulder joint. With slight modification, the sling and swathe can be used for fractures to the ribs (see Chapter 12). A sling and swathe should be applied after splinting fractures of the arm.

1st A sling and swathe are forms of soft splinting. Typically, when you splint, you are trying to immobilze the fracture site and the bones above and below the site, or you are trying to immobilize a joint and all the bones making up that joint. It is not practical to rigidly splint the shoulder girdle. Soft splinting with a sling and swathe does not completely immobilize the bones and the joint, but it does restrict movement and serves to remind the conscious patient to avoid moving and using the arm on the injured side.

Go over the following steps for applying a sling and swathe. After doing so, use Scansheet 10–2 to review and study the process.

1st To construct and apply a sling and swathe, you should:

1. Use a commercial sling, or make one from a piece of cloth, clothing, towel, or sheet. Fold or cut this material so that it is in the shape of a triangle. The ideal sling should be about 50 to 60 inches long at its base and 36 to 40 inches long on each of its sides.

2. Position the triangular material on top of the patient's injured side and chest as shown in Scansheet 10–2. Fold the patient's arm across the chest. If the patient cannot hold the arm, have a bystander assist you, or provide support for the patient's arm until you are ready to tie the sling. Note in Scansheet 10–2 that one point of the triangle should extend behind the patient's elbow on the injured side.

3. Take the bottom point of the triangle and bring this end up over the patient's arm. When you are finished, this bottom point should be taken over the patient's injured shoulder.

4. Draw up on the ends of the sling so that the patient's hand is about 4 inches above the elbow (see the illustration). Tie the two ends of the sling together, making sure that the knot does not rest against the back of the patient's neck (use dressing or a handkerchief to pad between the knot and the patient). Make certain that the patient's fingertips are exposed so you can see any color changes and feel for the temperature changes that may indicate a lack of circulation.

5. Take the point of material located at the patient's elbow and fold it forward, pinning it to the front of the sling. This forms a pocket for the patient's elbow. If you do not have a pin, twist the excess material and tie a knot in the point to form this shallow pocket. If you are going to tie a knot to form the pocket, it is best done before applying the sling.

6. A swathe is formed from a second piece of material folded in the shape of a triangle or folded as a 4-inch wide band. This swathe is tied around the chest and injured arm of the patient, over the sling. *Do not* place this swathe over the patient's arm on the uninjured side.

Sling and Swathe

A sling is a triangular bandage used to support the shoulder and arm. Once the patient's arm is placed in a sling, a swathe can be used to hold the patient's arm against the side of the chest. Commercial slings are available. Roller bandage can be used to form a sling and swathe. Velcro straps can be used to form a swathe. Use whatever materials you have on hand, provided that they will not cut into the patient. Remember, shirts, ties, and wide belts can be used to make both sling and swathe.

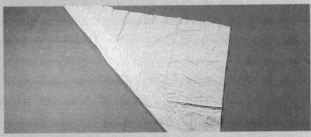

1 Make a sling from a piece of cloth, clothing, towel or sheet. Fold or cut this material into the shape of a triangle. The ideal sling should be about 50 to 60 inches long at its base and 36 to 40 inches long on each of its sides.

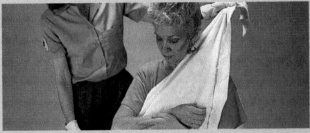

2 Position the triangular material over top of the patient's injured chest as shown in the figure. Fold the patient's arm across the chest. If the patient cannot hold her own arm, have someone assist you, or provide support for the patient's arm until you are ready to tie the sling. Note that one point of the triangle should extend behind the patient's elbow on the injured side.

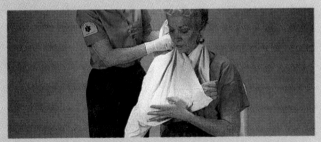

3 Take the bottom point of the triangle and bring this end up over the patient's arm. When you are finished, this bottom point should be taken over the top of the patient's injured shoulder.

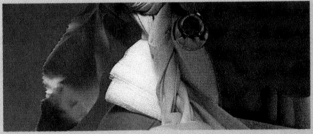

4 Draw up on the ends of the sling so that the patient's hand is about 4 inches above the elbow (exceptions are discussed later). Tie the two ends of the sling together, making sure that the knot does not press against the back of the patient's neck. Leave the patient's fingertips exposed to see any color changes that indicate lack of circulation. Check for a radial pulse. If the pulse has been lost, take off the sling and repeat the procedure.

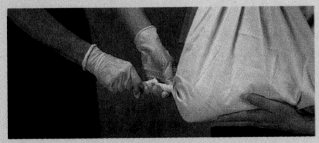

5 Take the point of material at the patient's elbow and fold it forward, pinning it to the front of the sling. This forms a pocket for the patient's elbow. If you do not have a pin, twist the excess material and tie a knot in the point. This will provide a shallow pocket for the patient's elbow.

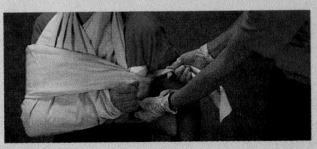

6 A swathe can be formed from a second piece of triangular material. This swathe is tied around the chest and the injured arm of the patient, over the sling. Do not place this swathe over the patient's arm on the uninjured side.

Roller bandage can be used to form a sling and swathe. Velcro straps or rope can be used to form a swathe. Use whatever materials you have on hand, provided that they will not cut into the patient. Remember, shirts can be used to make both sling and swathe.

NOTE: Using the sling and swathe in combination is better than using only a sling. However, for fractures to the breastbone or shoulder blade, you may apply only a sling if you do not have materials to make a swathe. For anterior dislocation of the shoulder, a sling and swathe should be applied, after inserting a pillow or pad between arm and chest.

Always assess distal pulse and capillary refill before and after applying a sling and swathe. Follow local care procedures or the emergency department physician's directions should circulation be reduced or interrupted.

1st WARNING: *Do not* try to straighten angulations or dislocations of the shoulder. Movement in this area may cause damage to blood vessels and nerves.

Injuries to the Upper Arm Bone

Injury to the bone of the upper arm (humerus) can take place at the end forming the shoulder joint (proximal end), along the shaft of the bone, or at the end forming the elbow joint (distal end). Deformity is the key sign used to detect fractures to this bone in any of these locations. In cases where deformity is not present, there is usually tenderness to indicate a possible fracture.

1st Rigid splinting is preferred, but a soft split may be done when necessary (p. 260). First Responder care for patients with upper arm fractures depends on the location of the fracture:

- Fractures near the shoulder—gently apply a sling and swathe. If you have only enough material for a swathe, bind the patient's upper arm to the body, taking great care not to cut off circulation to the lower arm.
- Fractures of the shaft—gently apply a sling and swathe. The sling should be modified so it supports only the patient's wrist.
- Fractures near the elbow—carefully apply a sling and swathe but *do not* draw the hand upward to a position that is 4 inches above the elbow. Instead, keep the elbow flexion to a minimum (90-degree angle).

FIGURE 10–11. The sling and swathe can be used for fractures to the shoulder and the upper arm bone.

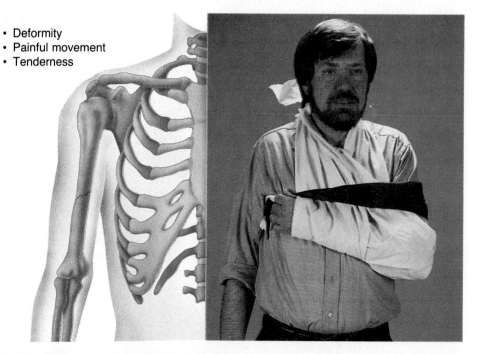

- Deformity
- Painful movement
- Tenderness

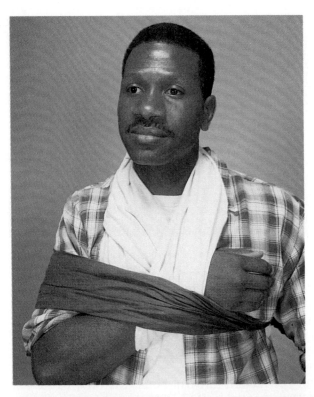

FIGURE 10–12. When providing care for upper arm bone shaft fractures, use rigid splints whenever possible; otherwise, gently apply a sling and swathe. The sling should be modified so that it supports the wrist only.

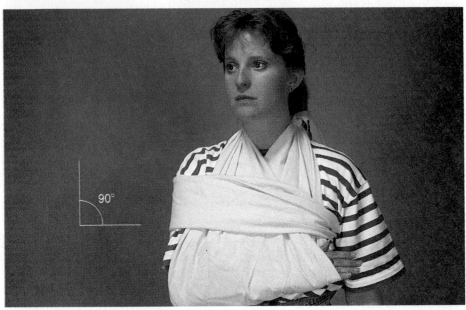

FIGURE 10–13. The sling and swathe can be used for fractures to the distal end of the upper arm bone.

Fractures of the upper arm often have an angulation. It does little good to try to correct this angulation if soft splinting is to be done. If you can, move the arm enough to allow for splinting. *Do not* pull on the arm in an effort to correct the angulation.

WARNING: Before applying a sling and swathe to care for upper arm injuries, feel for a radial pulse. If you do not feel a pulse, attempt to straighten any slight angulation in the upper arm bone if allowed to do so in your EMS System. *Do not* pull on the arm. This should be attempted only once. Stop the procedure if there is resistance or the patient complains of severe pain. Should straightening of the limb fail to restore a radial pulse, the patient will need to have a rigid splint applied as soon as possible (see Chapter 11). After applying a sling and swathe, check for a radial pulse. If there is no sign of circulation, remove the sling and swathe and apply a long board splint (see Chapter 11).

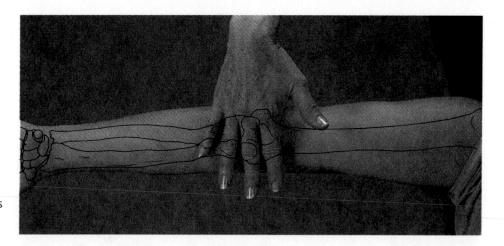

FIGURE 10–14. Consider this area to be the site of elbow injuries.

Injuries to the Elbow

When you begin care for a patient with an injured elbow, make sure that the injury is to the elbow only and not to the shafts of the upper or lower arm bones. The location of deformity and tenderness will help you determine if the injury is to the elbow, the elbow end of the upper arm bone, or the elbow end of the lower arm bone.

Since the elbow is a joint and not a bone, it is made up of part of the upper arm bone and part of the medial forearm bone (the ulna). You will have to decide if the injury is truly to the elbow. Place your hand over the back of your own elbow. Consider the elbow to be all the structures that can be covered by the palm of your hand. If the injury is above this area, you are dealing with a fractured upper arm bone. If the injury is below this area, it is a fractured forearm bone.

1st If the elbow is injured and found in a flexed (bent) position natural for the joint, a full sling and swathe can be applied. However, if the elbow is injured and the arm is in a straight position or the elbow is bent at an angle too great or too small to be easily positioned for a sling, *do not* move the patient's arm. If the elbow appears to be dislocated or it is in an unnatural position, *do not* move the patient's arm. Elbow injuries will require rigid splinting if the arm is straight, at the wrong angle to allow for easy application of a splint and swathe, or at an unnatural angle.

1st For cases requiring splinting of the elbow, the patient's elbow **must be immobilized in the position in which it is found.** If you change this position, you may cause severe damage to the blood vessels and nerves located in the patient's elbow. Some jurisdictions allow the First Responder to attempt, one time only, to straighten the limb if there is no radial pulse (check with your instructor). The attempt should not force the limb. If resistance is met, or if the procedure causes the patient extreme pain, the attempt should be stopped.

Injuries to the Forearm

1st If the injury is to the elbow end of the forearm, and you can check for a radial pulse, fold a pillow or rolled blanket around the patient's forearm, and apply a sling and swathe. Check circulation after the splinting is completed. Any apparent fractures to the shaft or the wrist end of a forearm bone will require rigid splinting (Chapter 11).

Injuries to the Wrist

1st Injuries to the wrist are best cared for with rigid splinting. However, you can place the hand into its position of function and tie the hand and forearm between two pillows. This soft splinting will do until more highly

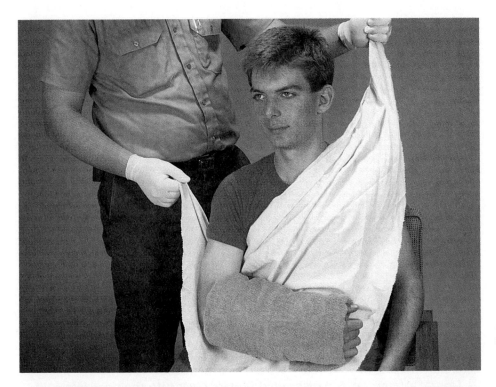

FIGURE 10–15. The sling and swathe can be modified for use in fractures to the elbow end of the forearm.

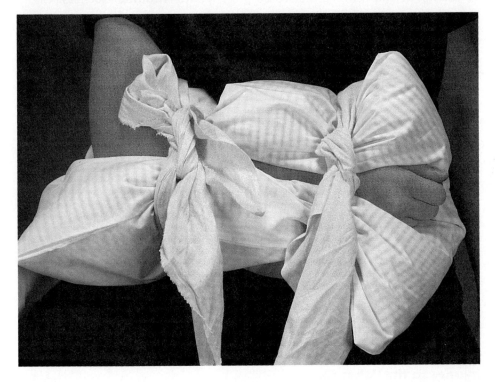

FIGURE 10–16. Soft splinting for wrist injuries.

trained personnel assume responsibility for the patient. The position of function for the hand is the position it would be in when picking up a small object, such as a ball. You can help maintain its position by placing a roll of gauze or cloth in the patient's palm.

Injuries to the Hand

Most injuries to the hand require rigid splinting; however, you can immobilize a fractured finger by taping the entire finger to an adjacent, uninjured finger.

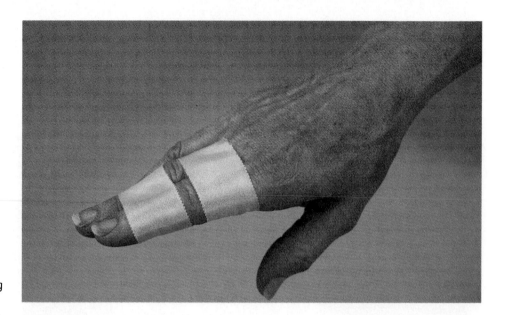

FIGURE 10–17. Immobilizing a fractured finger.

Some emergency department physicians request that the injured finger be wrapped in a soft bandage with no finger splint or adjacent finger taping. This may be part of your EMS System's care procedures.

Do not attempt to pop dislocated fingers back into their sockets.

INJURIES TO THE LOWER EXTREMITIES

Total Patient Care

In the preceding section dealing with injuries to the upper extremities, total patient care was covered. In cases where you find obvious injury to a lower extremity, you are still required to conduct a primary survey, and a secondary survey with an interview. Respiration, pulse, and bleeding are your first concerns. Care for neck, spinal chest, and abdominal injuries before fractures. Shock and serious burns are also to be cared for before fractures.

As in all First Responder care, providing emotional support to the patient is a significant part of total patient care.

REMEMBER: Always assess pulse and nerve function before and after care.

WARNING: Do NOT move or roll a patient who may have lower extremity injuries.

Injuries to the Pelvic Girdle

1st Fractures to the pelvic girdle (pelvis and hip joints) may be indicated if:

- The patient complains of pain in the pelvis or hips.
- The patient complains of pain when pressure is applied to the sides of the hip (never apply pressure over an obvious injury site).
- The patient has not been able to lift the legs while lying face up. *Do not* ask the patient to try to lift the legs.
- The foot on the injured side turns outward.
- There is noticeable deformity of the pelvis or at the hip joint.

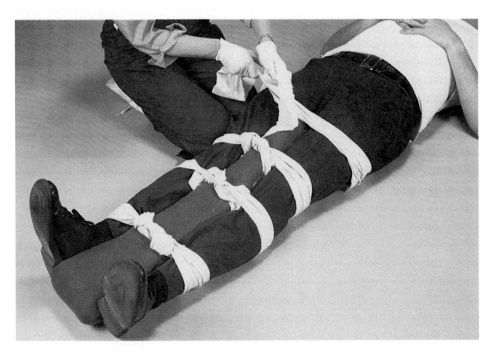

FIGURE 10–18. Tying the patient's legs together is used during the care for fractures to the pelvic girdle.

Pelvic girdle fractures are best treated at the scene by EMTs using special techniques such as pressurized garments (MAST), long board splints, and spineboards. When possible, wait for the EMTs to arrive.

1st As a First Responder, you can care for patients with fractures to the pelvic girdle by tying the patient's legs together. This should be done *only* if there will be a long delay before the EMTs arrive at the scene.

Place a folded blanket or some other padding between the patient's legs. Use wide strips of dressings, blankets, towels, or other similar materials to tie the patient's legs together. Ties should be placed at the top of the thighs, above the knees, below the knees, and at the ankles. Try not to lift the patient's legs. Attempt to slide strips of cloth (cravats) under the legs at the knees. A flat stick or a coat hanger will help (see pp. 201–202). Once a cravat is in place under the knees, gently slide it into position. After tying the patient's legs together, *do not* move the patient. Tying the patient's legs together does not offer any rigid support to the site of injury.

If you must raise a patient's legs in order to place the ties, raise them only slightly. If you suspect that the patient has injuries to the neck or spine, or that there may be fractures to the leg, *do not* raise the legs. Wait for EMT assistance.

It is difficult to tell a hip fracture from a hip dislocation. However, you must remember certain signs that indicate a possible hip dislocation. This is important because you should *never* attempt to move the leg on the injured side if there is the possibility of a hip dislocation. *Never* attempt to correct angulated fractures of the upper leg bone if the hip appears to be dislocated.

1st Assume the patient to have a dislocated hip if you find any signs of:

- Anterior hip dislocation—the patient's let is rotated outward, from the thigh (not just the foot rotated outward). This sign also may be present in cases of hip fracture. In the case of hip fracture, the injured limb may appear to be shortened.
- Posterior hip dislocation (most common)—the patient's leg is rotated inward and the knee is bent.

1st In cases of hip dislocation, wait for more highly trained personnel to arrive. While waiting, attempt to immobilize the injured leg with pillows,

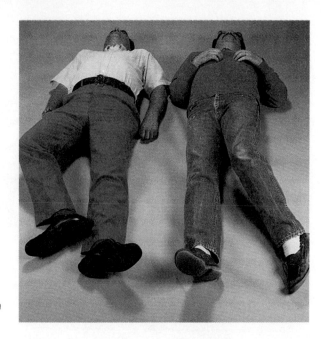

FIGURE 10–19. Classical signs of anterior hip dislocation and posterior hip dislocation.

rolled blankets, towels or clothing. Your purpose is to prevent the patient's leg from shifting. Some sources recommend that you secure these pillows in place by using straps. This is not recommended here because the use of such straps may require you to lift the patient's legs. *Do not* move the patient's leg.

Injuries to the Upper Leg

Many fractures of the upper leg bone (femur) are open fractures. Even in cases where the fracture is closed, bleeding can be life-threatening. The deformity produced with upper leg fractures can be remarkable. Often the leg below the fracture site will be angulated. Sometimes the rest of the leg will appear to twist below the fracture site. Care for patients with fractures to the thigh requires rigid splinting (see Chapter 11) or a special form of splinting (traction splinting) applied by the EMTs. Any other procedures, used in place of splinting, are discouraged.

Injuries to the Knee

1st In most cases, you will not be able to tell if the knee is fractured, dislocated, or both. For this reason, it is recommended that you immobilize an injured knee in the position in which it is found. *Do not* attempt to reposition or straighten the knee. Rigid splinting is the best course of action to use when immobilizing an injured knee. In place of standard procedures, the DOT suggests that you can wrap a pillow around the injured knee and tie this pillow in place using straps, dressing materials, roller bandage, or cord. This should only be done if the injury is obviously minor. Severe injury, including dislocation, will require rigid splinting (see Chapter 11).

Some EMS Systems allow First Responders to make one attempt to straighten the limb if there is no distal pulse. Check with your instructor.

If the kneecap (patella) has been dislocated and repositions itself spontaneously, soft splint or rigid splint and arrange for EMT transport.

Injuries to the Lower Leg

Injuries to the lower leg bones are best cared for using standard rigid splinting procedures. If you lack splints, you can tie pillows or rolled blankets, towels, or clothing around the lower leg, from knee to ankle. If the patient

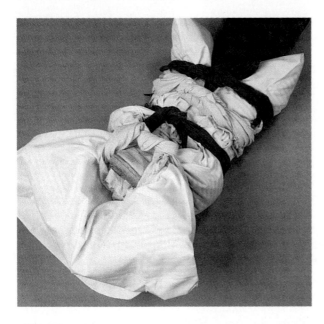

FIGURE 10–20. Care procedures for an injured ankle or foot.

has no distal pulse after applying these pillows or rolled materials, loosen the ties and resplint.

Injuries to the Ankle and Foot

1st If a patient has an injury to the foot or ankle, and you cannot feel a distal pulse, *do not* reposition the ankle. Immobilize the ankle in the position in which it is found. If you do not have splints, wrap a pillow or thick folds of blankets around the patient's ankle and foot. Tie the pillow or folded materials in place with cravats, dressing material, roller bandage, or clothing. Many EMS personnel believe this procedure is superior to rigid splinting.

SUMMARY

As a First Responder, you should never become so preoccupied with fractures that you forget to conduct a primary survey and a secondary survey with an interview. Remember that breathing, circulation, and bleeding are your first priorities. Neck injuries, spinal injuries, chest injuries, abdominal injuries, head injuries, shock, and serious burns are all to be cared for before fractures.

Remember, soft tissues are damaged when bones are injured. This includes damage to nerves and blood vessels.

The skeletal system is involved with body **support,** body **movement,** organ **protection,** and certain aspects of **blood cell production.** There are two major divisions to the skeletal system, the **axial skeleton** and the **appendicular skeleton.** The upper and lower extremities are part of the appendicular skeleton.

Each upper extremity consists of the **shoulder blade** (scapula), **collarbone** (clavicle), **upper arm bone** (humerus), **two forearm bones** (ulna and radius), **wrist bones** (carpals), **hand bones** (metacarpals), and **finger bones** (phalanges).

Each lower extremity consists of the **thigh bone** (femur), **kneecap** (patella), **two lower leg bones** (tibia and fibula), **ankle bones** (tarsals), **foot**

bones (metatarsals), and **toe bones** (phalanges). Each leg connects to the **pelvis.**

If a part of a fractured bone tears through the skin, the injury is called an **open fracture.** If the fractured bones do not tear through the patient's skin, the injury is called a **closed fracture.** You should apply sterile dressings, when possible, to all open fractures of the extremities.

When a bone is broken, it will often bend or twist to form an **angulated fracture.**

Any break to a bone is a **fracture.** A **dislocation** occurs when a bone is pulled out from a joint. Partially torn ligaments produce **sprains.** Stretching or minor tearing of muscles produces **strains.** Care for sprains and strains the same as fractures.

The symptoms and signs of fractures include **deformity, swelling, discoloration, tenderness, pain, loss of use, loss of distal pulse** or **slow capillary refill, grating, the sound of breaking bone,** and **exposed bone.** Dislocation usually has deformity, swelling, pain, and loss of use. Sprains usually have swelling, discoloration, and pain on movement. Pain is usually the only sign of strain.

There are some **special signs** you need to know as a First Responder. They are:

- "Knocked down" or "dropped" shoulder—shoulder fracture
- Top of upper arm bone out of socket—anterior dislocation of the shoulder
- Pelvic pain when you compress the patient's hips—pelvic fracture
- Pelvic injury with patient's foot turning outward—pelvic fracture
- Leg rotates outward—possible anterior dislocation of the hip. This also may indicate a hip fracture (usually limb appears shortened).
- Leg rotates inward and knee is bent—possible posterior dislocation of the hip

The care procedures for injuries to the extremities often require splinting. However, the following can be done by First Responders without splints:

- Fractured collarbone or shoulder blade: apply sling and swathe
- Dislocated shoulder: apply sling and swathe
- Anterior dislocation of the shoulder: place *pad* between patient's arm and chest and apply sling and swathe
- Upper arm bone fracture (shaft): apply sling and swathe. Apply a wrist sling if the fracture is to the shaft. If the fracture is near the elbow, apply a sling and swathe but do not raise the hand above the elbow.
- Elbow fracture: full sling and swathe if possible. If not, use rigid splints.
- Forearm fracture (elbow end, wrist pulse present): fold *pillow* around patient's entire forearm and apply a sling and swathe.
- Fractured wrist: tie the hand and forearm between two pillows.
- Fractured finger—tape the fractured finger to an adjacent uninjured finger
- Fractured pelvis or hip—place *pad* between patient's leg and tie the legs together
- Dislocated hip: immobilize limb with rolled blankets, towels, clothing, or dressings
- Fractured thigh: do not attempt soft splinting.
- Injured knee: leave knee in position in which it is found, fold pillow around knee and tie in place.
- Lower leg bone fracture: straighten angulation and apply rolled blankets, towels, or clothing around injured lower limb from knee to ankle; tie in place
- Ankle and foot fractures—fold pillow around ankle and foot; tie in place.

CHAPTER 11

Splinting

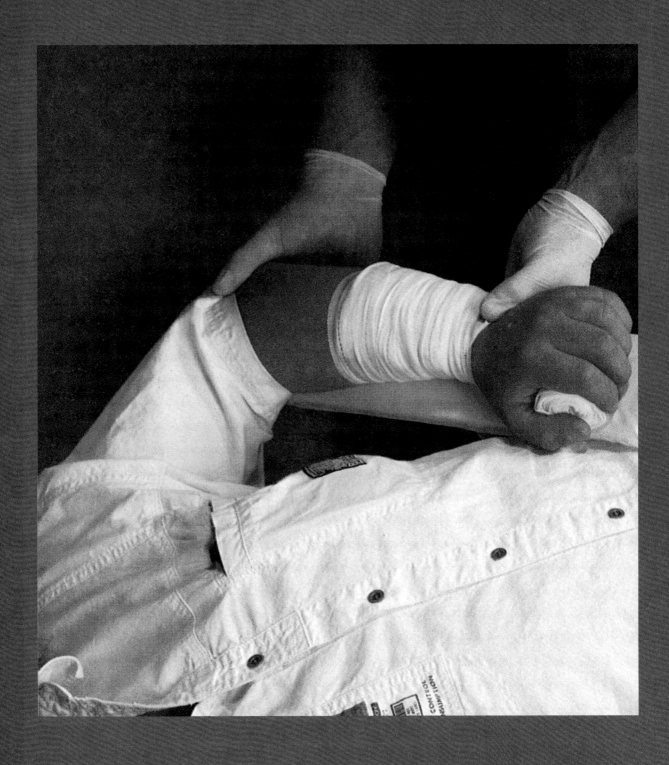

■ OBJECTIVES

By the end of this chapter, you should be able to:

1. Define splinting. (p. 250)
2. State the primary reason for splinting. (p. 251)
3. List five complications related to fractures and dislocations. (p. 251)
4. State when rigid splinting should be used as part of the care provided for a patient. (p. 252)
5. List the general steps to follow in all cases requiring the application of splints. (pp. 252–255)
6. Define traction and describe how traction is applied to an extremity prior to splinting. (pp. 256–257)
7. (*Optional*) Describe the procedures for straightening angulated closed fractures. (p. 257)
8. List objects that can be used as splints when commercial splints are not available. (p. 259)
9. Describe the rigid splinting procedures for possible fractures to the bones of the extremities. (pp. 260–270)

SKILLS

Upon completing this chapter and your class lectures and skills labs, you should be able to:

1. Evaluate simulated patients and determine if splinting is to be part of their care.
2. Perform splinting procedures, using noncommercial splints, for fractures to the bones of the extremities.
3. Use the commercial splints provided for First Responders in your area.

THE PROCESS OF SPLINTING

What Is Splinting?

Splinting—the application of a device that will immobilize a fractured bone and the joints above and below this bone.

1st Splinting is the process used to **immobilize** fractures and dislocations. Technically, any object that can be used for this purpose is called a splint.

In Chapter 10, pillows, blankets, towels, and dressings were listed for use in caring for patients with injuries to the extremities. These items are examples of **soft splints.** Soft splinting is not always very effective. It does a poor job of fully immobilizing the injured part and cannot immobilize the joints above and below the injury. Much of the effectiveness of soft splinting is dependent on patient cooperation. However, soft splinting does provide some support to the injured bone and will help to partially immobilize fractures and dislocations.

Soft splint—a device such as a pillow or sling that can be applied to immobilize a fracture.

It is easier to understand splinting when you consider **rigid splints.** These splints are stiff, with very little give or flexibility. They are applied along an injured bone to immobilize it and any joints directly above and below the injury site. In this way, the application of rigid splints helps to stabilize the injured bone and will keep the patient from moving the injured part. Rigid splints will allow for repositioning and transferring the patient without causing unwanted movement of bones and joints that might aggravate existing injuries.

Rigid splint—any stiff splinting device that has very little flexibility. Such a device must be long enough to immobilize the fractured bone and the joints above and below this bone.

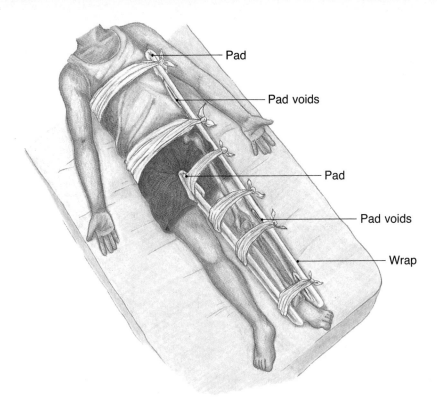

Labels on figure:
- Pad
- Pad voids
- Pad
- Pad voids
- Wrap

FIGURE 11–1. Splinting immobilizes fractures and dislocations.

Why Splint?

1st Splinting immobilizes fractured bones and dislocated joints, and reduces the movement of bone ends and fragments. By doing this, splinting helps to prevent or decrease the severity of the complications that accompany fractures and dislocations. These complications include:

1. Pain—in most cases, much of the patient's pain will be reduced after a splint is applied. Splinting helps to prevent the bone edges and fragments from rubbing against nerves and sensitive tissues. In cases of dislocation, splinting immobilizes bone ends to reduce pressure on these same tissues.
2. Damage to Soft Tissues—the processes of fracturing and dislocating cause soft tissue injuries. If the injured bone or dislocated joint is not immobilized, there will be additional damage to blood vessels.
3. Bleeding—dislocated bones, the ends of fractured bones, and bone fragments can damage blood vessels, producing serious bleeding. Splinting reduces this risk.
4. Restricted Blood Flow—dislocated bones, ends of fractured bones, and bone fragments can press against blood vessels, shutting off the flow of blood. The likelihood of this happening is greatly reduced by splinting.
5. Closed Fractures Becoming Open Fractures—the sharp edges of fractured bones can rip through the skin to produce an open fracture. Immobilizing fractured bones helps prevent this.

First Responder Responsibilities

NOTE: Some First Responder courses do not teach rigid splinting. If this is the case for your course, please understand that you *cannot* learn splinting skills by reading this book. You *must* be trained by a qualified instructor and you *must* practice splinting procedures under the guidance of this instructor.

Most First Responder courses teach the basics of rigid splinting. Since the majority of First Responders do not carry splints, or often find themselves

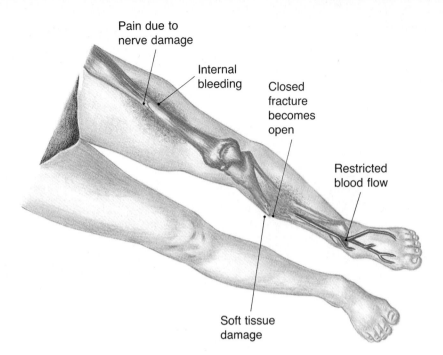

Pain due to
nerve damage

Internal
bleeding

Closed
fracture
becomes
open

Restricted
blood flow

Soft tissue
damage

FIGURE 11–2. Splinting can help prevent or lessen the severity of the complications associated with fractures.

providing care when away from their source of splints, noncommercial splints will be covered as part of your training. As a First Responder, you must be able to make and apply your own splints at the emergency scene.

In the majority of cases, EMTs will arrive before you have an opportunity to apply splints. Your primary duties will consist of detecting life-threatening problems and using your skills to control these problems. Since neck and spinal injuries, open head wounds, open chest wounds, open abdominal wounds, shock, and serious burns are cared for before fractures to the extremities, the EMTs will probably arrive at the scene before you start immobilizing fractures. In some situations, you will not be able to splint because you have to wait for the EMTs to arrive and provide care that must be done before splinting can be started. This would be true if a patient had possible neck or spinal injuries as well as possible fractures to his limbs. The splinting process could cause serious complications by moving the patient or the limb of the patient.

1st NOTE: For all cases involving possible fractures, have someone alert dispatch.

1st When you are in a situation where you must apply splints, you should:

- Use a sling and swathe or soft splint when the type of injury indicates their use.
- Apply rigid splints for cases of fractures to the shaft or wrist end of forearm bones, the thigh bone, and lower leg bones.
- Use soft or rigid splinting for injuries to the elbow end of the upper arm bone, the elbow, wrist, and hand (rigid splints are preferred).
- Splint when in doubt. If you are not certain if a fracture has occurred, go ahead and splint. Usually, the mechanism of injury and what signs you can detect will provide you with enough information to know if splinting is necessary. If you cannot determine if the patient has a probable hip fracture (upper end of the thigh bone) or a dislocated hip, *do not splint*. Wait for the EMTs to arrive.

For all cases of splinting, you should:

1. Reassure the patient, and say what you are doing and what you plan to do.
2. Control all serious bleeding, taking great care whenever possible not to apply pressure directly over a fractured bone or dislocated joint. Expose the injury site if necessary.

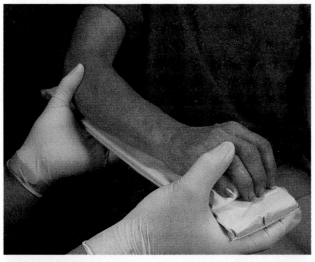
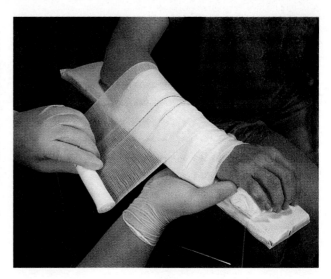
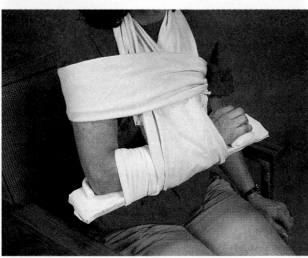

FIGURE 11–3. Applying a rigid splint.

3. Completely expose the injury site. Cut away clothing over the injury. In some cases, it may be possible to remove or fold back the clothing. Remove jewelry from the injured limb, if this can be easily done and you do not have to reposition the patient or the limb.

4. Dress open wounds (sterile dressings are highly recommended). *Do not* push bone ends back into an open fracture wound. *Do not* try to pick bone fragments from the wound. If the bone ends recede, report this to the EMTs.

5. Check for a distal pulse, capillary refill, and nerve function.

6. Have ready all the materials for splinting. Always use a padded splint. To do so will provide greater comfort to the patient and should improve the contact made between the patient's limb and the splint. If you are working with an unpadded splint, wrap it in dressing material or cloth to provide minimal padding.

7. If necessary, *gently* attempt to properly reposition the limb to apply the splint. Situations where this is not recommended will be discussed later in this chapter.

8. Where possible, immobilize the injured bone and the joints directly above and below the bone.

9. Splint firmly, but do not restrict circulation.

10. Secure the splint starting at the distal end. Leave fingertips and toes exposed.

11. Check for distal pulse, capillary refill, and nerve function after the splint is applied.

12. Provide care for shock.

■ SCAN 11–1.

Splinting

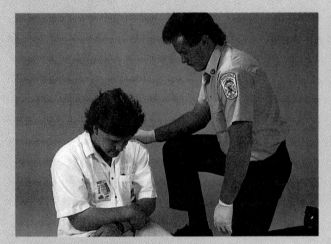

1 Reassure patient.

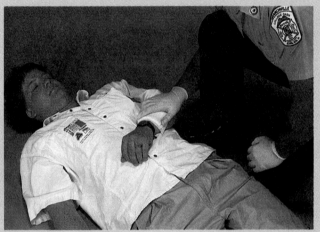

2 Control bleeding.

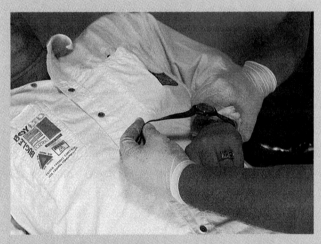

3 Completely expose site.

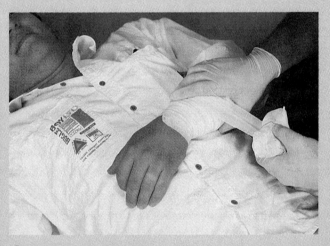

4 Dress open wounds.

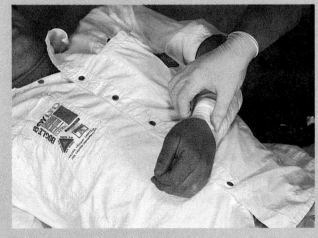

5 Check distal pulse, capillary refill, and nerve function.

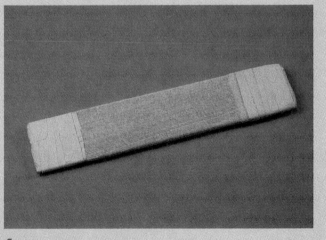

6 Use padded splint.

Splinting (continued)

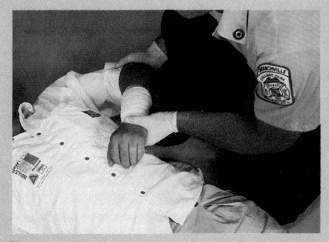

7 Reposition limb if appropriate.

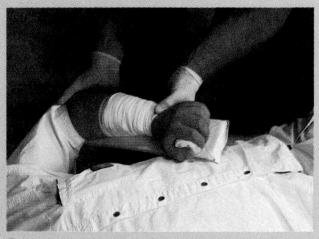

8 Immobilize joints above and below site.

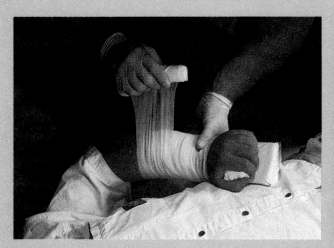

9 Splint firmly.

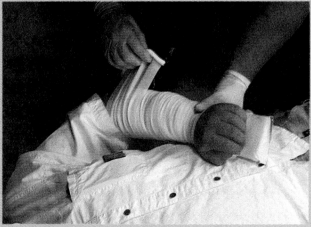

10 Secure splint.

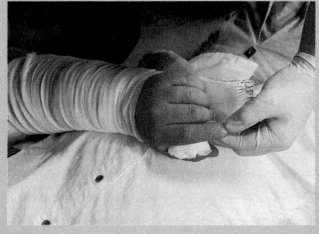

11 Reassess distal pulse, capillary refill, and nerve function.

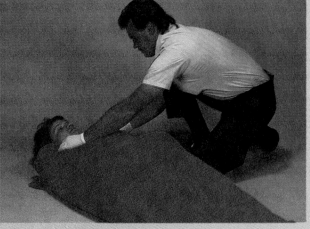

12 Provide care for shock.

Applying Manual Traction

NOTE: Not all EMS Systems have their First Responders apply manual traction when splinting. They permit them only to *gently* reposition a limb to allow for the application of a splint. Follow your local guidelines. When in doubt, contact your emergency department physician.

1st The results of splinting to immobilize fractures are improved if gentle tension is applied to the injured bone during the splinting process. In First Responder care, this tension is applied by pulling gently on the injured limb. The process is called *manual traction*. It will help to stabilize the fractured bones. In your EMS System, you may be limited to using manual traction to possible closed fractures that are not angulated. You should not apply manual traction to open fractures or angulated fractures.

WARNING: *Do not* apply manual traction if the injury is at or involves the shoulder, elbow, wrist, hand, pelvis, hip, knee, ankle, or foot. *Do not* apply manual traction to a lower limb if there is an angulated or open fracture of the thigh. Splint all dislocations in the position in which they are found.

Manual traction always causes a temporary increase in pain for the patient when it is first applied. You should tell the patient that there will be an increase in pain while you are applying traction, but that the pain caused by the fracture will probably lessen once the splint has been applied.

Traction is of little use if it is not maintained. A rigid splint, when secured to the patient, helps maintain traction. However, if you are working alone and apply manual traction to fractures and then release this tension to apply a splint, you have probably done little more than cause the patient additional pain.

If you have trained help at the scene, you can work with them to apply and maintain manual traction while a splint is secured to the patient. You may be able to have bystanders help you secure a splint while you maintain the traction.* Should you find yourself working alone, do not try to apply traction unless you cannot feel a distal pulse.

To apply manual traction, you should:

1. Be totally prepared to carry out the complete splinting process.
2. Grasp the patient's limb, placing one hand above the injury site and the other hand at the patient's uninjured hand or foot. Even though better tension can be applied if you place a hand just below the injury,

Manual traction—the stabilizing procedure that precedes the application of a rigid splint. Tension is applied by pulling gently along the long axis of the injured limb. The tension is maintained until the splint is fully applied.

*Follow your EMS System's guidelines.

FIGURE 11–4. Apply traction, whenever possible, before splinting.

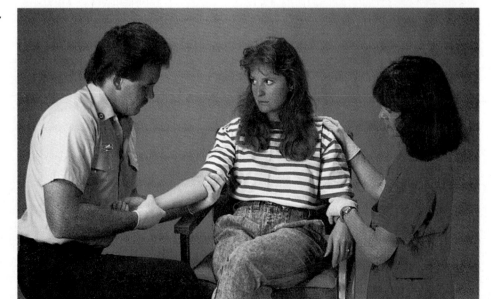

you must position your hands so that the splint can be applied without having to release manual traction.

3. *Gently* apply steady tension by pulling with your lower hand. The direction of pull should be along the natural line of the patient's limb. If you feel resistance, stop the procedure.

4. Maintain manual traction throughout the splinting process.

Straightening Angulated Fractures (*Optional*)

WARNING: Most EMS Systems do not allow their First Responders to straighten angulated fractures. Do only what you have been trained to do and what is allowed in your EMS System.

Angulated closed fractures can be straightened to improve circulation and ease the splinting process. If you are allowed to straighten angulated fractures, *follow your local guidelines* and:

- Do not attempt to straighten open angulated fractures.
- Do not attempt to straighten angulated fractures and dislocations of the wrist or shoulder.
- Angulated closed fractures of the elbow, knee, and ankle may be straightened if there is no distal pulse. In these cases, no tension is applied to the limb. This is simple repositioning for splinting.
- Make only one attempt to straighten the angulation.
- Stop if the limb offers resistance or the patient experiences additional pain.
- Do not attempt to straighten angulations if the injury involves the shoulder, pelvis, hip, thigh, wrist, hand, foot, or a joint immediately above or below the injury site.

The procedure for straightening angulated closed fractures is the same as for applying manual traction. Both should be done as one move.

SPLINTS

Commercial Splints

A wide variety of commercial splints are available for emergency care. These splints are made of wood, aluminum, compressed wood fibers, cardboard, foam, wire, or plastic. Some come with their own washable pads; others require padding to be applied before being secured. Most splints are either solid, rigid pieces, or inflatable plastic splints (air splints). Figure 11–5 shows some of the commercially available splints you might use in First Responder care.

Inflatable Splints

Very few First Responders carry commercial splints. Even fewer First Responders carry plastic inflatable splints (air splints). However, your area may train First Responders in the use of the inflatable splint. If so, your instructor will provide you with the details to apply the inflatable splints used in your locality. Typically, air splints are used when caring for patients with fractures of the arm or lower leg bones. When using inflatable splints, begin with an uninflated splint. Slip it over your forearm before you apply traction to the patient's injured limb. Once you have applied traction, you can easily slide the splint from your forearm onto the patient's injured limb. The splint can then be smoothed out and inflated by mouth (some areas prefer that you use a pump provided by the manufacturer). The splint is fully inflated for use when you can make a slight surface indentation with your fingertip.

■ SCAN 11–2.

Air-inflated Splints

WARNING:
Air-inflated splints may leak. Make certain that the desired pressure is maintained. When applied in cold weather, an inflatable splint will expand when the patient is moved to a warmer place. Variations in pressure also occur if the patient is moved to a different altitude. Occasionally monitor the pressure in the splint with your fingertip. Air-inflated splints may stick to the patient's skin in hot weather.

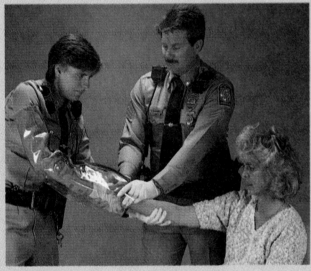

1 Slide the uninflated splint up your forearm, well above the wrist. Use this same hand to grasp the hand of the patient's injured limb as though you were going to shake hands.

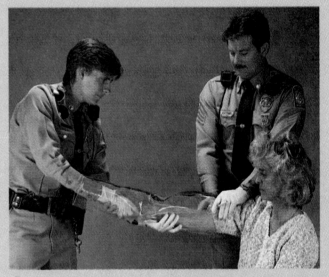

2 While holding her hand in this fashion, gently slide the splint over your hand and onto her limb. The lower edge of the splint should be just above her knuckles. Make sure the splint is properly placed and free of wrinkles.

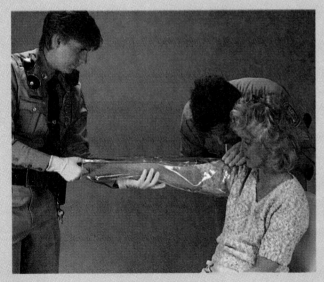

3 Continue to hold the patient's hand while you have your partner inflate the splint by mouth to a point where you can make a slight dent in the plastic when you press your thumb against the splint surface.

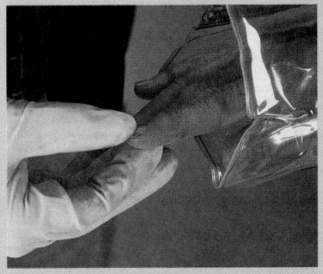

4 Monitor the patient's fingernail beds and fingertips for indications of circulation impairment. Continue to assess nerve function.

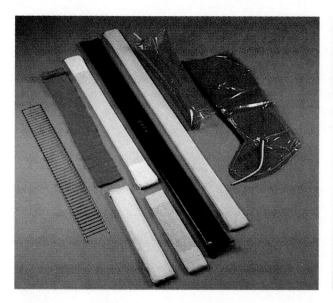

FIGURE 11–5. There are many types and sizes of commercial rigid splints.

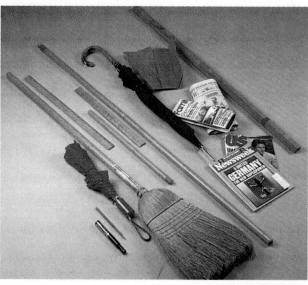

FIGURE 11–6. A First Responder must know how to make emergency splints.

If the patient is moved to a warmer or colder location, you will have to periodically recheck the pressure in the splint. Sometimes it is necessary to remove increased pressure by deflating the splint slightly. Do not leave the patient's splinted limb exposed to direct sunlight. Heat can build up in and under the plastic splint and cause serious burns. The pressure in the splint will change if the patient is moved to a different altitude. Always monitor the pressure in the splint. Old inflatable splints may leak.

Once an inflatable splint is applied, it is impossible to properly assess distal pulse. Instead, an evaluation of capillary refill is done. This limitation, the problems stated earlier, and the fact that some patients suffer significant pain when the splint is removed have led to some EMS Systems dropping inflatable splints from their approved equipment lists.

Making Emergency Splints

More often than not, First Responders arrive at the scene of an accident without any splints. Since this could happen to you, or you may find that you have used your splints before caring for all the patients at a scene, it is required that you learn how to make splints from materials at the scene. Your emergency splints may be soft splints (see Chapter 10) or they might be rigid splints made from a variety of materials.

1st Rigid splints can be made from pieces of lumber, plywood, compressed wood products, cardboard, rolled newspapers or magazines, umbrellas, canes, broom handles, shovel handles, sporting equipment (a catcher's or hockey goalee's shin guards have been used), and wire or tongue depressors (for fractured fingers). Most of these items can be found at the scene of a typical accident. Many people carry some of these items in the trunk of their car. Ask people at the scene to help you find something that can be used as a splint. Give them suggestions and ask if they have any ideas. Basically, you want something that is stiff and long enough to hold the fractured bone and the joints above and below this bone.

SPLINTING THE UPPER EXTREMITIES

The Shoulder Girdle

It is not practical to use a rigid splint for injuries to the collarbone, shoulder blade, and shoulder joint. Use a sling and swathe (see Chapter 10), remembering to add a pad between the patient's injured arm and chest if you are dealing with an anterior dislocation of the shoulder.

The Upper Arm

A sling and swathe are recommended for fractures to the shoulder end of the upper arm bone. Fractures to the shaft of the upper arm bone can be cared for with a wrist sling and swathe or a padded rigid splint and sling. A padded rigid splint and sling are recommended when the patient has a fracture to the elbow end of the upper arm bone.

If a sling is used, it is a good idea to add a swathe. This will secure the injured arm to the body, helping to immobilize the joints above and below the fracture sites.

1st When applying a splint in cases of upper arm fracture, you should try to work with a helper, even though the procedure can be carried out by one person. To apply a splint for injuries to the upper arm bone, you should:

1. Make sure that the splint is long enough and pad the splint before it is used.
2. Apply traction to the injured bone.
3. Place the splint alongside the injured bone.
4. Tie the splint to the patient using roller bandage, dressing material, handkerchiefs, cravats, or cloth strips. Start your ties at the distal end of the splint. Keep the hand in the position of function by placing a roll of dressing or cloth in the patient's palm.
5. Check for a distal pulse, capillary refill, and nerve function.
6. Apply a sling when possible. Adding a swathe will improve immobilization. Before applying a sling or swathe, place a pad between the side of the patient's chest and the splinted arm (small pillow, folded towel, and the like). After applying the sling or swathe, check once more for a pulse, capillary refill, and nerve function.

FIGURE 11–7. Splinting an injured upper arm.

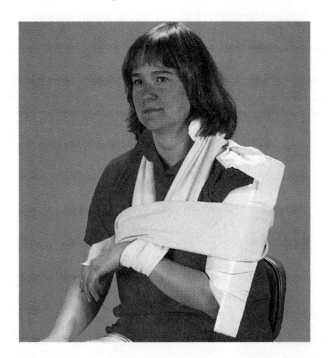

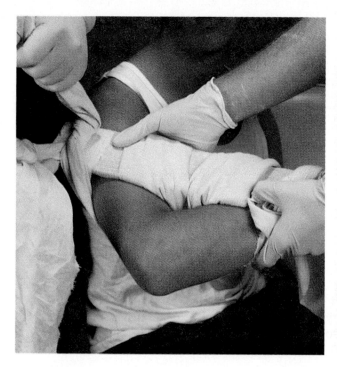

FIGURE 11–8. Applying a rigid splint for an injured elbow.

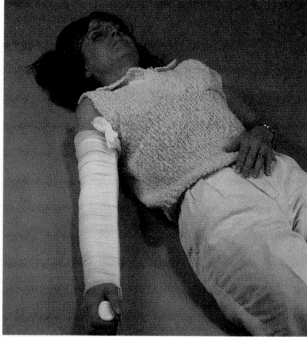

FIGURE 11–9. Splinting an injured elbow—arm straight.

The Elbow

Remember to immobilize the elbow in the position in which is was found. If the arm is in a straight position, you have to use a padded splint that will extend from the patient's armpit past the fingertips. If the patient's elbow is in a bent position, a splint can be applied as shown in Figure 11–8.

NOTE: Some EMS Systems allow their First Responders to make one gentle attempt to straighten the limb when there is no radial pulse. Perform this move only if you are allowed to do so. Check with your instructor. *Do not try to force the arm into its normal anatomical position.* Stop if the limb offers resistance or if the patient complains of increased pain.

The Forearm, Wrist, and Hand

1st Any fracture occurring to the forearm, wrist, or hand can be splinted using a padded, rigid splint that extends from above the elbow, past the fingertips. The patient's elbow, forearm, wrist, and hand should all receive support from the splint. The hand should be in the position of function.

FIGURE 11–10. The rigid splinting of an injured forearm.

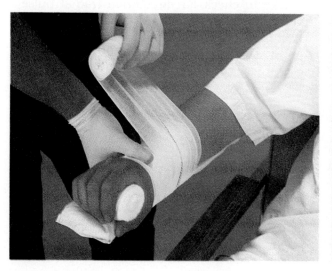

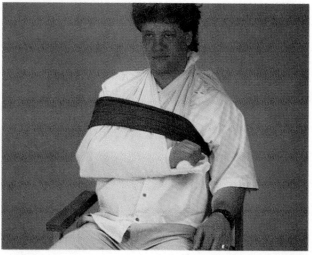

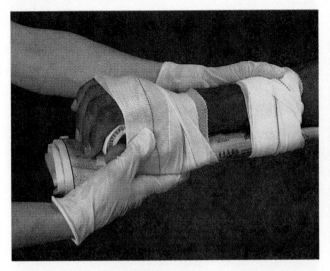
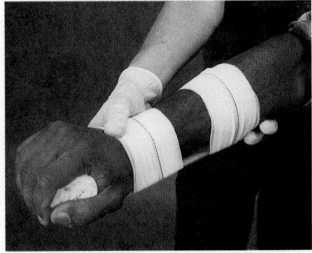

FIGURE 11–11. Rigid splints can be made from rolled newspapers, rolled magazines, or cardboard.

WARNING: If the injury is to the wrist, *Do not* attempt to straighten the wrist or hand. To do do could cause severe damage to blood vessels and nerves. Apply the splint while keeping the wrist in the position in which it was found.

1st Rolled newspapers, magazines, and creased cardboard make effective rigid splints for fractures to the forearm or wrist. Padding is still recommended. A sling should be applied after splinting. The addition of a swathe will improve immobilization of the elbow.

The Fingers

You can simply apply a soft bandage wrap, tape the injured finger to an adjacent, uninjured finger (as described in Chapter 10), or use a tongue depressor as a finger splint. The splint should be secured with roller bandage, cloth strips, or tape if no cloth is available. Care is improved if you apply a sling to reduce the movements of the patient's arm and hand.

Resplinting

1st After splinting, you will have to check for circulation (radial pulse), capillary refill, and nerve function (reaction to touch). Instead of removing the entire splint, first try loosening the ties. If there is any doubt about circulation and nerve function, maintain traction, remove the splint, and resplint the injured limb.

SPLINTING THE LOWER EXTREMITIES

WARNING: Do not use a log roll to move patients who may have lower extremity injuries. Wait for the EMTs to respond.

The Pelvic Girdle

1st As noted in Chapter 10, it is best to wait for more highly trained personnel to arrive in cases where a patient has fractures to the pelvis. Be prepared for the patient to go into shock. Take great care. If the force producing

■ SCAN 11–3.

Splinting: The Upper Extremity

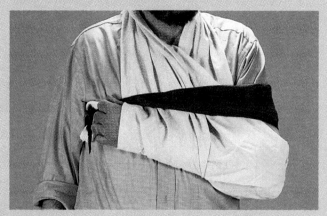

Shoulder: Apply a sling and swathe. Lift wrist 4 inches.

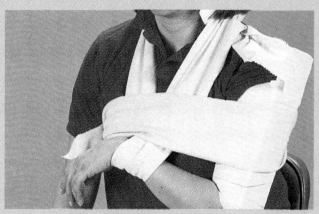

Arm: Immobilize with a rigid splint from shoulder past elbow. Apply sling and swathe.

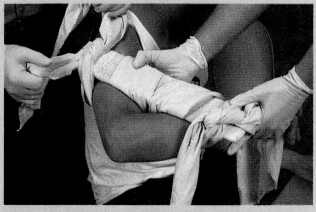

Elbow: Place splint from shoulder to wrist. Secure wrist first.

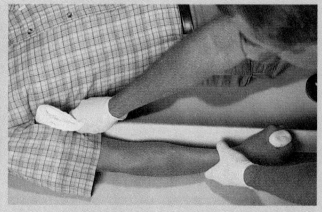

Elbow (limb straight): Pad armpit. Splint should extend from armpit, past hand. Secure with roller dressing, hand to shoulder.

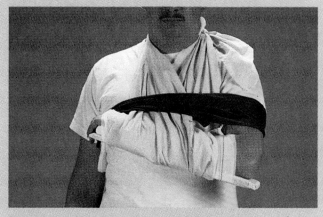

Forearm, wrist, or hand: The splint should extend from past the elbow to past the hand.

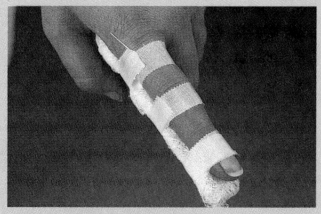

Finger: Splint with tongue depressor or tape to adjacent uninjured finger.

NOTE: When possible, place a roll of dressing in the hand of the injured limb. This will keep the hand in the position of function, the position the hand would be in if the patient were to reach out and pick up a small rubber ball.

the injury was great enough to severely injure the pelvis, there is a good chance that there are spinal injuries.

1st If the patient has fractures to the hip (upper end of the thigh bone), you may tie the legs together or apply a long board splint. If you tie the legs together, be certain to pad between the patient's legs. If you apply a splint, the splint must be long enough to extend from the patient's armpit past the foot. It must be rigid, with very little flexibility, and it must be well padded (add additional padding at the armpit). To secure the splint to the patient, ties must be made around the patient's trunk and the leg of the injured side. Applying these ties can require you to slightly reposition the patient several times. For this reason, you would do better to wait for EMTs to arrive or to use the simpler approach of tying the patient's legs together.

NOTE: If the hip is dislocated or you are not sure if the injury is a fracture or dislocation of the hip, **wait for the EMTs to arrive.**

1st If you know that EMTs will arrive quickly at the scene of an accident, *do not* splint for fractures to the thigh bone. To do so will complicate the care the EMTs need to provide at the scene. If their arrival is delayed and you must splint, use a long board splint that is rigid and well padded. When splinting is complete, the patient should appear like the person shown in Figure 11–12. Be certain to pad between the patient's armpit and the splint. *Do not* place a tie over the fracture site.

FIGURE 11–12. Using a long board splint for hip injuries.

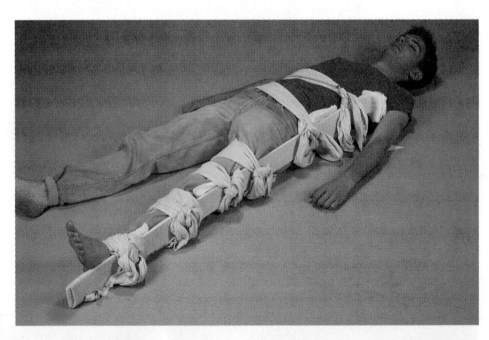

FIGURE 11–13. Use a coathanger flat splint to push cravat under void. B. Reposition the cravat over the proper site.

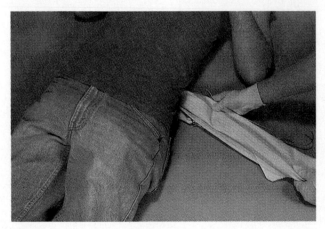

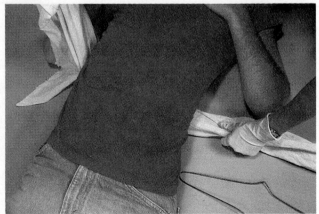

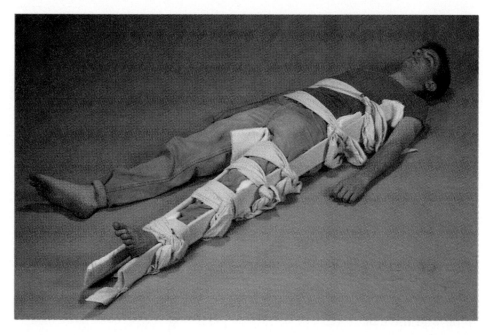

FIGURE 11–14. Splinting injuries to the thigh bone.

An even better approach is to splint with one long splint from the patient's armpit, extending past the foot and a shorter splint that will extend from the top of the inside thigh (crotch) to beyond the foot. This is shown in Figure 11–14. Whenever possible, push the ties under the patient's trunk and legs at the natural voids (lower back, knees) using a thin splint or cardboard, to reduce patient movement. Be certain to pad the patient's armpit and groin. *Do not* place a tie over the fracture site. For that part of the thigh, place one tie above, and one tie below the injury.
REMEMBER: Fractures to the thigh bone can produce profuse bleeding. Provide care for shock and monitor the patient.

The Knee

Unless there is no distal pulse, splint an injured knee in the position in which it is found. If the patient's leg is straight or you must straighten the leg because there is no distal pulse, you should secure a long splint from the patient's armpit to beyond the foot. If you cannot find a splint that long, use a splint that will extend from the patient's waist to beyond the foot. In cases where the patient's leg will remain flexed at the knee, you can use a shorter splint, as shown in Figure 11–15.

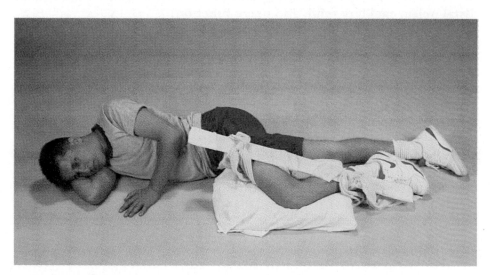

FIGURE 11–15. Splinting an injured knee in the position in which it was found.

If there is no distal pulse, some EMS Systems allow their First Responders one attempt to move the leg into the anatomical position. This must be done gently. *Do not force the leg* into the anatomical position. Stop if there is resistance or if the patient experiences an increase in pain.

The Lower Leg

1st Splinting of the lower leg can be done with two rigid splints. The application of these splints can be done as recommended for fractures of the thigh bone. Scansheet 11.6 shows the patient splinted using two splints. A single splint method can be used to immobilize possible lower leg fractures. The procedure is shown in Scansheets 11.4 and 11.5.

After splinting is complete, you MUST check for circulation and nerve function. If either is absent, you will have to resplint.

The Ankle and Foot

Soft splinting is recommended for injuries to the ankle or foot (see page 247). If you apply long splints, extend them from above the patient's knee to beyond the foot.

Resplinting

Resplint if there is a loss of distal pulse, slowed capillary refill, or a loss of nerve function after the splinting process. Begin by loosening the ties. If this does not work, stabilize the leg and remove the splint.

SUMMARY

Splinting is used to **immobilize** fractures. The process can be carried out using **soft splints** or **rigid splints.**

The application of a splint can help to prevent or reduce the severity of complications such as **pain, soft tissue damage, bleeding, restricted blood flow,** and closed fractures becoming **open fractures.**

When in doubt, splint.

Remember to cut away, remove, or lift clothing from the injury site before splinting. Control bleeding and dress open wounds. Check for a **distal pulse, capillary refill,** and **nerve function.**

All rigid splints should be padded before they are secured to the patient.

A rigid splint should immobilize the **injured bone** and the **joints** directly above and below the bone.

Manual traction is applied by pulling gently on an injured limb along its natural line. If traction is applied, it must be maintained until the rigid splint is secured.

As a First Responder, you must be able to use noncommercial splints. Consider lumber, plywood, rolled newspapers and magazines, compressed wood products, sporting equipment, canes, umbrellas, cardboard, and tool handles when you need to make an emergency splint.

Soft and rigid splinting for various injuries to the extremities is summarized in Scansheet 11–7.

■ SCAN 11–4.

The Ankle Hitch

The ankle hitch can be used with a single padded board splint to immobilize injured knees and legs. It is made with a 3-inch-wide cravat.

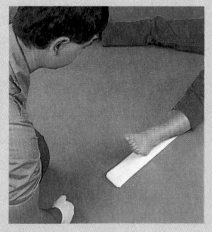

1 Kneel at distal end of injured limb.

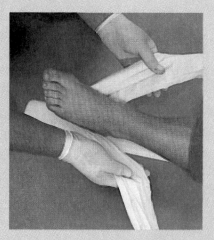

2 Center the cravat in arch.

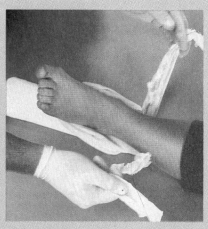

3 Place cravat along sides of foot and cross cravat behind ankle.

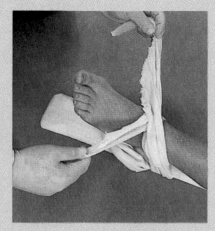

4 Cross the cravat ends over top of ankle.

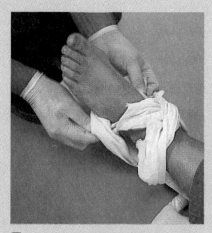

5 A stirrup has been formed.

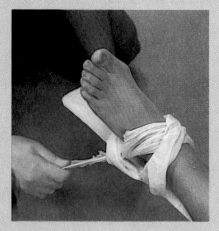

6 Thread ends through stirrup.

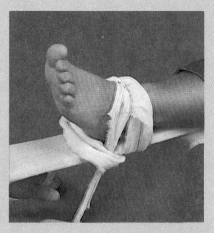

7 Pull ends downward to tighten.

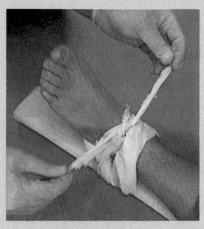

8 Pull upward and tie over ankle wrap.

Leg Injuries: Single-splint Method

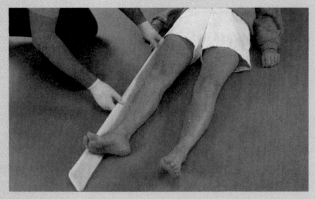

1 Measure splint—it should extend from mid thigh to 4 inches below ankle.

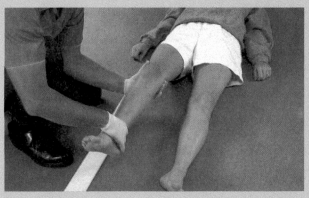

2 Apply manual traction and lift limb 10 inches off ground.

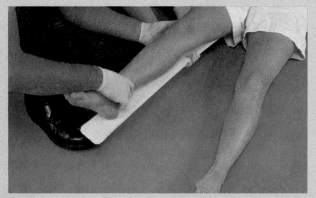

3 Place splint along the posterior of the limb, at mid thigh.

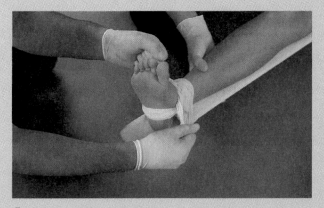

4 Apply ankle hitch (see Scansheet 11–4).

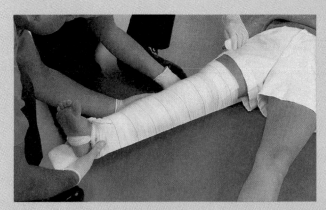

5 Secure, distal to proximal.

NOTE: Reassess distal pulse, capillary refill, and nerve function. Elevate the splinted injured limb and care for shock.

■ SCAN 11–6.

Splinting: The Lower Extremity

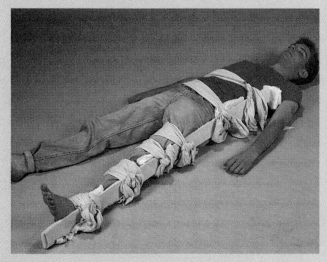

Hip

If possible, wait for the EMTs. If you must immobilize, tie the lower limbs together or apply a long rigid splint:

- Splint from armpit to past the foot.
- Pad armpit and splint surface.
- Tie around trunk and injured limb.

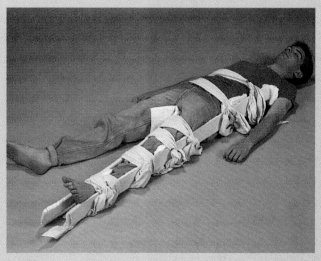

Thigh

If possible, wait for the EMTs. Otherwise, apply two splints:

- Long: armpit to past foot.
- Short: crotch to past foot.
- Pad armpit, crotch, and between patient and splints.
- Tie around trunk, above and below fracture, below knee, and at ankle.

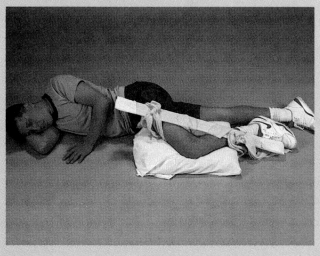

Knee

- Distal pulse: splint as found. No distal pulse: move gently to straight position (if allowed).
- Knee bent: secure splint to thigh and lower leg. Knee straight: use long splint from armpit past the foot.

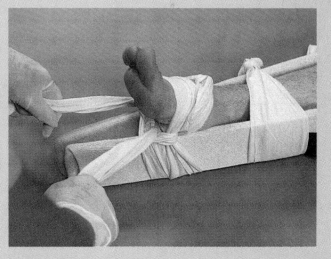

Lower Leg

Apply two rigid splints, one lateral, one medial. A single splint can be applied to the back of the leg and secured with an ankle hitch and dressing or cravats.

NOTE: Pillows can be used to splint injured ankles, and feet. REMEMBER: Check for distal pulse, capillary refill, and nerve function before and after splinting an injured extremity.

■ SCAN 11–7.

Care for Injuries to the Extremities

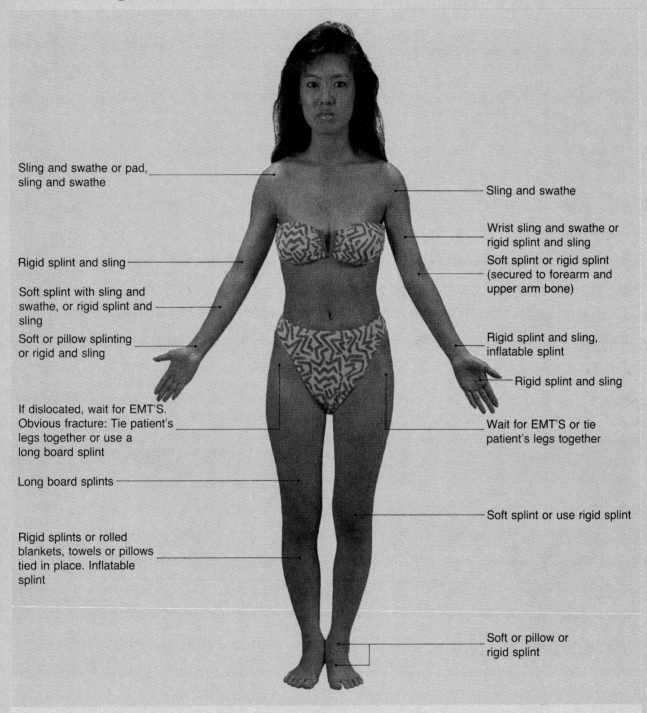

Sling and swathe or pad, sling and swathe

Sling and swathe

Wrist sling and swathe or rigid splint and sling

Rigid splint and sling

Soft splint or rigid splint (secured to forearm and upper arm bone)

Soft splint with sling and swathe, or rigid splint and sling

Soft or pillow splinting or rigid and sling

Rigid splint and sling, inflatable splint

Rigid splint and sling

If dislocated, wait for EMT'S. Obvious fracture: Tie patient's legs together or use a long board splint

Wait for EMT'S or tie patient's legs together

Long board splints

Soft splint or use rigid splint

Rigid splints or rolled blankets, towels or pillows tied in place. Inflatable splint

Soft or pillow or rigid splint

REMEMBER: YOU MUST CHECK FOR A DISTAL PULSE AND NERVE FUNCTION BEFORE AND AFTER SPLINTING. IF THERE IS A DISTAL PULSE, SPLINT THE ELBOW OR KNEE AS IT IS FOUND. WHEN POSSIBLE, A SPLINT SHOULD IMMOBILIZE THE INJURED BONE AND THE JOINTS ABOVE AND BELOW THIS BONE. IF A JOINT IS INJURED, IMMOBILIZE THE JOINT AREA AND THE BONES THAT MAKE UP THE JOINT.

CHAPTER 12

Injuries—3:
Skull, Spine,
and Chest

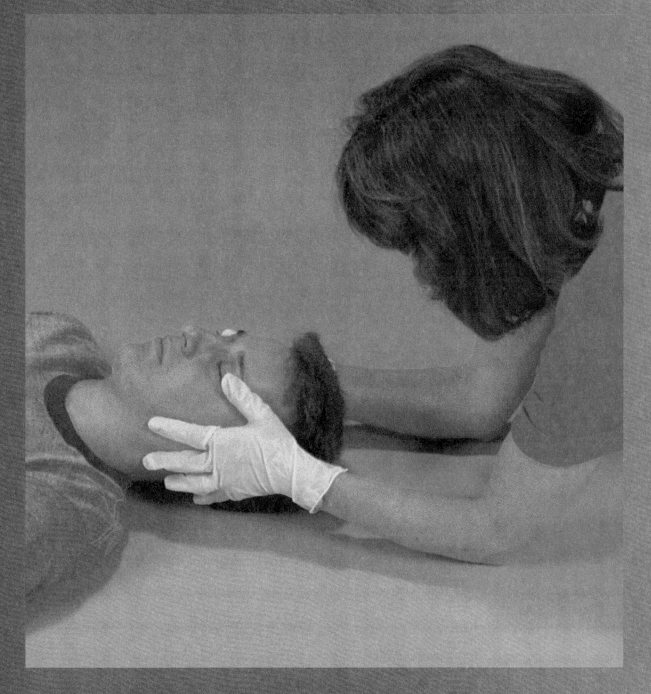

■ OBJECTIVES

By the end of this chapter, you ahould be able to:

1. Define axial skeleton using the terms: skull, cervical spine, spine, and rib cage. (p. 272)
2. Classify the brain and spinal cord as part of the central nervous system. (p. 275)
3. List the major injuries to the skull and brain. (pp. 276–277)
4. List the symptoms and signs of skull injury and brain injury. (pp. 277–279)
5. Describe what to do and what not to do when caring for patients with injuries to the skull or brain. (pp. 279–281)
6. List the steps for surveying the conscious and the unconscious patient to detect possible spinal injury and relate these methods to the secondary survey. (pp. 282–285)
7. Describe the common mechanisms of neck and spine injuries. (p. 281–282)
8. List the principles of emergency care for the neck and spine, telling what a First Responder should and should not do. (pp. 283–286)
9. List the symptoms and signs of chest injuries. (pp. 287, 289, 290, 291–292)
10. Describe how the First Responder should care for rib fractures, flail chest, and penetrating chest wounds. (pp. 288–293)

SKILLS

Upon completing this chapter and your class lectures and skills labs, you should be able to take situations presented by your instructor and:

1. Identify injuries to the skull, neck, spine, and chest.
2. Act out an assessment of a conscious patient to detect neck and spinal injuries.
3. Act out an assessment of an unconscious patient to detect neck and spinal injuries.
4. Perform emergency care procedures for simulated cases of skull, neck, and spine injuries.
5. Perform emergency care procedures for simulated cases of fractured ribs, flail chest, and penetrating chest wounds.

THE AXIAL SKELETON

Axial (AK-si-al) skeleton—the bones and joints of the skull, spine, and chest.

The axial (AK-si-al) skeleton consists of the skull, spine, and chest. It makes up the long axis of the body. The pelvis and shoulders are not part of the axial skeleton. They are part of the extremities or appendicular (AP-en-DIK-u-ler) skeleton, which was covered in Chapter 10.

Injuries to the axial skeleton can be very serious. The problems resulting from such injuries relate not only to the skeletal system, but also to the structures protected by the bones of the axial skeleton. Your major concern is not with the bones, but with the brain, spinal cord, airway, lungs, and heart. When the skull, spine, or chest is injured, carefully and gently assess the patient for more serious injuries, rather than caring immediately for possible fractures.

Cranium (KRAY-ni-um)—the bones that form the forehead and the floor, back, top, and upper sides of the skull. Usually, the term *skull fracture* refers to a break in one or more of the cranial bones.

The Skull

The skull is divided into two major structures, the cranium (KRAY-ni-um) and the face. Flat, irregularly shaped bones make up the cranium. They are fused together to produce immovable joints, which form a rigid, protec-

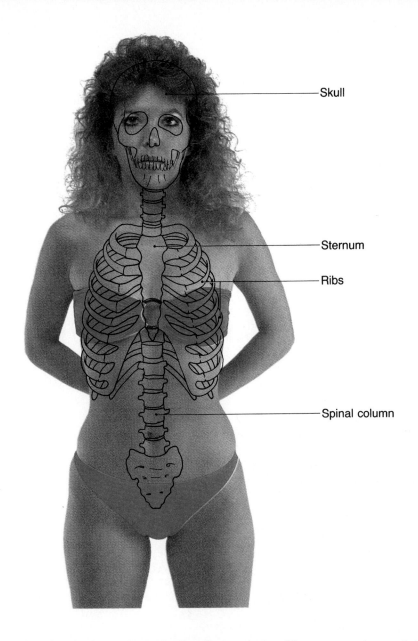

- Skull

- Sternum

- Ribs

- Spinal column

FIGURE 12–1. Axial skeleton.

tive housing for the brain. In infants, this process of fusion is not complete, causing "soft spots" to exist in a baby's skull. Therefore, you should never apply pressure to the skull of an infant. When you hold the head, spread out your fingers to reduce pressure and be alert so that your fingers do not rest over any "soft spots."

The cranium makes up the back and top of the skull, the sides of the upper skull, and the forehead.

The human face is made up of strong, irregularly shaped bones. These bones, just as in the case of the cranium, are fused into immovable joints, except for the lower jaw bone or mandible (MAN-di-bl). The face bones include part of the eye sockets, the cheeks, the upper part of the nose, the upper jaw, and the lower jaw.

Mandible (MAN-di-bl)—the lower jaw bone.

The Spine

The spine includes the neck bones and the back bones. The neck bones are known as the cervical (SER-ve-kal) spine. The rest of the spine is commonly known as the backbone. The spine protects the spinal cord as it runs from the brain down through the back. Many of the body's major nerves run into and out of the spinal cord, connecting most areas of the body to the brain. In addition, the spine acts as a support for the entire body. The skull, shoulders, ribs, and pelvis all connect to the spine.

Cervical (SER-ve-kal) spine— the neck bones.

SKULL

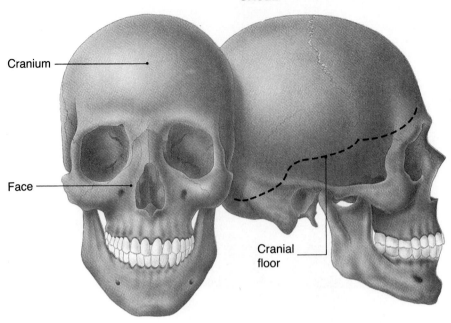

Cranium

Face

Cranial
floor

FIGURE 12–2. The skull.

FIGURE 12–3. The spine.

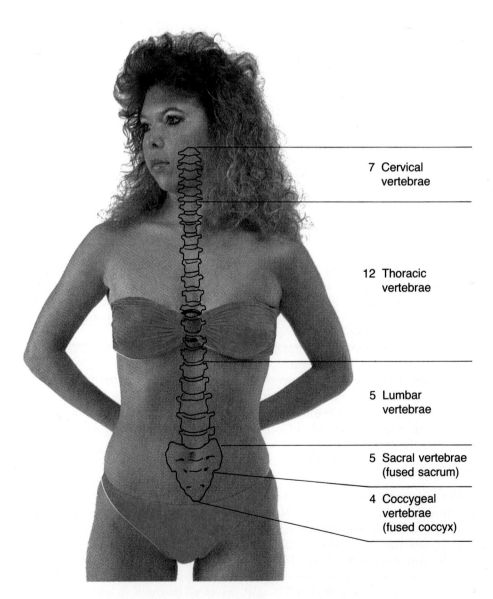

7 Cervical
vertebrae

12 Thoracic
vertebrae

5 Lumbar
vertebrae

5 Sacral vertebrae
(fused sacrum)

4 Coccygeal
vertebrae
(fused coccyx)

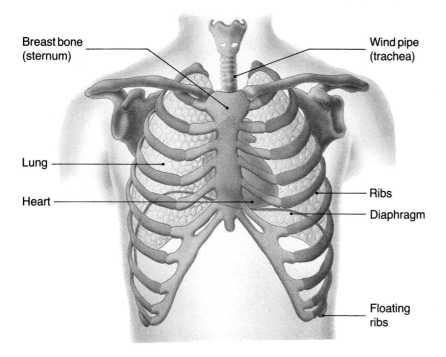

Breast bone
(sternum)

Wind pipe
(trachea)

Lung

Heart

Ribs

Diaphragm

Floating
ribs

FIGURE 12–4.   The chest.

The Chest

The ribs protect the structures found in the chest. All the ribs connect with the spine. Most of the ribs have pieces of cartilage that connect directly to the sternum (breastbone) in the front of the body. Some of the ribs connect to other ribs by way of cartilage strips. The bottom two ribs on each side do not connect to the breastbone or to other ribs. They are some-times called "floating" ribs. Since these lower ribs are held in place by muscles and their attachments to the spine, they do not really float. Men and women both have the same number of ribs, 12 on each side of the chest.

The lower ribs help to protect the liver, gallbladder, stomach, and spleen.

The center of the chest is occupied by the heart and the major blood vessels leading into and out of the heart. The trachea (windpipe), leading to the lungs, and the esophagus, leading to the stomach, pass through the center of the chest. The lungs occupy most of the remaining space found in the chest. The muscles of the back and chest, along with the muscles found between the ribs, give added strength to the spine and the ribs, helping to protect the heart and lungs.

The Central Nervous System

Remember, injuries to the head and spine can involve much more than just the bones making up these structures. The brain, spinal cord, and certain major nerves make up what is known as the central nervous system. The brain not only takes care of thinking, it also controls many of our most basic functions, including heart activity and breathing. The brain tells muscles when to contract and relax so that we can move. It receives messages from all over the body and decides how the body will respond to these messages. Any injury to the skull could injure the brain, causing vital body functions to fail.

The spinal cord takes messages from the brain to most of the body and from most of the body to the brain. Injury to the spine could cause damage to the spinal cord and isolate a part of the body so that it no longer has contact with the brain. If the damage is serious enough, a part of the body may never again be able to move or function. In addition to

Central nervous system—the brain and spinal cord. Sometimes referred to as the CNS.

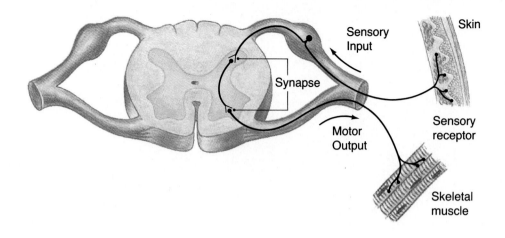

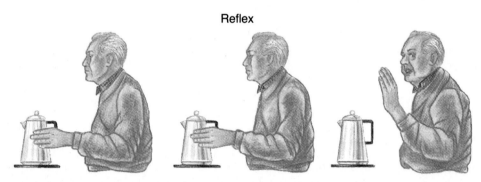

FIGURE 12–5. Reflexes allow for a swift reaction.

this, the spinal cord is also the site of many reflexes. Reflexes allow us to react quickly to such things as pain and heat (see Figure 12–5). Damage to the spinal cord can take away reflexes in certain areas of the body.

INJURIES TO THE SKULL

Types of Injuries

1st Injuries to the skull can include fractures to the cranium and face, direct injuries to the brain, and indirect injuries to the brain. In addition, there can be cuts to the scalp and other soft tissue injuries, as covered in Chapter 9.

1st Normally, when you hear the term "fractured skull," the person is really talking about fractures to the cranium. (Fractures to the facial bones are called facial fractures.) Any time the bones of the cranium are broken or cracked, the patient is said to have an **open head injury.** If the cranium is intact, that is, it is free of fractures, the term **closed head injury** is used. This is true even if the scalp has been cut or torn open.

Fractures to the skull can be simple cracks (linear), many cracks radiating out from the center of a wound (comminuted), depressed fractures where bone is pushed inward, or fractures to the base of the skull (basal).

Facial fractures can be very serious. Of main concern is the fact that many facial fractures cause airway obstructions. Blood, blood clots, bone, and teeth may cause partial or full airway obstruction. Often missed with facial fractures is the possibility of fractures to the base of the skull. This is not the back of the head, where head and neck meet. It is the floor of the cranium that makes up the lower wall of the brain cavity (see Figure 12–2).

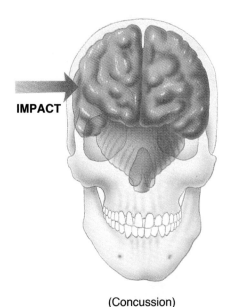

(Concussion)

Bruised brain
(contusion)

FIGURE 12–6. Closed head
injuries.

1st Injuries to the brain can be direct or indirect. Direct injuries often occur in open head injuries. The brain may be cut, torn, or bruised by broken bones of the skull or by foreign objects. In cases of closed head injuries and certain types of open head injuries, damage to the brain can be indirect. The patient's brain is injured by the force of something striking the skull. Indirect injuries to the brain include:

- *Concussion*—when a blow to the head does not cause an open head injury and damage to the brain is so minor that it is not easily detected, the patient is said to have a concussion. Patients may or may not become unconscious. If they do, the unconsciousness lasts for a short while and usually does not recur. Most patients with a concussion will be a little "groggy." Headache is common. Not so common is the temporary loss of short-term memory (recent events, including the accident). In rare cases, long-term memory may be lost temporarily. The symptoms and signs of a concussion indicate the possibility of serious injury.
- *Bruising* (contusion)—a bruised brain can occur with closed head injuries. The force of the blow can be great enough to rupture blood vessels on the surface of the brain or deep within the brain. Often, this bruising takes place on the side of the brain opposite the point of impact.

Concussion—a closed head injury producing minor brain damage. The patient may or may not become unconscious. The presence of a concussion indicates the possibility of more severe injury.

Symptoms and Signs of Skull Injury

1st Many skull fractures are obvious. Edges or fragments of bones can be seen. In some cases, the brain or pieces of the brain may be visible. Some skull fractures are difficult to detect. You should consider a cranial fracture as a possibility whenever you note:

- Unconsciousness or a decrease in level of awareness
- An injury that has produced a deep cut, tear, or bruise to the scalp or forehead
- Any pain or swelling at the site of a head injury
- Deformity of the skull—depressions in the cranium, large swellings ("goose eggs"), or anything that looks wrong with the shape of the cranium
- Any bruise behind the ear (usually a late sign)
- Black eyes or discoloration under the eyes

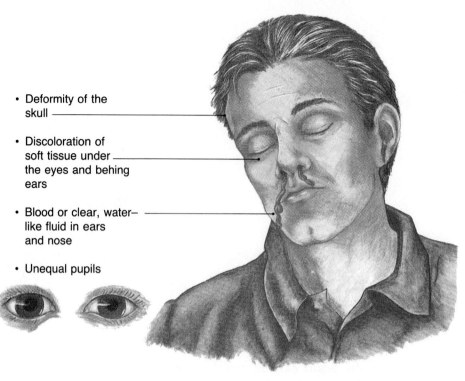

- Deformity of the skull
- Discoloration of soft tissue under the eyes and behing ears
- Blood or clear, water–like fluid in ears and nose
- Unequal pupils

FIGURE 12–7. Signs of skull fracture

- One or both eyes appearing to be sunken
- Unequal pupils
- Bleeding from the ears and/or the nose
- Clear or bloody fluid flowing from the ears and/or nose—this could be cerebrospinal (ser-e-bro-SPIN-nal) fluid, also called CSF. This fluid surrounds the brain and spinal cord. It cannot be released through the ears or nose unless the cranium has been fractured.
- Deterioration of vital signs—each time you assess the patient's pulse and respirations, the results are progressively worse.

1st Consider the possibility of fracial fractures when you note:

- Blood in the airway
- Facial deformities
- Black eyes or discoloration below the eyes
- Swollen lower jaw or poor jaw function
- Teeth that are loose or have been knocked out (or dentures that are broken)
- Large bruises on the face
- Any indication of a severe blow to the face

Symptoms and Signs of Brain Injury

1st In cases of head injury, you should consider the possibility of a brain injury if you note:

- Headache (mild to severe) following an accident
- Any signs of a skull fracture
- Loss of consciousness or altered states of awareness
- Confusion or personality changes
- Unequal or unresponsive pupils
- Paralysis—often, this will be paralysis to one side of the body. This can

Cerebrospinal (ser-e-bro-SPI-nal) fluid—the clear, watery fluid that surrounds the brain and spinal cord. It may be referred to as CSF.

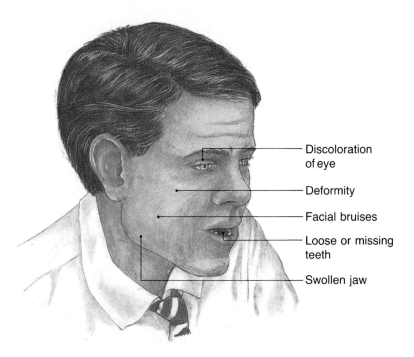

FIGURE 12–8. Signs of facial fracture.

be opposite the side of the head that has been injured. Paralysis of the facial muscles may interfere with speech.

- Loss of sensations—this may be limited to one body part on one side of the body
- Disturbed or impaired vision, hearing, and/or equilibrium (sense of balance)
- Pulse rate that is slow and full, then becoming fast and weak
- Changing patterns of respiration, usually becoming labored, then rapid, then stopping for a few seconds.

NOTE: Since many of the signs of head and brain injury can be produced by drug or alcohol abuse, take great care in assessing the patient. *Never assume alcohol or drug abuse and rule out possible injuries.*

CARE FOR HEAD INJURIES

Injuries to the Cranium

1st When caring for patients with injuries to the cranium, assume that neck or spinal injuries also exist and:

1. Maintain an open airway—if injuries are open or if skull fracture is obvious, use the jaw-thrust technique.
2. Provide resuscitative measures if needed.
3. Keep the patient at rest—this can be a critical factor. Do not let the patient move or change position.
4. Control bleeding—do not apply pressure if the injury site shows bone fragments or depression of the bone, or the brain is exposed. A bulky dressing will have to be loosely applied. *Do not* attempt to stop the flow of blood or CSF from the ears or the nose. For such cases, loosely secure a dressing to help prevent further contamination.

5. Talk to the conscious patient—try to keep the person alert.
6. Dress and bandage open wounds, stabilizing any penetrating objects (*do not* remove any objects or fragments of bone).
7. Provide care for shock—avoid overheating the patient. Remember, the patient is not to be given anything by mouth.
8. Monitor vital signs.
9. Provide emotional support.
10. Be prepared for vomiting.

WARNING: It is a serious sign when an unconscious patient regains consciousness and then loses consciousness again. Make certain you report this to the EMTs.

Do not reposition any patient with an open head wound or any other possible serious injury to the skull, unless you must do so to provide CPR or pulmonary resuscitation. If there is any chance of neck or spinal injuries, the patient should not be repositioned. For conscious patients with minor closed head injuries, with no signs of neck or spinal injuries, you have two choices for positioning the patient. Both methods are suitable for patients with facial fractures. The methods are:

1. Head elevated—do not simply elevate the patient's head and neck. This could partially obstruct the airway. Also, this is a dangerous position for the patient if vomiting should occur. It is best to place the patient's upper body at a 45-degree angle.
2. Side placement—the patient with no open head injuries or possible neck and spine injuries can be placed on one side with the head turned to allow for drainage of blood and mucus from the mouth and nose.

FIGURE 12–9. Head and shoulders elevated position for patients having mild head injuries.

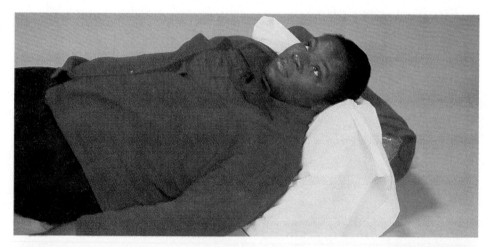

FIGURE 12–10. Side position for patients having mild head injuries.

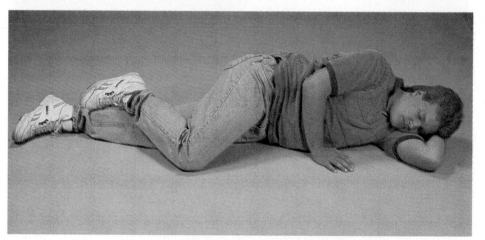

Facial Fractures

1st As in all cases of facial injury, make certain that the patient has an open airway. If any resuscitative measures must be taken, it is better to use the jaw-thrust method whenever possible in case there is injury to the neck and spine. Take care in applying direct pressure in cases of bleeding. Try not to apply any pressure over a possible fracture site. Care for soft tissue injuries as directed in Chapter 9.

The lower jaw is the site of many facial fractures. Since it is a movable joint, dislocation is possible. The indications of possible fracture or dislocation include:

- Pain
- Swelling
- Facial distortion
- Discoloration
- Loss of use or difficulty with speech
- Bleeding around the teeth

To care for possible fracture or dislocation of the lower jaw:

1. Maintain an open airway.
2. Control bleeding and dress any open wounds. *Do not* tie the patient's mouth shut, since there may be vomiting.
3. Keep the patient at rest and provide care for shock.
4. Closely monitor the patient, staying alert for vomiting.

Injuries to the face can damage teeth, crowns (caps), bridges, and dentures. Always look for and remove avulsed (dislodged) teeth and parts of broken dental appliances. Be careful not to push these down the patient's airway.

When a tooth is avulsed, there is bleeding from the socket. Tell the conscious patient to bite down on a pad of gauze placed over the socket.*For the unconscious patient, hold the gauze over the socket or place a small piece of gauze into the socket. *Do not* place cotton packets or bits of cotton into the socket.

Wrap the avulsed tooth in a dressing. If you have a source of clean water, keep the dressing moist (milk can be used if no water is available.) *Do not* attempt to clean the tooth. Your efforts could damage microscopic structures needed to replant the tooth.

INJURIES TO THE NECK AND SPINE

Types of Injuries

Soft tissues of the neck can be injured in a number of ways, as discussed in Chapter 9. In addition to these types of injuries, the patient may have injuries to the bones and spinal cord running through the neck. The neck portion of the spine is called the cervical (SER-ve-kal) spine. Damage to this portion of the spine can be one of the most serious of all injuries. Improper care of cervical spine injuries can lead to paralysis or death. Injuries along the rest of the spinal column also can be as serious as those to the cervical spine.

Neck and spinal injuries can occur from blows to the head, neck, back, chest, pelvis, or legs. Often, you will find patients with head injuries who also have neck injuries. Fractures to the upper leg bones or to the pelvic

---

* Leave several inches of the gauze outside the patient's mouth to allow for quick removal.

bones may also indicate a strong possibility of spinal injury. Certain types of emergencies such as motor vehicle accidents (including those producing whiplash), falls, diving board accidents, and skiing accidents often cause neck and spinal injuries.

Should a patient have numbness, loss of feeling, or paralysis in the legs, with no problems in the arms, the injury is probably, but not always, below the neck. If numbness, loss of feeling, or paralysis involves the arms and the legs, the injury probably involves the neck and perhaps other areas of the spine. Numbness, loss of feeling, and paralysis may be limited to only one side of the body, but usually both sides are involved.

Injuries to the spine can include swelling, bones being pressed on nerves, fractured vertebrae (spinal column bones), and damaged nerves. All these can produce the same symptoms and signs. In many cases, the loss of function associated with spinal injuries will be temporary. For others, even the best surgery and care cannot restore function.

Symptoms and Signs of Spinal Injury

1st In general, the symptoms and signs of spinal injury include:

- Weakness, numbness or tingling sensations, or loss of feeling in the arms or legs
- Paralysis to arms and/or legs
- Painful movement of arms and/or legs
- Pain and/or tenderness along the back of the neck or the backbone.
- Burning sensations along the spine or in an extremity
- Deformity—the angle of the patient's head and neck may appear odd to you. You may feel pieces of bone that have broken off the neck and back bones. Such findings are rare.
- Injuries to the head or bruises on the shoulders, back, or sides
- Loss of bladder and bowel control
- Difficult breathing, with little or no chest movements. There will only be a slight movement of the abdomen.
- Positioning of the arms over the head—you may find the patient lying face up with arms stretched out above the head (see Figure 12–11). This could indicate damage to the cervical spine.
- A persistent erection of the penis, indicating possible spinal injury affecting nerves to the external genitalia. This is called priapism (PRY-ah-pizm).

FIGURE 12–11. Patients found in this position may have spinal injuries.

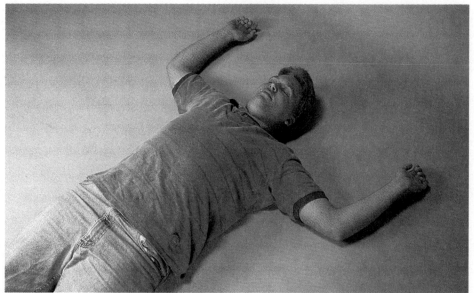

Assessing Patients for Spinal Injury (cont'd)

Unconscious patients: Test the responses to painful stimuli (pinching) applied to the distal limb. If removal of shoes may aggravate existing injuries, apply the stimuli to the skin around the ankles.

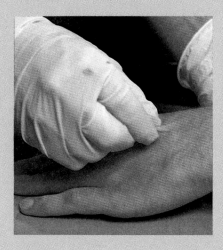 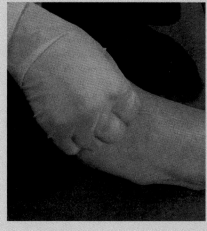

Remember: It is difficult to survey the unconscious patient with accuracy. A deeply unconscious patient will not pull back from a painful stimulus. Should the mechanism of injury indicate possible spinal damage, or if the trauma patient is unconscious, assume that spinal injury is present.

Results: Slight pulling back of foot: cord usually intact. No foot reaction: possible damage anywhere along the cord. Hand or finger reaction: usually no damage to cervical cord. No hand or finger reaction: possible damage to the cervical cord. Assume damage to the spinal cord if you find negative results, the failure to perform any test, limited performance, or performance with pain.

Summary of Observations and Conclusions

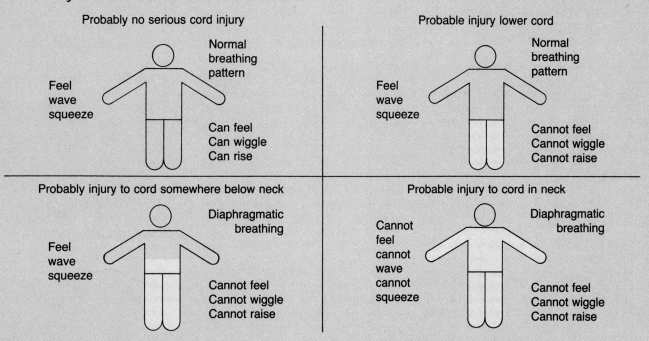

Probably no serious cord injury

Feel wave squeeze

Normal breathing pattern

Can feel
Can wiggle
Can rise

Probable injury lower cord

Feel wave squeeze

Normal breathing pattern

Cannot feel
Cannot wiggle
Cannot raise

Probably injury to cord somewhere below neck

Feel wave squeeze

Diaphragmatic breathing

Cannot feel
Cannot wiggle
Cannot raise

Probable injury to cord in neck

Cannot feel cannot wave cannot squeeze

Diaphragmatic breathing

Cannot feel
Cannot wiggle
Cannot raise

WARNING: If the patient is unconscious or the mechanism of injury indicates possible spinal injury, assume that spinal injury is present.

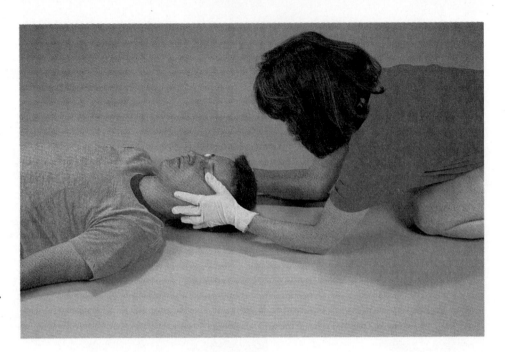

FIGURE 12–12. If necessary, in-line stabilization may be applied to the patient's head and neck.

Stabilizing the Patient's Head and Neck

Assume that a patient with neck injuries also has spinal injuries. Also, assume that a patient with apparent spinal injuries below the neck has some sort of injury to the cervical spine. This means that you should try to immobilize the patient so that head, neck, trunk, and limb movements are restricted.

To immobilize the patient, work as gently as possible. Do not try to apply traction to the patient's head and neck. You will not be able to hold steady traction while waiting for the EMTs to respond. Do not try to position an extrication collar and spineboard unless you have had special training in using these items and you have enough trained helpers (the use of cervical collars, extrication collars, and spineboards is not considered to be part of most First Responder training programs).

A patient with neck or spinal injuries may be able to move the head, neck, arms, trunk, or legs. Movement can cause more injury to occur. For this reason, you should keep the patient from moving and try to stabilize the head and neck. Stabilizing is best done by gently holding the patient's head.

When you must stabilize a patient's head and neck, you should:

1. Kneel at the top of the patient's head.
2. Place one of your hands to each side of the head and position your fingers under the lower jaw.
3. Keep the patient's head and neck stable. *Do not* apply traction or turn or lift the patient's head.
4. Maintain your position until a rigid cervical or extrication collar is properly applied.

1st WARNING: It is best not to try to apply traction to the patient's head and neck. If at all possible, stabilize the head and neck and wait for the EMTs to respond.

INJURIES TO THE CHEST

Types of Injuries

The majority of soft tissue injuries to the chest are the same as those that occur in other areas of the body and will receive the same basic type of care. Typically, these injuries are cuts, bruises, and shallow puncture wounds. These are often seen in motor vehicle accidents, usually because the occupants were not wearing seat and lap belts.

Serious soft tissue wounds to the chest include deep puncture wounds, penetrating wounds, and impaled objects. Care for objects impaled in the chest requires that you stabilize the object. Wounds may go through the chest, requiring you to care for both an entrance and an exit wound. Any deep penetrating or perforating wound opening the chest cavity is a very grave injury and will require special care.

Injury to the chest may also damage the lungs and the heart. In many cases, there is little the First Responder can do. However, there are times when First Responder care will undoubtedly save the patient's life.

Ribs can be fractured or crushed. The sternum (breastbone) may become fractured or completely broken off from the ribs. The section of the spine in the upper body may be injured.

Sternum (STER-num)—the breastbone.

Fractured Ribs

1st The symptoms and signs of fractured ribs include:

- Pain at the site of the fracture
- Tenderness over the site of the fracture
- Increased pain at the site upon moving or inhaling deeply
- Shallow breathing, sometimes with the patient reporting a crackling sensation at or near the site of fracture
- Characteristic stance—often, the patient will lean toward the side of the fracture, with a hand or forearm pressed over the site of injury

If only one or two ribs are fractured, as determined by the number of injury sites, no immediate action need be taken, other than keeping the patient at rest. However, providing additional care for this patient will often relieve pain. If there are signs that the lungs have been damaged by the

FIGURE 12–13. Rib fractures and flail chest.

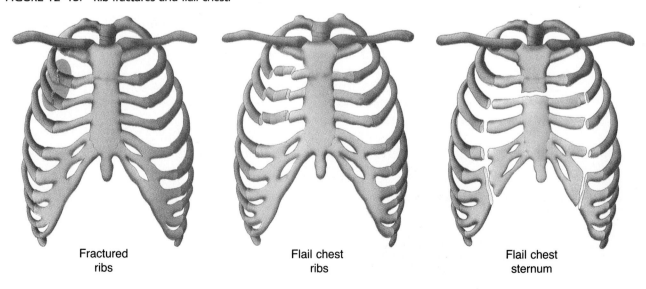

Fractured ribs   Flail chest ribs   Flail chest sternum

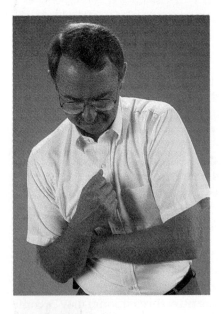

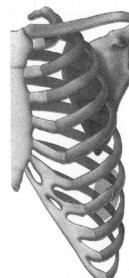

- Tenderness
- Local pain
- Deformity
- Shallow breathing
- Coughing
- Painful movement
- "Crackling" sensation in skin if lung is punctured

FIGURE 12–14. Signs of rib fracture.

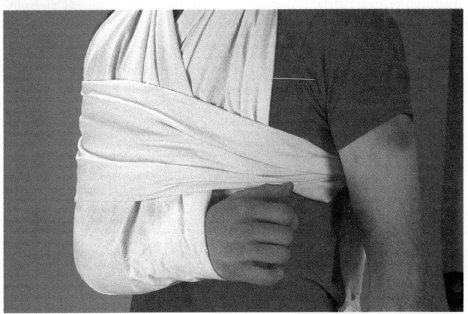

FIGURE 12–15. Care for simple rib fractures. Apply a sling and swathe to hold the arm against the injured side of the chest.

fractured rib (for example, frothy blood in the mouth) or several ribs are apparently fractured, you must provide additional care for the patient.
1st The care for fractured ribs requires you to:

1. Place the forearm of the injured side in a sling so that it rests across the patient's chest.
2. Apply a swathe to provide additional support.
3. Keep the patient at rest and monitor breathing.
4. Make certain to alert dispatch and have the patient examined by more highly trained personnel.

Flail Chest

Flail chest—the condition where multiple rib fractures and/or breastbone fractures produce a loose section of the chest wall that does not move with the rest of the wall during breathing.

If three or more consecutive ribs on the same side of the chest are fractured in two places, this produces a section of chest wall that will not move with the rest of the chest wall. The same problem occurs when the breastbone is broken away from' the ribs. Both of these conditions are called a **flail**

chest. First Responders see flail chests most often at motor vehicle accidents, usually caused by the patient being forced against a steering wheel. Most flailed sections are found on the side of the chest.

1st The symptoms and signs of flail chest include:

- The symptoms and signs of fractured ribs
- The failure of a section of the chest wall to move with the rest of the chest when the patient is breathing. Usually the flail section will move in the opposite direction to the rest of the chest wall.

A flail chest must be cared for differently than simple rib fractures. It will do little to help the patient if you bind the injured section of ribs or the breastbone involved in the flail chest. Instead, you must try to hold the flail section in place.

FIGURE 12–16.   Flail chest.

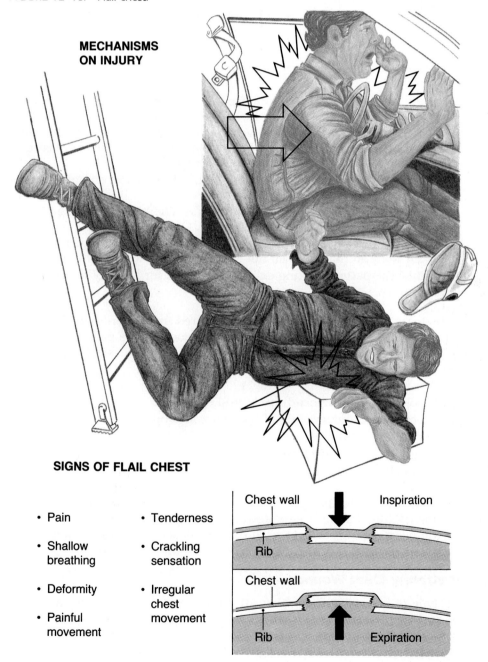

MECHANISMS ON INJURY

SIGNS OF FLAIL CHEST

- Pain
- Shallow breathing
- Deformity
- Painful movement

- Tenderness
- Crackling sensation
- Irregular chest movement

Chest wall   Inspiration

Rib

Chest wall

Rib   Expiration

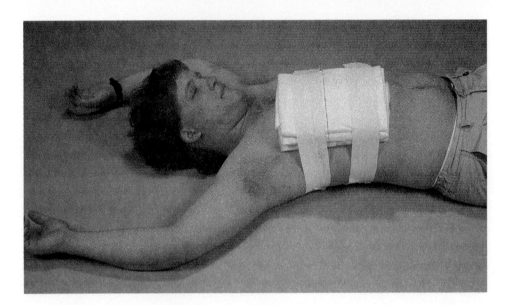

FIGURE 12–17. Emergency care for flail chest.

1st To care for a flail chest, you should:

1. Locate the flail section by gently feeling the injury site. In the majority of cases, the injury will be on the side of the chest.
2. Apply a thick pad of dressings over the site. This pad should be several inches thick. A small pillow can be used in place of the pad of dressings. Whatever is used should be soft and lightweight.
3. Use large strips of tape to hold the pad in place. If you do not have tape:
    *   Have the patient lie on the injured side. The body weight against the surface will help splint the injury. Or . . .
    *   Hold the pad by hand. When doing so, take care in how you position your body so that you will not shift your weight and move the pad.
4. Monitor the patient, taking extra care to look for signs of heart or lung injury.

The lungs and the heart also can be injured in accidents involving the ribs and breastbone. Always look for frothy blood in the patient's mouth. This is an indication of possible injury to the lungs. In cases of flail chest, make certain to examine the patient for the following:

*   Blue coloration of the head, neck, and shoulders
*   Blue coloration and swelling of the lips and tongue
*   Bulging, bloodshot eyes
*   Bulging (distended) neck veins
*   Obvious chest deformity

These signs indicate that the heart has been injured and that blood has been forced into its right side and up through the major veins leading into the heart. Such patients need oxygen as soon as possible and must be transported by EMTs to a medical facility immediately.

Penetrating Chest Wounds

This type of wound occurs when an object tears or punctures the chest wall and exposes the chest cavity. The object may remain impaled in the chest or the wound may be completely open. As explained in Chapter 4, breathing requires pressure changes to take place in the chest cavity. When the chest cavity is open, the lungs will collapse due to the extra pressure

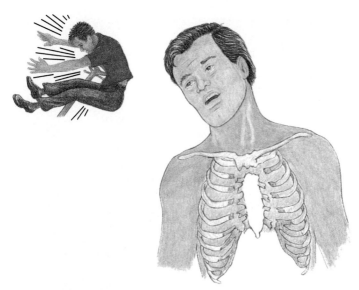

- Distended (bulging) neck veins
- Head, neck and shoulders appear dark blue or purple
- Eyes may be bloodshot and bulging
- Tongue and lips may appear swollen and blue (cyanotic)
- Chest deformity may be present

FIGURE 12–18. Chest injuries may involve the heart.

being exerted on them. The wound must be sealed to prevent lung collapse or to allow the lungs to re-expand.

In some cases, the lung will be penetrated. As the patient inhales, air from this lung will enter the chest cavity. If the wound has been tightly sealed, pressure will build as air continues to enter the cavity. Unless this pressure is released, it may interfere with heart and lung actions.

1st You will be able to tell if a puncture wound is a penetrating wound by noting:

- A severe chest wound, where the chest wall is torn or punctured
- A sucking sound being made each time the patient breathes. This is why these wounds are sometimes called "sucking" chest wounds.

Sucking chest wound—an open chest wound in which air is sucked through the wound opening and into the chest cavity each time the patient breathes.

FIGURE 12–19. Penetrating chest wounds.

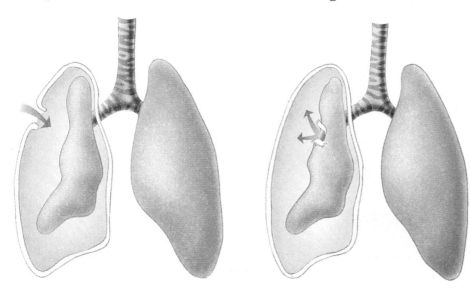

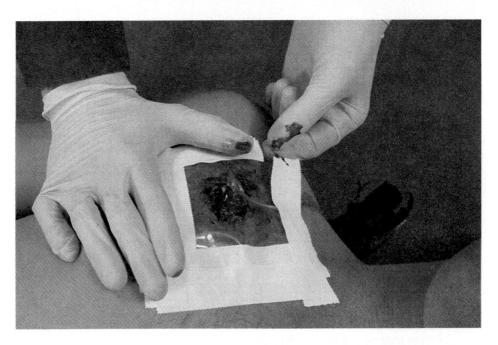

FIGURE 12–20. Penetrating chest wound—punctured lung.

1st You should suspect that the patient's lung is punctured if you notice:

- A penetrating chest wound
- The patient is coughing up bright red, frothy blood

If you find that a penetrating chest wound has both an entrance and an exit wound through the chest, assume that at least one of the lungs of the patient has been punctured.

1st The following method is recommended for *all* penetrating chest wounds free of impaled objects. If there is no puncture to the lung, the method will work. If there is a punctured lung, this method will allow for the release of air entrapped in the chest cavity.

1. Seal the patient's wound with the palm of your gloved hand. *Do not* unseal the wound to find dressings. Have others at the scene help you prepare the dressing.

FIGURE 12–21. Create a flutter valve to release entrapped air.

On inspiration, dressing seals wound, preventing air entry

Expiration allows trapped air to escape through untaped section of dressing

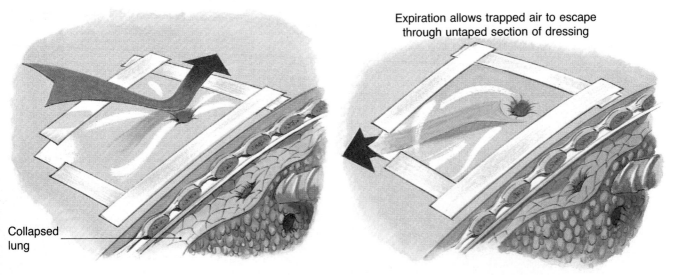

Collapsed lung

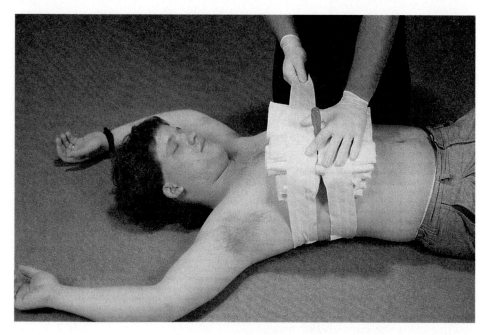

FIGURE 12–22. Never remove an object impaled in the chest. Stabilize the object.

2. Apply an occlusive dressing, sealed by tape on three edges. This produces a "flutter valve" effect. When the patient inhales, the free edge will seal against the skin. As the patient exhales, the free edge will break loose from the skin and allow any build-up of air in the chest cavity to escape.
3. Provide care for shock.
4. Make certain that someone alerts the EMS System dispatcher.

A commercial occlusive dressing is the best choice for open chest wounds. Plastic wrap can be used, but it must be folded over several times so that it will not be sucked into the wound. The occlusive dressing should extend beyond the edge of the wound by 2 or more inches.

If blood or perspiration prevent the tape from sticking to the patient's skin, apply bulky dressings over the occlusive dressing and secure this in place with cravats. In cases where the EMTs will not be delayed in their arrival and tape will not hold the dressing, it is best to wait and hold the occlusive dressing in place with the palm of your hand. If the patient's condition declines, periodically release one edge of the seal to allow trapped air to escape.

REMEMBER: If there is an entrance wound and an exit wound, both will need a dressing.

Penetrating wounds of the chest may also penetrate the heart. When this occurs, there is little that the First Responder can do other than provide care for shock, care for the open chest wound, and provide basic life-support measures as they are needed.

1st *Impaled Objects*

As covered in Chapter 9, an impaled object should be left in place. The object must be stabilized with bulky dressings or pads. Begin by placing these materials on opposite sides of the object, along the vertical line of the body or affected limb. Place the next layer perpendicular to the first. Use tape to hold all dressings and pads in place. If tape will not hold, carefully apply cravats according to local protocols.

SUMMARY

The skull is made up of the **cranium** (CRAY-ni-um) and the **face.** The spine connects to the skull. That portion of the spine running through the neck is called the **cervical** (SER-ve-kal) **spine.** The ribs are attached to the spine. The **skull, spine, ribs,** and **breastbone** form the **axial skeleton.**

The brain is protected by the skull. The spinal column (backbone) protects the spinal cord. The **brain** and **spinal cord** are parts of the **central nervous system.**

Injuries to the skull include **open head injuries** and **closed head injuries.** If the cranium remains intact, the injury is classified as a closed head injury.

Open head injuries involve **fractures of the cranium** (skull fractures). There can be **direct injury to the brain** in open head injuries. Closed head injuries include **indirect injuries to the brain,** such as **concussions** and **contusions** (brain bruises).

Skull fractures may be obvious or they may be difficult to detect. Always look for wounds to the head, **deformity** of the skull, bruises behind the ear, black eyes, sunken eyes, **unequal pupils,** and **bloody** or **clear fluids** flowing from the ears and/or nose.

Brain injury can occur with head injuries. Look for signs of skull fracture, loss of awareness, confusion, unequal pupils, and paralysis.

When caring for a patient with injuries to the cranium, maintain an open airway using the **jaw-thrust** technique. Use resuscitative procedures, if needed.

Keep the head injury patient at rest and talk to the patient. Control bleeding, but avoid pressure over the site of a fracture. *Do not* remove impaled objects, bone fragments, or any other objects from skull wounds.

Facial fractures often cause **airway obstruction.** You should maintain an open airway using the **jaw-thrust** technique.

Neck and spinal injuries can be very serious. **Keep the patient from moving.** The **secondary survey** is very important in determining if the patient has neck or spinal injuries. Always look for **weakness, numbness, loss of feeling, pain,** or **paralysis** to the limbs of a patient. Remember that you will have to probe or pinch the feet and hands of the unconscious patient. Consider **all unconscious injury patients to have spinal injuries.** If the mechanism of injury indicates possible neck and spinal injuries, assume the injuries are present.

You must follow certain rules when caring for a patient who may have neck or spinal injuries. Even though a patient has neck or spinal injuries, provide **resuscitation,** if needed, and **control serious bleeding. Always** consider the unconscious injury patient to have neck or spinal injuries. *Do not* attempt to splint fractures. **Never move** a patient with neck or spinal injuries unless absolutely necessary. Do your best to **stabilize** the patient's head and neck and as much of the body as possible. **Continuously monitor** the patient.

Injuries to the chest can include **soft tissue injuries, fractured ribs, flail chest, spinal injuries, lung injuries,** and **heart injuries.**

If pain at the site indicates **rib fractures,** you should apply **a sling and swathe,** placing the forearm of the injured side across the chest. If rib or breastbone movements indicate **flail chest,** apply a **thick pad** over the site and **tape** this **pad** into place.

Objects **impaled** in the chest should not be removed. **Stabilize** these objects with **pads** and **tape** the **pads** into place.

Penetrating chest wounds require an **occlusive dressing.** Seal three edges of the occlusive dressing and leave the fourth edge free to act as a flutter valve.

This is a self-test. It has been designed for you to take on your own to evaluate your progress. After you have completed Chapters 9 to 12 and believe that you have met all the objectives listed for these chapters, take this test to see if you have any weaknesses in a specific area of study. Answers are listed at the end of the test. Page references are provided for each question so you can go back to the text to restudy any questions missed in the test.

If you wish to check your knowledge in more detail, note that the objectives listed at the beginning of each chapter can be read as questions and exercises. Go back to these objectives and see if you can list, describe, name, and so on, as directed in the objective statements.

Circle the letter of the best answer to each question.

1. A bruise the size of a man's fist equals an internal blood loss of about (p. 199)

    A. 2%
    B. 5%
    C. 10%
    D. 15%

2. The first step in caring for an open wound is to (p. 200)

    A. Clear the wound surface
    B. Expose the wound
    C. Stop bleeding
    D. Prevent contamination

3. You may remove impaled objects from the (p. 208)

    A. Cheek
    B. Eye
    C. Pelvis
    D. Chest

4. For open wounds to the eye, you should (p. 209)

    A. Apply a pressure dressing
    B. Remove all objects, probing the socket, if necessary
    C. Apply loose dressing
    D. Encourage the patient to rotate his eyes to remove any loose objects

5. If dark blood is flowing from a wound in a patient's neck, you should (p. 216)

    A. Use direct pressure only
    B. Use a carotid artery pressure point
    C. Apply bulky dressings
    D. Apply an occlusive dressing

6. If a patient shows bleeding from the ear canal, you should (p. 212)

    A. Pack the ear canal
    B. Apply an external dressing and bandage
    C. Apply an occlusive dressing
    D. Do nothing to the ear

7. A simple nosebleed is best controlled by (p. 213)

    A. Pinching the nostrils shut
    B. Facial pressure points
    C. Packing the nostrils with gauze
    D. Tilting the head back

8. Your first concern with injuries to the mouth should be (p. 213)

    A. An open airway
    B. Avulsed lips
    C. Bleeding
    D. Loosened teeth

9. If an open wound to the abdomen has exposed organs, you should (p. 219)

    A. Gently push the organs back into the abdominal cavity
    B. Apply a loose dressing or a towel
    C. Apply bulk dressings and pressure
    D. Apply an occlusive dressing

10. Bleeding from cuts to the genitalia should be controlled by (p. 219)

    A. Occlusive dressings
    B. Loose dressings
    C. Pelvic pressure points
    D. Direct pressure

11. Which of the following is *not* part of the axial skeletal system? (pp. 228 and 272)

    A. Breastbone (sternum)
    B. Pelvic bones
    C. Backbone (vertebrae)
    D. Skull bones

12. Which of the following is *least* likely to produce deformity? (p. 234)

    A. Fracture
    B. Strain
    C. Dislocation
    D. Sprain

13. The main purpose of splinting is to (p. 251)

    A. Immobilize fractured bones and injured joints
    B. Apply tension to a broken bone
    C. Allow for the realignment of broken bones
    D. Set broken bones in their normal position

14. Shoulder injuries are best cared for by applying a (p. 236)

    A. Long rigid arm splint
    B. Air splint (inflatable splint)
    C. Sling and swathe
    D. Sling

15. For fractures to the shaft of the upper arm bone (humerus), you should (p. 240)

    A. Only apply a sling

B. Modify the sling to hold the wrist and apply a swathe
C. Apply a standard sling and swathe
D. Use a rigid splint with no sling (for all cases)

16. You should reposition a fractured arm bone in order to splint for cases of (p. 241, p. 257)

A. Open fractures
B. Severe, closed angulated fractures
C. Dislocated shoulders
D. Mild, closed angulated fractures

17. When treating an angulated fractured elbow, you should immobilize the joint (p. 242)

A. Only after correcting angulations
B. And then correct angulations
C. After extending the arm and taking a radial pulse
D. In the position in which it is found

18. Always assume the patient has a hip dislocation if you (p. 245)

A. See that the patient's leg has rotated outward or inward
B. Cannot find a distal pulse
C. See that the patient's foot turns inward or outward
D. Cannot find a femoral pulse

19. Rigid splinting of an injured knee requires you to (p. 265)

A. Straighten the patient's entire leg
B. First apply a soft splint
C. Reposition the knee into a "natural" position
D. Keep the knee in the position in which it is found

20. After applying a rigid splint to a patient having a fractured lower leg bone, you notice that he no longer has a distal pulse. You should (p. 266)

A. Transport immediately
B. Unsplint, applying traction, and splint again
C. Unsplint and keep the leg protected
D. Loosen the splint

21. The best course of action to take for a fractured rib is to (p. 288)

A. Tape over the injury site
B. Apply a sling and swathe on the injured side
C. Tape and apply a sling
D. Apply cravats and a swathe

22. Clear fluids flowing from the nose usually indicate (p. 278)

A. Facial fractures
B. Lung injuries
C. Skull fractures
D. Upper airway injury

23. You find a patient lying on his back with his arms stretched out above his head. You should suspect (p. 282)

A. Severe chest injuries
B. Shoulder dislocation
C. Spinal injuries
D. Flail chest

24. You are providing care for a patient having a penetrating chest wound. You should (pp. 292–293)

A. Apply an occlusive dressing, sealed on three edges
B. Transport immediately
C. Completely seal with an occlusive dressing
D. Wait for the EMTs

25. A victim of an automobile accident has a flail chest. You should (p. 290)

A. Provide care for shock and wait for the EMTs
B. Stabilize the flail with an object or pad
C. Tape his chest and apply a swathe
D. Tape his arm over the flail

ANSWERS

Each question is worth 4 points.

1.	C	10.	D	19.	D
2.	B	11.	B	20.	B
3.	A	12.	B	21.	B
4.	C	13.	A	22.	C
5.	D	14.	C	23.	C
6.	B	15.	B	24.	A or C (as to local protocol)
7.	A	16.	D	25.	B
8.	A	17.	D		
9.	D	18.	A		

Start with 100 points. Subtract four points for each wrong answer. If you scored below 70, you should see your instructor for additional help or new study methods. A score from 70 to 79 indicates you still need to do much more work on these chapters. You have done very well if you scored 80 or above; however, you should go over the text sections dealing with the questions that you missed.

CHAPTER 13

Medical Emergencies

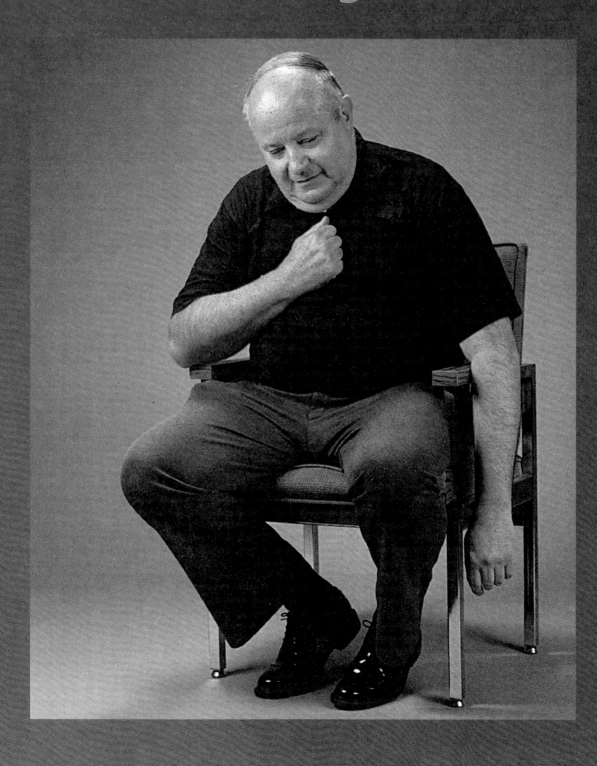

By the end of this chapter, you should be able to:

1. Define medical emergency. (p. 299)
2. List the major symptoms and signs associated with medical emergencies. (What do you look for to see if someone is ill?) You should be able to relate these to the secondary survey and the patient interview. (pp. 299–300)
3. List the symptoms and signs of a heart attack and describe First Responder care for possible heart attack patients. (pp. 301–302, 303)
4. List the symptoms and signs of congestive heart failure and describe First Responder care for possible congestive heart failure patients. (pp. 304–305)
5. List the symptoms and signs of stroke and describe First Responder care for possible stroke patients. (pp. 305–306, 307)
6. List the symptoms and signs of respiratory distress and describe First Responder care for possible respiratory distress patients. (pp. 306, 308, 311)
7. List the symptoms and signs of chronic obstructive pulmonary disease (COPD) and describe First Responder care for possible COPD patients. (pp. 309–310)
8. Define hyperventilation, listing the symptoms and signs of this condition. State how a First Responder cares for patients who are hyperventilating. (pp. 308–309)
9. List the symptoms and signs of a convulsive seizure and describe First Responder care for seizure patients. (pp. 310–313)
10. List the symptoms and signs of diabetic coma and describe First Responder care for diabetic coma patients. (pp. 313–314, 315)
11. List the symptoms and signs of insulin shock and describe First Responder care for insulin shock patients. State the main differences between this list and the list for diabetic coma. (pp. 314, 315)
12. State what a First Responder should do if it is unclear if the patient is in diabetic coma or insulin shock. (pp. 314, 315)
13. Define acute abdomen and list the more common symptoms and signs that may be associated with this problem. (pp. 314, 316)
14. State the basic First Responder-level care that should be provided for the acute abdomen patient. (p. 316)
15. List the symptoms and signs of ingested poisoning and describe First Responder care for patients who have ingested a poison. Are there any exceptions to these procedures? (pp. 320–321)
16. List the symptoms and signs of inhaled poisoning and describe First Responder care for patients who have inhaled a poison. (p. 322)
17. List the symptoms and signs of absorbed poisoning and describe First Responder care for patients who have absorbed a poison. (pp. 322–323)
18. List the symptoms and signs of an injected poisoning (not snakebite) and describe First Responder care for patients who have been injected with a poison. (p. 323)
19. List the symptoms and signs of snakebite and describe First Responder care for patients who have been bitten by a snake. (pp. 324–325)
20. List the ways in which an infectious agent can be passed (transmitted) from person to person. (p. 325)
21. State what a First Responder should do if exposed to an infectious disease while providing care. (p. 326)

SKILLS

Upon completing this chapter and your class lectures and skills labs, you should be able to:

1. Conduct a secondary survey, stating what information can be gained in relation to medical emergencies.

2. Determine, in practice sessions, if a patient is having a medical emergency and the nature of the emergency.
3. Demonstrate proper care for patients having heart attack, congestive heart failure, stroke, respiratory distress, COPD, hyperventilation, seizure, diabetic coma, insulin shock, and acute abdomen.
4. Act out the procedures you would follow for ingested, inhaled, absorbed, and injected poisonings.
5. Act out how to care for a patient who has been bitten by a snake.
6. Demonstrate the proper personal protection equipment, supplies, and methods require by your EMS System (or the Centers for Disease Control).

MEDICAL EMERGENCIES

What Are Medical Emergencies?

Medical emergencies include a wide variety of illnesses and conditions. These may be brought about by germs, the failure of body organs and systems, or by some outside agent, such as a poison. In most cases, the problem is not the result of an accident causing damage to the body.

Medical emergencies may be hidden because of an accident. Someone with diabetes may collapse and be injured from the fall. As a First Responder, you will have to treat the injuries received by the patient. However, the medical problem should not go unnoticed. Proper surveying and interviewing of the patient should indicate that there is also a medical emergency. **REMEMBER:** Part of the patient assessment is to look for medical identification devices.

Accidents may produce medical emergencies. The stress of an accident may be enough to set off a heart attack, stroke, or seizure. First Responder-level patient assessment will enable you to detect some of the more common medical emergencies. You must conduct both primary and secondary patient surveys, including an interview with the conscious patient. While the patient is under your care, continue to gather information and monitor the patient. **WARNING:** Always wear the appropriate personal protection when providing care for possible medical emergency patients. Avoid direct contact with the patient's blood, body fluids, vomitus, wastes, and mucous membranes. Universal precautions are recommended (see pages 4 and 326).

SYMPTOMS AND SIGNS

Your training as a First Responder may not always allow you to know what the problem is, but you should be aware that the patient is having some sort of medical emergency. There are several ways of recognizing this type of emergency. The patient or a bystander may tell you of a known disease or condition. You may detect a medical identification device. However, in most cases, what you observe and what the patient describes will probably be your only clues.

Symptoms are what the patient tells you about the problem. The patient might complain of chest pains or bloody bowel movements over the last few days. **Signs** are what you detect when examining the patient. A rapid pulse rate might be the sign of a medical emergency.

Assessment Signs

This information is gained during the primary and secondary patient surveys. Review this information in Chapter 3, pages 54–78. To detect a medical emergency, you will have to be aware of unusual:

- Altered states of awareness or consciousness
- Pulse rate and character—remember that a pulse rate above 120 beats per minute or below 50 beats per minute indicates a true emergency for an adult patient.
- Breathing rate and character—remember that a breathing rate above 30 breaths per minute indicates a true emergency for an adult patient.
- Skin temperature, condition, and color
- Pupil size and response
- Color of the lips
- Breath odors
- Abdominal tenderness or rigidity
- Vomiting
- Muscular activities—spasms and paralysis
- Bleeding or discharges from the body

None of these signs is new information. All this is part of the secondary patient survey.

NOTE: If you are a First Responder who determines blood pressure, realize that blood pressure is a vital sign and a diagnostic sign. Remember that a systolic pressure greater than 140 mm Hg or a diastolic pressure above 90 mm Hg indicates a high blood pressure reading. If you detect a low or a falling blood pressure, assume the patient is developing shock.

When surveying the patient, remember:

1st RULE: If the patient appears or feels unusual in any way, assume that there is a medical emergency.

1st RULE: If the patient has atypical (unusual) vital signs, assume that there is a medical emergency.

Assessment Symptoms

A patient may complain of:

- Pain
- A "temperature" or fever, or chills
- An upset stomach and/or vomiting
- Dizziness or feeling faint
- Shortness of breath
- Feelings of pressure or weight on the chest or abdomen
- Unusual bowel or bladder activity
- Thirst, hunger, or odd tastes in the mouth
- Burning sensations

1st RULE: Consider all patient complaints to be valid. If the patient is not feeling normal in any way, assume that the patient is having a medical emergency.

SPECIFIC MEDICAL EMERGENCIES

Heart Attack

Many conditions can give the appearance of being a heart attack. Indigestion can cause chest pains and nausea that may be the same as those produced by a heart attack. Excessive sneezing, as found in patients with allergies, may cause chest pains. Stress may tighten chest muscles, causing pain that is very much like a heart attack. As a First Responder, you will not be able to tell the difference between these problems and what may be a true heart attack.

1st RULE: If a patient is having chest pains, assume that the patient is having, or is about to have, a heart attack.

1st RULE: Whenever you suspect the patient is having, or is about to have, a heart attack, alert the EMS dispatcher. Report the symptoms and signs gathered. It may be possible for dispatch to send an advanced cardiac life-support unit.

Many terms are used in reference to heart attacks and problems with the heart. They include coronary, angina, angina pectoris, coronary thrombosis, coronary occlusion, myocardial infarction (MI), and acute myocardial infarction (AMI). You need not worry about these terms. Being able to tell one condition from another requires advanced medical training. Just realize that the heart is a muscle, with its own blood vessels. Any damage to the muscle or to the vessels can lead to a heart attack. As a First Responder, treat all chest pain as a possible heart attack.

Heart attack—a general term used to indicate a failure of circulation to the heart muscle that damages or kills a portion of the heart.

Symptoms and Signs

1st Any or all of the following can indicate a heart attack:

- Chest discomfort—this may take the form of pain or the feeling of tightness, fullness, pressure, or squeezing sensations in the chest. The patient may indicate this by holding a fist over an area of the chest rather than point to the location of the discomfort. Sometimes the pain is not in the chest, but displays itself in the arms or the jaw. Often the pain radiates (spreads out) from the chest to the neck and arms. Usually, the pain radiates down the left arm, and lasts more than 2 minutes.
- Recent chest pains—these are reported as having occurred hours to days before the attack.
- Nausea
- Shortness of breath
- Sweating
- Weakness
- Restlessness

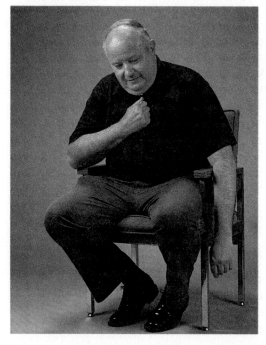

FIGURE 13–1.
Chest pain is the primary sign of a heart attack.

NOTE: Pain that is described by the patient as being "sharp twinges" or "stabbing pains" usually does not indicate a heart attack. See Scansheet 13–1.

1st RULE: If any of the symptoms or signs of a heart attack are present, assume the patient is having, or is about to have, a heart attack.

Many patients who are having, or are about to have, a heart attack will deny that they are having pain or any other discomfort. Usually, these patients will appear very frightened. If there are other signs of a heart attack, or if bystanders report the pain or other discomforts, provide care for a heart attack.

WARNING: *Do not* assume the cause of a patient's chest pains, even if your assumption is based on the patient's past problems (history). Should the patient have a history of heartburn or of pain from the condition caused by stomach acid moving up into the esophagus (hiatal hernia), *do not* rule out possible heart attack.

Emergency Care

If the patient is in cardiac arrest, perform CPR and have someone notify dispatch. Otherwise, complete the patient survey and interview as required, carefully noting the patient's vital signs. Should the patient be unconscious when you arrive, gain what information you can from witnesses. If there are no witnesses, assume the possibility of the patient being a heart attack victim.

NOTE: If you are a First Responder who is allowed to administer oxygen (see Appendix 3), follow your EMS System's protocols for chest pain patients. Sometimes the patient's pain will decrease once supplemental oxygen is provided. If this occurs, do not be fooled into believing that the patient's problem has grown any less serious.

1st Upon gathering symptoms and signs indicating a heart attack or the possibility of a heart attack, you should:

1. Make certain that the EMS System dispatcher has been alerted. *Do not* abandon the patient. While you are away, cardiac arrest may occur.
2. Provide emotional support. It is very important that you reassure the patient.
3. Keep the patient at rest.
4. *Place* the patient into a comfortable position. You should do all the work for the patient. This position should be one that allows for easiest breathing. Many patients with the symptoms and signs of a heart attack are most comfortable in a semisitting position. If the patient is also an accident victim, do not cause additional problems through incorrect or inappropriate repositioning.
5. Loosen any restrictive garments.
6. Cover the patient to prevent chill, but *do not* overheat the patient.
7. Continue to monitor vital signs.

It is very important that you conduct all the above activities in a calm, professional manner. Patients with the symptoms and signs of a heart attack are very anxious. Their chances for survival may be lessened if they remain alarmed and restless.

The patient may ask if this is a heart attack. It is best to say, "It could be a lot of things, but let's not take any chances." Do all you can to keep the patient still. Do not argue with the patient and do not try physical restraint. The stress caused by such efforts could be very harmful. Remain calm and talk to the patient, keeping eye contact whenever possible. Let the patient know that more harm could be done by refusing to remain at rest. Do not be surprised to find that many patients will want to try to

■ SCAN 13-1.

Heart Attack

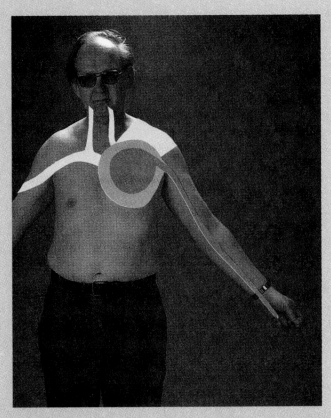

Symptoms and Signs may include:

- Early symptoms are often mistaken for indigestion
- As an attack worsens, pain originates behind the sternum and radiates to either of the upper extremities (usually the left) with pain radiating to the shoulder, arm, and elbow. In some cases, the pain may extend down the limb to the little finger.
  The neck, jaws, and teeth
  The upper back
  The superior, medial abdomen
  The pain may not originate under the sternum. Some patients have pain only in the jaw or the teeth.
- Shortness of breath
- Nausea
- Pain lasts throughout the attack
- Patient usually remains still
- Pain may diminish when physical or emotional stress ends or when nitroglycerin is taken

Additional signs may include sweating, increased pulse rate, and, on rare occasions, a shock-level blood pressure. Patients who have taken repeated dosages of nitroglycerin may have low blood pressure as a result of blood vessel dilation.

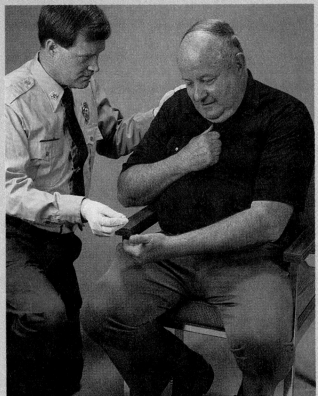

Emergency Care

- Provide emotional support—keep the patient calm and reassured.
- Keep the patient at rest—*do not* allow the patient to move himself.
- Place the patient in a restful, comfortable position.
- Ensure an open airway.
- Cover to conserve body heat, but do not allow overheating.
- Find out if patient takes nitroglycerin and when the last dose was taken and how much was taken over what period of time.
- Contact medical facility and let them know:
  1. You have a patient with chest pain
  2. Patient's history
  3. When last medicated
- Assist the patient with the prescribed dose of medication (nitroglycerin).
- Do not leave the patient unattended.
- Monitor vital signs.

get up and walk around. Some may even wish to do exercises. Know that a patient may act this way and be prepared to talk the patient into remaining at rest.

Continue to comfort the patient as long as you provide care. Say that highly trained help is on the way. Tell the patient that you are a trained First Responder and that you will stay with him. *Do not* tell the patient that you can perform CPR, if need be. How reassured would you be if someone implied that you may become clinically dead?

Medications

Normally, a First Responder does not have to worry about medications. However, some patients with a history of heart problems have been given medications to take when having an attack. Always ask if a physician has given the patient any medications for the condition. If medications have been prescribed, then *assist* the patient in taking them.

Patients suffering from angina pectoris (An-ji-nah PEK-to-ris) will usually have nitroglycerin tablets to take when having an attack (nitroglycerin ointment and tablets meant to be swallowed are not prescribed for anginal attacks). An angina attack indicates that the heart muscle needs more oxygen. Placing a nitroglycerin tablet under the patient's tongue will allow the drug to rapidly enter the bloodstream. Nitroglycerin will provide for greater circulation of blood to the heart muscle and reduce the workload of the heart.

1st Help all patients with the symptoms and signs of a heart attack to take their own prescribed medications given by a doctor unless they have taken the prescribed limit prior to your arrival. If the symptoms and signs of a heart attack are present, provide care as if the patient is having, or is about to have, a heart attack. This includes those patients with known angina pectoris. Continue to monitor the patient and provide care, even if the pain stops. *Do not* cancel your request for an EMT response.

Congestive Heart Failure

Congestive heart failure—the condition in which the heart cannot properly circulate the blood. This causes a back-up of fluids in the lungs and other organs.

Heart failure is not the same thing as a heart attack or cardiac arrest. For a number of reasons, often associated with chronic lung problems, the heart cannot pump blood properly. This causes fluids to build up in the lungs and other body organs. Respiratory distress occurs because of the inefficient air exchange in the lungs.

1st The symptoms and signs of congestive heart failure include:

- Rapid pulse rate—the rate can often be greater than 120 beats per minute. This is a true emergency.
- Shortness of breath—breathing will be labored, often rapid and shallow. Unusual breathing sounds may be heard. The rate of breathing can often be greater than 30 breaths per minute. This is a true emergency.
- Swelling can occur, usually at the ankles.
- Neck veins may appear engorged and pulsating.
- The abdominal region may appear swollen—this is most frequently seen in the region of the liver.
- Skin, lips, and nail beds may turn blue.
- The patient may act confused or anxious.

1st The emergency care for a patient in congestive heart failure is the same as for most patients in respiratory distress (see page 306). Maintain an open airway and keep the patient at rest. Make certain that someone calls the dispatcher. Position the patient to provide the greatest ease when breathing. Keep the patient covered to conserve body heat, but do not overheat.

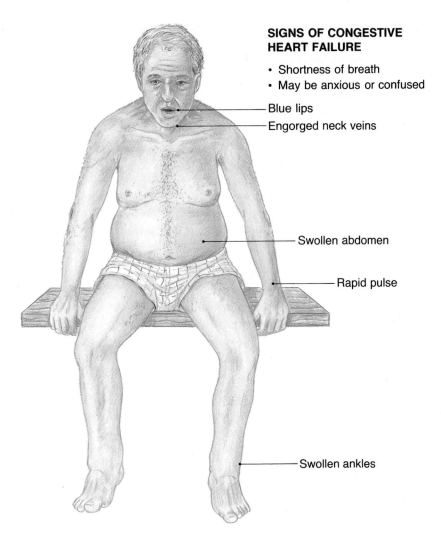

**SIGNS OF CONGESTIVE
HEART FAILURE**

- Shortness of breath
- May be anxious or confused

— Blue lips
— Engorged neck veins

— Swollen abdomen

— Rapid pulse

— Swollen ankles

FIGURE 13–2. Signs of
congestive heart failure.

Stroke

If a blood vessel supplying blood to the brain is obstructed, or if the
vessel ruptures, a *stroke* has occurred. During a stroke, the brain is damaged. Additional damage takes place as areas of the brain fail to receive
enough oxygen. This damage may be so great as to cause death.

Stroke—the blocking or
bursting of a vessel that
supplies blood to the brain. A
portion of the brain is damaged
or killed by this event.

Strokes are also called cerebrovascular (SER-e-bro-VAS-cu-ler) accidents,
or CVAs for short. A stroke and a CVA are the same thing.

Symptoms and Signs

1st There are many symptoms and signs for stroke, including:

- Headache—this may be the only symptom at first
- Collapse
- Altered states of consciousness
- Numbness or paralysis—usually to the extremities and/or to the face
- Difficulty with speech or vision
- Confusion
- Convulsions
- Difficulty in breathing
- Unequal pupils
- Loss of bowel and bladder control

1st RULE: If a patient has any of the symptoms or signs of a stroke, including nothing more than a headache, assume that the patient may be having, or is about to have, a stroke. Remember, the risk of having a stroke increases with age.

Emergency Care

1st When caring for a possible stroke victim, you should:

1. Maintain an open airway and be prepared to provide artificial respirations or CPR if needed.
2. Keep the patient at rest.
3. Protect all paralyzed parts.
4. Provide emotional support. Be certain to make an effort to understand everything that the patient says. Remember, the speech centers of the brain may be affected.
5. Position the patient so that the head, neck, and shoulders are slightly elevated. Be certain to allow for drainage from the patient's mouth by turning the head slightly to one side.
6. *Do not* allow the patient to become overheated.
7. *Do not* administer anything by mouth.
8. Continue to monitor the patient. Shock or respiratory or cardiac arrest is possible.

Respiratory Distress

Respiratory distress—any difficulty in breathing. Sometimes the problem is severe enough to require emergency care. Once distress begins, it is difficult to predict the short-term course of the problem.

People may experience difficulty in breathing for a number of reasons. A patient may be unable to stop breathing too rapidly (hyperventilation). Spasms may be occurring along the airway (asthma). There may be a disease or condition such as bronchitis or pneumonia. Perhaps the heart and lungs can no longer function properly for circulation and gas exchange (congestive heart failure). The patient's difficulty in breathing may stem from being exposed to a poison or something to which the patient is allergic.

Signs and Symptoms

1st For most cases of respiratory distress, any or all of the following symptoms and signs may be noticed:

- Labored breathing
- Unusual breathing sounds
- Rapid or slowed rate of breathing
- Unusual pulse rate and character
- Changes in the color of the lips, skin, and nail beds—usually, the color will change to blue or gray
- Confusion, hallucinations, or the patient feels that people want to hurt him—this is sometimes seen in advanced cases

Emergency Care

1st When caring for most cases of respiratory distress, you should:

1. Have someone call the EMS System dispatcher. *Do not* abandon the patient, since respiratory arrest might develop.
2. Maintain an open airway.
3. Make certain that the problem is not caused by an airway obstruction.

■ SCAN 13-2.

Stroke: Cerebrovascular Accident

Causes of Cerebrovascular Accidents: Stroke

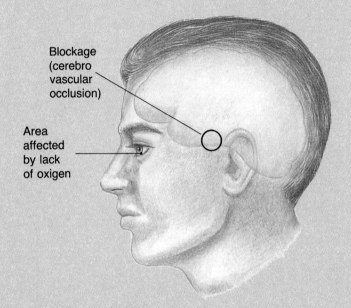

Blockage (cerebro vascular occlusion)

Area affected by lack of oxigen

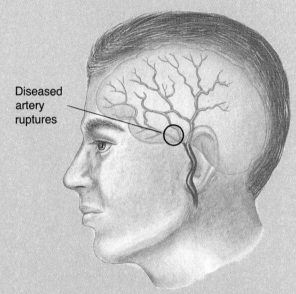

Diseased artery ruptures

Cerebral Thrombosis: Blockage in arteries supplying oxygenated blood will result in damage to affected parts of the brain.

Cerebral Hemorrhage: An aneurysm or other weakened area of an artery ruptures. This has two effects:
1. An area of the brain is deprived of oxygenated blood.
2. Pooling blood puts increased pressure on the brain, displacing tissue and interfering with function. Cerebral hemorrhage is often associated with arteriosclerosis and hypertension.

Symptoms and Signs of Stroke

- Headache
- Confusion and/or dizziness
- Loss of function or paralysis of extremities (usually on one side of the body)
- Numbness (usually limited to one side of the body)
- Collapse
- Facial flaccidness and loss of expression (often to one side of the face)
- Impaired speech
- Unequal pupil size
- Impaired vision
- Rapid, full pulse
- Difficult respiration, snoring
- Nausea
- Convulsions
- Coma
- Loss of bladder and bowel control

Emergency Care of Stroke Patients

- Ensure an open airway.
- Keep the patient calm.
- Monitor vital signs.
- Give nothing by mouth.
- Treat for shock.
- Properly position the patient.
  CONSCIOUS PATIENT: Keep in semireclined position. Sit in front of patient, keep eye contact, and speak slowly and clearly.
  UNCONSCIOUS PATIENT: Keep in lateral recumbent position. Keep affected limbs underneath patient. Use protective padding.

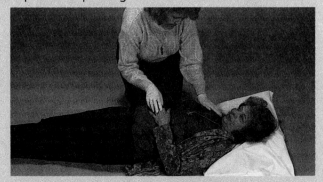

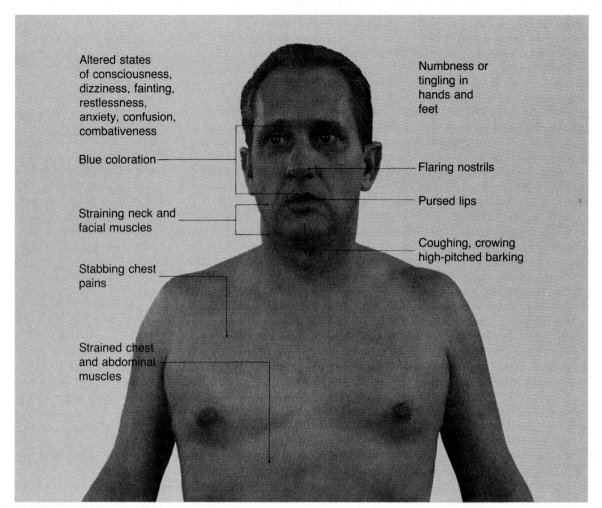

Altered states
of consciousness,
dizziness, fainting,
restlessness,
anxiety, confusion,
combativeness

Blue coloration

Straining neck and
facial muscles

Stabbing chest
pains

Strained chest
and abdominal
muscles

Numbness or
tingling in
hands and
feet

Flaring nostrils

Pursed lips

Coughing, crowing
high-pitched barking

FIGURE 13–3. The symptoms
and signs of respiratory distress.

4. Make certain that the patient is not allergic to substances at the scene. If this is the case, move the substance or move the patient.
5. Keep the patient at rest.
6. Place the patient in a sitting position, allowing for proper drainage from the mouth. It often helps if the patient can support himself by the forearms when in a sitting position. This eases the patient's efforts in expanding the chest.
7. Cover the patient to conserve body heat, but do not allow the patient to overheat.
8. Provide emotional support.
9. Continue to monitor the patient.

Hyperventilation

Hyperventilation
uncontrolled rapid, deep
breathing that is usually self-
correcting. This may occur by
itself or as a sign of a more
serious problem.

When someone is hyperventilating, breathing is too rapid and too deep. Since fear or stress can set off an attack of hyperventilation, the person may appear to be frightened. Unless the patient tells you that hyperventilation problems have happened before, you may be fooled into believing that it is some other emergency. Sometimes a hyperventilating patient will have sharp chest pains. Rarely, he or she may have chest pains and many of the other signs of a heart attack. Even when you believe that you are dealing with simple hyperventilation, stay alert for the signs of a possible heart attack and changes in vital signs that may indicate medical problems that are more serious than simple hyperventilation. If the patient's breathing is rapid and shallow rather than rapid and deep, assume that the problem

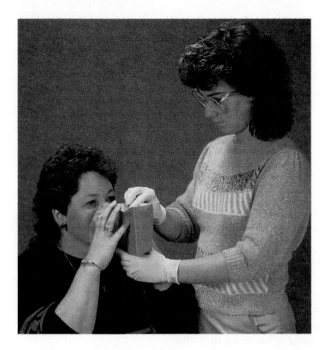

FIGURE 13–4.
Care for simple hyperventilation by having the patient rebreathe his exhaled air.

is more serious than simple hyperventilation. Do not rule out impending heart attack, poisoning, or other serious medical problems.

Hyperventilating patients do not show a blue coloration to the skin, lips, or nail beds. This clue can be used to separate hyperventilation from the latter stages of most severe forms of respiratory distress. In addition to this, many hyperventilating patients will complain of tingling sensations or numbness in their limbs and a cramping of the fingers.

1st Have the hyperventilating patient breathe into a paper bag (not plastic). The bag should be positioned over the patient's mouth and nose so that the patient rebreathes exhaled air. This process will increase the carbon dioxide in the blood, allowing the respiratory centers of the brain to establish proper control over the patient's breathing. Normal breathing should return within a few minutes.

1st WARNING: Hyperventilation can be a sign of possible respiratory distress or an impending heart attack. If you are unable to control a patient's hyperventilation, there may be a more serious medical condition. Alert the EMS System dispatcher and provide care for respiratory distress. Monitor vital signs and be prepared in case the patient has a heart attack or respiratory arrest.

Chronic Obstructive Pulmonary Disease

A variety of respiratory conditions can be classified as a chronic obstructive pulmonary disease (COPD). These include emphysema, chronic bronchitis, black lung, and unknown conditions that have symptoms and signs like emphysema. Usually the patient is middle aged or older, but COPD can occur in children and teenagers.

Chronic obstructive pulmonary disease (COPD)—a variety of lung problems related to disease of the air passageways or exchange levels. The patient will suffer difficulties in breathing.

1st The symptoms and signs of COPD may include:

- The patient is usually an older person. Often there is a history of heavy cigarette smoking, respiratory problems, or allergies.
- There may be a persistent cough.
- There is usually shortness of breath. Sometimes the patient breathes through pursed lips and tries to breathe easier by sitting and pushing up with the hands or elbows.

- The patient tires easily.
- The patient may complain of a tightness in the chest.
- The patient may have periods of dizziness (in a few cases).

In advanced cases there may be:

- Irritability
- Rapid pulse, sometimes irregular
- Barrel-chest appearance
- Strong desire to remain sitting, even when asleep
- Blue coloration to the skin, lips, and nail beds
- Swelling of the lower extremities
- Apparent congestive heart failure

1st To care for COPD patients:

1. Ensure an open airway, making certain that the problem is not due to obstruction by the tongue or some form of mechanical obstruction.
2. Have someone alert the EMS System dispatcher and report the problem as a possible COPD patient who is in distress.
3. Provide emotional support for the patient.
4. Monitor vital signs.
5. Help the patient into a position to ease respirations.
6. Loosen any restrictive clothing.
7. Cover the patient to conserve body heat, but *do not* overheat the patient.
8. Encourage coughing when necessary.
9. Do what you can to reduce stress.

NOTE: If you are a First Responder who may administer oxygen, take great care with COPD patients, especially if they are in respiratory distress or show the advanced signs of COPD. Provide 24% oxygen (2 liters) by Venturi mask or nasal cannula (see Appendix 3). *Do not* withhold the amount of oxygen needed by a patient. When in doubt, radio or phone the emergency department physician for specific orders.

Seizures

Seizure—in general, any event in the brain that causes uncontrolled muscle contractions (convulsions).

The most common form of seizure seen by the First Responder is caused by the condition known as epilepsy. Epileptic seizures may produce convulsions (grand mal seizure) or they may not produce convulsions or any other outward sign of a problem (petit mal seizure). Abnormal brain activity causes an attack to occur in individuals having the disorder. This is an organic disorder, *not* a mental illness.

First Responders are seldom involved with the less serious form of epilepsy (petit mal). Convulsions and other outward signs are not apparent in this form of epilepsy. The patient having a petit mal seizure has a sudden, but short, loss of consciousness. During this loss of contact, the patient may appear dazed and usually has a loss of speech. It is quite common for this type of seizure to go unnoticed by everyone but the patient. As a First Responder, you should be more concerned with those seizures that produce convulsions.

1st Symptoms and Signs
In cases of severe seizures, such as the grand mal epileptic seizure, any or all of the following may be present:

- Sudden loss of consciousness with the patient falling to the ground.

■ SCAN 13-3.

Respiratory Disorders

RESPIRATORY
DISTRESS

CHRONIC OBSTRUCTIVE
PULMONARY DISEASE

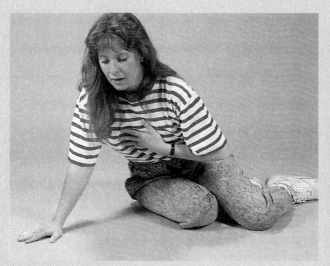

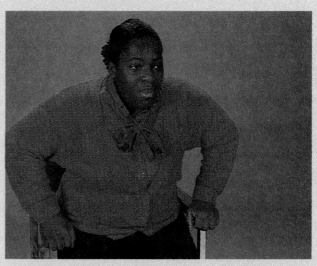

Symptoms and Signs

- Difficult breathing
- Shortness of breath
- Temporary cessation of breathing
- Rapid deep breathing
- Noisy breathing
- Faintness of unconsciousness
- Dizziness
- Restlessness, anxiety, or confusion
- Strained muscles: face, neck, chest, abdomen
- Stabbing chest pains
- Numbness or tingling in limbs (hands or feet)
- Pursed lips or mouth
  open wide to aid breathing
- Blue discoloration (cyanosis)

Symptoms and Signs

Usually the patient will have emphysema or chronic
bronchitis

- History of respiratory problems or allergies
- Cough
- Shortness of breath
- Tightness in chest
- Swelling in lower extremities (advanced cases)
- Rapid pulse (some cases)
- Barrell chest (some cases)
- Dizziness (some cases)
- Blue discoloration (cyanosis)
- Desire to sit upright at all times. May use hands or
  elbows to push up on chair arms.

Emergency Care

1. Do not abandon patient. Have someone call EMS
   dispatch.

2. Ensure an open airway. Check for airway obstructions.

3. Check to see if the patient is allergic to anything at
   scene (remove substance or move patient).

4. Keep patient at rest. Conscious patient may desire
   to sit upright.

5. Cover to conserve body heat.

6. Monitor patient and provide emotional support.

Emergency Care

Provide the same care as you would for respiratory
distress. Be certain not to overheat the patient. Do what
you can to reduce stress. If appropriate, encourage
coughing.

WARNING: IF YOU ARE ALLOWED TO
PROVIDE OXYGEN, YOU MUST FOLLOW
LOCAL GUIDLINES FOR THE COPD.

The patient may report a bright light, bright colors, or the sensation of a strong odor prior to losing consciousness.

- The patient's body will stiffen.
- Sometimes the patient will temporarily stop breathing and lose bladder and bowel control.
- The patient will go into convulsions, jerking all parts of the body. Breathing will be labored and there may be frothing at the mouth.
- After convulsions, the patient's body completely relaxes.
- The patient becomes conscious, but is very tired and confused. The patient may complain of a headache.

Emergency Care

1st The basic emergency care for seizures producing convulsions is to:

1. Place the patient on the floor or the ground.
2. Loosen restrictive clothing.
3. *Do not* try to hold the patient still during the convulsions. Your primary job as a First Responder is to protect the patient from injury. Keep the patient from striking any nearby objects.
4. After convulsions have passed, keep the patient at rest, with the head positioned to allow for drainage in case of vomiting.
5. Protect the patient from embarrassment by asking onlookers to give the patient some privacy.
6. If the patient says that this is the first attack, alert the EMS System dispatcher. If the patient is aware of the problem and has had other attacks, ask if you may phone the patient's doctor. It is possible that the doctor may wish to see the patient, change medications, or have the patient transported to a medical facility. Remember, the patient has the option to refuse additional care.

After any seizure, it is best to keep the patient at rest. Provide emotional support for the patient and witnesses. If you arrived after the seizure, interview the patient and perform a secondary survey to check for injuries. Call the EMS System dispatcher. Should the patient refuse additional care, strongly recommend that he wait to be examined by the EMTs. Should the patient refuse to wait, caution against driving a car or operating any

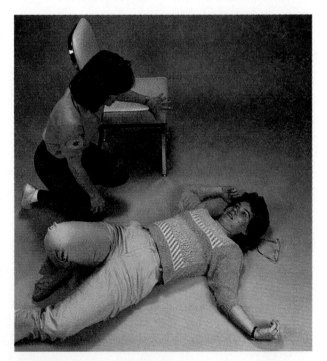

FIGURE 13–5. During a seizure, protect the patient from injury.

machinery. If need be, arrange for transportation so that the patient will not attempt to drive. If you are a police officer or an industrial First Responder, follow standard procedures in regard to letting the patient drive or operate machinery.

NOTE: You may have heard that you should place an object between the teeth of a convulsing patient. This is very poor practice. Many objects can be broken and obstruct the patient's airway (for example, a pencil). "Bite sticks" can be used. They are made from padded tongue depressors. A "bite stick" should be used only if the patient is biting the tongue. Even in this case, you should not use a bite stick unless you have been properly trained to do so. Most agencies studying convulsions do not report favorably on the use of bite sticks. Beware of placing objects such as a small wallet between the patient's teeth. It is possible for a convulsing patient to swallow rather large objects. Never force anything into a convulsing patient's mouth. Never place your fingers into the patient's mouth during a seizure.

Diabetes

The main source of energy for the cells of the body is sugar. This sugar, usually in the form of glucose, is carried to the cells by the way of the bloodstream. Even though all the cells need this "blood sugar," it is most critical for the cells of the brain and nervous system.

The pancreas produces insulin. Body cells cannot take up blood sugar unless insulin is present. If there is not enough insulin produced, the cells will starve for sugar even if there is plenty of sugar in the bloodstream. Diabetes is a disease that prevents individuals from producing enough insulin. Some cases of diabetes can be managed by diet. Others require the patient to take doses of insulin. If a diabetic person does not have enough insulin, a **diabetic coma** may result.

When diabetics take in too much insulin, they will force all their blood sugar into muscle and organ tissues, robbing the brain cells of the sugar they need. If diabetics have too much insulin in their blood for the sugar present, they may go into **insulin shock.***

1st REMEMBER: Check for medical identification devices.

Diabetic Coma

Diabetic coma usually is a gradual event, taking several days to develop. Should the individual not take enough insulin, or eat too much sugar for the amount of insulin being taken, or if the diabetes has not been diagnosed, diabetic coma may occur.

1st The symptoms and signs of diabetic coma are:

- Difficult breathing—typically the patient will take deep, rapid breaths, often heaving or sighing. This may appear to be hyperventilation.
- Dry, warm skin—sometimes the skin will take on a red coloring.
- Rapid, weak pulse
- In some cases, the eyes will appear "sunken."
- A sweet or fruity odor will be on the patient's breath, called "acetone breath," which smells like fingernail polish remover.
- The patient may complain of having a dry mouth.
- The patient may be restless and in a stupor.
- The patient may become unresponsive and go into a coma.

Diabetes—usually refers to diabetes mellitus. This is the condition in which there is a decrease or absence of insulin produced by the pancreas. The glucose level of the blood will increase and the movement of this sugar into the cells will decrease as the insulin level falls.

Diabetic coma—severe hyperglycemia. The sugar (glucose) level increases in the blood and decreases in the tissue cells. The problem can be serious enough to produce coma.

Insulin shock—severe hypoglycemia. A form of shock usually caused by too high a level of insulin in the blood, producing a sudden drop in blood sugar. The causes are too much insulin injected by the diabetic or too little food taken in for the amount of insulin injected or produced by medication.

---

* Diabetic coma and insulin shock are terms used in prehospital emergency care. Diabetic coma is the end result of severe hyperglycemia (high sugar in the blood, low in the tissues). Insulin shock is part of severe hypoglycemia (too little available sugar). Technically, some of the patients you will see are hyperglycemic or hypoglycemic. It is best for you to make use of the general terms and say patients are probably suffering from insulin shock or developing diabetic coma.

WARNING: Some patients who are about to go into deep stages of diabetic coma may appear to be drunk, at first. Do not assume someone is drunk unless there is obvious alcohol abuse and you have ruled out diabetic coma. Keep in mind that an alcoholic may also be diabetic.

1st The emergency care for diabetic coma consists of:

1. Having someone alert the EMS System dispatcher—this patient will have to be transferred to a medical facility.
2. Keeping the patient at rest. If the patient is alert, try to gain additional information. Ask if the patient is diabetic. Find out if the patient has taken insulin and has eaten recently.
3. If you are not certain if you are dealing with diabetic coma or insulin shock, give the patient sugar, candy, orange juice, or soda (make certain that the substance contains real sugar, not an artificial sweetener). *Do not* give any liquids to patients unless they are fully alert. Granulated sugar can be placed under the tongue of an unconscious patient; however, you *must* sprinkle a few granules at a time from your fingers and constantly monitor the patient to ensure an open airway. Follow your local EMS System guidelines.

Insulin Shock

The diabetic who has taken too much insulin, has eaten too little sugar, or is overexerted may go into insulin shock. Insulin shock, unlike diabetic coma, comes on suddenly.

1st The symptoms and signs for insulin shock include:

- Pale, moist skin, often cold and "clammy"
- A full and rapid pulse
- Dizziness—the patient may become disoriented, faint and go into convulsions or a coma.
- Headache
- Normal or shallow breathing with no unusual odors
- Being very hungry
- Some patients will develop convulsions if they do not receive early care.

1st The emergency care for insulin shock consists of:

1. Keeping the patient at rest.
2. Providing sugar for the patient in the form of granulated sugar, sugar cubes, candy, orange juice, soda, syrup, or honey. Make certain that the substance contains sugar and not an artificial sweetener. *Do not* give liquids or foods to the patient who is not fully alert.
3. Having someone alert the EMS System dispatcher. If you are not sure that you are dealing with insulin shock, if the patient does not respond to sugar, if this is the patient's first case of insulin shock, or if the patient went into convulsions or coma, be sure that the dispatcher has this information.

REMEMBER: When in doubt, follow the "sugar for everyone" rule.

Acute Abdomen

Acute abdomen—the sudden onset of severe abdominal pain. Abdominal distress related to one of many medical conditions or specific injury to the abdomen.

1st The sudden onset of severe belly pain is called acute abdomen or acute abdominal distress. The presence of pain alone is enough to indicate that the patient must be seen as soon as possible by someone with more advanced training.

The cause of the pain may be anything from simple indigestion to a

■ SCAN 13-4.

Diabetic Emergencies

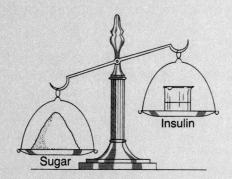

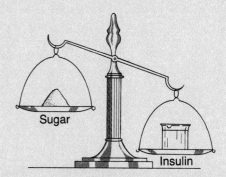

Diabetic Coma (Hyperglycemia)

Causes:

- The diabetic's condition has not been diagnosed and/or treated.
- The diabetic has not taken his insulin.
- The diabetic has overeaten, flooding the body with a sudden excess of carbohydrates.
- The diabetic suffers an infection that disrupts his glucose/insulin balance.

Emergency care:

- Immediately transport to a medical facility

Symptoms and signs:

- Gradual onset of symptoms and signs, over a period of days.
- Patient complains of dry mouth and intense thirst.
- Abdominal pain and vomiting common.
- Gradually increasing restlessness, confusion, followed by stupor.
- Coma, with these signs:
  - Signs of air hunger—Deep, sighing respirations.
  - Weak, rapid pulse.
  - Dry, red, warm skin.
  - Eyes that appear sunken.
  - Breath smells of acetone—Sickly sweet, like nail polish remover.

Insulin Shock (Hypoglycemia)

Causes:

- The diabetic has taken too much insulin.
- The diabetic has not eaten enough to provide his normal sugar intake.
- The diabetic has overexercised, or overexerted himself, thus reducing his blood glucose level.
- The diabetic has vomited a meal.

Emergency care:

- Conscious patient—administer sugar, granular sugar, honey, lifesaver or other candy placed under the tongue, or orange juice.
- Avoid giving liquids to the unconscious patient. Provide "sprinkle" of granulated sugar under tongue.
- Turn head to side or place on side.
- Transport to the medical facility.

Symptoms and signs:

- Rapid onset of symptoms and signs, over a period of minutes.
- Dizziness and headache.
- Abnormal, hostile, or aggressive behavior, which may be diagnosed as acute alcoholic intoxication.
- Fainting, convulsions, and occasionally coma.
- Full rapid pulse.
- Patient intensely hungry.
- Skin pale, cold, and clammy; perspiration may be profuse.
- Drooling.

Special Notes: Diabetic Coma and Insulin Shock

When faced with a patient who may be suffering from one of these conditions:

- Determine if the patient is diabetic. Look for medical alert medallions or information cards; interview patient and family members.
- If the patient is a known or suspected diabetic, and insulin shock cannot be ruled out, assume that it is insulin shock and administer sugar.

Often a patient suffering from either of these conditions may simply appear drunk. Always check for other underlying conditions—such as diabetic complications—when treating someone who appears intoxicated.

very serious medical problem. Your role is to assess the patient and provide the needed care, making certain that the EMS dispatcher has been alerted. *Do not* attempt to diagnose the patient's problem. If the pain is severe enough for the patient to seek emergency care, then his or her problem must be considered to be serious. This approach must be taken until modified by a physician's diagnosis.

Many medical problems are associated with severe abdominal pain. Some examples include appendicitis, ulcers, inflamed abdominal cavity membranes, pancreas, gallbladder, or internal reproductive organs, obstruction of the intestine, serious liver disease, gallstones, and kidney stones. Female patient's may have severe abdominal pain related to problems with pregnancy. Detecting the exact nature of the pain is not possible at the First Responder level of care.

NOTE: Do not assume that pain over the top of a specific organ means that this organ is the location of the patient's problem. Abdominal pain is usually spread out over one or more areas. The pain may not be over the top of or near the sick or damaged organ (see Figure 13–6).

1st The symptoms and signs associated with acute abdomen may include:

- Abdominal pain
- Back pain
- Nausea and vomiting
- Fear
- Rapid pulse
- Rapid and shallow breathing
- Fever
- Signs of developing shock
- Guarding the abdomen (The patient's arms are folded across the belly and the knees are drawn up. Usually, the patient tries not to move.)
- Bulging (distention) and/or rigid abdominal wall
- Abdominal tenderness
- A protrusion, lump, or mass is seen or felt
- Rectal bleeding, blood in the urine, or nonmenstrual vaginal bleeding

As you gather symptoms and signs, be sure to look over the patient. Does the person appear ill? Does he or she continue to guard the abdomen? Is the person reluctant to move?

1st The basic care for acute abdomen patients requires you to:

1. Maintain an open airway. Stay alert for vomiting.
2. Provide care for shock.
3. Make certain that EMS dispatch is alerted.
4. Keep the patient at rest. Sometimes, the patient's pain may be reduced if he or she is positioned on the back with the knees flexed. Do not force the patient to assume this position.
5. Save all vomitus. Avoid contact with the vomitus, discharges, mucous membranes, and body fluids.
6. Reassure the patient and continue to gather information. Ask if the pain came on suddenly, the nature of the pain (sharp, dull, stabbing), if there were any fevers or chills, any unusual bowel movements (dark, light, tarry, bloody, loose, or hard), or any problems with urination (unable to go, frequent urination, or blood in the urine). Ask the patient when he or she last ate and what was consumed.

1st WARNING: Do not give the patient anything by mouth. To do so may cause the patient to vomit or may set off organ or gland activity that could prove harmful.

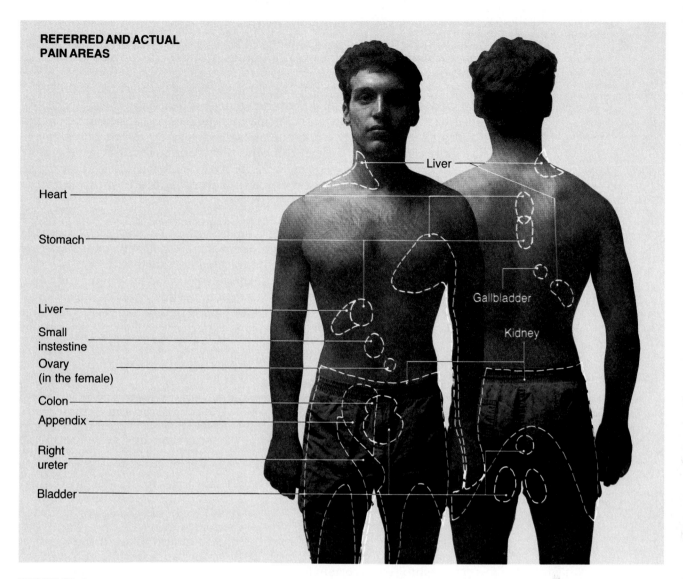

REFERRED AND ACTUAL PAIN AREAS

Heart

Stomach

Liver

Small instestine

Ovary (in the female)

Colon

Appendix

Right ureter

Bladder

Liver

Gallbladder

Kidney

FIGURE 13–6.
Patterns of abdominal pain.

Poisoning

A great number of substances can be considered poisons. In fact, any chemical that can damage the body is a poison. Associated with this damage are symptoms and signs that indicate the patient is having a medical emergency. Different people will react differently to various poisons. In some cases, what may be a dangerous poison to one person may have little effect on another. For most poisonous substances, the reactions seen in children are more serious than adult reactions.

Poisons can be taken into the body by way of the mouth (ingestion), by breathing (inhalation), through the skin (absorption) and through body tissues and the bloodstream (injection). Ingested poisons can include various household and industrial chemicals, certain foods and improperly prepared foods, plant materials, petroleum products, and poisons made specifically to control rodents, insects, and crop diseases.

Inhaled poisons take the form of gases, vapors, and sprays, including carbon monoxide (from car exhaust, kerosene heaters, and wood burning stoves), ammonia, chlorine, volatile liquid chemicals (including many industrial solvents), and insect sprays.

Poisons absorbed through the skin may or may not damage the skin. Many contact poisons will do harsh damage to the skin and then be slowly absorbed into the bloodstream. Some insecticides and agricultural chemicals can be absorbed through the skin. Corrosive chemicals may damage the skin and then be absorbed by the body. Contact with a wide variety of plant materials and certain forms of marine life can cause damage to the skin, with the poison (toxin) being absorbed into tissues under the skin.

Insects, spiders, snakes, and certain marine life forms are able to inject poisons into the body. Injection might be self-induced by way of a hypodermic needle. Unusual industrial accidents producing cuts or puncture wounds also can be a source of poisons being injected into the body.

In this chapter, we will consider general symptoms and signs and some basic courses of action. Table 13-1 lists some of the types of poisons you may see that require emergency care. This information is provided so that you may learn more about various poisons as part of your continued training.

TABLE 13-1 COMMON POISONS

Poison	Helpful Signs and Symptoms
Acetaminophen (Tylenol, Comtrex, Bancap, Datril, Excedrin P.M.)	Nausea, vomiting, heavy perspiration. The victim is usually a child.
Acids	Burns on or around the lips. Burning in the mouth, throat and stomach, often followed by heavy vomiting.
Alkalis (ammonia, bleaches, detergents, lye, washing soda, certain fertilizers)	Check mouth to see if the membranes appear white and swollen. There may be a soapy appearance in the mouth. Abdominal pain is usually present. Vomiting may occur, often full of blood and mucus.
Arsenic (rat poison)	"Garlic breath," with burning in the mouth, throat and stomach. Abdominal pain can be severe. Vomiting is common.
Aspirin	Delayed reactions, including ringing in the ears, rapid and deep breathing, dry skin, and restlessness.
Chloroform	Slow, shallow breathing with chloroform odor on breath. Pupils are dilated and fixed.
Corrosive agents (disinfectants, drain cleaners, household acids, iodine, pine oil, turpentine, toilet bowl cleaners, styptic pencil, water softeners, strong acids)	(See Acids)

The table is not meant to be memorized as part of your basic course. Note that drugs and alcohol will be covered in Chapter 14.

1st Poison Control Centers

In most localities, a poison control center can be reached 24 hours a day. The staff at the center can tell you what should be done for most cases of poisoning. Your instructor will tell you which center serves your area and give you the phone number for this center. Carry this number with you at all times.

In some EMS Systems, rescuers must receive directions for the care of poisoning patients from a physician. This is not always the case for every poison control center. If directions must come from a physician, the First Responder should phone or radio the emergency department or EMS dispatch. This is termed seeking help from medical command. You are to follow the method used by your EMS System. Remember, a nurse or the dispatcher may relay the physician's directions. You may not have a chance to speak directly to a physician.

To aid the poison control center or medical command, note and report any containers at the scene of the poisoning. Let them know if the patient has vomited and describe the vomitus. When possible, and if it can be

TABLE 13–1 CONTINUED

Poison	Helpful Signs and Symptoms
Food poisoning	Difficult to detect since signs and symptoms vary greatly. Usually, you will note abdominal pain, nausea and vomiting, gas and bowel sounds, and diarrhea.
Iodine	Upset stomach and vomiting. If a starchy meal has been eaten, the vomitus may appear blue.
Metals (copper, lead, mercury, and zinc)	Metallic taste in mouth, with nausea and abdominal pains. Vomiting may occur. Stools may be bloody or dark.
Petroleum Products (some deodorizers, heating fuel, diesel fuels, gasoline, kerosene, lighter fluid, lubricating oil, naphtha, rust remover, transmission fluid)	Note characteristic odors on patient's breath and clothing or in vomitus.
Phosphorus	Abdominal pain and vomiting.
Plants: Contact (poison ivy, poison oak, poison sumac)	Swollen, itchy areas on the skin, with quickly forming blisterlike structures
Plants: Ingested (azalea, castor bean, poison elder, foxglove, lily of the valley, mountain laurel, mushrooms, nightshade, oleander, mistletoe and holly berries, rhododendron, rhubarb leaves, rubber plant, some wild cherries)	Difficult to detect, ranging from nausea to coma. Always question in cases of apparent child poisoning.
Strychnine	The face, jaw and neck will stiffen. Strong convulsions occur quickly after ingesting.

done quickly, gather information from the victim or from bystanders before you call the center.

Ingested Poisons

In cases of possible ingested poisoning, you must gather information quickly. If at all possible, do so while you are making a primary survey. Note any containers that may hold poisonous substances. See if there is any vomitus. Check if there are any substances on the patient's clothes or if the patient is wearing clothing that may indicate the nature of work (farmer, miner, and so on). Can the scene be associated with certain types of poisonings? Question the patient and any bystanders.

1st The symptoms and signs for ingested poisons can be gathered during the primary and secondary surveys. They can include any or all of the following:

- Burns or stains around the patient's mouth
- Unusual breath odors, body odors, or odors on the patient's clothing or at the scene
- Abnormal breathing
- Abnormal pulse rate and character
- Sweating
- Dilated or constricted pupils
- Excessive saliva formation or foaming at the mouth
- Pains in the mouth or throat, or painful swallowing
- Stomach or abdominal pain
- Upset stomach or nausea
- Vomiting
- Diarrhea
- Convulsions
- Altered states of awareness, including unconsciousness

1st *Always* call the poison control center, even if you know what the ingested poison is and what you are to do in such cases. Methods of care for various poisons often change. Even the information on the container label may not be the most recent care procedure. Make sure that the EMS System dispatcher is alerted.

1st In most cases, emergency care will consist of diluting the poison in the patient's stomach and then inducing the patient to vomit. Never attempt to dilute the poison or induce vomiting if the patient is unconscious.

1st WARNING: *Do not* induce vomiting if the patient is not fully conscious, has been convulsing, or if the source of the poison is a strong acid, alkali, or petroleum product. Included in these groups of substances are oven cleaners, drain cleaners, toilet bowl cleaners, lye, ammonia, bleaches, kerosene, and gasoline. Always check for burns around the patient's mouth and the odor of petroleum products on the patient's breath. Some poison control centers allow vomiting to be induced for cases of petroleum product poisoning if this action can be started soon after the ingesting of the poison. Usually, this means no more than 10 minutes after ingesting. Follow your local guidelines and the instructions given by the poison control center.

1st For conscious patients, the typical procedures for care include:

1. Maintain an open airway.
2. *Call the poison control center* or *medical command.* If directed to do so . . .
3. Dilute the poison by having the patient drink one or two glasses of

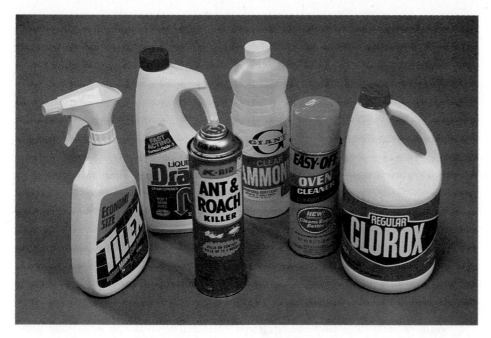

FIGURE 13–7.
If the patient has taken certain poisons, vomiting is usually not induced.

water or milk. The poison control center or medical command may tell you to have the patient consume the fluids in sips to prevent vomiting. *Do not* give anything by mouth if the patient is having convulsions, unless otherwise directed by a physician or poison control center.

4. If supplies are available and you are allowed to do so, induce vomiting by giving the patient two tablespoons of syrup of ipecac followed by no less than 8 ounces of water (one full glass). You will obtain a better dilution if you can have the patient take 16 ounces of water. If the patient is a child under the age of 10, give only one tablespoon of syrup of ipecac, followed by at least 8 ounces of water.

5. Position the patient so that no vomitus will be aspirated (breathed in) (on one side or in a semisitting position with the head turned to the side). Wait 15 to 20 minutes for the patient to vomit. If the patient does not vomit after this time, give another dose of ipecac and water. Instead of inducing vomiting, you may be directed to give the patient two tablespoons of activated charcoal mixed vigorously into 8 ounces of water. If you are directed to induce vomiting and then give charcoal, give the patient ipecac and water, followed by charcoal after the patient has vomited.

6. Save all vomitus.

7. Provide care for shock, keeping the patient positioned to drain the mouth should vomiting occur.

In cases of ingested poisons, be realistic about the limits to emergency care. Some poisons kill instantly. Some patients can be helped only by very special antidotes. There are no antidotes for some poisons. You may do your best as a First Responder and the patient will still die from the ingested poison.

Controversies exist in the emergency care of ingested poisons. One such controversy is inducing the patient to vomit by using the patient's finger or a blunt object to irritate (tickle) the back of the patient's throat. This is useful when no ipecac is available. This method should *never* be used unless you are directed to do so by the poison control center or medical command.

Another controversy exists as to when mouth-to-mouth ventilations should not be performed. If the patient has taken a highly concentrated dose of certain poisons, such as arsenic or cyanide, and if deposits remain on the patient's lips, there is a chance the rescuer may be harmed. Your instructor may wish to describe certain types of poisonings where you are not to perform mouth-to-mouth ventilations in accordance with EMS guidelines. The current recommendation is to use a pocket face mask (see Chapter 4) on all patients who need rescue breathing. Keep in mind that patients receiving a high dose of these poisons usually die within seconds.

Inhaled Poisons

Gather information from the patient and bystanders as quickly as possible. Look for indications of inhaled poisons. Possible sources can be automobile exhaust systems, stoves, charcoal grills, industrial solvents, and spray cans. **1st** The symptoms and signs of inhaled poisons vary depending on the source of the poison. Shortness of breath and coughing are good indicators. Pulse rate is usually too fast or too slow. Often, the patient's eyes will appear irritated.

1st WARNING: *Do not* attempt to rescue the victim of an inhaled poisoning unless you are *absolutely* certain that the scene is safe. This is true even when the accident occurs outside or in a well-ventilated area. Hazardous materials experts will have to approve your entry into the area (see page 401). Unless you are trained to enter such a scene and have the proper equipment, *do not* try to provide care for a patient in a poisonous atmosphere. Do only what you have been trained to do.
1st Emergency care consists of safely removing the patient from the source of the inhaled poison, maintaining an open airway, providing needed life-support measures, contacting the poison control center or medical command, and making certain that the EMS System dispatcher has been notified.

It may be necessary to remove contaminated clothing from the patient. Take care to avoid touching this clothing since it may cause skin burns. Wear latex or vinyl gloves to protect yourself.

Absorbed (Contact) Poisons

As mentioned earlier in this chapter, absorbed poisons usually irritate or damage the skin. However, there are cases where a poison can be absorbed through the skin with little or no damage being done to the skin. The patient, bystanders, and the scene will help you determine if you are dealing with such rare cases. In First Responder care, most cases of absorbed poisoning will be detected because of skin reactions related to chemicals or plants at the scene.
1st The symptoms and signs of absorbed poisoning include any or all of the following:

- Skin reactions—ranging from mild irritations to chemical burns
- Itching
- Eye irritation
- Headache
- Increased skin temperature
- Allergy shock

1st Emergency care for absorbed poisoning includes moving the patient from the source of the poison (when safe to do so) and immediately flooding with water all the areas of the patient's body that have been exposed to the poison. After flooding with water, remove all contaminated clothing (including shoes) and jewelry, and wash the affected areas of the patient's skin with soap and water. If no soap is available, continue to flood the exposed areas of the patient's skin. Be certain to have someone contact the poison control center and the EMS System dispatcher or medical command. More specific directions for chemical burns appear in Chapter 14. **NOTE:** You are responsible for clothing or jewelry removed from the patient. Obtain a receipt for these items once they are turned over to the proper authorities.

Injected Poisons

Insect stings, spider bites, marine life form stings, and snakebites can all be sources of injected poisons. Some of these poisons cause true emergencies for all patients. Others are only problems for those patients sensitive to the poison. In all cases of injected poisons, be alert for allergy shock.

Poisons can also be injected into the body by way of a hypodermic needle. Drug overdose and drug contamination can produce serious medical emergencies. This will be covered in Chapter 16.

1st Gather information from the patient, bystanders, and the scene. The symptoms and signs of injected poisoning may include:

- Noticeable stings or bites to the skin
- Puncture marks to the skin—pay careful attention to the fingers and hands, forearms, toes and feet, and lower legs
- Pain at or around the wound site
- Itching
- Weakness, dizziness, or collapse
- Difficult breathing and unusual pulse rate
- Headache
- Nausea
- Allergy shock

1st Since a patient may go into allergy shock, alert the poison control center and the EMS System dispatcher or medical command as soon as possible for all cases of injected poisoning. Emergency care for injected poisons (except snakebite) includes:

1. Provide care for shock—this is done even if the patient does not show any of the signs of shock.
2. Scraping away bee and wasp stingers and venom sacs—*do not* pull out stingers, always scrape them from the patient's skin. A plastic credit card works well as a scraper.
3. Placing an ice bag or cold pack over the bitten or stung area.

Some patients sensitive to stings or bites carry medication to help prevent allergy shock. Help all such patients to take their medications. (Your First Responder course may include training in how to administer injectable medications for cases when the patient cannot do so. *Do only what you have been trained to do.*) Remember to look for medical identification devices.

Snakebites

Nearly 50,000 people in the United States are bitten by poisonous snakes each year, with fewer than 10 deaths being reported annually.* The symptoms and signs of poisoning may take several hours to develop. Death from snakebite is usually not a rapidly occurring event unless allergy shock also occurs. Most victims of poisonous snakebite take one to two days to

---

* In the United States, more people die each year from bee and wasp stings than from snakebites.

die from the bite. Staying calm and keeping the patient calm is critical. There is time to alert the EMS System dispatcher and to provide care for the patient.

Consider all snakebites to be from poisonous snakes. The patient or bystanders may indicate that the snake was not poisonous. They could be mistaken. If you see the live snake, *do not* approach it to gather information for determining its species. If safe to do so, note its size and coloration. Unless you are an expert in capturing snakes, do not try to catch the snake. **1st** The symptoms and signs of snakebite may include:

- A noticeable bite to the skin—this may appear as nothing more than a discoloration.
- Pain and swelling in the area of the bite—this may be slow to develop, taking 30 minutes to several hours.
- Rapid pulse and labored breathing
- Weakness
- Vision problems
- Nausea and vomiting

1st The emergency care for snakebite includes:

1. Keep the patient calm and lying down.
2. Have someone alert the EMS System dispatcher.
3. Locate the fang marks and clean this site with soap and water.
4. Remove from the bitten extremity any rings, bracelets, and other constricting items.
5. Keep any bitten extremities immobilized—the application of a soft splint will help. A rigid splint may cause problems if there is swelling at the site of injury. Try to keep the bitten area at the level of the heart, or when possible, below the level of the heart.
6. Provide care for shock, conserve body heat, and monitor vital signs.

If you know that the patient will not reach a medical facility within 5 hours after having been bitten, or if the symptoms and signs of the patient begin to worsen, apply a constricting band above and below the fang marks. Each band should be about $1\frac{1}{2}$ to 2 inches wide, placed about 2 inches from the wound, or above and below the swelling. (*Never* place one band on each side of a joint, such as above and below the knee.) The constricting bands should be from a snakebite kit or made of wide soft rubber. If only one band is available, place it above the wound (between the wound and the heart). If no bands are available, use a handkerchief.

FIGURE 13–8.
Constricting bands should not be too tight.

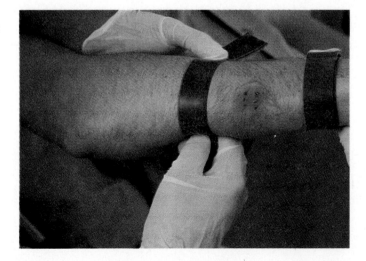

NOTE: The coral snake has a small mouth. Usually, its bites are limited to the patient's finger or toe. When the bite is known to be from a coral snake, apply one constricting band above the wound site.

The constricting bands should be placed so that you can slide your finger underneath them. Do not place them so that they cut off arterial flow. Monitor for a pulse at the wrist or ankle, depending on the extremity involved.

Many EMS Systems recommend constricting bands for *all* cases of snake-bite. Check with your instructor.

Do not place an ice bag or cold pack on the bite unless you are directed to do so by a physician or the poison control center. Do not cut into the bite and apply suction unless you are directed to do so by a physician. *Never* suck the venom from the wound using your mouth.

Infectious Diseases

An infectious disease can be passed from person to person. The agent (germ) causing the disease may be transmitted in water, food, air, body fluids, blood, and wastes. In some cases, the agent may be carried from one person to another by bites from an insect or some arthropod such as a tick or mite.

1st During the rendering of emergency care, the First Responder must be careful of diseases transmitted by direct contact, indirect contact, droplets, and airborne droplets.

Infectious disease—any disease that is directly caused by a microorganism (germ). In general, this is a disease that may be transmitted to another person.

- *Direct contact*—the germs are in the patient's body fluids, blood, or wastes and can be picked up through a cut or transferred from the rescuer's hands to his or her mouth, nose, eyes, or breaks in the skin. An example of a disease that can be transmitted this way is infectious hepatitis.
- *Indirect contact*—the infectious agents have contaminated items at the scene such as clothing, handkerchiefs, thermometers, and diapers. If the rescuer touches the contaminated item, germs may enter through breaks in the skin or be carried to the rescuer's mouth, nose, or eyes. Staphylococcus (staph) infections can be transmitted this way.
- *Droplet contact*—items at the scene and the patient's clothing are contaminated by droplets carrying the microorganisms. Usually this comes from saliva and mucus released during coughs and sneezes. Influenza is transmitted this way.
- *Airborne*—microscopic droplets (droplet nuclei) contain infectious agents. They are released into the air when the patient talks, laughs, sneezes, or coughs. These droplets can travel several feet from the patient and remain suspended in the air. Tuberculosis can be transmitted this way.

As a First Responder, you may be confronted with a patient who has an infectious disease. The patient may not display any symptoms or signs of illness or the illness may be noticeable because the patient shows any of the following symptoms and signs:

- Fever
- Profuse sweating
- Vomiting or diarrhea
- A rash or obvious skin changes
- Indications of a headache, chest, or abdominal pains
- Coughing or sneezing

1st By now, you know the major indications of someone being "sick." Use this knowledge to consider if the patient may have an infectious disease.

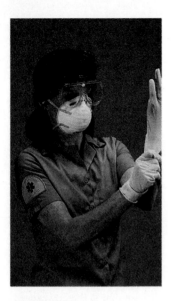

FIGURE 13–9.
Wear the appropriate protective gear to avoid contact with the patient's blood and body fluids.

Keep the patient warm and at rest. Provide care as you would for shock, monitoring vital signs. Wash your hands and face with soap and water after caring for the patient. **Avoid coming into direct contact with the patient's vomitus, wastes, body fluids, blood, or mucous membranes.** The risk of catching the patient's disease is minor; however, always report to your local hospital if you have been exposed to a patient who may have an infectious disease.

It is recommended by the Centers for Disease Control that all emergency care personnel wear approved latex or vinyl gloves while rendering care. These gloves should be changed after contact with each patient or items that may have been contaminated by a patient. When possible, you should follow the rules of universal precautions that were described in Chapter 3 (see p. 54). Wash your hands or other skin surfaces that come into contact with blood, body fluids, vomitus, mucous membranes, or wastes.

1st REMEMBER: You must wear vinyl or latex gloves every time you assess and care for a patient. Always change gloves between patients.

Acquired immune deficiency syndrome (AIDS) is a deadly disease that is of great concern to emergency care personnel. The HIV virus that causes the disease can be transmitted through sexual contact with a person having AIDS or infected by the HIV virus, by blood transfusion from a donor who has AIDS or carries the HIV virus, by sharing needles with someone having the disease or carrying the HIV virus, or by passage of the virus from an infected mother to her unborn child.

Being near someone who has AIDS will not give you the disease. There has to be direct contact with the patient's blood, semen, or other body fluids. Even though there is no hard evidence of saliva being a source of transmission, contact with this fluid should be avoided. The use of gloves while providing care, a pocket face mask with one-way valve during resuscitation, and avoiding all contract with the patient's syringes and needles should be enough to keep the rescuer safe. Remember, a patient who has AIDS is in need of your professional care.

1st REMEMBER: Dispose of used gloves in accordance with local guidelines. Always wash your hands after removing your gloves.

SUMMARY

Various illnesses and conditions can bring about a medical emergency. The **symptoms** and **signs** gained from patient surveys and interviews will help you determine if you are dealing with a possible medical emergency.

Abnormal pulse, breathing, temperature, skin color, and skin condition are all important signs in determining a medical emergency. Be certain to check pupil size and response. Note lip coloration and any odors on the breath. Abdominal tenderness, spasms or paralysis of muscles, nausea, vomiting, and bleeding and discharges are also important signs. Many medical emergencies produce altered states of consciousness.

Listen to the patient and bystanders for reports of pain, fever, nausea, dizziness, shortness of breath, problems with bowel and bladder activities, burning sensations, thirst, hunger, and odd tastes in the mouth. All these are important symptoms in medical emergencies.

If there is no accident-related injury, and the patient **appears or "feels" unusual,** assume that there is a medical emergency. If there is no accident-related injury and the patient has **unusual vital signs,** assume that there is a medical emergency. If the patient says that he is **not feeling normal,** assume that there is a medical emergency.

REMEMBER: An accident may mask a medical emergency or problem that caused the accident. Always check for medical emergencies.

Consider that any patient with **chest pain** is having, or is about to have, a **heart attack.** Look for chest, arm, neck and jaw pains. Nausea, shortness of breath, sweating, weakness, and restlessness also may indicate a heart attack. If cardiac arrest occurs, it may be due to a heart attack.

In cases of possible heart attack, alert the EMS System dispatcher. **Keep the patient at rest.** Position the patient comfortably to ease breathing difficulties, loosen any restrictive clothing, and keep the patient from becoming chilled. **Monitor vital signs** and provide **emotional support.**

Look for medical identification devices and question the patient. There may be medication that should be taken during medical emergencies.

A patient having, or about to have, a **stroke** may complain of nothing more than a **headache.** Consider all headaches to be a serious complaint. In cases of stroke, you may notice collapse with altered states of consciousness, numbness or paralysis, difficulty with speech or vision, confusion, convulsions, difficulty in breathing, and **unequal pupils.**

Maintain an **open airway** and **keep the patient at rest.** Slightly elevate the patient's head, neck, shoulders, and back. Protect all paralyzed limbs. Be sure to provide **emotional support.** Monitor the patient's vital signs.

Respiratory distress, including that seen in congestive heart failure, may produce the same signs and symptoms, regardless of the cause of the distress: Always check for labored breathing, unusual breath sounds, rate, and character. Make sure that the problem is not caused by an airway obstruction. **Skin color** changes are an important sign in serious cases of respiratory distress. Be prepared for the patient to be confused or to have changing states of consciousness. In cases of **congestive heart failure,** you may also note abdominal swelling, swelling at the ankles, and engorged neck veins.

For all cases of respiratory distress, have someone call the EMS System dispatcher. Except for hyperventilation, care for all respiratory distress cases the same way. Maintain an open airway and check to be sure that there is not something at the scene causing an allergic reaction. Place the patient in a **sitting position** and **keep the patient at rest.** Conserve the patient's body heat. Provide **emotional support.**

When dealing with **hyperventilation** *that is not a sign of more serious illness,* have the patient **breathe into a paper bag.**

Individuals with **diabetes** may have trouble with **diabetic coma** or **insulin shock.** Diabetic coma comes on slowly, while insulin shock occurs suddenly. In both cases, the patient may become unresponsive and go into a coma.

In **diabetic coma,** expect to find labored breathing with a **fruity** or **sweet odor** on the patient's breath. The patient's **pulse** will be **rapid** and **weak.** The **skin** will be **dry** and **warm.** Alert the EMS System dispatcher and **keep the patient at rest.**

In **insulin shock,** there is no labored breathing and no fruity odor. The patient's **pulse** will be **full** and **rapid.** The **skin** will be **cold** and **moist.** **Keep the patient at rest** and **give sugar.**

When in doubt as to whether you are dealing with insulin shock or diabetic coma, **give sugar** to the conscious patient.

Patients having **seizures** will often have a sudden **loss of consciousness** and **collapse.** The body will stiffen and there may be a loss of bowel and bladder control. **Convulsions** usually occur, followed by the body going limp. On regaining consciousness, the patient is usually very **confused** and tired.

As a First Responder, your primary role in caring for patients having seizures is to **protect the patient** from physical harm during the seizure and embarrassment after the seizure. After any seizure, **keep the patient at rest.**

Severe abdominal pain is noted in cases of **acute abdomen.** You should keep the patient at rest, as comfortable as possible. Monitor the patient for vomiting. Give nothing by mouth. Make certain that EMS dispatch is alerted.

If you are dealing with a possible **poisoning,** always look for evidence at the **scene** that may indicate poisoning and the nature of the poison. Learn to make use of your local **poison control center** or **medical command.**

There are many symptoms and signs associated with **ingested poisons.** Always look for **burns** or **stains** around the patient's **mouth.** Expect unusual breathing, pulse rate, and sweating. Abdominal pain, nausea, and vomiting are common. Be sure to **save all vomitus.**

Inhaled poisons can cause **shortness of breath** or **coughing.** Often, the patient will have **irritated eyes, rapid** or **slow pulse rate,** and changes in **skin color.**

Reactions to **absorbed poisons** can be severe. These poisons usually **irritate** or **damage the skin.** Look for **irritated eyes.**

Injected poisons usually cause **pain and swelling** at the site. **Difficult breathing** and **unusual pulse rate** are often seen.

If possible, contact the **poison control center** and **medical command** (follow your EMS guidelines). If directed to do so, **dilute ingested poisons with water or milk. Induce vomiting** with ipecac and water or as directed. **Charcoal** and **water** may be given when vomiting is not called for or after vomiting has occurred.

WARNING: *Do not* induce vomiting if the poison is a strong acid, alkali, or petroleum product (follow local guidelines and directions). *Do not* induce vomiting if the patient is unconscious or has been convulsing.

In cases of **inhaled poisons, remove the patient from the source** (when safe to do so). Provide **life-support** measures as needed. It may be necessary to **remove contaminated clothing.**

Remove the patient from the source of an **absorbed poison** and **flood with water** all areas of the body that have come into contact with the poison. **Remove contaminated clothing and jewelry.** Continue to flood the exposed areas of the patient's skin.

When providing care for **injected poisons** other than snakebite, **care for shock, scrape** away stingers and venom sacs, and place an **ice bag** or **cold pack** over the area. For **snakebite,** you should **keep the patient calm** and **lying down, clean the site,** and keep any bitten extremities **immobilized.** Alert the **EMS System dispatcher** and **provide care for shock.** If necessary, apply **constricting bands.**

Always consider the possibility that a patient may have an **infectious disease.** Use the symptoms and signs you already know to consider if infection is the cause of the patient's problem. **Keep the patient at rest and provide care as you would for shock.** Avoid contact with the patient's mucous membranes, blood, wastes, and body fluids. If you think you have been exposed to an infectious disease, report to your local hospital and give the details of your First Responder care and why you think you may have been exposed.

CHAPTER 14

Burns, Smoke, Heat, and Cold

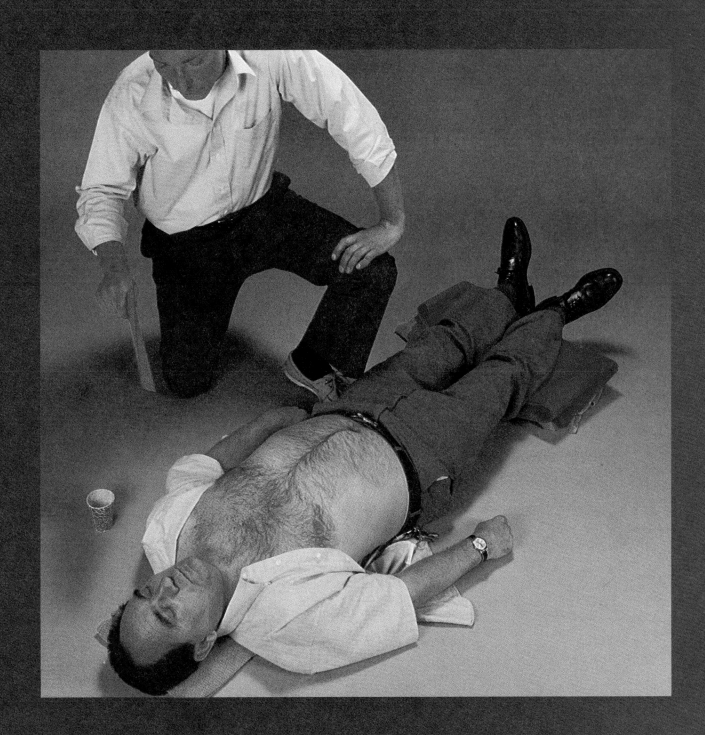

■ OBJECTIVES

By the end of this chapter, you should be able to:

1. Define first, second, and third degree burns. (p. 331)
2. Label an adult's and a child's body in terms of the "Rule of Nines." (pp. 332–333)
3. State the rules of First Responder care applying to burns. (p. 333)
4. Describe proper care for thermal, chemical, and electrical burns. (pp. 333–338)
5. Describe the care given to smoke inhalation victims. (pp. 339–340)
6. Use symptoms and signs to distinguish between heat cramps, heat exhaustion, and heat stroke. (p. 343)
7. List the steps in caring for heat cramps, heat exhaustion, and heat stroke. (p. 343)
8. State how to distinguish between hypothemia, frostnip, frostbite, and freezing. (pp. 344–345, 347)
9. Describe the care given to patients with hypothermia, frostnip, frostbite, and freezing. (pp. 345, 347)

SKILLS

Upon completing this chapter and your class lectures and skills labs, you should be able to:

1. Classify burns as first, second, or third degree and determine their extent.
2. Demonstrate First Responder care for thermal, chemical, and electrical burns.
3. Demonstrate the care for a patient with smoke inhalation.
4. Classify problems due to exposure to cold in terms of hypothermia, frostnip, frostbite, and freezing.
5. Demonstrate methods of care used for patients with problems due to various levels of exposure to cold.

BURNS

Classifying Burns

When most people think of burns, they think of injury to the skin. Burns can injure much more than the skin. Structures below the skin, including muscles, nerves, blood vessels, and bones, may be injured. The eyes can be injured beyond repair when burned. Respiratory system structures can be damaged, perhaps to the point of airway obstruction or respiratory arrest. In addition to the physical damage caused by burns, patients also may suffer emotional and psychological problems.

1st Burns are classified in a number of ways. One approach is to name the agent causing the burn, or the source of the burn. This information should be gathered and passed on with the patient when you are relieved by more highly trained personnel. Burns may be caused by:

- Heat (thermal)—this includes fire, steam, and hot objects
- Chemicals—this includes various caustics, such as acids and alkalis
- Electricity (including lightning)
- Light—this includes burns to the eye caused by intense light sources and burns to the skin or eyes by ultraviolet light (including sunlight)
- Radiation—usually from nuclear sources.

Never assume the source of a burn. What may appear to be a thermal burn could be from radiation. You may find minor thermal burns on the patient's face and forget to consider light burns to the eyes. Patient and bystander interviews, observations of the incident scene, and a proper physical examination will help you to determine the source of the burn.

1st Most often, burns are classified as to their severity as well as their source. This system uses the term *degree*, with burns considered as first, second, or third degree. The least serious burn is the first degree burn, while the most serious is the third degree.

- *First degree burn*—only the outer layer of the skin is burned. There will be a reddening of the skin and perhaps some swelling. The patient will usually complain about pain at the site. Since the skin is not burned through, this type of burn is sometimes called a **mild partial thickness burn.**

  First degree burn—a mild partial thickness burn involving only the outer layer of skin (epidermis).

- *Second degree burn*—the first layer of skin is burned through and the second layer is damaged. You will see intense reddening, blisters, and a spotted (mottled) appearance to the skin. Burns of this type can cause considerable swelling within 48 hours of the injury. A second degree burn does not burn through all the layers of skin and is thus called a **partial thickness burn.** Severe pain will always accompany this type of burn. First degree burns often surround second degree burn sites.

  Second degree burn—a partial thickness burn in which the outer layer of skin is burned through and the second layer (dermis) is damaged.

- *Third degree burn*—this is a **full thickness burn,** where all the layers of the skin are damaged. Fat, muscles, nerves and even bones may be involved. Some third degree burns are difficult to distinguish from second degree burns; however, third degree burns usually have areas charred black or that appear dry white. Patients may complain of severe pain or, if enough nerves are damaged, they may not feel any pain at all. First and second degree burns will usually be found adjacent to third degree burns, often causing severe or additional pain.

  Third degree burn—a full thickness burn involving all the layers of skin. Muscle layers below the skin and bones may also be damaged.

FIGURE 14–1. Burns are classified according to degree.

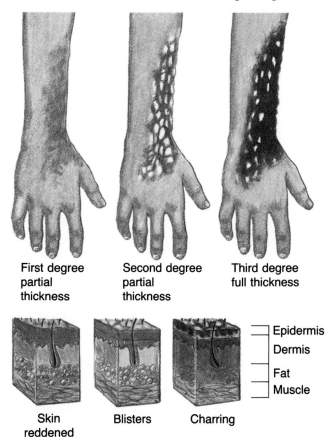

First degree partial thickness

Second degree partial thickness

Third degree full thickness

Skin reddened

Blisters

Charring

Epidermis
Dermis
Fat
Muscle

EVALUATING THE EXTENT OF A BURN

1st *The Rule of Nines*

Rule of Nines—a system used for estimating the amount of skin surface that is burned. The body is divided into 12 regions. Each of 11 regions equals 9% of the body surface and the genital region is classified as 1%.

The Rule of Nines is a system for estimating the amount of skin surface burned. For an adult patient, the head and neck, chest, abdomen, each arm, the front of each leg, back of each leg, the upper back, and the lower back and buttocks are each considered equal to 9% of the body surface. This gives a total of 99%. The remaining 1% is assigned to the genital area.

The emergency department Rule of Nines used for infants and children is too complicated for field use in First Responder-level care. A simpler approach is to assign 18% to the head and neck, 9% to each upper limb, 18% to the chest and abdomen, 18% to the entire back, 14% for each lower limb, and 1% to the genital region. This adds up to 101%, but does give you a way of making approximate determinations. When in doubt, use the adult Rule of Nines, but remember the 18% for the head and neck. This must be done because the head of an infant or a child is much larger in proportion to the rest of the body than what is typical for an adult.

By adding up the areas affected by a certain degree of burn, you can state how much of the patient's body has been injured by the burn. For example, if an adult patient has third degree thermal burns to the chest and the front of one leg, this is 9% + 9% or 18%. You would report the

FIGURE 14–2. The Rule of Nines.

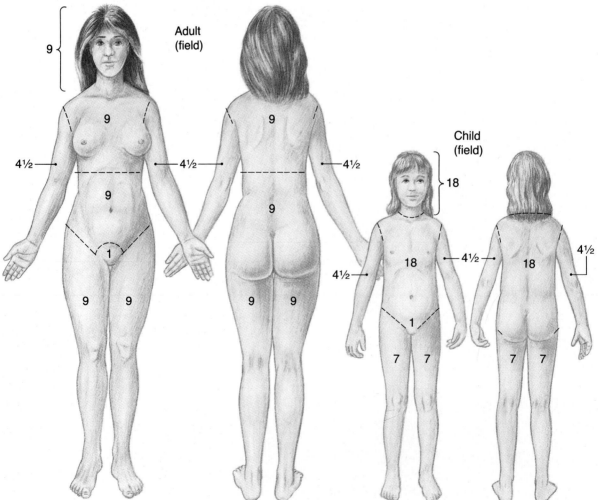

patient as having third degree thermal burns to 18% of the body. This would be a very serious injury.

Most First Responder courses are short in terms of time. Since you will treat *all* burns and you will alert dispatch for *all* burns, or at least *all* serious second degree burns and *all* third degree burns, you may not be required to learn the Rule of Nines. In most field situations, this kind of evaluation will not be necessary in order for you to carry out your duties. Should you be involved in a disaster requiring you to phone or radio information and you cannot remember the Rule of Nines, the staff at the emergency department will know what questions to ask you so that they can determine the extent of a patient's burns.

Rules for the First Responder

Regardless of the system used to evaluate burns, you should follow these rules:

1st RULE 1: Always perform a primary and secondary survey. Provide basic life support as needed.

1st RULE 2: Always continue to monitor vital signs, checking to see if the heat or smoke has affected the patient's respiratory system. Thermal, electrical, and chemical burns can cause life-threatening injury to the airway and the lungs. Tissue swelling may cause airway obstruction that could lead to respiratory arrest.

1st RULE 3: Provide care for all burns, including the most minor of first degree burns.

1st RULE 4: Alert the dispatcher for all cases involving burns unless directed to do otherwise in your EMS System. Regardless of the region in which you practice your First Responder duties, call dispatch for any chemical, radiation, or electrical burns, all third degree burns, or any serious second degree burn. Consider as serious any second degree burn of the face, hands, feet, a major joint, groin, medial thigh, buttocks, an entire part of the body, or what you believe to be 15% or more of the patient's body. Make sure the dispatcher knows the severity and extent of the burn.

1st RULE 5: Any burn, other than mild sunburn, involving the hands, feet, face, groin, buttocks, medial thighs, or a major joint should be seen by someone in the EMS System above the level of First Responder.

1st RULE 6: Any burn, other than mild sunburn, involving a whole area of the body (an arm or leg, chest or back, and so on) should be seen by someone in the EMS System above the level of First Responder.

1st RULE 7: When in doubt, consider serious first degree burns to be second degree and serious second degree burns to be third degree.

1st RULE 8: Always consider the effects of a burn to be more serious if the patient is a child, elderly, the victim of other injuries, or someone with a respiratory disease. If the patient is over 50 or under 10 years of age, any second or third degree burn involving more than 10% of the skin surface must be assessed as being very serious.

Caring for Thermal Burns

WARNING: *Do not* attempt to rescue people trapped by fire unless you have been trained to do so. The simple act of opening a door could cost you your life. In some fires, opening a door or window may greatly intensify the fire or even cause an explosion. See Chapter 17 for more information.
1st Your first course of action when caring for thermal burns is to ensure

that the burning process has been stopped. This may require you to smother flames or to smother, wet down, or remove smoldering clothing. If the agent of the burn is hot tar, you should cool the area with water. *Do not* attempt to remove the tar. *Do not* apply any burn ointments. Remember to wear latex or vinyl gloves when caring for burn patients.

1st *Minor Burns*—A first or second degree burn involving a small portion of the patient's body is a minor burn unless it includes the respiratory system, face, hands, feet, groin, buttocks, or major joint. If these areas show heavy first or second degree burns, treat the patient for major burns. For minor burn care, you should:

Minor burn—a first or second degree burn involving a small portion of the body with no damage to the respiratory system, face, hands, feet, groin, medial thigh, buttocks, or major joints.

1. Have someone alert dispatch. In some EMS Systems, First Responders are directed not to request EMT support and transport if the problem is a minor first degree burn. In some systems, the dispatcher may ask questions to see if an EMT response is needed. Often, small second degree burns, such as a steam burn to part of one finger, can be cared for by the patient. If, for example, the patient has a second degree burn involving the entire forearm, play it safe and request an EMT response.

2. If the skin is unbroken, soak the burned area with cool water or use running cool water over the site. It is best to submerge the affected part to avoid additional damage to areas injured by second degree burns. Keep cool water on the burn for several minutes. The exception is if you are providing care in a cold environment. For such cases, do not apply water to the burn site. If the burn is active, you must use water to stop the burning process.

FIGURE 14–3. First Responder supplies for the care of burns.

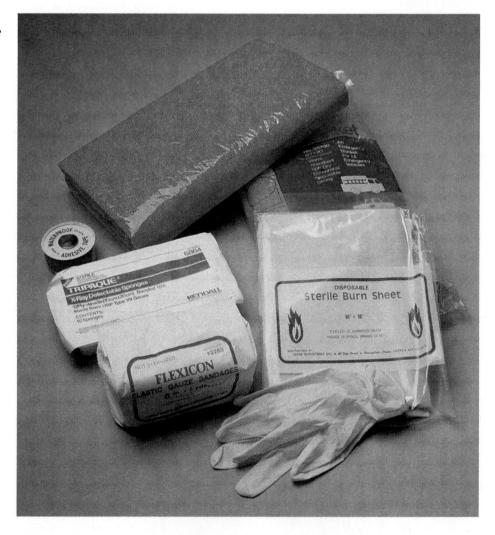

3. Wrap the burn with a sterile or clean, loose dressing. If the skin is not broken, the dressing can be kept moistened to help relieve pain, *only* if the total burn involves less than 9% of the skin surface and the patient will not remain in a cold environment while awaiting transport.

1st *Major Burns*—Any burn to the face, other than simple (mild) sunburn, is to be treated as a major burn by First Responders. Be on the alert for respiratory problems. First degree burns, other than simple sunburn covering large areas of the body, must be considered to be a major burn. Second degree burns covering an entire area of the body, the hands, feet, groin, buttocks, or a major joint are major burns. Any third degree burn is a major burn. Consider any third degree burn to the face, hands, or feet to be critical. When providing care for a major burn, you should:

1. Stop the burning process.
2. Have someone alert dispatch. Request an EMT response.
3. Maintain an open airway—make certain that the patient is breathing. Check respiratory rate and character. If there are any indications of airway obstruction, be prepared for the patient to worsen.
4. Cover the entire burn—use a loose sterile or clean dressing. *Do not* obstruct the mouth and nose *Do not* apply any burn ointments. *Do not* use a blanket or towel as a dressing.
5. Give special care to the eyes—if the eyelids or eyes have been burned, cover the eyelids with sterile or clean pads. If sterile water is available, moisten the pads before applying them to the patient's eyelids.
6. Give special care to the fingers and toes—never dress fingers or toes having serious second degree or any third degree burns without first inserting sterile or clean pads between each finger or toe. A slight elevation of the legs in cases of burns to the feet and a slight elevation of the arms if burns are to the hands is recommended.
7. *Do not* moisten the dressings (if required in your area) unless the burn involves less than 9% of the skin surface, you are using sterile dressings, you have sterile water for application, and the patient will not remain in a cold environment while awaiting transport.
8. Provide care for shock.
9. Make certain that dispatch was alerted.

NOTE: If you have to remove a piece of the patient's clothing to evaluate and care for burns, *never* pull it off. To avoid inflicting more damage to the burned tissues, cut away the clothing in contact with the patient's burns.

Caring for Chemical Burns

NOTE: All cases of chemical burns require you to alert dispatch.
WARNING: Some scenes where chemical burns take place can be very hazardous. Always evaluate the scene. There may be large pools of dangerous chemicals around the patient. Acids could be spurting from containers. Toxic fumes may be present. If you believe there are hazards at the scene that will place you in danger, *do not* attempt a rescue unless you have been trained for such a situation and have the necessary equipment, personnel, and support (see Chapter 17).
1st The major way to care for chemical burns is by washing away the chemical with water. A simple wetting of the burn site is not enough. Flood the area of the patient's body that has been exposed. Continue to wash the area for at least 20 minutes; remove contaminated clothing, shoes, socks, and jewelry from the patient. Remember to wear latex or vinyl gloves.
1st Once you have washed the burned areas, apply a sterile or clean dressing, render care for shock, and make certain that dispatch has been alerted.

■ Scan 14-1.

Care for Thermal Burns

Type of Burn	Tissue Burned			Color Changes	Pain	Blisters
	Outer Layer of Skin	Second Layer of Skin	Tissues Below Skin			
1st DEGREE	Yes	No	No	Red	Yes	No
2nd DEGREE	Yes	Yes	No	Deep red	Yes	Yes
3rd DEGREE	Yes	Yes	Yes	Charred black or white	Yes	No

Minor first and second degree:

- Have someone alert dispatch
- Immerse in cold water 2–5 minutes
- Cover entire burn with dry, sterile dressing
- Moisten—only if burn is less than 9% of skin surface

Major burns:

- Stop burning process
- Have someone alert dispatch
- Maintain open airway
- Wrap area with dry clean dressing*
- Provide care for shock

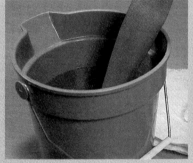

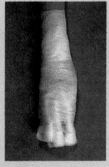

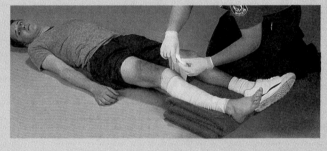

*Moisten if less than 9% of skin surface is affected

If hands or toes are burned:

- Separate digits with sterile gauze pads
- When appropriate, elevate the extremity

Burns to the eyes:

- Do not open eyelids if burned
- Be certain burn is thermal, not chemical
- Apply moist, sterile gauze pads to both eyes

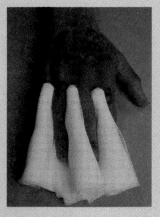

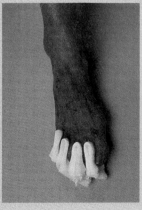

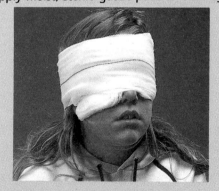

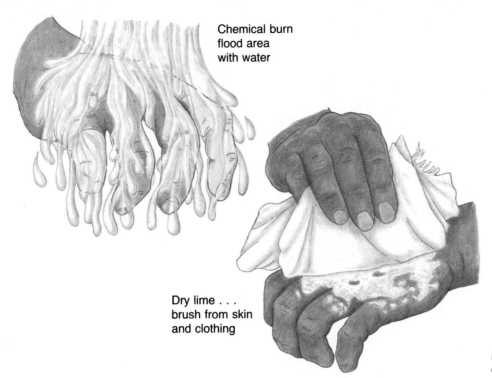

Chemical burn
flood area
with water

Dry lime . . .
brush from skin
and clothing

FIGURE 14–4.   Care of
chemical burns.

Be on guard for delayed reactions that may interfere with the patient's ability to breathe.

1st If the patient complains of increased burning or irritation, rewash the burned areas with water for several minutes. Avoid removing dressings once they are in place.

1st NOTE: If dry lime is the agent causing the chemical burn, *do not* begin by washing the burn site with water. Instead, brush the dry lime from the patient's skin, hair, and clothing. Remove all jewelry and contaminated clothing from the patient and use water to flush the areas exposed to the lime. Apply the wash for at least 20 minutes.

1st Chemical burns to the eyes require immediate action. Always assume that both eyes are involved. When caring for chemical burns to the eyes, you should:

1. Have someone alert the dispatcher.
2. Immediately flood the eyes with water.
3. Keep running water from a faucet, low pressure hose (small diameter, garden), bucket, cup, bottle, or other such source flowing into both eyes. You may have to hold the patient's eyelids open to ensure a complete washing. If you must alternate washing each eye, do so quickly, turning the patient's head to the side so that you can pour the water from the nasal corner, across the surface of the eyeball.
4. Continue washing the eye for the following time periods:

    Acid burns—at least 5 minutes
    Alkali burns—at least 15 minutes
    Unknown caustic—at least 20 minutes

    These are standard guidelines. It is good policy to *wash all chemical eye burns for at least 20 minutes.*
5. After washing the patient's eyes, cover both eyes with moistened pads.
6. Remove the pads and wash the patient's eyes for 5 more minutes if the patient begins to complain about increased burning sensations or irritation.

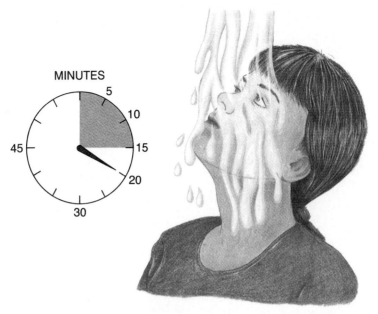

FIGURE 14–5.   Care of chemical burns to the eyes. Immediately flood the eyes with water.

Caring for Electrical Burns

NOTE: Alert dispatch for *all* cases involving electrical burns.

WARNING: The scene of an electrical burn is often very hazardous. If the source of electricity is still active, *do not* attempt a rescue unless you have been trained to do so and have the necessary equipment. See Chapter 17 for more details.

When a patient is the victim of an electrical accident, burns usually are not the most serious problem. Cardiac arrest, nervous system damage, and injury to internal organs may occur with electrical accidents. Care for the whole patient, not just the burns.

If you have to provide care for a patient with an electrical burn, you should:

1.   Have someone alert dispatch.
2.   Make certain that you and the patient are in a *safe zone.*
3.   Check breathing and pulse—electrical energy passing through a patient's body will often cause cardiac arrest. Many patients who have received an electrical shock will have partial airway obstruction due to swollen tissues along their airway. Even if the patient appears stable, be prepared for complications involving the airway or heart. Play it safe and provide care for the patient as if a heart attack is about to occur.
4.   Evaluate the burn—look for at least two burn sites. One will be where the patient came into contact with the energy source (most often, it will be the hand). The other will be where the patient came into contact with a ground. This is where the energy has left the patient's body (most often, this will be a foot or hand). Remember to wear latex or vinyl gloves during assessment and care.
5.   Apply dry sterile or clean dressings to the burn sites. If transport will be delayed, the burn involves less than 9% of the skin surface, and the patient will not be kept in a cold environment, you may moisten the dressings with sterile water.
6.   Provide care for shock.
7.   Make certain that dispatch has been alerted.

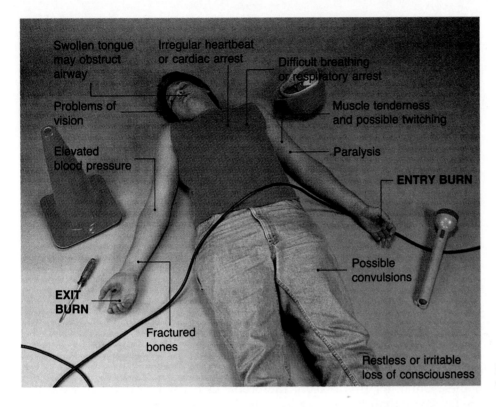

Swollen tongue
may obstruct
airway

Irregular heartbeat
or cardiac arrest

Difficult breathing
or respiratory arrest

Problems of
vision

Muscle tenderness
and possible twitching

Elevated
blood pressure

Paralysis

ENTRY BURN

EXIT
BURN

Possible
convulsions

Fractured
bones

Restless or irritable
loss of consciousness

FIGURE 14–6. Injuries due to
electrical accidents.

SMOKE INHALATION

Fire presents problems other than thermal burns. One such problem is
smoke inhalation. The smoke from any fire source contains poisonous substances. Modern building materials and furnishings often contain plastics
and other synthetics that release toxic fumes when they burn or are overheated. It is possible for the substances found in smoke to burn the skin,
irritate the eyes, injure the airway, cause respiratory arrest and, in some
cases, cause cardiac arrest. Do not attempt a rescue unless you have been
trained to do so and have all the required personnel and equipment.

As a First Responder, you will probably see irritation to the eyes and
injury to the airway associated with smoke. Irritations to the skin and
eyes may be treated by simple flooding with water. Your first priority will
be the patient's airway. In cases of smoke inhalation, you should:

1. Move the patient to a safe, smoke-free area.
2. Do a primary survey and supply life-support measures as needed.
3. If conscious and without signs of neck or spinal injury, place the patient
    in a sitting or semisitting position. The patient may find it easier to
    breathe in a different position. Let the patient assume the position
    that proves best. Always provide support for the back and be prepared
    if the patient loses consciousness.
4. Provide care for shock.

NOTE: The body's reaction to toxic gases and foreign matter in the airway
often can be delayed. It is good First Responder practice to alert dispatch
for all cases of smoke inhalation.

Carbon monoxide poisoning is often seen at fire scenes. This gas enters
the patient's bloodstream, where it is picked up by red blood cells that
should be carrying oxygen. The typical patient complains of headache and
dizziness. In a short time, the patient shows the classic signs of respiratory
distress and may develop blue coloration (cyanosis) of the skin, lips, nailbeds,

tongue, or earlobes. Some individuals with dark complexions will show a discoloration of the whites of the eyes, inner surface of the eyelids, or tissues in the corners of the eyes.

Proper care requires moving the patient away from the source and the same basic procedures as would be provided for any smoke inhalation or inhaled poison victim. EMT-level care and transport are required in all cases of carbon monoxide poisoning.

EXCESSIVE HEAT

Emergencies can be brought about by exposure to too much heat. Moist heat usually tires individuals very quickly. This fact often prevents people from harming their bodies, forcing them to quit exerting themselves before any real harm is done. Some people, however, continue to push themselves, running the risk of placing their bodies into a state of emergency.

Dry heat can often fool individuals, causing them to continue work or exposure to the heat far beyond the point that can be accepted by their bodies. Often, for this reason, the problems caused by dry heat exposure are far worse than those seen in moist heat exposure.

When dealing with problems created by exposure to excessive heat, keep in mind that you must do patient surveys and interviews. Collapse due to heat exposure may break bones. A history of blood pressure or heart or lung problems may have quickened the effects of heat exposure. What may appear to be a problem related to heat exposure could be a heart attack. Remember the basics of total patient care and always consider the problem to be greater if the patient is a child, elderly, or injured or has a chronic disease.

Heat Cramps

Heat cramps—muscle cramps in the lower limbs and abdomen associated with the loss of fluids and possibly salts while active in a hot environment.

Heat cramps are brought about by long exposure to heat. The amount of heat does not have to be that much greater than what you would consider to be a "normal" environmental temperature. The individual sweats, often drinking large quantities of water. As the sweating continues, water and salts are lost by the body, bringing on painful muscle cramps. Medical authorities are not yet certain as to the cause of these cramps. Evidence seems to indicate that it is the loss of water, not salts, that produces conditions that lead to the cramps.

1st The symptoms and signs of heat cramps are:

- Severe muscle cramps, usually in the legs and the abdomen
- Exhaustion, often to the point of collapse
- Sometimes dizziness or periods of faintness

1st The emergency care procedures for heat cramps require that you:

1. Move the patient to a nearby cool palce.
2. The patient should be given water at the rate of one-half glass every 15 minutes for one hour. Even though the problem may not be due to the loss of salts, better results may be obtained if you give the patient salted water to drink. This is a "play it safe" measure in case you have

underassessed the severity of the patient's heat-related problem. The salted water can be prepared by adding one teaspoon of salt to one quart of water.* You may use Gatorade or other commercial electrolyte (salted) fluid diluted to half-strength with water in place of the salted water. (Do not delay providing the patient with water in order to find salt and make the preparation.) The muscle cramps should ease shortly after the patient drinks the salted water.

3. Help ease the patient's cramps by massaging cramped muscles. Such action cannot be recommended for patients with a history of circulatory problems that form blood clots in the veins of the lower limbs. Since these problems are seen with many elderly patients, caution is advised. If there is no history of circulatory problems, massage very gently.

4. Warm moist towels applied to the patient's forehead and over the cramped muscles provide added relief for some patients.

NOTE: You should alert dispatch for all cases of possible heat cramps. As soon as you arrive at the scene, have someone phone the EMS System.

Heat Exhaustion

The typical heat exhaustion patient is a healthy individual who has been exposed to excessive heat while working or exercising. The circulatory system of the patient begins to fail, related to fluid and salt loss. This problem is often seen with fire fighters, construction workers, dock workers, and those employed in poorly ventilated warehouses. Obviously, heat exhaustion is more of a problem during the summer.

Heat exhaustion—a failure of the circulatory system that is related to the loss of fluids and salts while active in a hot environment.

1st The symptoms and signs of heat exhaustion are:

- Rapid and shallow breathing
- Weak pulse
- Cold and clammy skin, with heavy perspiration
- Sometimes the skin appears pale
- Total body weakness
- Dizziness, sometimes leading to unconsciousness

1st To care for a heat exhaustion patient, you should:

1. Move the patient to a nearby cool place.
2. Keep the patient at rest.
3. Remove as much of the patient's clothing as is necessary to cool the patient without causing him or her to become chilled.
4. Fan the patient.
5. Give the patient salted water made by adding one teaspoon of salt to one quart of water, or provide a commercial electrolyte solution diluted to half-strength with water. If no salted fluids are available, give the patient water at the rate of one-half glass every 15 minutes for one hour. *Do not* try to administer fluids to an unconscious patient or one who displays problems with swallowing. Do not delay giving the patient water in order to find salt and mix the preparation.
6. Provide care for shock, but do not cover the patient to the point of overheating.
7. If the patient is unconscious, fails to recover rapidly, has other injuries, or has a history of medical problems, be prepared for the patient to worsen.

* Some medical authorities are questioning the concentration of salted water used for heat-related emergencies. Follow the recommendation of your EMS System medical advisor.

NOTE: Alert dispatch for all cases of heat exhaustion. As soon as you arrive at the scene, have someone phone the EMS System.

Heat Stroke

Heat stroke—a life-threatening emergency resulting from the failure of the body's heat-regulating mechanisms. The body cannot cool itself.

When a person is exposed to excessive heat and stops sweating, heat stroke will shortly follow. Most cases of heat stroke are reported on hot, humid days; however, many cases occur from exposure to dry heat. Do not be fooled by the fact that some people call heat stroke by the name of sunstroke. Heat stroke can be caused by excessive heat other than exposure to the sun. This condition is a **true emergency,** requiring the cooling of the patient and EMT transport to a medical facility. ALL cases of heat stroke are serious, requiring the patient to be sent to a medical facility as quickly as possible.

1st The symptoms and signs of heat stroke include:

- Deep breaths, followed by shallow breathing
- Rapid, strong pulse, followed by a rapid, weak pulse
- *Dry*, hot skin (sometimes red in color)
- Large (dilated) pupils
- Loss of consciousness—the patient may go into a coma
- Convulsions or muscular twitching may be seen

1st To care for heat stroke:

1. Make absolutely certain that someone has called dispatch.
2. Cool the patient—do this in any manner possible and do it rapidly. Move the patient out of the sun or away from the heat source. Remove the clothing and wrap him or her in wet towels and sheets. Pour cold water over these wrappings. The patient's body heat must be lowered rapidly or brain cells will die!
3. If cold packs or ice bags are available, wrap them and place one bag or pack under each of the patient's armpits, one on each wrist and ankle, one on the groin, and one on each side of the patient's neck. These areas are rich in blood lying close to the surface of the skin.
4. Alert the dispatcher that transport is required *as soon as possible*.
5. Should transport be delayed, find a tub or container and immerse the patient up to the neck in cooled water (if recommended by your EMS System). Even a partial covering of the patient with cooled water will help. Otherwise, keep the patient wrapped and continue to soak with cool water. Use a low pressure hose if necessary.
6. Continue to monitor the patient's vital signs.

WARNING: If you immerse an unconscious patient, you must monitor the patient continuously. Failure to do so could result in the patient drowning.

1st Recent studies have shown that immersing a heat stroke patient is an extreme measure. The cold water shuts down circulation to the skin and allows for a build up of heat in the deeper tissues. This is the opposite of what you desire: to rid the patient of excess heat. If your EMS System recommends you immerse the patient, then do so. If they do not, then your best course of action would be to keep the patient wrapped in wet sheets, continue to apply cooled water, use ice packs if available, and wait for the EMTs to respond.

■ SCAN 14-2.

Heat-related Emergencies

Condition	Muscle Cramps	Breathing	Pulse	Weakness	Skin	Perspiration	Loss of Consciousness
Heat cramps	Yes	Varies	Varies	Yes	Moist, warm, no change	Heavy	Seldom
Heat exhaustion	No	Rapid, shallow	Weak	Yes	Cold, clammy	Heavy	Sometimes
Heat stroke	No	Deep, then shallow	Full rapid	Yes	Dry, hot	Little or none	Often

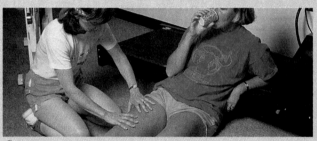

1 Heat cramps

Signs and symptoms: Severe muscle cramps (usually in the legs and abdomen), exhaustion, sometimes dizziness or faintness

Emergency care procedures:

- Move patient to a nearby cool place.
- Give patient salted water to drink or half-strength commercial electrolyte fluids.
- Help ease cramps by muscle massage. Massage with pressure is more effective than light rubbing action.
- Apply warm, moist towels to the forehead and over cramped muscles for added relief.
- Alert EMS dispatch.

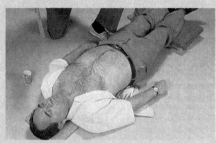

2 Heat exhaustion

Signs and symptoms: Rapid, shallow breathing, weak pulse, cold clammy skin, heavy perspiration, total body weakness and dizziness leading to unconsciousness

Emergency care procedures:

- Move the patient to a nearby cool place.
- Keep the patient at rest.
- Remove enough clothing to cool the patient without chilling him.
- Give patient salted water to drink or half-strength commercial electrolyte fluids. Do not administer fluids to unconscious patient.
- Provide care for shock, but do not cover to the point of overheating patient.
- If unconscious, fails to recover rapidly, has injuries or a history of medical problems, make certain that dispatch is informed of need for immediate transport.

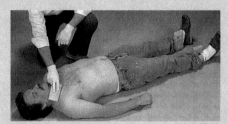

3 Heat stroke

Signs and symptoms: Deep breaths, then shallow breathing, rapid, strong pulse, then rapid weak pulse; dry, hot skin, dilated pupils; loss of consciousness (possible coma) convulsions or muscular twitching

Note: All heat-related emergencies require alerting EMS dispatch.

Emergency care procedures:

- Cool patient in any manner, rapidly. Move patient out of sun or away from heat source. Remove clothing. Wrap in wet towels or sheets. Pour cold water over wrappings. Body heat must lower rapidly or brain cells die!
- Wrap cold packs or ice bags, if available, and place one under each armpit, each wrist, each ankle, and each side of patient's neck.
- If transport is delayed, find tub or container. Immerse patient up to face in cooled water. Monitor in order to prevent drowning.
- Monitor vital signs throughout process.
- Provide care for shock.

EXCESSIVE COLD

If you live in an area where cold weather is never a problem, this part of your First Responder training may be limited. It is a good idea to know a little about treating patients exposed to excessive cold, regardless of the area in which you live. Refrigeration accidents do occur. Some cold-related problems are seen even in "mild" environments, especially if the patient is elderly or has abused drugs or alcohol. In addition to problems you may deal with in your home community, your travels may take you through a cold environment where an emergency may require you to help the local EMS System. Those in First Responder training hope that you will not only be a local First Responder, but that you will be a national First Responder. Should time limitations during training make it necessary for your instructor to limit coverage of excessive cold, continue your own education by reading this section after completing your training.

General Cooling

Hypothermia (HI-po-THURM-i-ah)—a general cooling of the body. Severe forms can lead to death.

The general cooling of the human body is known as **hypothermia** (HI-po-THURM-i-ah). Exposure to cold reduces body heat. With time, the body is unable to maintain its proper internal temperature. If allowed to continue, hypothermia will lead to death.

Hypothermia is becoming a serious problem of the aged. During the winter months, many older citizens attempt to live in rooms that are kept too cool. Failing body systems, poor diets, and a lack of exercise combine with this cold environment to bring about hypothermia.

1st The signs and symptoms of hypothermia include:

- Shivering—seen in early stages
- Feelings of numbness—increases as hypothermia worsens
- Drowsiness and lack of interest in even the simplest activities
- Slow breathing and pulse rates—seen in cases of prolonged hypothermia
- Failing eyesight—seen in cases of prolonged hypothermia
- Unconsciousness, usually with the patient having a "glassy stare"—seen in extreme cases
- Freezing of body parts—seen in the most extreme cases. Action taken must begin immediately, for the patient may be near death.

1st The care of MILD hypothermia patients (alert, shivering, perhaps some numbness) requires you to:

1. Do patient surveys and interviews to determine the extent of the problem.
2. Keep the patient dry.
3. Use heat to raise the patient's body temperature. Move the patient to a nearby warm environment, if at all possible. Apply heat to the patient's body in the form of heat packs, hot water bottles, electric heating pads, hot air, radiated heat, and your own body heat and that of bystanders. A warm bath is very helpful, but you must guard the patient so that drowning does not occur. Constant monitoring is necessary for unconscious patients. *Do not warm the patient too quickly.*
4. If the patient remains alert, give warm liquids. Do not administer alcoholic beverages.

NOTE: You will not be providing very much help to patients with mild general cooling if you simply wrap them in blankets. Their bodies can no longer generate enough heat to make such care useful. External heat sources must be used to **slowly** rewarm the body. If there is any doubt as to the severity of the hypothermia or if the patient's condition worsens, **do not rewarm the patient.**

WARNING: Alert dispatch for *all* cases of hypothermia. There is no way that you can tell if the patient's condition will improve or grow worse. If you rewarm a patient successfully and do not arrange for EMT transport, the patient will probably remain in or return to the same cold environment. Hypothermia will probably return.

Do not rewarm the severe hypothermia patient. To do so may cause the heart to develop a lethal rhythm (ventricular fibrillation). Consider the patient to have severe hypothermia if you note any of the following:

- Unconsciousness
- Slowed respirations or respiratory arrest
- Slowed pulse or cardiac arrest
- Irrational or stuporous state
- Muscular rigidity

Care for severe hypothermia includes:

1. Handle the patient very gently. Rough handling will set off lethal heart rhythms.
2. Place the patient's head in a down position. Reposition if resuscitation is needed.
3. Ensure an open airway.
4. Wrap the patient in blankets.
5. Continuously monitor the patient's vital signs.
6. Make certain that dispatch has been alerted. This is a *true emergency* requiring advanced life support.

Some cases of hypothermia are extreme. The patient will be unconscious and not show any vital signs. The patient will be cold to your touch. (In fact, the body core temperature is probably below 80°F.) This patient is still alive and may respond to resuscitation. You cannot assume that this patient is dead. You must provide basic life support. The emergency department staff will continue resuscitation and rewarm the patient. They will not pronounce biological death until the patient is rewarmed.

Local Cooling—Frostnip

Frostnip can be brought about by direct contact with a cold object, cold temperatures, the combined effect of cold temperatures and wind (wind-chill), and the combined effect of cold temperatures and contact with moisture. This condition is not a serious one. Damage to tissues is minor and the response to care is good. As a First Responder, you must never confuse frostnip (incipient frostbite) with frostbite (superficial frostbite) and freezing (deep frostbite).

1st The signs and symptoms of frostnip include:

- Slow onset—frostnip usually takes some time to develop
- Unawareness on the part of the patient—most people with frostnip are not aware of the problem until someone indicates that there is something unusual about their skin color.
- The area of the skin affected becomes white (blanches)—this color change can take place very quickly.
- The affected area will feel numb to the patient.

Frostnip—minor damage to the outer layer of skin caused by excessive cold. This is incipient frostbite.

The emergency care for frostnip is simple. *Gently* warm the affected area. Have the patient apply warmth from his own bare hands. Blowing warm air on the site of the frostnip will help. The patient may find quick relief for frostnipped fingers by placing the hands between the upper arms and chest. If the condition does not respond to this simple care, begin to treat for frostbite. During recovery from frostnip, the patient may complain about "tingling" or burning sensations. This is normal.

Local Cooling—Frostbite

There are two serious types of frostbite, superficial and deep. Another term for deep frostbite is freezing. Freezing will be covered later in this chapter. Remember that all cases of superficial and deep frostbite are serious and will require the patient to be taken to a medical facility for completion of care. EMT response and transport should be done as soon as possible.

NOTE: There are times when it is very difficult to tell superficial frostbite from freezing, since both involve the formation of ice crystals in the skin. When in doubt, assume freezing has occurred and inform dispatch of this possibility.

1st The symptoms and signs of superficial frostbite are:

- The affected area of the skin appears white and waxy.
- The affected area will feel frozen on the surface. The tissue below the surface *must* still be soft and have its normal "bounce." If it also feels frozen, then you are dealing with a case of freezing.

1st To care for superficial frostbite, you must:

1. Protect the frostbitten area by covering the site of injury and handling the affected part as gently as possible. *Do not* rub the site.
2. Apply a steady source of external warmth to the site of injury. *Never* use a heat source that is uncomfortable for you to hold with your bare hand.
3. Arrange for transport to a medical facility or do the above two steps during immediate transport. Your instructor will tell you the policy for your area. If at all possible, keep the patient warm and at rest. Avoid having the patient do any walking if any part of the feet are frostbitten. Strongly discourage the use of alcoholic beverages.
4. If transport is delayed, you must rewarm the affected body part. To do so, you will need a container for warming water and a container of proper size to immerse the entire site of injury. Warm some water, but do not allow it to become too hot. It must be at a temperature that is warm, but will still allow you to keep your finger in the water without experiencing discomfort (100° to 105°F). Place the water into the container to be used for immersion. Fully immerse the injured body part. (Do not allow the affected part to touch the bottom or sides of the container.) Continue to heat additional water. Remove some cooled water and add warm water to the immersion container. *Do not* allow the water used in treating the patient to become cool. The patient may complain of some pain as the affected area rewarms. Often, the more severe the frostbite, the more severe the pain.
5. If you complete rewarming the part (it no longer feels frozen and is turning red or blue in color), dry the affected area and apply a clean dressing. Place pads of dressing materials between fingers and toes before dressing hands and feet. Next, cover the site with clothing, towels, blankets, or whatever you have available to keep the affected area warm. If the frostbite involves a limb, gently place the limb in a slightly elevated

■ SCAN 14-3.

Cold-related Emergencies

Condition	Skin surface	Tissue under skin	Skin color
Frostnip	Soft	Soft	White
Frostbite	Hard	Soft	White and waxy
Freezing	Hard	Hard	Blotchy, white to yellow-gray to blue-gray

Frostnip: Slow onset with numbing of affected part. Have the patient rewarm the part with his own body heat. Tingling and burning sensations are common during rewarming.

Frostbite: Tissues below the surface will still have their normal bounce. Protect the entire limb. *Handle gently.* Keep the patient at rest and provide external warmth to injury site.

Freezing: Tissue below the surface will feel hard. Provide the same care you would for superficial frostbite. Immediate EMS transport is recommended.

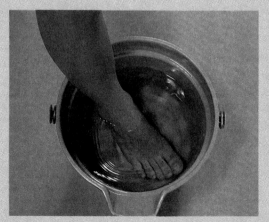

Rewarming: If transport is delayed in case of frostbite or freezing, rewarm the affected part by immersing it in warm water (100 to 105 degrees Fahrenheit). *Do not* allow the body part to touch the container bottom or side. After rewarming, gently dry the part and pad between fingers or toes. Dress the affected area, cover and elevate the limb, and keep the patient warm.

position. Make certain that the entire patient is kept as warm as possible without overheating. Continue to monitor and keep the patient at rest.

Local Cooling—Freezing

Local freezing, or deep frostbite, requires careful handling to avoid further injury to the affected body parts.

1st The symptoms and signs of freezing include:

- The skin will turn spotted (mottled) or blotchy. The color will turn to white, then grayish yellow, and finally a grayish blue.
- At the site of the freezing, the surface of the skin will feel frozen and the layers of tissue below the surface will also be hard.

When caring for patients with frozen body parts or areas, you should:

1. Arrange for immediate EMT response and transport. If your locality has you provide transport for this type of patient, have someone else drive so that you can render care during transport.
2. Provide the same care as you would for superficial frostbite.
3. If transport is delayed, rewarm the affected body parts the same as you would for superficial frostbite. Be very gentle with frozen tissues. Do not allow the limb to refreeze.

NOTE: As a First Responder, never listen to bystanders' myths and folktales as to the care of frostbite. *Never* rub a frostbitten or frozen area. *Never* rub snow on a frostbitten or frozen area. Politely tell people such procedures will cause serious damage to the already injured tissues.

SUMMARY

Burns can be caused by heat (thermal), chemicals, electricity, light, and radiation.

As a First Responder, you must be able to classify burns in terms of first, second, and third degree. Scansheet 14–1 shows the factors involved in this classification.

Care for all burns, keeping in mind that burns are more serious for children, the elderly, injured patients, and those with a chronic illness. Always monitor **vital signs,** since the respiratory system may be involved and also the circulatory system.

Any burn to the hands, feet, buttocks, groin, medial thigh, major joints, or the face is to be considered as a serious burn (exception: simple sunburn). If a whole area of the body is involved, such as the chest, consider this to be a serious burn. Always *alert* the dispatcher for:

- Extensive first degree burns
- Serious second degree burns
- All third degree burns
- Burns of the face, hands, feet, groin, medial thigh, buttocks, or major joints
- Burns involving the respiratory system
- Burns involving at least a whole section of the body

When in doubt, **overclassify.** Consider a questionable first degree burn to be second degree and a questionable second degree burn to be third degree.

Provide care for **minor burns** with **cold water** and a sterile or clean dressing. Do not soak **major burns** in cold water. Wrap the affected areas in sterile or clean dressings. Your EMS System may require you to moisten the dressings (the water must be sterile; distilled water is not sterile water) if the burn is to less than 9% of the skin surface. Provide care for shock and make certain that dispatch has been alerted.

If the patient's eyes or eyelids are burned, cover the eyelids with sterile or clean pads. Moisten with sterile water. Use sterile or clean pads to separate burned fingers and toes before dressing.

The care for **chemical burns** involves **flooding with water** for at least **20 minutes.** Do not use water if the cause of the burn is **dry lime.** Instead, **brush away** the chemical from the patient's skin and clothing. Remove contaminated clothing and flood the site with water. After washing, apply dressings, provide care for shock, and make certain that dispatch has been alerted.

When the **eyes** are involved in cases of **chemical burns,** take immediate action and **flood with water.** Use **running water** for 5 minutes in acid burns, 15 minutes in alkali burns, and 20 minutes in cases of unknown agents. A simple method is to wash all eye burns for 20 minutes.

In the care for patients with **electrical burns,** your primary concern should be with **breathing** and **pulse.** For the actual care of the burn, remember to look for at least **two burn sites.** One will be where the electricity entered the patient's body and the other will be the site where the electricity left to a ground. Apply sterile or clean dressings, provide care for shock, and make certain that dispatch has been alerted.

Smoke contains many poisonous substances. Move the patient to a safe atmosphere and help place him in a position that is best for unlabored breathing. Make certain that someone alerts the dispatcher.

Exposure to excessive heat can bring about **heat cramps, heat exhaustion,** or **heat stroke.** Heat cramps are seldom a serious problem. Some cases of heat exhaustion can turn serious. All cases of heat stroke are serious. **Heat stroke is a true emergency.** Scansheet 14–2 compares the symptoms and signs of all three conditions. You must be able to tell one condition from the others.

Care for heat cramps includes cooling the patient, giving salted water or half-strength commercial electrolyte solution, and gently massaging cramped muscles. In cases of heat exhaustion, you must cool the patient, give salted water or half-strength commercial electrolyte solution, and provide care for shock. Dispatch must be alerted for all cases of heat-related emergencies.

Heat stroke requires that you **cool the patient as rapidly as possible.** Use ice bags, cold packs, or cool running water. Arrange for immediate transport.

Excessive cold can bring about **hypothermia.** Shivering, feelings of numbness, and drowsiness are most frequently seen in hypothermia. Care for mild hypothermia involves using **external heat sources** to raise the patient's body temperature. Hypothermia can be very serious. If the patient becomes unconscious, experiences problems with breathing, has a slowed pulse rate, has frozen body parts, or does not respond to external heat, arrange for EMT transport as soon as possible. **Do not rewarm the severe hypothermia patient.**

Exposure to cold can cause **frostnip, frostbite** (superficial frostbite), or **freezing** (deep frostbite). The signs for each of these conditions are given in Scansheet 14–3.

The patient can use body heat to warm frostnipped areas of the body. Frostbite requires an external heat source on the site (avoid hot sources), gentle handling of the affected part, keeping the patient warm, dressing the site, and transport to a medical facility. If transport is delayed, the affected area will have to be rewarmed by immersing it in warm water (100° to 105°F). Keep the water warm, but still comfortable to your touch. The same basic care also applies to freezing.

CHAPTER 15

childbirth

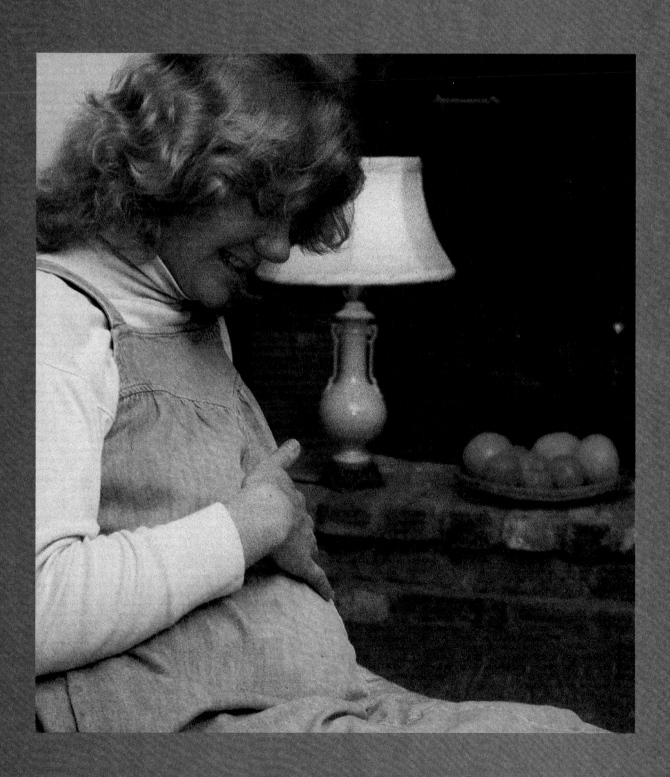

■ OBJECTIVES

SKILLS

Upon completing this chapter and your class lectures and skills labs, you should be able to:

1. Go through the steps of preparation, delivery, and postdelivery care ultilizing an obstetrical manikin.
2. Act out how you would comfort parents during both a normal and abnormal delivery.

UNDERSTANDING CHILDBIRTH

You may have noted that this chapter is called "Childbirth" and not "Emergency Childbirth." As a culture, we have arrived at the point where any birth away from a hospital delivery room is considered an emergency. This simply is not true. Worldwide, most babies are born away from modern medical facilities. Birth is a natural process. The anatomy of the human female, babies, and the structures formed during pregnancy allow for the process to occur with few immediate problems. Assistance from the medical community reduces the chances of problems for mother and child. However, in most deliveries all this medical skill and equipment are not needed.

1st NOTE: First Responders do not deliver babies . . . mothers do! Your role will be one of helping the mother as she delivers her child.

The presence of a First Responder at the scene of a birth that takes place away from a medical facility can prove to be the key factor in a baby's survival should something go wrong. First Responder-level care skills may be needed to ensure safe delivery if there are complications. The care provided after delivery is just as important. The first hour of life after birth can be a difficult time for some babies and their mothers. Your participation in birthing and the care you provide can make a difference.

Anatomy of Pregnancy

A baby developing and growing inside of its mother is called a **fetus** (FE-tus). The fetus develops inside of a muscular organ called the womb or **uterus** (U-ter-us). The uterus will contract during labor and push the baby down through the neck of the uterus known as the **cervix** (SUR-viks). During

Fetus (FE-tus)—the developing unborn child. It is an embryo until the eighth week after fertilization, when it becomes a fetus.

Uterus (U-ter-us)—the womb. The muscular structure in which the fetus develops.

Cervix (SUR-viks)—the neck of the uterus. The lower portion of the uterus, where it enters the birth canal (vagina).

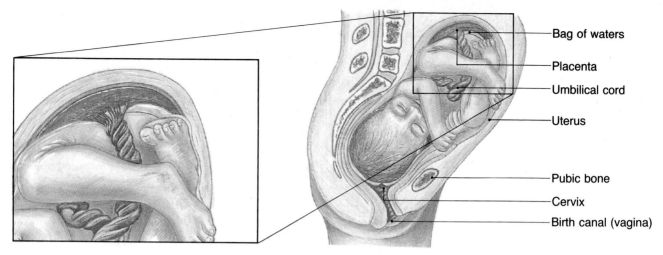

Labels on figure:
- Bag of waters
- Placenta
- Umbilical cord
- Uterus
- Pubic bone
- Cervix
- Birth canal (vagina)

FIGURE 15–1. *The structures of pregnancy.*

delivery, the fetus passes through the cervix and enters the birth canal or **vagina** (vah-JI-nah), from which it is carried to the outside world to be born.

The fetus is not the only thing developing inside the womb. A sac of fluids, sometimes called the "bag of waters" or **amniotic** (am-ne-OT-ic) **sac,** forms to surround and protect the fetus. This sac usually breaks during labor.

A special organ is forming in the womb during pregnancy. This organ, known as the **placenta** (plah-SEN-tah), is made up of tissues from the mother and the fetus. Oxygen and nourishment from the mother's blood pass through this organ and enter the fetus's blood. The fetus is connected to the placenta by way of the **umbilical** (um-BIL-i-kal) **cord.**

Vagina (vah-JI-nah)—the birth canal.

Amniotic (am-ne-OT-ic) sac the "bag of waters." The fluid-filled sac that surrounds the developing embryo and fetus.

Placenta (plah-SEN-tah)—an organ of pregnancy that is composed of maternal and fetal tissues. Exchange between the circulatory systems of the mother and fetus can take place without the mixing of blood.

Umbilical (um-BIL-i-kal) cord—the structure that connects the body of the fetus to the placenta. It contains fetal blood vessels.

Stages of Labor

There are three stages of labor:

1. First stage—starts with contractions and ends when the cervix fully dilates to allow the baby to enter the birth canal.
2. Second stage—covers the time from when the baby is in the birth canal until it is born.
3. Third stage—begins when the baby is born and ends when the afterbirth (placenta, umbilical cord, some tissues from the amniotic sac, and some tissues from the lining of the uterus) is delivered.

A significant feature of labor is the contractions of the uterus. These contractions occur as cycles consisting of contraction and relaxation periods. At first, the contractions are far apart. As birth approaches, the time between contractions becomes shorter. In most cases, the contractions will take place every 30 minutes down to 3 minutes or less. Labor pains and discharges from the vagina accompany these contractions.

The discharges should be a watery, bloody mucus during the first stage of labor. After this stage, the discharge will appear as a watery, bloody fluid. This is not the same as bleeding. If there is blood flowing from the vagina prior to delivery, rather than the expected bloody fluids, then something is wrong. The problem could be very serious and will require EMT assistance and transport as soon as possible.

Pain during labor is normal. Labor pains usually start as an ache in the lower back and then can be felt as lower abdominal pain as labor continues. The intensity of the pain will increase as labor progresses. As the uterus contracts, the pain will begin. When the muscles of the uterus relax, there should be relief from the pain.

Labor pain should come at regular intervals, lasting for 30 seconds to 1 minute. It is not unusual for these pains to start, stop for a period of time, then start again.

As a First Responder, you will have to time labor pains for two characteristics:

Contraction time—the period of time a contraction of the womb lasts during labor. It is measured from the start of the uterus contracting until it relaxes.

Interval—during labor this term means the time from the start of one contraction until the beginning of the next.

- Contraction time—this is how long it takes from the time the uterus begins to contract until it relaxes.
- Interval—this is the time from the start of one contraction to the beginning of the next.

About 4 weeks prior to delivery, the uterus begins to change its size and shape. Some women experience pain and the sensation that labor has begun. This is known as *false labor*. False labor pains do not display the same regular interval pattern of true labor pain. The pain is limited to the lower abdomen, with no back involvement.

It is difficult to tell some false labors from true labor. In most cases, before you have the evidence to declare a false labor, the EMTs have arrived. Even when you are certain that the patient is having false labor, it is still recommended that you have the EMTs respond and make the decision regarding transport.

DELIVERY

Preparing for Delivery

Always begin by introducing yourself and letting the mother know that you are a trained First Responder. Have someone alert the dispatcher. Let the mother know that this has been done and that you will stay with her to help if she starts to deliver the baby. Provide emotional support throughout the entire process of birth. Remind the mother that birth is a natural process. Suggest, as needed, that she remain calm. If she complains that she feels as if she needs to go to the bathroom, tell her that this is normal, caused by pressure on her bladder and intestine. Do not let her leave the scene in order to find a bathroom. She probably is not in need of a bathroom. Her body is simply reacting to all the changes taking place in her body cavities. It is important that you keep her calm and begin assessing the situation as soon as possible.

The fear of a delivery away from a hospital can cause some people to try to find a way to delay the process. The mother and onlookers may suggest that she try holding her knees together. This should not be allowed. To do so will not slow down delivery and may complicate the process. The sooner you have unneeded onlookers leave the scene, the easier it will be for you to reassure the mother and begin with the assessment.

1st Begin to evaluate the mother by asking:

1. Her name and age.
2. If she has been seeing a physician during the pregnancy. If so, have someone phone the doctor's office or service. The doctor's familiarity with the patient will help in making the decision to transport.
3. If this is her first pregnancy. The typical first delivery usually lasts about 16 hours. The time in labor is considerably shorter for each subsequent baby.

4. How long she has been having labor pains and if the bag of waters has broken.
5. If she feels strain in her pelvis or lower abdomen, if she feels as if she needs to move her bowels, and if she can feel the baby beginning to move out through her vaginal opening.

If the mother says she feels the baby trying to be born, birth of the baby will probably occur before more highly trained personnel arrive. If the mother is having labor pains from contractions about 2 minutes apart, birth is very near. Should she also be straining, crying out, and complaining about having to go to the bathroom, birth will probably occur very shortly.

Give the woman some credit for knowing what is going on. Even if this is her first experience with birthing, when she tells you that she feels the baby coming, believe her.

Find out if she has had a childbirth preparation or natural childbirth class. Tell her that you will help her to follow the procedures taught in her class. Keep in mind that you must follow standard EMS System practices for assisting with the physical delivery of the infant and providing care after the delivery. However, you will be able to help the trained mother with her breathing and timing contractions as she was taught in her classes. In addition to these activities, you can offer the encouragement and support she will need throughout labor. If you are well versed in the proedures of natural childbirth, this is not the time to try to teach the patient. You may make some suggestions on how she can breathe and how she can reduce strain, but do not try to give her a "crash course."

1st After evaluating the mother and finding that birth may occur shortly, you must immediately examine her and prepare her for delivery. To do so, you should:

1. Control the scene so that the mother will have privacy. Ask unneeded bystanders to leave. If you are outdoors, request that they turn their backs to help shield the mother. If she appears to be in early labor, this is her first child, and labor pains are typical, you may opt to move her a short distance to a more private place. It is best to avoid moving her whenever possible.
2. Have the mother lie down on her back. Her knees should be bent, her feet flat, and her legs spread wide apart.
3. Feel for contractions. If the mother says that she can feel the baby starting to be born, skip this step. Obviously, feeling for contractions may have to be delayed until the patient says she is having labor pains. Explain what you are going to do and place the palm of your hand on her abdomen, above the navel. This should be done without removing any of the patient's clothing. As birth nears, the uterus and the tissues between it and the skin will feel more rigid. Do not delay other procedures to wait for a contraction. Do the procedure and repeat as necessary to help determine if birth is near.
4. Tell the mother that you need to see if her baby has entered the birth canal. Remove any clothing or underclothing that obstructs your viewing her vaginal opening. Use clean cloth, sheets, towels, or table cloths to cover the mother as shown in Figure 15–2. If you have an obstetrical pack (OB pack), use the materials provided. If the mother's bag of waters has broken or there is evidence of vaginal bleeding, stop to put on latex or vinyl gloves.
5. Look to see if any part of the baby is visible at the vaginal opening (crowning). If it is, or if part of the baby's head becomes visible with each contraction, birth is probably near. Do not assume that birth is not about to happen shortly if the baby is not visible or if the area of the baby seen is "less than a fifty-cent piece." Do not transport the mother. You should wait for the EMTs to respond.

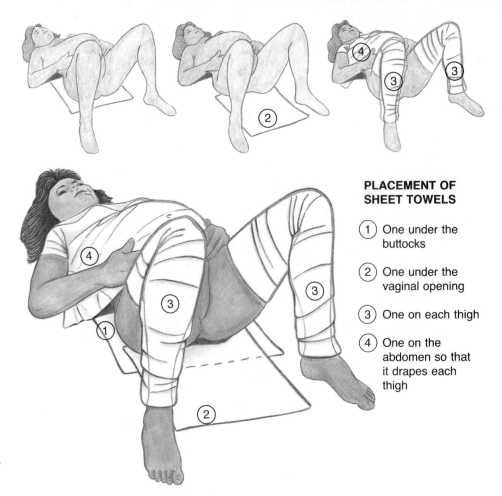

PLACEMENT OF SHEET TOWELS

① One under the buttocks

② One under the vaginal opening

③ One on each thigh

④ One on the abdomen so that it drapes each thigh

FIGURE 15–2. Preparing the mother for delivery.

During the entire process of assessment and delivery, you should be wearing the necessary items supplied for personal protection. Latex or vinyl gloves should be worn to avoid contact with blood, body fluids, and mucous membranes. A gown is strongly recommended to help reduce the chance of the forearms coming into contact with these substances. Protection for the eyes should be worn in the form of goggles or a faceshield since the process of birth will sometimes spray blood and fluids.

You may choose to assist in a birth without using any of these items; however, you do so at your own risk. Again, the major concern is the transmission of infectious diseases.

Normal Delivery

During delivery, talk to the mother. Ask her to relax between contractions. If her bag of waters breaks, remind her that this is normal. Consider the delivery to be normal if the baby's head appears first.

1st The steps for assisting the mother with a normal delivery are:

1. Keep the mother draped and in the examination position, but place a folded blanket, towels, or sheets under her buttocks so that her pelvis is lifted about 2 inches above the supporting surface. One or two pillows can be used to elevate her head and shoulders.

2. If you have not done so, put on sterile gloves if you have an OB pack (Figure 15–3), or wash your hands with soap and water if possible at the scene (wearing gloves is *strongly* recommended).

3. Place someone near the mother's head to reassure her, offer encouragement, and to turn her head in case she vomits. If no one is on hand to help, be alert for vomiting.

4. Place one hand below the baby's head as it is delivered. Spread your fingers evenly around the baby's head (see Scansheet 15.1). Support the baby's head, but avoid pressure to the soft areas of the baby's skull. Maintain slight pressure on the baby's head in case you need to control an explosive delivery. Use your other hand to help cradle the baby's head. **Do not pull on the baby!**

5. If the umbilical cord is wrapped around the baby's neck, gently loosen the cord. If the bag of waters does not break, use a clamp (OB kit) or a **blunt** object to puncture the membrane. Do not delay this process. Tear the bag with your fingers, if need be. Pull the membranes away from the baby's mouth and nose.

6. Most babies are born face down and then begin to rotate to the right or left. The upper shoulder (usually with some delay) delivers next, followed quickly by the lower shoulder. You should continue to support the baby throughout the entire birth process. If you can gently guide the baby's head downward, you will assist the mother in delivering the baby's upper shoulder.

7. Once the baby's feet are delivered, lay the baby on its side with its head slightly lowered. This is done to allow blood, fluids, and mucus to drain from the mouth and nose.

8. Note the exact time of birth.

NOTE: Standard procedures call for clearing the baby's airway once its head is exposed; however, most First Responders do not carry the rubber bulb syringe needed for this procedure. Even when you have such a syringe, do not try to stop the birthing process or release your support of the baby in order to clear its airway. Since you will not be aiding in the delivery of babies every day, it will not be surprising to find that you lack the confidence needed to try to assist with the birth and clear the airway at the same time. The vast majority of babies can wait to have their airways cleared.

CAUTION: Babies being born are slippery! Make certain that you offer proper support. Some deliveries are explosive. Do not squeeze the baby, but do provide adequate support. Remembering that an explosive delivery can be controlled by using one hand to maintain a slight pressure on the baby's head. Again, do not squeeze the baby.

FIGURE 15–3. Contents of a disposable obstetric kit.

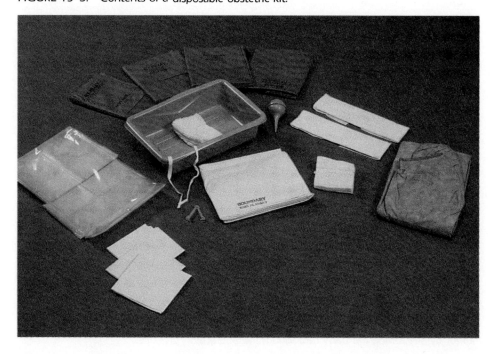

■ SCAN 15-1.

Normal Delivery

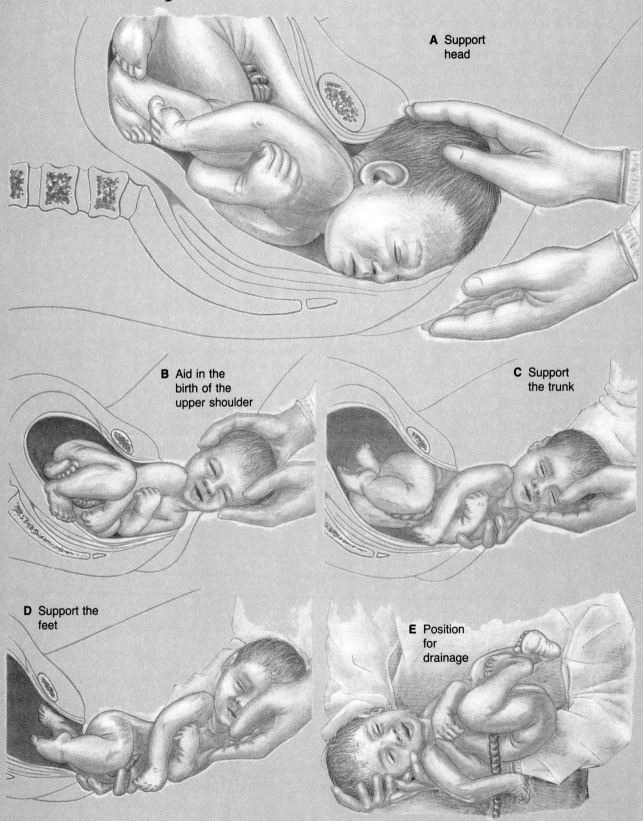

A Support head

B Aid in the birth of the upper shoulder

C Support the trunk

D Support the feet

E Position for drainage

Assist the mother by supporting the baby throughout the entire birth process.

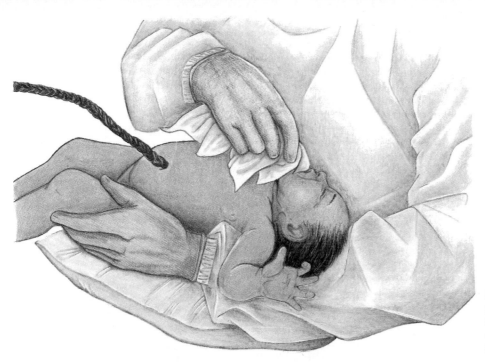

FIGURE 15–4. Use a sterile pad or a clean handkerchief to clean blood and mucus from around the baby's mouth and nose.

Caring for the Newborn

1st Each step in the care of the newborn is essential for the infant's survival. Upon assisting the mother with the delivery of her baby, you should:

1. Clear the baby's airway—use a sterile gauze pad or a clean handkerchief to clear mucus and blood from around the baby's nose and mouth. If you have an OB kit, use the rubber bulb syringe. Squeeze the bulb of the syringe and insert the tip about 1 inch into the baby's mouth.

FIGURE 15–5. Suctioning the mouth of the newborn is accomplished by squeezing the bulb, then inserting the tip into the infant's mouth. The bulb is released to suction, then the tip is removed from the mouth and the bulb is squeezed to remove its contents.

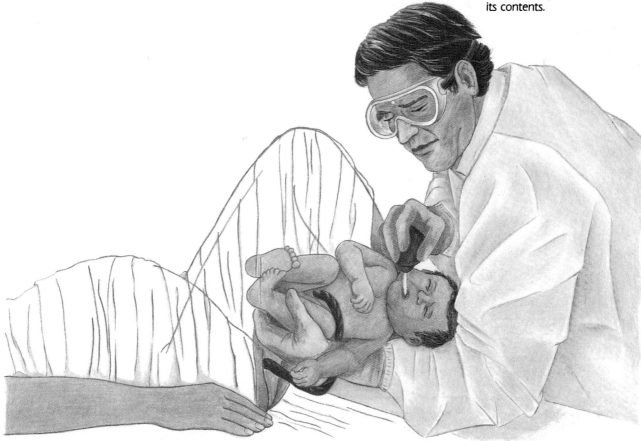

Continue to hold the bulb as you gently release pressure to allow the syringe to take up fluids from inside the baby's mouth. Remove the tip of the syringe from the baby's mouth and squeeze out any fluids. Repeat this process two or three times and then once for each nostril. Throughout the remainder of care, make certain that the baby's nose is clear. Babies breathe through their nostrils.

2. Make certain that the baby is breathing—usually the baby will be breathing on its own by the time you clear the airway (within 30 seconds). If it is not then you must "encourage" the baby to breathe. Begin by rigorously but gently rubbing the baby's back. If this fails to stimulate breathing, snap one of your index fingers against the soles of the baby's feet. Do not hold the baby up by its feet and slap its bottom! Care for the nonbreathing infant will be covered later in this chapter.

3. Clamp or tie off the cord (directions will be given later in this chapter).

4. Keep the infant warm—wrap the baby in a clean towel, sheet, or baby blanket and place it on its mother's abdomen. Keep the top of the baby's head covered. This will help to reduce heat loss. The mother may wish to put the baby to her breast. This is to be encouraged.

5. If tape is available, write the mother's last name and the time of delivery on a piece of the tape and form it into a loop. The tape must be folded back onto itself so the adhesive does not come into contact with the baby's skin. Place it loosely around the baby's wrist.

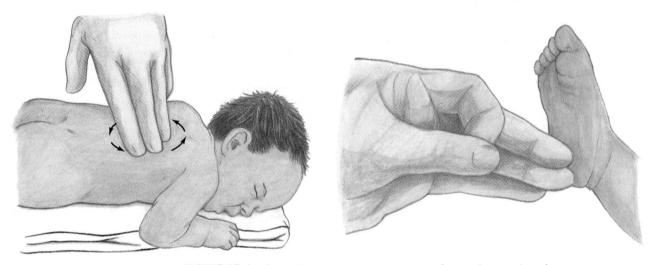

FIGURE 15–6.   It may be necessary to encourage the newborn to breathe.

FIGURE 15–7.   Wrap the baby and place it on its mother's abdomen. Be sure to make a wrist identification tape.

Loosely secure tape to the baby's wrist, with mother's name and time of birth

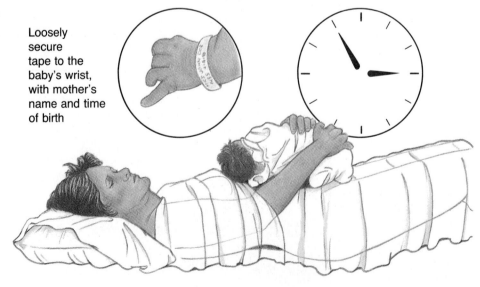

The Nonbreathing Infant

Should you fail in your efforts to "encourage" the baby to breathe, provide two gentle but adequate breaths mouth-to-mask or mouth-to-mouth and nose (at your own risk) and assess breathing and brachial pulse. Make certain that any breathing adjunct used is approved for infants. Be careful not to hyperextend the head and neck, closing off the airway. If you cannot feel a brachial pulse, begin CPR. If there is a pulse, provide pulmonary resuscitation, checking every several minutes for a pulse. Continue resuscitation until the infant has spontaneous heart and lung actions or you are relieved by more highly trained personnel. Have someone alert dispatch to the fact that the infant will require advanced cardiac life support.

Once you have begun resuscitation procedures, transport to a medical facility is critical. If it is impossible to contact dispatch or the EMS System is unable to respond, arrange to transport the mother and child as a unit, with the mother kept on her back. Do not stop resuscitation to provide for transport. Do not stop resuscitation to tie and cut the umbilical cord. The effectiveness of CPR will be higher if the cord has been tied and cut. However, this will have to be done by someone else while you provide CPR.

If you are involved in transport, keep in mind that the mother may still be in labor. This is the case if she has not delivered the afterbirth. She still carries the placenta and a portion of the umbilical cord if you have tied and cut the cord. You must exercise extreme care in moving the mother. Both ends of the cut cord must be monitored for bleeding. If you have not tied and cut the cord, both mother and infant are a unit that has to be moved with great care.

NOTE: First Responder transport of mother and child is an extreme measure that is not advised unless there is no other choice. If EMTs can respond, the First Responder should provide basic life support while awaiting their arrival.

Umbilical Cord Care

In most cases, if dispatch has been alerted, clamping or tying off the cord will not be necessary. Some EMS Systems recommend that First Responders tie off the cord. Cutting of the cord is usually not recommended unless a medical facility is more than 30 minutes away. In such cases, a sterile pair of scissors or single-edged razor blade is required. Soaking these items in alcohol for 20 minutes can be done if no sterile items are available.

Your instructor will tell you if tying off or clamping of the cord is done by First Responders in your area. There may be special cases (cord was around baby's neck during delivery) when First Responders in your area are always to tie the cord. If you are to tie off the cord, then you should:

1. Use sterile clamps or umbilical tape found in the OB kit. If you do not have a kit, then clean shoelaces may be used (never wire or string). Ties should be made using a square knot. It is recommended that you wait until pulsations of the cord have stopped before you begin tying or clamping.
2. Apply one tie or clamp to the cord about 10 inches from the baby's belly.
3. Place a second tie or clamp about 3 inches closer to the baby.
4. If cutting is to be done, it must be done between the two ties or clamps. *Never* untie or unclamp a cord once it is cut. Should bleeding continue, apply another tie or clamp as close to the original as possible.

WARNING: Never tie, clamp, or cut the cord of a baby who is not breathing

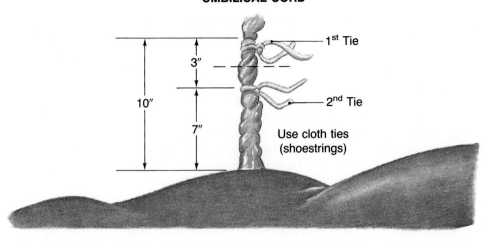

TYING THE UMBILICAL CORD

1st Tie

3″

10″

2nd Tie

7″

Use cloth ties (shoestrings)

FIGURE 15–8. Tying of the cord is recommended in some EMS Systems.

on its own, unless the cord has been damaged and there is excessive bleeding, or CPR must be initiated.

CAUTION: If you cut the cord, both ends must be monitored for bleeding. If you have an OB kit, umbilical tape can be used to tie the baby's *clamped* cord after cutting.

Should the placenta deliver and you are not able to cut the cord, it has been recommended that the placenta be placed at the same level as the baby, or in a slightly higher position. Once the placenta is delivered, the cord should be tied or clamped and cut.

Caring for the Mother

Care for the mother involves helping her deliver the afterbirth, controlling vaginal bleeding, making her as comfortable as possible, and providing reassurance.

Delivering the Afterbirth

The afterbirth is usually delivered a few minutes after the baby is born. In some cases, it may take 20 minutes or longer. Some women wish to get up or assume a seated position after they deliver their babies. You may have to remind some mothers that they will have to remain at rest until they deliver the afterbirth. Make her as comfortable as possible and wait for the delivery.

1st The afterbirth must be saved. It is critical that the afterbirth be examined by a physician. Try to catch the afterbirth in a container. Think this out before the afterbirth is delivered. It may be very difficult to place the container you have selected for use. After collecting the afterbirth, wrap the container in a towel, paper, or plastic. If no container is available, catch the afterbirth in a towel, paper, or a plastic bag.

Control of Vaginal Bleeding After Delivery

Bleeding from the uterus, discharged through the vagina, always occurs after the mother has delivered the afterbirth. Seldom is this a problem.

1st To help control vaginal bleeding after delivery, you should:

1. Place a sanitary napkin, clean towel, or clean handkerchief over the mother's vaginal opening. Do not place anything in the vagina.
2. Have the mother lower her legs and keep them together (she does not have to squeeze them). Elevate her legs.
3. Feel the mother's abdomen until you find a "grapefruit-size" object. This is the uterus. Gently, but firmly rub this area of her abdomen, using a circular motion.

COLLECT AND SAVE THE AFTERBIRTH

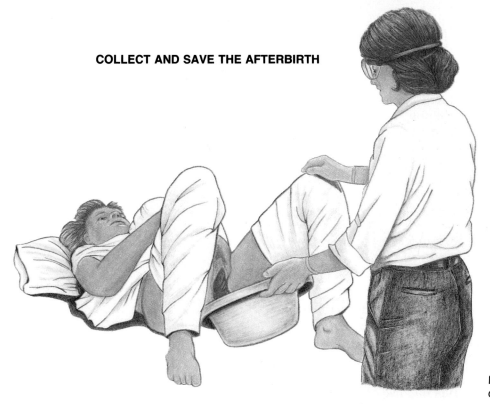

FIGURE 15–9. You must collect and save the afterbirth.

CONTROL BLEEDING

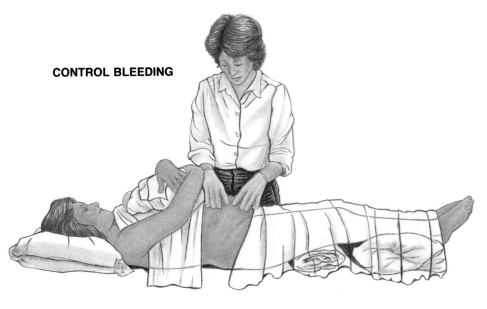

FIGURE 15–10. Control vaginal bleeding that follows the delivery of the afterbirth.

Providing Comfort to the Mother

1st Keep contact with the mother throughout the entire birth process and after she has delivered. Once you have completed your duties with the afterbirth, replace any wet towels or sheets. If possible, wipe and dry the mother's face and hands. Make sure that both she and the baby remain warm. When delivery occurs at home, ask a member of the family or a trusted neighbor to help clean up.

Remember, birth is an exciting and joyous event. Talking to the mother and paying attention to her and her new baby are very important parts of First Responder care.

COMPLICATIONS

Prebirth bleeding and other predelivery emergencies, miscarriages, prolonged (protracted) labor, abnormal deliveries, premature deliveries, multiple births, and stillbirths make up some of the more common complications in childbirth. Keep in mind that most births are normal. Those births that produce complications often do not have immediate problems at the scene. Some difficulties with unusual deliveries can be cared for by First Responders. However, there are severe complications that must be handled by advanced life-support and immediate EMT transport to a medical facility.

The risk of complications before, during, and after delivery increases dramatically when a woman is:

- A teenager
- Over age 35
- Suffering from high or low blood pressure
- Diabetic
- Displaying predelivery bleeding
- Suffering from infections
- Drug dependent (including alcohol)
- Taking certain medications (lithium carbonate, magnesium, reserpine), or
- Has had five or more pregnancies

Gathering this information requires a patient interview. As you proceed with the assessment of the patient, ask her the questions necessary to see if she is a high-risk group.

1st Some pregnant patients develop problems long before they are ready to deliver. Many cases require care before the patient may show any dramatic outward signs of pregnancy. You may improperly assess the patient if you do not know she is pregnant. Be certain to ask if the patient is pregnant when you note any of the following:

- Vaginal bleeding
- Swelling of the face, hands, and feet
- Headache, visual problems, apprehension, and shakiness associated with upper abdominal pain
- Severe abdominal pain that had a sudden onset

Pregnant women with any of these symptoms and signs require immediate EMT response. Make certain that someone alerts dispatch.

PREDELIVERY EMERGENCIES

1st Prebirth Bleeding

When a pregnant woman has excessive vaginal bleeding early in pregnancy, it is probably due to a miscarriage. Should the bleeding occur late in pregnancy or while the patient is in labor, the problem is probably related to the placenta. Regardless of the cause of bleeding, you should:

1. Make certain that someone alerts dispatch, telling them of the excessive bleeding.
2. Place the patient on her left side, but do not hold her legs together.
3. Provide care for shock.
4. Place a sanitary napkin or bulky dressings over the vaginal opening.
5. Replace napkins or dressings as they become soaked. Do not place anything in the vagina.

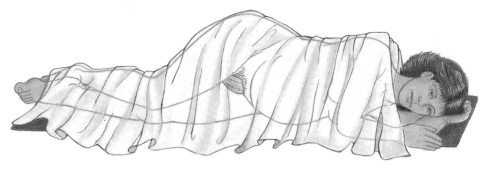

FIGURE 15-11. Attempt to control excessive pre-birth bleeding.

6. Save all blood-soaked napkins and dressings.
7. Save all tissues that are passed.
8. Monitor and reassure the patient and wait for the EMTs to respond.

Miscarriage and Abortion

A miscarriage occurs if the fetus is delivered before it can survive on its own (before the 28th week). The correct term for a miscarriage is a spontaneous abortion. However, since the word abortion has other meanings in our society, *never* use the word with women having a miscarriage or premature signs of labor.

When specific actions are taken to stop a pregnancy, the term induced abortion is used. This may be done legally by a physician as a medical procedure, or it may be done by the woman or someone else as an illegal act. Usually, an illegal abortion is attempted by taking excessive dosages of medications or other chemicals. This type of patient will require care for the overdose or poisoning. Some illegal abortions are attempted by inserting objects into the womb through the vagina. This type of patient often has excessive internal and external bleeding.

1st The miscarriage and the abortion patient typically have abdominal cramps and pains. Vaginal bleeding will usually occur, ranging from mild to severe. In many cases, there will be vaginal discharges of bloody mucus and tissue particles.

1st When caring for a woman having a miscarriage, or an abortion, you should:

1. Provide care for shock, placing the patient on her side.
2. Place a sanitary napkin or other clean pad over the opening to the vagina. Do not place anything into the vagina.
3. Save all blood-soaked pads and any tissues that are passed.
4. Provide emotional support.

NOTE: Regardless of the cause of the emergency, the patient will be in need of emotional support. Professional care, a show of concern, and reassurance must be provided by the First Responder.

Prolonged Labor

Consider the patient to be in a prolonged labor when contractions have been 2 to 3 minutes apart for 20 minutes. This patient requires transport by the EMTs as soon as possible.

ABNORMAL DELIVERY

Breech Birth

In a breech birth, the buttocks or both feet (not just one leg) are delivered first. Often, the baby will still manage to be born without any major complications. The buttocks and trunk of the infant will be delivered together, requir-

Miscarriage—the natural loss of the embryo or fetus before the twenty-eighth week of pregnancy. A spontaneous abortion.

Abortion—typically used to mean the induced loss of the embryo or fetus.

Breech birth—a birth in which the buttocks or both feet are delivered first.

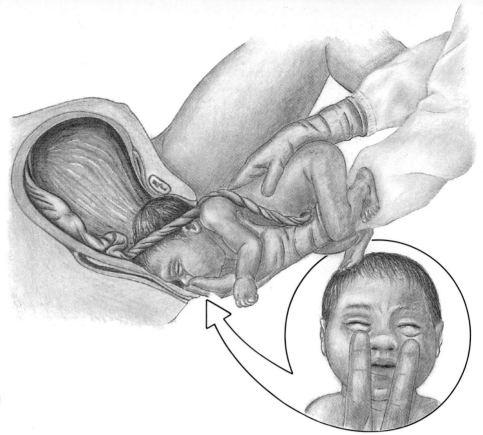

FIGURE 15–12. Provide and maintain an airway during breech births.

ing you to place one hand and forearm under the baby's trunk. The head will deliver last, also requiring you to provide support.

1st In cases where the baby's head does not deliver within **3 minutes** of its buttocks and trunk, you must:

1. Create an airway for the baby—flow through the umbilical cord has been shut off. Tell the mother what you must do and why. Insert your hand into the vagina, with your palm toward the baby's face. Form a "V" by placing one finger on each side of the baby's nose. Push the wall of the birth canal away from the baby's face. If you cannot complete this process, then try to place one finger tip into the infant's mouth and push away the birth canal wall with your other fingers.
2. Maintain the airway—once you have provided an airway for the baby, you must keep this airway open. **Do not pull on the baby.** Allow delivery to take place, maintaining support for the baby's body and head.
3. Allow 3 minutes for delivery after you have established an airway. If delivery of the head does not take place, EMT transport to a medical facility is critical. Maintain the airway throughout *all* stages of care until you are relieved by more highly trained personnel.

NOTE: The presentation of an arm or a leg is not a breech birth. This is a limb presentation and requires immediate EMT transport to a medical facility. Do not pull on the limb or try to place your hand into the birth canal. Do not try to place the limb back into the vagina. Place the mother in the knee–chest position (see Figure 15–13) to help reduce pressure on the fetus and the umbilical cord, or keep her in the typical delivery position (follow local guidelines).

Prolapsed Cord

Prolapsed cord—a birth in which the umbilical cord is delivered first. In all cases, this is a very serious emergency.

1st When the umbilical cord is delivered first, this is known as a prolapsed cord. Immediate EMT transport to a medical facility is required. Do not try to push the cord back into the birth canal. Do not try to place your hand into the mother's vagina. Place the mother in a knee–chest position

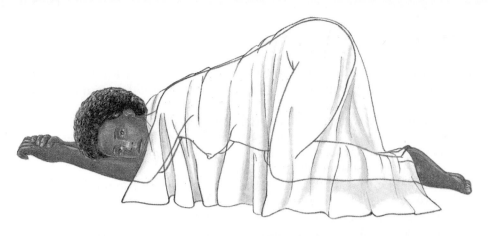

to reduce pressure on the cord (your EMS System's guidelines may call for the mother to remain in the typical delivery position). Wrap the cord in a towel or dressings. It must be kept warm.

NOTE: The baby's chances for survival are greatly improved if you can keep its head from applying pressure to the umbilical cord. Some EMS Systems are considering if they should permit First Responders to insert several fingers into the mother's vagina and gently push up on the baby's head to keep pressure off the cord. Check with your instructor to see if this procedure is part of First Responder-level care in your state.

Multiple Births

In cases of multiple birth, labor contractions will start again shortly after the birth of the first child. Ask the mother if she has been told to expect a multiple birth. The procedures for assisting the mother remain the same. It is recommended that you tie or clamp the cord of the first child before the second child is born.

Premature Births

Any baby weighing less than 5½ pounds at birth is to be considered premature. Any baby born before the thirty-seventh week or prior to the ninth month of pregnancy is to be considered premature. If the mother tells you the baby is early by more than two weeks, play it safe and consider the baby to be premature.

In addition to the procedures for normal births, you must take special steps to keep a premature baby warm. Wrap the newborn in a blanket, sheets, towels, or aluminum foil (fold the edges to avoid cutting the infant). A combination of a blanket and aluminum foil is ideal. Cover the baby's head, but keep its face uncovered. As quickly as possible, transfer the baby to a warm environment (90° to 100′F). Do not place a heat source too close to the baby.

Premature baby—a baby that is born before the thirty-seventh week or prior to the ninth month of pregnancy. Any baby with a birth weight of less than 5½ pounds.

Stillborn Deliveries

Some infants are born dead or die very quickly after they are born. Such events are very sad. You should be prepared for stillbirths so that you can act professionally, providing comfort to the mother, father, and other members of the family who may be present.

Should a baby be born dead or go into respiratory or cardiac arrest, provide resuscitation measures. Do not stop resuscitation until the baby regains lung and heart activity, until you are relieved, or until you are too exhausted to continue.

There are cases when a baby has died hours or longer before it is born. Do not attempt to resuscitate any stillborn baby that has large blisters and a strong unpleasant odor. Sometimes these stillborns will have very soft heads, swollen body parts, or obvious deformities.

SUMMARY

Always begin by letting the mother know that you are a First Responder. Make sure that dispatch has been alerted and the mother is made aware of this fact.

Evaluate the mother to see if she is about to deliver. Consider if this is her first labor, how far apart the contractions are, if she feels pressure or feels as if she may have a bowel movement, if her bag of waters has broken, or if she feels the baby moving into her vagina.

If you believe that birth will occur shortly, provide the mother with as much privacy as possible, position her on her back, with her knees bent, feet flat, and legs spread apart. Ensure your own safety by wearing gloves, eye protection, and a gown. Remove any clothing obstructing your view of the vaginal opening. See if any part of the baby is visible or becomes visible during contractions (crowning).

Assist the mother as she delivers her baby. Carefully support the infant's head as it is born. Provide support for its entire body and head as birth proceeds.

If the umbilical cord is around the baby's neck, gently loosen the cord with your fingers. If the bag of waters does not break, puncture it and pull it away from the baby's mouth and nose.

If caring for the newborn, clear the airway and make certain that the baby is breathing. If it is not breathing, "encourage" it to do so by rubbing its back, and if necessary, by snapping your index finger on the soles of its feet. For nonbreathing babies, provide mouth-to-mask (if available) or mouth-to-mouth and nose ventilations (at your own risk). Check for breathing and a brachial pulse. If there is no pulse, provide CPR. If there is a pulse but no breathing, continue respiratory resuscitation, monitoring for lung and heart action.

Wrap the newborn and keep it warm.

Your state guidelines may require you to tie or clamp the cord. Do not tie, clamp, or cut a cord until the baby is breathing on its own (unless there is profuse bleeding or you must start CPR).

Assist the mother as she delivers the afterbirth and save all tissues for transport. Help control vaginal bleeding with clean pads over the vaginal opening and a massage of her abdomen over the site of the uterus. Remove all wet towels and sheets. Wipe clean the mother's face and hands.

REMEMBER: Throughout the entire birth process, provide emotional support to the mother.

Be ready for complications during a delivery. Provide an airway with your fingers in cases of breech birth. Maintain this airway until the baby is born or until you turn the mother over to more highly trained professionals. The EMS System should transport mothers with prolapsed umbilical cords, and those with limb presentations, to a medical facility as soon as possible. If there is severe bleeding before delivery, pad the vaginal opening, provide care for shock, and arrange for transport as soon as possible.

Expect a multiple birth if contractions continue after the first baby is born. When possible, tie or clamp the umbilical cord of the first child before the next child is born.

Keep all babies warm. It is especially critical that premature babies be kept warm.

In cases of miscarriage, be certain to provide emotional support to the mother. Pad her vaginal opening if there is bleeding. Save all blood-soaked pads and any passed tissues. Provide care for shock.

In cases of stillborns, remain professional and provide emotional support to the mother, father, and other members of the family.

SELF-TEST III

This is a self-test. It has been designed for you to take on your own to evaluate your progress. After you have completed Chapters 13 to 15 and believe that you have met all the objectives listed for these chapters, take this test to see if you have any weaknesses in a specific area of study. Answers are listed at the end of the test. Page references are provided for each question so you can go back to the text to restudy any questions missed in the test.

If you wish to check your knowledge in more detail, note that the objectives listed at the beginning of each chapter can be read as questions and exercises. Go back to these objectives and see if you can list, describe, name, and so on, as directed in the objective statements.

**Circle the letter of the best answer
to each question.**

1. A 70 year-old man is found with slow, snoring respirations. His face is flushed and warm. The pupils of his eyes are uneven. He has probably had (p. 305)

   A. A stroke (CVA)
   B. Congestive heart failure
   C. A heart attack
   D. An epileptic seizure

2. Which of the following indicates the main course of action to be taken when caring for a patient having convulsive seizures? (p. 312)

   A. Induce vomiting
   B. Provide oxygen
   C. Transport at once
   D. Protect the patient from injury

3. A man in his early fifties suddenly has pain in his chest that radiates down his left arm. He is short of breath and very restless. He is probably having (p. 303)

   A. A stroke (CVA)
   B. Congestive heart failure
   C. A heart attack
   D. Insulin shock

4. In which of the following will a patient have "acetone breath?" (p. 315)

   A. Stroke (CVA)
   B. Diabetic coma
   C. Heart attack
   D. Insulin shock

5. Stroke patients should be placed so that their (p. 306)

   A. Legs are elevated
   B. Head, neck, and shoulders are slightly elevated
   C. Head and neck are lower than their trunk
   D. Any of the above, as long as the patient is comfortable

6. If you cannot determine if a conscious diabetic is in diabetic coma or insulin shock, you should (p. 315)

   A. Give insulin
   B. Give insulin and sugar
   C. Give sugar
   D. Do nothing and wait for EMS transport

7. Which of the following is a sign of a snakebite? (p. 324)

   A. Weakness
   B. Nausea
   C. Vision problems
   D. All of the above

8. You have administered 1 tablespoon of syrup of ipecac followed by 1 full glass of water. Your patient, a victim of ingested poisoning, does not vomit in 20 minutes. You should (p. 321)

   A. Administer charcoal and water
   B. Administer mineral oil
   C. Repeat the syrup and water
   D. Continue to wait for vomiting and give charcoal and water

9. Which of the following usually should *not* be eliminated by vomiting? (p. 320)

   A. Oven cleaner
   B. Bleach
   C. Acid drain cleaner
   D. All of the above

10. Once you have located the fang marks on a snakebite patient, you should (p. 324)

    A. Clean the site with soap and water
    B. Scrape the site with a knife blade
    C. Immediately apply constricting bands below the site
    D. Cut open and suction the wound

11. An unknown chemical burn to the eyes should be flooded with water for at least (p. 337)

    A. 30 minutes
    B. 20 minutes
    C. 10 minutes
    D. 5 minutes

12. At an industrial scene, a man collapses. As you are questioning him, he becomes unconscious. His skin is hot and dry. His pulse is rapid and weak, and respirations are shallow. He is probably suffering from (p. 343)

    A. Heat stroke
    B. Heat exhaustion
    C. Heat cramps
    D. Heart failure

13. In the care for heat stroke, it is critical that you (p. 343)

    A. Immediately transport the patient.
    B. Cool the patient as rapidly as possible
    C. Provide salted water
    D. Massage the patient's thigh muscles

14. Which of the following may be soaked in water *prior* to dressing? (p. 336)

    A. Third-degree burn to the foot

B. Second-degree burn to the hand
C. First-degree burn to the forearm
D. All of the above

15. A chemical burn to the skin was caused by contact with dry lime. You should (p. 337)

A. Wash the skin with soap and water
B. Flood the skin with water for 15 minutes
C. Apply petroleum jelly directly over the lime
D. Brush the lime from the skin and clothing

16. A conscious patient has mild hypothermia. You must (p. 344)

A. Wrap him in blankets
B. Apply heat
C. Give salted liquids
D. Any one of the above

17. A patient has superficial frostbite of the right lower leg. Transport will be delayed. You should (p. 346)

A. Rewarm the leg with warm water
B. Rub snow or melting ice on the leg
C. Rigorously rub the leg with your hands
D. Simply keep the leg covered with a blanket

18. You are caring for a case of frostbite. Which of the following color changes in the patient's skin is a good indication that you are providing proper care? (p. 346)

A. White to yellow
B. Yellow to gray-blue
C. Blotchy to red
D. Blotchy to yellow-gray

19. A patient has a deep red burn to his hand. Blistering is starting to take place. He complains of severe pain. His burn may be classified as (p. 331)

A. First degree
B. Second degree
C. Third degree
D. Fourth degree

20. If a woman is having her first baby, labor will usually last (p. 354)

A. 2 hours
B. 5 hours
C. 11 hours
D. 16 hours

21. Which of the following includes all three stages of labor? (p. 353)

A. Contractions, baby enters birth canal, baby is born, afterbirth is delivered
B. Contractions, baby is born, afterbirth is delivered
C. Contractions, baby enters birth canal, baby is born
D. Baby enters birth canal, contractions, baby is born, afterbirth is delivered

22. To make a final decision about how close an expectant mother is to delivering her child, you should (p. 355)

A. Time her contractions
B. See if any part of the baby is visible
C. Feel for pelvic movement
D. Check for bleeding

23. After delivery, a newborn should begin breathing on its own (spontaneous respiration) within (p. 360)

A. 30 seconds
B. 1 minute
C. 2 minutes
D. 5 minutes

24. Which of the following is the correct distance from the baby when placing the first tie or clamp on the umbilical cord? (p. 361)

A. 2 inches
B. 5 inches
C. 10 inches
D. 12 inches

25. During a breech delivery, the baby's head does not deliver in 3 minutes of its buttocks and trunk. You should (p. 366)

A. Create an airway for the baby by inserting your fingers into the mother's vagina
B. Transport immediately
C. Wait 5 minutes as your massage the mother's abdomen
D. Gently pull on the baby's legs, attempting to turn its body and free the umbilical cord

ANSWERS

Each question is worth 4 points.

1.	A	10.	A	19.	B
2.	D	11.	B	20.	D
3.	C	12.	A	21.	A
4.	B	13.	B	22.	B
5.	B	14.	C	23.	A
6.	C	15.	D	24.	C
7.	D	16.	B	25.	A
8.	C	17.	A		
9.	D	18.	C		

Start with 100 points. Subtract four points for each wrong answer. If you scored below 70, you should see your instructor for additional help or new study methods. A score from 70 to 79 indicates you still need to do much more work on these chapters. You have done very well if you scored 80 or above; however, you should go over the text sections dealing with the questions that you missed.

CHAPTER 16

Special Patients

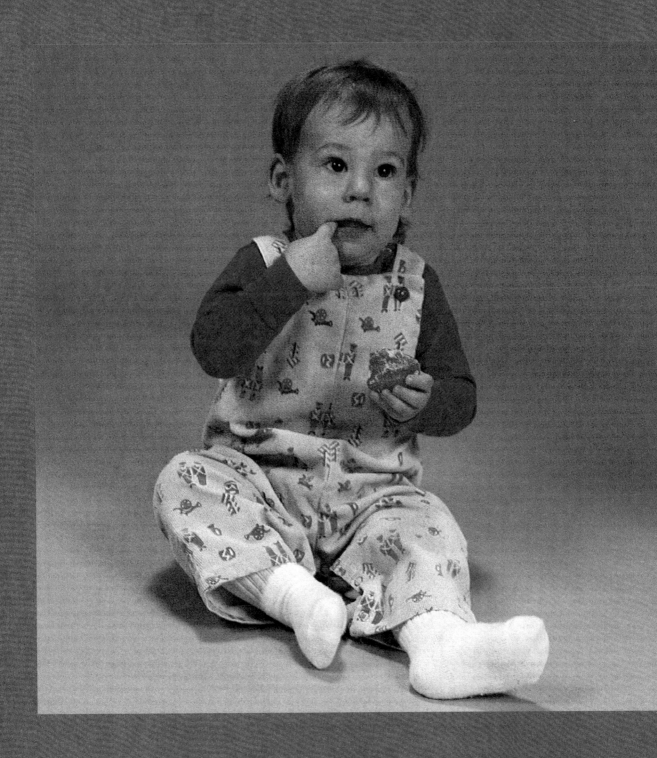

◼ OBJECTIVES

By the end of this chapter, you should be able to:

1. State the special problems faced when caring for the child patient. (pp. 373, 375)
2. Describe the changes in the approach to care that you will have to take when dealing with children. (pp. 373–375)
3. State the special problems faced when caring for elderly patients. (p. 377)
4. Describe the changes in the approach to care that you will have to make when dealing with elderly patients. (p. 377)
5. State how a First Responder should deal with patients who are blind or deaf. (pp. 377–379)
6. State the special problems faced when caring for physically disabled patients. (p. 379)
7. State the special problems faced when caring for mentally retarded or developmentally disabled patients. (pp. 379–380)
8. **1st** Define "personal interaction" and tell why this is the best approach to take when caring for patients having emotional emergencies. (p. 380).
9. **1st** Describe the special problems faced when dealing with a patient under the influence of alcohol. (p. 381–382)
10. **1st** Define uppers, downers, and mind-affecting drugs (hallucinogens). (p. 382)
11. **1st** Describe, in general, a patient under the influence of each of the above substances. (p. 383)
12. **1st** Summarize the care given to patients who are the victims of drug abuse (use local rules and regulations provided by your instructor). (p. 384)
13. State some of the special problems faced when the patient is also a victim of crime. (p. 385)

SKILLS

Upon completing this chapter and your class lectures and skills labs, you should be able to:

1. Act out how you would gain information from:
   A. Young patients
   B. Deaf patients
2. Act out how you would provide care for a given situation involving:
   A. Elderly patients
   B. Blind patients
   C. Physically disabled patients
   D. Mentally retarded patients

1st 3. Act out how you would deal with a patient having an emotional emergency.

1st 4. Act out how you would deal with a patient under the influence of alcohol.

1st 5. Act out how you would determine that a patient is the victim of drug overdose and simulate the steps you would take in the care of this patient.

6. Act out how you would care for a patient at a simulated crime scene.

NOTE: Most of this chapter is optional in the typical First Responder course. Knowing how to deal with special patients is very important, but coverage of this topic usually is limited because of time restrictions. After you have completed your training, come back to any parts of this chapter not covered in your course. Those portions that are part of major First Responder courses have been marked in the objectives list.

THE PROBLEM OF AGE

The Child Patient

Everyone is somewhat afraid of the unknown. Since so many things are unknowns to a child, it is easy to see why emergencies can be so frightening for children. For most children, security comes from their parents. Any problems experienced by the child will be intensified if the parents are not at the scene. Wanting the parents may be a child's first priority, even above having you help or relieve pain.

When you are dealing with a child, you should:

- Let him know that someone will call his parents.
- If the child has a toy on the scene and wants it, make certain the child receives the toy.
- Sit with the child. If you stand, you will tower over him, inducing fear.
- Let the child see your face and speak directly to him. Speak clearly and slowly, making sure that the child can hear you. Try to maintain eye contact.
- Stop occasionally to find out if the child has understood what you have said or asked. Even if you communicate easily with your own children, never assume that a child has understood you. Find out by questioning the child.
- Determine as quickly as you can if there are any life-threatening problems and care for these problems (see Scansheet 16-1). If there are no problems of this nature, continue with patient survey and interview at a relaxed pace. When possible, do not move the child. To do so may cause additional injury or cause severe reactions if the child has a respiratory or heart problem. A fearful child cannot take the pressure of a rapidly paced examination and a lot of "meaningless" questions all being controlled by a stranger. An alert young child may become very frightened if you start to examine his head and face. Should a child show fear as you reach out to touch him, it might prove wiser to begin the secondary survey physical examination at the feet and slowly work your way up to the head. This survey is done looking for the same signs of illness and injury as would be done for the adult patient. However, you should take the time to consider special survey needs based on the anatomy of the child (see Figure 16–2).
- Always tell the child what you are going to do during a patient survey. Do not try to explain the entire procedure at once. Explain one step, do the procedure, then explain the next step.
- **Never lie to the child.** Tell the child when there might be pain during the physical examination. If a child asks if he or she is sick or hurt, tell the truth, but give reassurance by saying that you are there to help and other people also will be helping. *Smile* at the child. This is one sign from an adult that carries a lot of weight with most children.
- Touch the child on the forehead and hold his hand. The child will let you know if he does not wish to be touched. How much you have been accepted by the child will often show in the reactions to your touch. Do not force the issue. Your smile and your words can provide comfort to the child.

If the child's parents are on hand, do not direct all your conversation to them. Talk to the child. Should you be at the scene of an accident where the parents have also been injured, let the child know that people are taking care of them.

■ Scan 16-1.

Pediatric Emergencies—Primary Survey and Basic Life Support

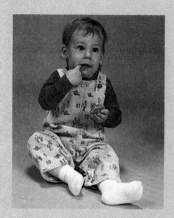

INFANTS

Birth to One Year

- Act as a professional—control your emotions and facial expressions. This may help reduce fear.
- Protect the head and spine. Remember, head and neck injuries are common because the infant's head is so large and heavy.
- Always ensure an adequate airway. When needed, provide adequate ventilations.
- Remember, even a small loss of blood may lead to shock.

Establishing unresponsiveness: The infant should move or cry gently when gently tapped or shaken.
Airway: Use the head-tilt, chin-lift. (The head-tilt, neck-lift may be needed to provide an adequate airway.)
Evaluating breathing: Use the *look, listen, feel* approach. If the infant is cyanotic or he is struggling to breathe, immediate transport is recommended.

Clearing the airway
- Use the mouth-to-mouth and nose or mouth-to-mask technique.
- Provide two adequate breaths.

If there is evidence of airway obstruction requiring action:
- Make certain that you have not overextended or underextended the neck.
- Straddle the infant over your arm face down and with the head lower than the trunk. Support the head by placing your hand around the jaw and chest. Add support by placing your forearm on your thigh.
- Rapidly deliver four back blows using the heel of your free hand. Strike directly between the shoulder blades.
- Place your free hand on the infant's back, sandwiching him between your two hands. Turn the infant over and place his back on your thigh. The head should be lower than the trunk.
- Rapidly deliver four chest thrusts as you would if providing external chest compressions for CPR.
- If the airway remains obstructed, but the patient is conscious, continue backblows and chest thrusts.
- If the airway remains obstructed, but the patient is unconscious, place your thumb into the patient's mouth, over the tongue. Wrap you other fingers around the lower jaw and look for an obstruction.
- Do *not* attempt blind finger sweeps. When removing an obstruction, use your little finger.
- If the patient is unconscious and the obstruction has not been dislodged, provide two breaths and repeat the procedure of back blows and chest thrusts, looking for and removing visible obstructions, and reattempting ventilations.

Rescue breathing
- Open the airway.
- Use mouth-to-mouth and nose or mouth-to-mask technique
- Provide two adequate breaths, noting the chest rise (take 1 to 1.5 seconds/ventilation).
- If airway is clear and patient is still not breathing, determine if there is a brachial pulse.

- If there is no pulse, provide CPR. Should there be a pulse, but no breathing, provide rescue breathing.
- Deliver one adequate breath every *three seconds*.
- Check for a pulse every few minutes.

CPR
- If patient is unresponsive and not breathing,—
  Open the airway.
  Provide two adequate breaths.
  Look, listen, and feel for breathing. If there is no indication of obstruction, but the patient is unconscious and is not breathing . . .
- Determine if there is a *brachial pulse*. If no pulse and no breathing, provide CPR.
  Apply compressions to the sternum, one finger width below an imaginary line drawn between the nipples.
  Use the tips of two or three fingers.
- Depress the sternum ½ to 1 inch.
- Deliver compressions at a rate of at least 100 per minute.
- Deliver a ventilation, mouth-to-mouth and nose or mouth-to-mask, *1 every 5 compressions* ("one, two, three, four, five"-breathe).
- Check for a brachial pulse every few minutes.

Bleeding
- Use direct pressure as a primary method.
- When necessary, use elevation, pressure points, or a blood pressure cuff. A tourniquet is a last resort.
- Consider a blood loss of 25 milliliters or more to be very serious.

Shock
- Consider the infant to be in shock if the blood loss is 25 milliliters or greater.
- Consider shock to be more severe if there is evidence of dehydration (vomiting, diarrhea, exposure to high temperatures, overheating, high skin temperature).
- Ensure adequate breathing and circulation, and control serious bleeding.
- Elevate the lower extremities, but avoid placing pressure on the cervical spine and head.
- Prevent the loss of body heat.
- Splint fractures.
- Avoid rough handling.
- Give nothing by mouth.
- Arrange for transport as soon as possible, monitoring vital signs.

Pediatric Emergencies—Primary Survey and Basic Life Support

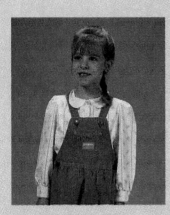

CHILDREN

1 to 8 Years

* Act as a professional—control your emotions and facial expressions. This may help reduce fear.
* Protect the head and spine. A child's head is proportionally large.
* Always ensure an open airway. When needed, provide adequate ventilations.
* Carefully evaluate blood loss.

Caution: The Size and Weight of the Child May Be More Important Than Age.

Establishing unresponsiveness: The child should move or cry when gently tapped or shaken.
Airway: Use the head-tilt, chin-lift or jaw-thrust to provide an adequate airway.
Evaluating breathing: Use the *look, listen, feel* approach. If the child is cyanotic or struggling to breathe, immediate transport is recommended. Should the child be in respiratory arrest, or is cyanotic and failing at attempts to breathe, make certain that the airway is open and clear of obstructions so you can begin rescue breathing efforts.

Clearing the airway
* Make certain that you have the proper head-tilt.
* Use the mouth-to-mask techniques or mouth-to-mouth and nose for small children and the mouth-to-mask or mouth-to-mouth techniques for large children.
* Provide two adequate breaths. Watch for the child's chest to rise.
If there is evidence of airway obstruction requiring action:
* Rapidly deliver six to ten abdominal thrusts.
* If the airway remains obstructed, but the patient is conscious, continue with sets of abdominal thrusts.
* If the airway remains obstructed, but the patient is unconscious, place the child on his back upon a hard surface. Provide support for his head and back as you move him. Place your thumb into the patient's mouth, over the tongue. Wrap your other fingers around the lower jaw and look for an obstruction. Do *not* attempt blind finger sweeps.
* If the patient is unconscious and the obstruction has not been dislodged, arrange for immediate transport, attempting two ventilations and repeating the procedure of abdominal thrusts, looking for and removing visible obstructions, and reattempting to ventilate.

Rescue breathing
* Open the airway without overextending the neck.
* Provide two adequate breaths, noting the chest rise.
* If airway is clear and patient is still not breathing, determine if there is a carotid pulse. If there is no pulse, provide CPR. Should there be a pulse, but no breathing, provide rescue breathing . . .
* Deliver one adequate breath every *four seconds.* Check for a pulse every few minutes.

CPR
* If the patient is unresponsive and not breathing,
Open the airway.
Provide two adequate breaths.
Look, listen, and feel for breathing. If there is no indication of obstruction, but the patient is still unconscious and is not breathing. . .

* Determine if there is a *carotid pulse.* If no pulse and no breathing, provide CPR.
* Apply compressions to the CPR compression site (locate the same way as you would an adult), using the tips of three fingers if the patient is a small child. For larger children, use the heel of one hand to apply compressions.
* Depress the sternum 1 to 1½ inches.
* Deliver compressions at a rate of 80 to 100 per minute.
* Deliver a ventilation as an adequate breath, mouth-to-mouth and nose or mouth-to-mouth or mouth-to-mask, *1 every 5 compressions.*
* Check for a carotid pulse every few minutes.

Bleeding
* Use direct pressure as a primary method.
* When necessary, use elevation, pressure points, or a blood pressure cuff. Use a tourniquet as a last resort.
* Consider a blood loss of 500 milliliters (½ liter or about 1 pint) or more to be very serious.

Shock
No one sign is absolute, but:
* Consider the child to be in severe shock if blood loss is 500 milliliters (about 1 pint) or more.
* Consider shock to be more severe if there is evidence of dehydration (vomiting, diarrhea, exposure to high temperature, overheating, high skin temperature).
* Ensure adequate breathing and circulation, and control serious bleeding.
* Evaluate uninjured lower extremities, but avoid placing pressure on the cervical spine and head.
* Prevent loss of body heat.
* Splint fractures.
* Avoid rough handling.
* Give nothing by mouth.
* Arrange for transport as soon as possible, monitoring vital signs.

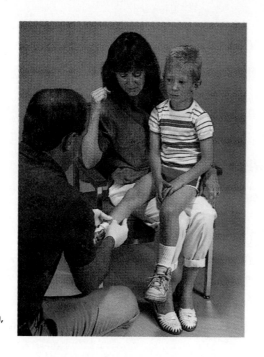

FIGURE 16–1.
When assessing young children,
do a "toes-to-head" survey.

When dealing with a possible case of child abuse, do not make any accusations. Provide whatever care is needed and follow the recommendations provided in the section of this chapter on patients who are crime victims.

Be a professional when dealing with the child patient. Do not allow your emotions to surface when dealing with an injured or seriously ill child. After your responsibilities are over, talk to your family and friends or to others in the EMS System to allow your own emotions to be released. Injuries to children can trigger emotions that should not be bottled up.

FIGURE 16–2.
Special survey considerations.

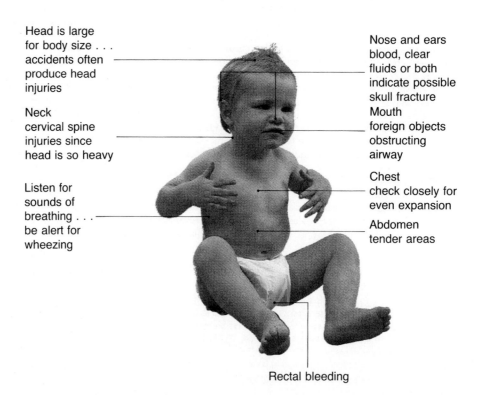

Head is large
for body size . . .
accidents often
produce head
injuries

Neck
cervical spine
injuries since
head is so heavy

Listen for
sounds of
breathing . . .
be alert for
wheezing

Nose and ears
blood, clear
fluids or both
indicate possible
skull fracture

Mouth
foreign objects
obstructing
airway

Chest
check closely for
even expansion

Abdomen
tender areas

Rectal bleeding

The Elderly Patient

As with any age group, those in late adulthood are individuals of all types and personalities. Never stereotype older patients. Deal with them as you would any adult. Find out the patient's name and use it frequently. Show respect by using "Mr.," "Mrs.," or "Miss." Never say "old timer," "pops," "grandma," or other such phrases.

Diminished hearing is a problem faced by some individuals as they age. Unresponsiveness to your questions may be due to a hearing problem, but do not assume that an older person cannot hear what you are saying. Avoid shouting whenever possible. Keep strong eye contact and speak directly to the patient. If need be, talk directly into the patient's ear.

As we grow older, words become more important. People in late adulthood spend more time thinking about what you say and what they are going to say back in response. This has been shown to have nothing to do with the mind slowing down. Older people, through experience, know that words can have many different meanings during a conversation and even more meanings after a conversation is over. Do not rush the speed of the conversation.

Many older people are isolated and this changes their speech patterns. You may find older patients changing topics or drifting slowly away from what you have questioned. In some cases, this may be due to changes in the circulation to the brain (hardening of the arteries); however, often this is simply because they are out of practice in the art of conversation.

As a First Responder, remember that your patient is an adult who has gone through other crises in life. Older patients know what works for them. Make certain that there are no life-threatening problems and then allow the older patient some control of the pace of the survey and interview.

If the patient's spouse or a close friend is at the scene, think of yourself as having more than one patient. You may be caring for a woman while her husband of 30 years watches in total fear that she may die. Provide emotional support to both individuals. Be watchful of partners and friends, for the stress of the situation could set off a heart attack or other medical emergency.

DEAF PATIENTS AND BLIND PATIENTS

The Deaf Patient

Seldom will you find a deaf person who is embarrassed about being deaf. Usually, it is the person who can hear who becomes embarrassed when trying to communicate with a deaf person. Unfortunately, most of us have little experience in communicating with the deaf. This is true despite the fact that several million people in our country are totally deaf and many others experience some serious degree of hearing loss.

Be aware that a patient might not be able to hear you. The patient may be able to speak clearly and still not be able to hear. In most cases, a deaf person will tell you of this condition or point to an ear and shake the head to indicate, "No, I cannot hear." Some patients may try to speak to you in sign, using the hands and fingers to make communicating gestures. When in doubt, write out, "Are you deaf?" on a card or piece of paper and give this to the patient.

Once you are aware of the patient's deafness, or hearing difficulty, see if the patient can read lips. Either write this out or ask, "Can you read lips?" When speaking to the lip-reading deaf patient, make certain your face is in bright light (use a flashlight if you have to). Speak slowly without distorting how you would normally form words. When you ask a question, point to your mouth to alert the person to read your lips. Never turn away from the deaf person while you are speaking.

Many deaf people cannot read lips. Your best methods of communication will be through writing and using gestures. If you point to an area on your body, gesture as if you are in pain, and point back to the individual, the patient will usually understand your question. During an examination, point to your own body before you attempt to do something to the patient's body.

Throughout the entire care of a deaf patient, try to keep face-to-face contact. Direct physical contact also helps. Hold hands, keeping one of your hands free to gesture or to gain attention by a gentle tap on the shoulder. When the dispatcher is alerted, make a gesture as if a phone call is being made. Point out the arrival of additional help.

Some deaf people can speak clearly, some can speak in a voice that may take a little practice to understand, and others may not be able to speak at all. If the patient cannot speak, use written communication. Should the deaf patient be able to speak, but you cannot understand something that was said, **do not pretend to understand.** This could be a serious mistake in gaining information and patient confidence. Always indicate that you do not understand by shrugging your shoulders as you place both hands in a palm-up position in front of your body. As you do this, you should say, "What did you say?"

The Blind Patient

Blind people are seldom embarrassed by their blindness. Again, it is the inexperienced person who usually becomes ill at ease when trying to communicate with the blind. Many individuals in emergency medicine claim that the survey and interviews of blind patients are really not that much different from those of sighted patients. If you remember to tell the blind patient what you are going to do before you do it, if you keep voice and touch contact throughout the period of care, and if you keep the blind person informed of what is happening (the source of strange noises, the arrival of additional help, and the like), you will find little extra difficulty in caring for the blind patient.

Try to remember three things when dealing with the blind. First, do not shout or speak loudly. Being blind does not mean that the person cannot hear. Second, do not change the words you would normally use in

FIGURE 16–3.
A blind person is led, not pushed.

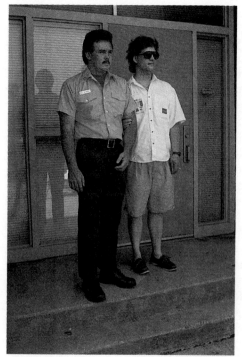

speaking to someone. People often become upset if they use the words "see" or "look" when they are with a blind person. Blind people also use these words. Your blind patients will know that you are not trying to embarrass them. As a third point, keep in direct contact with the patient through speech or touch.

Should you have to move a blind or vision-impaired patient who can walk, allow the person to hold on to your arm, standing slightly behind you, off to your side. Warn of steps and other hazards. *Never* push or pull the blind patient, always lead.

DISABLED PATIENTS

The Physically Disabled Patient

Most First Responder interaction with disabled patients will be with those who have muscle and skeletal or nervous system disabilities. Your biggest problem when dealing with these patients will be in conducting accurate physical assessments. These patients have body parts that function improperly or not at all. When such patients are injured, it is often impossible for the First Responder to evaluate the disabled limb or body part. You will have to assume there is injury and provide the standard form of care. A physician will have to determine if there is an injury.

Should an accident victim have a physical handicap, then you must ask questions about this handicap. This is the only way you may be able to detect injury to a disabled body part. For example, if the patient could move the left arm slightly before the accident and now finds that the arm won't move at all, then the possibility of direct injury to the limb, nerve damage, or spinal damage exists. This is not conclusive, but it is certainly better than assuming that the patient had no movement in the arm before the accident.

Ask questions about the specific nature of the patient's disability. Use terms such as "handicap" or "disability." Never use the terms "lame," "cripple," or "crippled." Gather as much information as possible through questions and the standard physical examination. If the patient tells you of a disability or of no longer having use of a limb, or reports a loss in function since the accident, do not grab the limb and try to move it yourself. To do so may cause additional injury if the accident has caused undetected fractures or dislocations.

As with most people, the physically handicapped like to do for themselves. If you want the typical patient to do something, then allow the handicapped patient capable of the task to have the same privilege. The exception is when you believe the patient has an injury to a disabled body part.

Mental and Developmental Disabilities

Some patients' disabilities do not involve body parts. These disabled individuals are handicapped by mental retardation or developmental disabilities. Your major task will be to establish relaxed, useful communications with the patient.

It is not always easy to detect mental retardation or developmental disability. At first, you may assume that you are dealing with the "typical" patient who may be a little confused. Whenever you suspect that the patient may be mentally retarded or developmentally disabled, you should:

1. Begin by treating the patient as you would any patient of the same age.
2. Ask questions that require a "yes" or "no" response and questions

that require a detailed response. Try some questions that require the patient to make a choice between answers. For example, "Would you like to sit here or over in that chair?" Find out if the patient knows where he is, the day of the week, and the date (at least the year).

3. Evaluate the patient's answers in terms of:
   • Understanding
   • What terms are familiar
   • What you may need to reexplain.

4. Listen carefully to everything the patient says, reassessing the level of understanding.

5. Slow the pace of the interview and examination. Be prepared for delayed responses and actions. Also, be prepared to reexplain the situation, your actions, and what you want the patient to do.

EMOTIONAL EMERGENCIES

What Are Emotional Emergencies?

Emotional emergency—a situation in which a patient's behavior is not typical for the occasion. The patient's emotions are strongly expressed, interfering with his or her thoughts and behavior.

Crisis—any event that the patient believes to be a turning point or crucial moment in life.

Emotional emergencies may be independent problems, or they may arise as the result of an accident, injury, illness, or disaster. As an independent event, the display of emotions you may find when you reach the patient might be due to depression, anxiety, or a psychiatric problem. If not independent, the problem could be the result of a crisis. Any crisis can cause a change in emotional state simply due to stress.

As a First Responder, always consider the emotional and mental health of the patient, family and friends, and the bystanders affected by the situation. Outward signs of depression, fear, hurt, and even hysteria may quickly go away once you begin to communicate with the patient. When someone loses control and is acting in a way that will cause harm or injury, you have a true emotional emergency.

Caring for the Patient

Personal interaction—a way of acting in a calm, professional manner to talk with and listen to a patient. During the process, emotional support can be accepted by the patient.

* Make certain that both you and the patient have clear access to the doorway of a room.

1st To evaluate and care for the patient having an emotional emergency, stay calm and act in a strictly professional manner. Observe the patient and attempt to narrow down the problem. Make certain that throughout the entire process of care you can eliminate the possibilities of head injury, stroke, insulin shock, and other medical emergencies.

Talk to the patient; have the patient talk to you. Listen to what the patient is saying and show that you have heard what was said. Do *not* threaten or argue with the patient (no matter what you may be called!). Reassure the patient that you are there to help. Speak in a calm, direct manner, maintaining eye contact whenever possible. This is personal interaction, your first line of action in trying to care for a patient having an emotional emergency.

If it seems that the patient may cause further harm or injury, make sure that dispatch is alerted to this fact and that the police are needed. Keep your distance from the patient and make certain that neither of you is "cornered."* Should a patient appear ready to become violent, move to a safe place and wait for police assistance. If you are a law enforcement officer, follow standard operating procedures.

As a First Responder, it is not your duty to restrain a patient. The law is very specific on who may restrain another person. Unless you are trained to do so and have proper help, **do not try to restrain a violent patient.** Not only might you hurt the patient or get hurt yourself, you may cause an even more violent reaction in the person.

Attempted Suicide

Whenever you have to care for a patient who has attempted suicide or is about to attempt suicide, your first concern is your safety. Make certain that the scene is safe and the patient does not have a weapon. Unless you are a trained law enforcement officer following standard operating procedures, do not try to deal with someone who has a weapon.

Make certain that dispatch is alerted to the problem and that the police are needed. If your own safety is secure, establish visual and verbal contact with the patient as soon as possible. Talk with the patient in a calm, professional manner. Make no threats and offer no indications of using force. Do not argue with or criticize the patient. Never joke about the situation. Ask if you can help. Find out if the patient is hurt. Stay calm and keep face-to-face contact whenever possible. Listen to the patient and let the patient know that you are paying attention. Do not place yourself in danger. If the patient gives any indications of wishing to harm others, make certain of your own safety and wait for police assistance.

ALCOHOL AND DRUGS

Alcohol Abuse

Alcohol is a drug, socially acceptable in moderation, but still a drug. Abuse of alcohol, as with any other drug, can lead to illness, poisoning of the body, antisocial behavior, and even death. A patient under the influence of alcohol is not funny. He or she may have a medical problem or an injury requiring your care. The patient may be injured or could hurt others while under the influence of alcohol.

As a First Responder, try to provide care for the patient suffering from alcohol abuse as you would any other patient. Quickly determine that the problem has been caused by alcohol and that alcohol abuse is the only problem. Remember, diabetes, epilepsy, head injuries, high fevers, and other medical problems may make the patient appear drunk. If the patient allows you to do so, conduct a primary and secondary survey that includes an interview. In some cases, you will have to depend on bystanders for meaningful information.

1st The signs of alcohol abuse in an intoxicated patient may include:

- The odor of alcohol on the patient's breath or clothing. This is not enough by itself unless you are sure that this is not "acetone breath" as experienced by the diabetic.
- Swaying and unsteady, uncoordinated movement.
- Slurred speech and the inability to carry on a conversation. Do not be fooled into thinking that the situation may not be serious because the patient jokes or clowns around.
- A flushed appearance, often with the patient sweating and complaining of being warm.
- Nausea and vomiting or the desire to vomit.

1st A patient suffering from alcohol abuse may be going through withdrawal from having been without alcohol. Delirium tremens (DTs) may result from sudden withdrawal. In such cases, look for:

- Confusion and restlessness

- Atypical behavior, to the point of being "mad" or demonstrating "insane" behavior
- Some DT patients will hallucinate
- Gross tremor (obvious shaking) of the hands

As you see, some of the signs displayed in alcohol abuse are similar to those found in medical emergencies. **Be certain** that the only problem is alcohol abuse. Remember, persons who abuse alcohol may also be injured or ill. The effects of the alcohol may mask out the typical symptoms and signs used in assessment. Also, be on the alert for other signs, such as depressed vital signs due to the patient mixing alcohol and drugs. Never ask if the patient has taken any "drugs." The patient may think that you are gathering evidence of a crime. Ask if any "medications" have been taken while drinking.

1st The basic care for the alcohol abuse patient consists of:

1. A proper survey and interview to detect any medical emergencies or injuries. Remember, alcohol may mask pain. Look carefully for mechanisms of injury and the signs of illness.
2. Monitoring of vital signs, staying alert for respiratory problems.
3. Talking in an effort to keep the patient alert.
4. Helping the patient when vomiting so that vomitus will not be aspirated (breathed in).
5. Protecting the patient from further injury without the illegal use of restraint.
6. Alerting dispatch and letting them decide if the police must be alerted or if EMTs are to respond on their own.

Drug Abuse

Upper—a stimulant that will affect the central nervous system to excite the user.

Downer—a depressant that will depress the central nervous system to relax the user.

Narcotic—a class of drugs that affects the central nervous system for the relief of pain. Illicit use is to provide an intense state of relaxation.

Hallucinogen—a mind-affecting or mind-altering drug that acts on the central nervous system to excite the user or to distort his or her surroundings.

Volatile chemicals—vaporizing chemicals that will cause excitement or produce a "high" when they are breathed in by the abuser.

1st Drugs may be simply classified as uppers, downers, narcotics, hallucinogens (mind-affecting drugs), or volatile chemicals. Uppers are stimulants affecting the nervous system to excite the user. Downers are depressants meant to affect the central nervous system to relax the user. Narcotics affect the nervous system and change many of the normal activities of the body. Often they produce an intense state of relaxation and feelings of well-being. Mind-affecting drugs act on the nervous system to produce an intense state of excitement or distortion of the user's surroundings. Volatile chemicals are depressants acting on the central nervous system.

Some courses that train rescuers, EMTs, and others in the EMS System have spent considerable time in the past teaching specific drug names and reactions. As a First Responder, you will not need such knowledge. For you, it is important to be able to detect possible drug abuse at the overdose level and to relate certain signs to certain types of drugs. Your care for the drug abuse patient will be basically the same for all drugs and will not change unless you are ordered to do something by a poison control or drug abuse center. Table 16–1 provides some of the names of common drugs being abused. Do not worry about memorizing this chart.

Signs of Drug Abuse

The symptoms and signs of drug abuse and drug overdose can vary from patient to patient, even for the same drug. The scene, bystanders, and the patient may be your only sources for finding out if you are dealing with drug abuse and the substance involved. When questioning the patient and bystanders, you will get better results if you ask if the patient has been taking any medications rather than using the word "drugs." If you have any doubts, then ask if the patient has taken drugs or is "using anything."

TABLE 16–1. COMMONLY ABUSED SUBSTANCES

Uppers	Downers	Narcotics	Mind-affecting Drugs	Volatile Chemicals
Amphetamine (Benzedrine, bennies, pep pills, ups, uppers, cartwheels) Biphetamine (bam) Cocaine (coke, snow, crack) Desoxyn (black beauties) Dextroamphetamine (dexies, Dexedrine) Methamphetamine (speed, meth, crystal, diet pills, Methedrine) Methylphemidate Preludin	Amobarbital (blue devils, downers, barbs, Amytal) Barbiturates (downers, dolls, barbs, rainbows) Chloral hydrate (knockout drops, Noctec) Ethchlorvynol (Placidyl) Glutethimide (doriden, goofers) Methaqualone (Quaalude, ludes, Sopor, sopors) Nonbarbiturate sedatives (various tranquilizers and sleeping pills: Valium or Diazepam, Miltown, Equanil, meprobamate, Thorazine, Compazine, Librium or chlordiazepoxide, reserpine, Tranxene or chlorazepate and other benzodiazepines) Paraldehyde Pentobarbital (yellow jackets, barbs, Nembutal) Phenobarbital (goofballs, phennies, barbs) Secobarbital (red devils, barbs, Seconal)	Codeine (often in cough syrup) Demerol Dilaudid Heroin ("H," horse, junk, smack, stuff) Methadone (dolly) Morphine Opium (op, poppy) Meperidine Paregoric (contains opium)	DMT LSD (acid, sunshine) MESCALINE (peyote, mesc) Morning glory seeds PCP (angel dust, hog, peace pills) Psilocybin (magic mushrooms) STP (serenity, tranquility, peace) ⎯⎯⎯⎯⎯ Nonhallucinogenic Mind-altering ⎯⎯⎯⎯⎯ Marijuana (grass, pot, weed, dope) Hash THC	Cleaning fluid (carbon tetrachloride) Furniture polish Gasoline Glue Hair spray Nail polish remover Paint thinner Amyl nitrate (snappers, poppers) Butyl nitrate (locker room, rush)

1st Some significant symptoms and signs related to specific drugs include:

- *Uppers*—excitement, increased pulse and breathing rates, rapid speech, dry mouth, dilated pupils, sweating, and the complaint of having gone without sleep for long periods.
- *Downers*—sluggish, sleepy patient lacking normal coordination of body movements and speaking with slurred speech. Pulse and breathing rates are low, often to the point of a true emergency.
- *Mind-affecting drugs*—fast pulse rate, dilated pupils, and a flushed face. The patient often "sees" things, hears voices or sounds that do not exist,

FIGURE 16-4.
Abused substances.

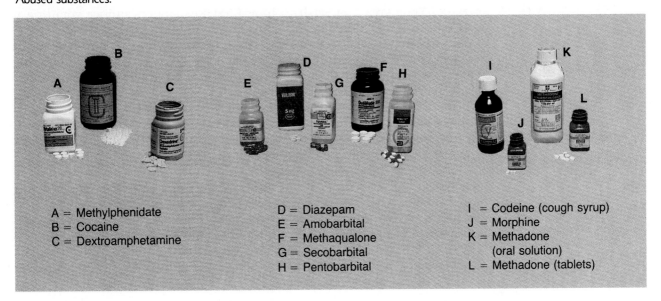

A = Methylphenidate
B = Cocaine
C = Dextroamphetamine

D = Diazepam
E = Amobarbital
F = Methaqualone
G = Secobarbital
H = Pentobarbital

I = Codeine (cough syrup)
J = Morphine
K = Methadone (oral solution)
L = Methadone (tablets)

has little concept of real time, and may not be aware of the true environment. Often, the patient makes no sense when speaking. Many show signs of anxiety and fearfulness. They have been described as "paranoid." Some patients become very aggressive, while others tend to withdraw.

- *Narcotics*—reduced rate of pulse and breathing, often seen with a lowered skin temperature. The pupils are constricted, muscles are relaxed, and sweating is heavy. The patient is very sleepy and does not wish to do anything. In overdoses, coma is a common event. Respiratory arrest may occur.
- *Volatile chemicals*—dazed or showing temporary loss of contact with reality. The patient may go into a coma. The inside of the nose and mouth may show swollen membranes. The patient may complain of a "funny numb feeling" or "tingling" inside the head or a headache. The face may be flushed and the pulse rate accelerated. There may be a chemical odor to the patient's breath, skin, or clothing.

These symptoms and signs have a lot in common with many medical emergencies. Never assume drug abuse or drug abuse occurring by itself. **NOTE:** Many drug abusers will abuse more than one drug, often mixing several at one time. Because of this, it may be impossible through simple physical examination to tell what drugs are causing the patient's problem. **1st** Withdrawal varies from patient to patient and from drug to drug. In most cases of drug withdrawal, you will see shaking, anxiety, nausea, confusion, irritability, sweating, and increased pulse and breathing rates.

Care for Drug Abuse Patients

1st When providing care for drug abuse patients, you should:

1. Provide life-support measures if required.
2. Alert dispatch as soon as possible. They should be informed that the problem may be caused by drugs.
3. Monitor vital signs and be alert for respiratory arrest.
4. Talk to the patient to gain confidence and to maintain the level of consciousness.
5. Protect the patient from further harm.
6. Provide care for shock.
7. Continue to reassure the patient throughout all phases of care.

NOTE: Your area may wish to have First Responders induce vomiting if an overdose was taken within 30 minutes of your arrival at the scene. Your instructor will give you the rules and exceptions for your area. In most cases, vomiting is induced the same as in cases of ingested poisons. For all cases of possible drug overdose, it is good practice to contact your local poison control center.
CAUTION: Many drug abusers may appear calm at first and then become violent as time passes. Always be on the alert and be ready to protect yourself. If the patient creates an unsafe scene and you are not a trained law enforcement officer, *get out* and find a safe place until the police arrive.
CAUTION: PCP is a dangerous drug that is being abused more and more each year. Patients on PCP can be very dangerous, even though they may appear calm when you arrive. If PCP is the cause of the problem, wait for police to arrive, unless the patient is unconscious or in need of life-support measures. PCP usage leads to aggressive behavior. The drug can build up in the body and cause a violent reaction without warning. Many patients on PCP no longer display the qualities considered "human." Always consider a PCP user to be dangerous.

VICTIMS OF CRIME

If a crime is in progress or if the criminal is still at the scene, do not attempt to provide care. Wait until the police arrive or until the scene is safe.

Your first duty as a First Responder is to provide emergency care to the patient. In addition, you must try to preserve the chain of evidence that will go from the crime scene to the courtroom. Touch only what you need to touch. Do not use private telephones unless you have no choice and must immediately alert the dispatcher. Move the patient only if there is danger or if the patient must be moved to provide proper care (for example, to a hard surface for CPR). If you touch or move anything, be certain to tell the police.

If the crime is a rape or child abuse, do not wash the patient or allow the patient to wash or use the bathroom. Do not let the patient change clothes. Do not allow any liquids or food to be taken. To do so may destroy evidence. Explain your actions to the adult patient. Comfort and distract the child patient while you wait for help to arrive.

When approaching a crime victim, make certain that you clearly identify yourself by name and say that you are a First Responder trained to help. Otherwise, you may be mistaken for the criminal returning to the scene. Do not burden the patient, especially the rape victim, with questions about the crime. Keep to your duties involving the care of the patient.

One of the most important things a First Responder can do when caring for a crime victim is to provide emotional support and reassurance.

SUMMARY

The child patient requires special care. Keep in mind that the child is frightened, wants his parents, and considers you a stranger. After making certain that there are no life-threatening problems, slow down your pace of examination and questioning. Make sure the child knows what you are asking and what you are doing. Remain professional with your emotions, smile, and talk to the child to provide comfort. Try to maintain eye contact.

Remember that patients in late adulthood have faced other emergencies. The elderly patient may set a pace of examination and interviewing different from your normal one. The older patient knows what works, so allow some control. Never assume that an older patient cannot hear you or cannot think clearly. Provide emotional support to the patient, family, and friends.

Always make certain that a patient can see and hear you. If the patient is deaf, establish this fact and then find out if the patient can read lips or if you will have to use writing and gestures for communication. Try to keep face-to-face contact with the deaf patient.

When dealing with blind patients, do not raise your voice. Talk as you would to any other patient, and keep both verbal and physical contact with the patient throughout all stages of care.

Take great care when assessing the physically handicapped patient who is involved in an accident. A disabled body part may have been injured. Ask the patient questions about the disability so that you can determine if the accident has caused any change. Let the physically handicapped patient do things when it is safe to do so.

If you believe a patient may be mentally retarded or developmentally disabled, take your time to assess the level of understanding. Keep the interview and examination slow-paced, staying on the alert for delayed answers and actions.

In cases involving emotional emergencies, maintain a professional manner and talk calmly with the patient. Show that you are listening. If the patient is violent, wait for police assistance. Never try to provide care for a conscious patient who has a weapon.

Patients suffering from alcohol abuse should receive the same professional level of care as any other patient. Be certain that the problem is due to alcohol or alcohol withdrawal. There may be a medical problem or injuries. Try to detect the odor of alcohol, slurred speech, swaying, and unsteadiness of movement. Find out if the patient is nauseated. Be alert for vomiting. In cases of alcohol withdrawal, look for hand tremors that may indicate the DTs. In all cases of alcohol abuse, monitor vital signs and be alert for respiratory arrest.

Drug abuse can show itself in many ways, depending on the drug, the patient, and whether you are dealing with withdrawal or overdose. Withdrawal from most drugs will produce shaking, anxiety, nausea, confusion, irritability, sweating, and increased pulse and breathing rates.

Uppers usually speed up activity, speech, pulse, and breathing and tend to excite the user. Downers do just the opposite. Mind-affecting drugs increase pulse rate, dilate pupils, and cause the patient to see things and lose touch with reality. Narcotics reduce pulse and breathing rates. The pupils usually will be constricted. The patient may appear sleepy and may not wish to do anything. Volatile chemicals act as depressants, causing the patient to be dazed.

In cases of drug overdose or drug withdrawal, provide life support as needed and alert the dispatcher. Monitor vital signs and talk to the patient. Protect the patient and provide care for shock. Reassure the patient through the entire care process.

If you are to provide care at the scene of a crime, make certain that the scene is safe. Your first priority is to provide care for the patient, but be careful not to break the chain of evidence.

Always clearly identify yourself when you approach the patient. Be certain to provide emotional support.

Do not allow rape and child abuse victims to wash, change clothing, use the bathroom, eat, or drink. Care for medical problems and injuries rather than asking a lot of questions about the crime.

CHAPTER 17

Gaining Access to Patients

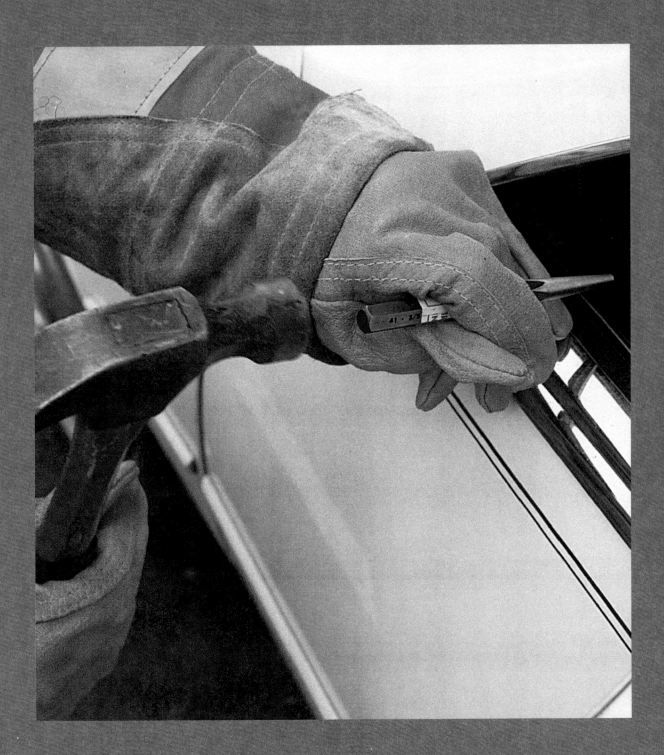

■ OBJECTIVES

By the end of this chapter, you should be able to:

1. State what factors you need to evaluate at the scene of a motor vehicle accident. (pp. 388–389)
2. Describe several ways in which you can make a motor vehicle accident scene safe so that you can gain access to the patients. (pp. 389–391)
3. List the four major ways to gain access to patients who are in a closed, upright vehicle. (pp. 391–392)
4. Describe how you might stabilize a vehicle that is on its side. (p. 396)
5. State how you would gain access to patients who are in a stabilized vehicle that is on its side. (p. 396)
6. State how you would free patients pinned by parts of vehicles or jammed inside of vehicles. (pp. 397–398)
7. Describe the basic ways in which to gain access to patients found in houses and buildings. (pp. 398–399)
8. List the rules of safety you should follow if there is a fire at the scene. (pp. 399–401)
9. State what you should do if electrical hazards or gas hazards exist at the scene. (p. 401)
10. State how to recognize a possible hazardous materials incident. (pp. 402, 404–405)

SKILLS

Upon completing this chapter and your class lectures and skills labs, you should be able to:

1. Demonstrate how you would evaluate and make safe the scene of an automobile accident.
2. Demonstrate how you would stabilize an upright vehicle and then gain access to patients.
3. Demonstrate how to stabilize an overturned, closed vehicle.
4. Act out the release of pinned and trapped patients.
5. Act out gaining access to patients when there is a fire at the scene. (This requires training beyond the typical First Responder course.)
6. Act out First Responder activities at a scene with electrical, natural gas, or propane gas hazards.
7. Demonstrate the safe gathering and reporting of information from a hazardous materials scene when such activities are appropriate for a First Responder.

FIRST RESPONDER SAFETY

Your first consideration at any emergency scene is your own safety. Professionals in the EMS System avoid taking chances. They do what they have been trained to do, using the proper equipment and the required number of trained persons needed to do a task. There are some risks, but most are controlled risks. For example, you have no control over the slight chance that a drunk driver could crash into you as you provide care at an accident scene. However, you do have control over the normal risks involved at such a scene by using the proper warning devices (for example, flares) to divert traffic, and by parking your own car properly away from the scene.

At any emergency scene, you should always:

1. Evaluate the scene—make certain that you will be safe. You may have to take steps to control potential dangers.
2. Wear the proper protective gear—use what is appropriate for the situation (goggles, gloves, and so on).
3. Do only what you have been trained to do—act as an EMS professional. If you attempt to do things beyond your training, you may injure yourself, cause harm to the patient, or cause an accident.
4. Get the help you need—have dispatch alerted to the situation and the personnel and equipment that may be required.

MOTOR VEHICLE ACCIDENTS

The Scene

As a First Responder, once certain of your own safety, the main duty at the scene of an accident is to provide patient care. If the accident involves motor vehicles, you may have other duties to perform before you can provide this care. Your responsibilities at the scene may include:

*   Making the scene safe
*   Evaluating the situation and calling for help
*   Gaining access to patients
*   Evaluating patients and providing emergency care
*   Freeing trapped patients
*   Removing and moving patients who are in danger from fire, potential explosion, and the like
*   Removing and moving patients, if necessary, to provide care or to reach another patient who is in need of life-saving care

Many individuals are injured each year when they attempt to help victims of motor vehicle accidents. Usually, these people are struck by another vehicle. Most often, this occurs because the scene was not safe. Assessment and care cannot be rendered until the scene is safe.

If you are a law enforcement officer, follow standard operating procedures. Likewise, if you are in the fire service and have been trained for such scenes, follow standard operating procedures. However, if you are a First Responder without a special course in accident scene procedures, use the items listed here as guidelines. Since each motor vehicle scene is unique, you will need to act as a professional, carefully observe the scene, and decide what actions to take to control the situation.

1st When arriving at the scene of a motor vehicle accident, you should follow local protocols. In most cases, the following are used:

1. Pull your vehicle completely off the road surface. If possible, park no closer than 50 feet from the scene. Turn on your vehicle's emergency flasher. If it is night and your vehicle is facing oncoming traffic, turn off the headlights.
2. Make certain that you have parked in a safe location. Look for fuel spills and fire. Are you downhill from the scene? If you are, fuel may run in your direction. Check the wind direction. Will it carry smoke or fire to where you have parked?
3. Turn off the engine, and set the parking brake.
4. Set emergency warning devices, such as flashing lights or flares, to warn others (see Scansheet 17.1). On high-speed roads, place one of these devices at least 250 feet from the scene. On low-speed roads, set

■ SCAN 17-1.

Warning Devices

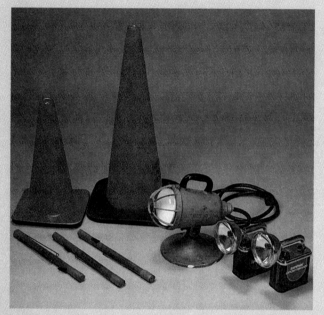

Use your vehicle's emergency flashers and set up highway use approved emergency warning devices. For low visibility and night use, you must have flashing lights or flares.

WARNING:
KEEP THE FLARE POINTED AWAY FROM YOUR BODY. WATCH OUT FOR SPILLED OR LEAKING FUEL, DRY GRASS, AND DEBRIS ON

Igniting Flares
Use one hand to grasp the flare near its base and your other hand to pry off the plastic cap to expose the scratching surface. Pull off the cap to expose the ignitor. Hold the flare in one hand and the cap in the other, keeping the scratching surface against the ignitor. Use a sharp movement so that the ignitor strikes against the scratching surface. Always move the flare away from your body.

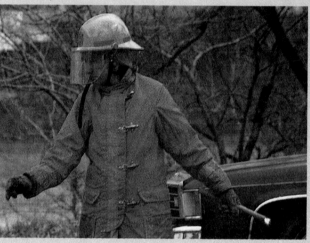

THE ROAD SURFACE. REMEMBER, LEAKING FUEL WILL FLOW DOWNHILL.

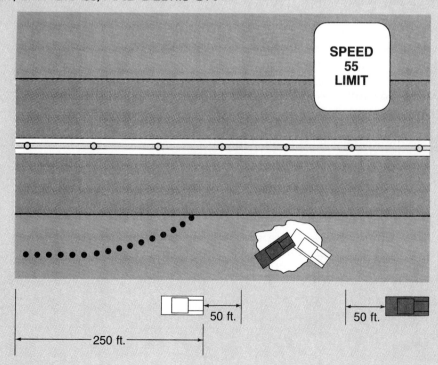

one of these devices at least 100 feet from the scene. Add at least 25 feet to these measurements if the scene involves a curve in the road. If appropriate, ask for help so that you can gather tools and supplies and put on protective gear.

NOTE: As a First Responder, you may ask citizens for help at an accident scene, but you cannot order them to assist you. If people wish to help, alert them to potential dangers. If you are a law enforcement officer, follow standard operating procedures.

5. Again, check the scene for safety. Is there fire, leaking fuel or gases, unstable vehicles, or downed electrical wires? If the scene involves such hazards, make certain that someone phones or radios for all the help you will need. You may need to request that electrical power be turned off. It may be necessary for the fire service and rescue squad to respond. Your area may have all services respond to motor vehicle accidents.

6. If it is safe to do so, see how many potential patients there are. Does it appear as if someone could have been thrown from a vehicle? Are there open doors that indicate that someone may have walked away from the scene? Do you see any signs of an infant or child having been in the vehicle (bottles, toys, and the like)? Are there any indications that a pedestrian or bike rider was involved? Have someone alert dispatch and report the number of possible patients.

7. If the scene is safe, gain access to the patients, do your surveys, and begin care. Surveys and care will be covered in Chapter 19.

Do not attempt to gain access to patients if the scene is too dangerous. If you cannot control traffic at the scene, you are in danger. If electric lines are down, you are in danger. If there is fire at the scene, you are in danger. Ask for help to control traffic. Follow the guidelines in this chapter regarding electrical hazards. Do *not* ignore fire. If you are not trained to deal with a vehicle fire, protect yourself and stay in a safe area.

1st REMEMBER: A First Responder's first priority is personal safety. Your primary duty is to provide patient care at a safe scene. Do only what you have been trained to do.

The Closed Upright Vehicle

In most traffic accidents, the vehicles involved remain upright. Vehicles found in this position are the easiest to approach and to work in and around. Usually, the vehicles are stable, with little chance of rolling or sliding away from their at-rest position.

Make certain that you evaluate the stability of the vehicle when you assess the scene. As you look for traffic hazards, electrical hazards, spilled fuel, and fire, also see if there is any chance that the vehicle(s) may begin to roll away or flip over. You may find the following situations:

- **Inclined surface**—the vehicle may have come to rest on a surface that slants enough to allow forward or backward roll. Wheel chocks (a wedge or block that can be placed against a wheel to prevent movement), spare tires, logs, rocks, or similar objects should be used to keep the vehicle from rolling.
- **Slippery surface**—ice, snow, or oil can produce a road surface that will allow a vehicle to slide as the door is opened. Chocking the wheels will reduce the chances of this happening.
- **Tilted vehicle**—even though a vehicle is upright, it may be tilted to one side, or possibly slanted down a steep hill. Do *not* work on the downhill side of the vehicle. Chocking the wheels may help. If strong rope or line is available, tie lines to the frame of the car (not the bumper) in front and back or to both sides and then secure the lines to strong trees, guardrails, or heavy, secured vehicles. If possible, wait for the rescue squad or fire department to arrive.

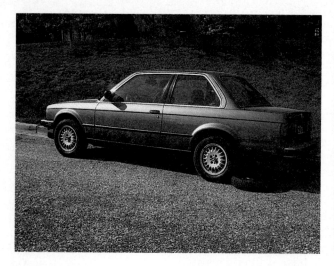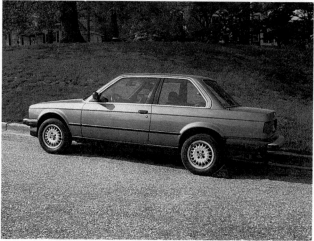

FIGURE17–1. Stabilize the vehicle before rendering care.

- **Stacked vehicles**—part of one vehicle may be resting on top of another vehicle. You will have to chock the wheels of both vehicles. You may have to insert tires, lumber, blocks, or other materials between the road surface and the part of the misplaced vehicle that is closest to the road surface. In some cases, you may have to use line or rope to tie and secure both vehicles.

1st REMEMBER: Never try to enter or work around a vehicle until you are certain that it is stable.

In most cases, you will approach an upright, stable vehicle. Usually, the doors and windows will be closed. There are four ways to gain access to the patients in such a situation:

1st 1. **Opening the doors**—many people drive without locking their doors. Be sure to check all the doors to a vehicle, including side and rear doors on vans and hatchbacks. If all the doors are locked, one of the patients may be able to assist you by unlocking a door.

1st 2. **Through a window**—locked or jammed doors will require you to gain access through a window. If the patient can roll down a side window, the problem of access is easily solved. Directions for breaking windows will be given later in this section.

3. **Prying doors open**—a pry bar or jack handle can be used to pry open the doors of most cars made before 1967. This method will not work for most cars made after this date. When it does work, the method is very time consuming. Prying open doors is not considered a First Responder skill. Access through windows is usually more practical.

4. **Cutting**—the process of cutting metal to gain access through vehicle roofs, trunks, and doors is not considered a First Responder skill. If you cannot gain access through a door or window, it is possible to cut around the lock of a door, using a sharp tool (chisel or strong screwdriver) and a hammer. This method will not work on most cars made before 1967.

Unlocking Vehicle Doors

Special tools are available for unlocking doors, but training in their use is not a part of most First Responder courses and few First Responders carry such tools. However, you can unlock many vehicle doors with a wire hook made from a coat hanger or with a bent oil dip stick. A piece of wire with a washer attached to one end can be used on "thief-proof" locking buttons. See Scansheet 17.2 for directions in unlocking a vehicle door.

■ SCAN 17-2.

Unlocking Vehicle Doors

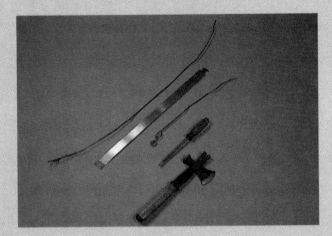

Various tools can be used to help unlock vehicle doors:
  wire hook (coat hanger)
  slim-jim® (or similar device)
  wire and washer
  screwdriver
  flat pry bar

An oil dip stick or a keyhole saw may be used to help force up a locking button

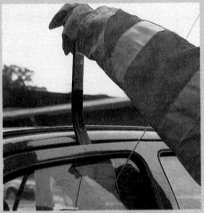

1 Framed windows. Pry frame away from vehicle body and insert wire hook

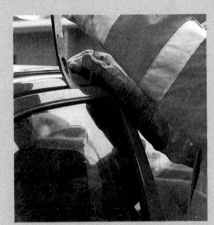

2 Snag the locking button and pull upward

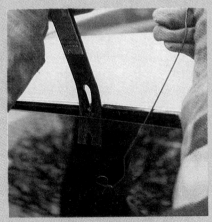

Unframed windows. Pry window and insert wire hook, screwdriver, keyhole saw, or dip stick to lift button

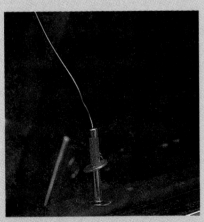

"Thief-proof lock." Insert washer on wire and drop over shank. Pull up and allow washer to cant and grab.

Keep in mind that speed is crucial. If you have to return to your vehicle or another location to retrieve tools, precious time will be lost. Take all the tools you may need. If you cannot unlock the door, you may have to break glass to reach the lock.

Before attempting to unlock the door, check if all the vehicle's doors are locked. If so, see if the people inside can safely help you by unlocking a door. Check the doors for damage. If a door is so severely damaged that it might not open, it would be foolish to try to unlock it. If all the doors are severely damaged (a rare happening), be prepared to break glass and gain access through the window. Note, too, if the car has hidden buttons or slot buttons in the armrest. You will not be able to easily open locked vehicle doors having such devices. Should the vehicle have electrically operated locks and windows, you may not be able to unlock the door if the battery is disabled.

Gaining Access through Vehicle Windows

At the scene of an accident, most people consider breaking the windshield of a vehicle if they cannot gain access through the doors. Unfortunately, this is the wrong approach. Windshields are made of laminated safety glass having great strength. Even when shattered, the glass will still cling to an inner plastic layer. All cars have laminated safety glass windshields. Many foreign cars have this type of glass in all the vehicle's windows.

Rear and side windows are usually made of tempered safety glass. When this glass is broken, there is no plastic layer to hold the pieces. Tempered safety glass will not shatter into sharp pieces or shards. Instead, this glass will shatter into rounded pieces about ¼ inch in size. Some of these pieces can cut the occupants trapped in the vehicle, but these cuts are seldom serious. If occupants can shield their faces or look away, there is little chance of any injury.

The real danger comes from glass entering open wounds. This risk is necessary if you must quickly enter a locked vehicle to render life-saving care or assess a patient who may not be breathing. Most of the time, this glass can be removed by the emergency department physician before it has a chance to cause additional harm. Always alert the EMTs to the possibility that glass may have entered the patient's wounds. They can pass this information on to the emergency department staff.

The risk of flying glass can be greatly reduced if you use a sharp tool (punch) and a hammer to tap the window until it breaks. To simply "bash" the glass with a hammer will probably send pieces throughout the entire passenger compartment. If you apply adhesive-backed contact paper or duct tape to the window before breaking the glass, you may reduce the number of pieces forced onto the victims.

1st When gaining access through a vehicle window, you should:

1. Make certain the vehicle is stable. If possible, have the driver turn off the ignition.
2. Be sure that access through a door is not possible.
3. Protect yourself by wearing gloves and protecting your eyes. Goggles, safety glasses, or a face shield should be worn. If you lack *either* gloves or eye protection, drape a coat, towel, or blanket over the glass before you attempt to break through the window, and position yourself so that you can shield your face with your shoulder and upper arm.

   REMEMBER: Never attempt to break through a tempered safety glass window by striking it with a blunt object unless you have no choice due to the patient's condition or the danger of the scene. If you must use a blunt object such as a hammer, warn the patients so they can cover their faces. In cases where you do not have eye protection, cover your head with a coat or blanket. Once you are properly positioned, you do not have to see the window in order to break it.

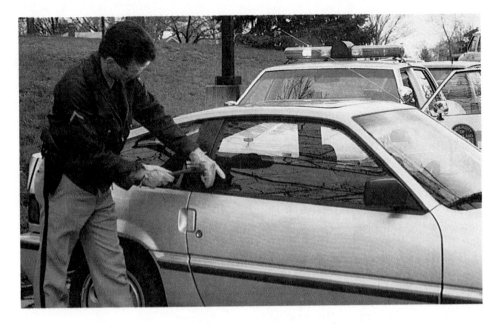

FIGURE 17–2.
Protect yourself when breaking glass.

4. If possible, select a window that is away from the patients. Use a sharp tool to break through a tempered safety glass window (a punch, Halligan tool, or the pike of a Pry-Axe or similar tool). *Begin in one of the lower corners, as close to the door as possible.* Deliver light taps to the tool with a hammer and increase the strength of each blow until the glass shatters. If no other tools are available, use a jack handle point.

5. Once you are through the window, try to open the vehicle door from the inside. You may only have to unlock the door to open it. Many jammed doors that will not open from the outside will open from the inside of the vehicle.

6. Make certain that the vehicle ignition is off and that its transmission is set in park. When safe to do so, engage the parking brake.

The Overturned Closed Vehicle

First Responders should *not* try "righting" a vehicle found in an overturned position. Before you try to reach the patients inside of such a vehicle, it must be stabilized. In addition, you must be alert for spilled fuel or battery acid leaking from an overturned vehicle.

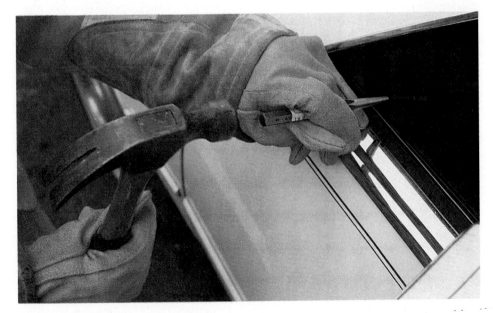

FIGURE 17–3.
Use a sharp object, positioned at a lower corner of the glass.

Unless you have special training and equipment, stabilizing overturned vehicles is not part of First Responder duties. If your area wishes you to know how to stabilize such a vehicle, this will be a special part of your course. Your instructor will inform you of your responsibilities and show you how to deal with this very hazardous situation.

The Vehicle on Its Side

1st If you find a vehicle on its side and are specifically trained to deal with this situation, you should:

1. Stabilize the vehicle by using tires, blocks, lumber, wheel chocks, rocks, or whatever materials are available. Place these stabilizers between the roof line and the road surface and between the wheels and the road surface (if possible). Note how this is done in Figure 17–4.
2. If time allows, or the vehicle is still unstable, use strong rope or line to tie the vehicle to secure objects.
3. Try to enter through a door.* If this is not possible, attempt to gain access to the patients by going through a window as described earlier. The rear window is the best approach to take.
4. Once you open a door, keep it tied open. Do not try to prop a door open. Props can slip or be knocked away, causing the door to slam on you or your patients.

* This is very dangerous since the door may be 7 feet or more off the ground. Also, your actions may *destabilize* the vehicle period.

Patients Pinned beneath Vehicles

In the vast majority of cases where patients are pinned beneath a vehicle, it is best to wait for the rescue squad to arrive. (Do *not* reach or crawl into where the patient is pinned.) However, if you believe that the scene is too dangerous, or life-saving measures require that the patient be freed from the trapped position, then certain procedures can be done by First Responders and bystanders working together. Any such procedures are

FIGURE 17–4.   Stabilize the vehicle before trying to gain access to the patients. This requires special training.

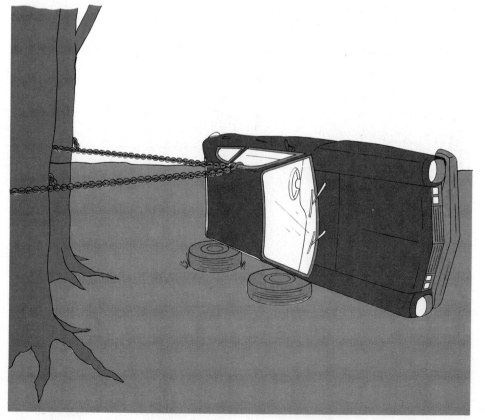

too dangerous if the vehicle is on its roof (*never* attempt to use a jack on vehicles in this position).

A vehicle can be raised to allow the patient to be moved from the pinned position. A jack or pry bar and blocks can be used, or you and the bystanders may be able to lift the vehicle or wreckage off of the patient. In all cases, you *must* shore up the vehicle as you work so that it will not slip or fall back onto the patient. Blocks, tires, lumber, or whatever else you can find at the scene should be used to make certain the vehicle remains shored up. Do *not* attempt any such procedures until the entire vehicle is stable.

Patients Caught in Wreckage

You may find patients with their arms, legs, or heads thrown through a window. Before trying to free them, you should:

1. Use dressing materials, towels, blankets, or clothing to protect the body part thrown through the window.
2. Use pliers, the claws of a hammer, or a knife to break or fold away glass trapping the patient. This requires very careful moves to avoid cutting the patient. Do *not* attempt this with glass that is impaled in the patient. Wait for the EMTs to arrive.

If you provide First Responder care at motor vehicle accident scenes on a regular basis, you will see cases where patients are jammed inside of their vehicle. In many cases, special power tools operated by skilled rescue personnel will be needed. Other times, the trapped patient can be easily set free.

1st As a First Responder working with patients pinned inside a vehicle, you will be able to free some patients by:

- Simply removing wreckage from on top of and around the patient
- Carefully moving a seat forward or backward
- Carefully lifting out a back seat
- Removing a patient's shoe in order to free a foot or cutting away clothing caught on wreckage
- Cutting seat belts, taking great care to properly support the patient during the cutting and after the tension has been released

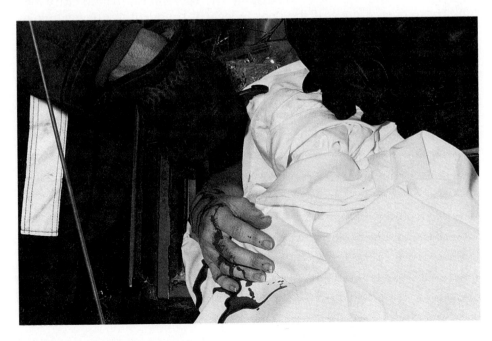

FIGURE 17–5. Protect the patient from injury while removing glass.

Unless you have no choice due to dangers at the scene, avoid the above procedures with any patient who might have neck or spinal injuries. If there is no immediate danger, leave the patient in place until more highly trained personnel respond to the scene. During the wait, keep bystanders away from the vehicles and do not allow smoking at the scene.

PATIENTS IN BUILDINGS

First Responder Responsibilities

Gaining access to a patient in a locked building may require special skills and tools outside the range of First Responder duties. There are many types of gates, doors, and windows, and an even wider variety of locks. In addition to these problems, there are the dangers associated with old buildings, the barriers presented by special security devices, and the hazard of dogs at the scene.

As a First Responder, you are not expected to know how to open or destroy locks, to have all the tools needed for the variety of windows, doors, and gates found in buildings, or to know how to enter and make your way safely around an abandoned building. No one expects the First Responder to go up against trained guard dogs.

1st What are your responsibilities in terms of gaining access to patients found inside of buildings? You will be expected to:

- Make certain that someone alerts dispatch
- Try opening doors
- Try opening windows
- Call bystanders and neighbors to see if they have a key
- Look quickly for a key under mats or in mailboxes
- Break glass to unlock doors or windows

The exception to these is when you know or can see that someone inside needs immediate care. Do not waste time trying to gain access before calling for help. Have someone alert the dispatcher. Your efforts to gain entry may fail. Try to open a door. If the door is locked, try opening a few windows on your way to finding a second door. If the second door is locked, do not start hunting for a third door or more windows. Break the glass in a window or a door and enter as quickly but as safely as possible.

Entering Buildings

When you find the doors to a building are locked and there is no quick access to a key, try to reach the person by way of a low window. Do not try climbing up walls or posts to reach a high window. Do not try to gain access to a window by walking across roofs. Should the windows at low level be locked, you will have to break glass in order to enter the building. Do *not* attempt to break through doors or windows made of large sheets of tempered glass. This glass is very strong and it is flexible enough to bounce a hammer back into your face.

REMEMBER: Wear gloves and have protection for your eyes.

1st To break window or door window glass, you should:

1. Make certain that the patient is not lying near the other side of the glass.

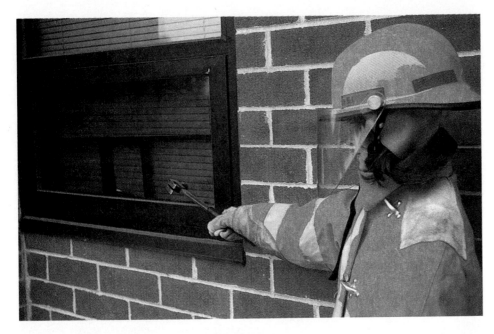

FIGURE 17–6.
When doors and windows are locked, break glass to gain access to the locks.

2. Use a hammer, jack handle, or pinch bar to break the glass near one of its edges. If you do not have tools, throw a rock or other suitable object through the glass. (A night stick or an aluminum "aircraft" flashlight will break most window glass.)

3. Carefully clear all glass from the frame and reach in to unlock the door or window. If your only point of entry is through a window that will not open, break and clear out all the glass and frames necessary for you to enter.

4. Make certain that you are stepping onto a safe floor if you are entering through a doorway. Be sure that you do not have an unusual drop and the floor is safe when entering through a window. Take a moment to visually inspect the floor for signs of weakness and damage.

HAZARDS

Fire

Television and movies have led people to believe that they should enter burning buildings or run up to burning vehicles in order to save victims. This is a very dangerous tactic. Those in the fire service are highly trained to do their jobs. They are given special equipment and use special strategies to fight fires at a minimum risk to their own safety. Fire fighting requires special training, protective clothing, the right equipment, and usually more than one firefighter.

If you are a member of the fire service, follow standard operating procedures for rescue involving vehicle and structural fires. If you are in law enforcement and have special training in rescue involving vehicle and structural fires, do only what you have been trained to do. Should you be a First Responder without fire fighting training, do not risk your life to provide care.

Motor vehicle accidents do not usually produce fire and most medical and injury emergency calls to buildings do not involve fire. However, these events do occur and you must be prepared to protect yourself. Your own safety is the first priority. The following rules should be followed by First Responders with no training or little experience at fighting fires:

- *Never* approach a vehicle that is in flames. Using blankets, sand, or a hand extinguisher is fine, if you know how to evaluate the fire and the

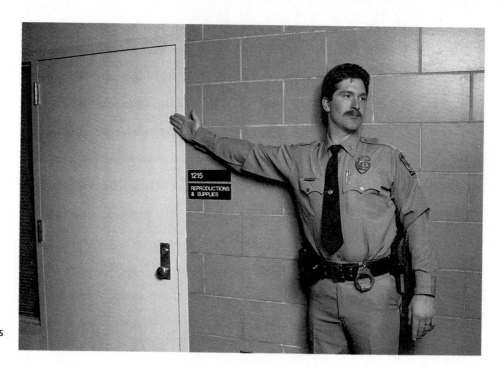

FIGURE 17–7.   If a door is hot, *do not open it.*

danger of explosion, and if you have protective clothing and know how to attack a fire. If you do not know these things and do not have the necessary protection, stay clear. Make sure that dispatch knows there is a fire or the possibility of a fire.

- *Never* attempt to enter a building that is on fire. Even a small fire can spread toxic fumes throughout the structure. Remember that most of the fire could be hidden within the walls, floors, and ceilings.
- *Never* enter a room or building if smoke is present or go through an area of dense smoke or possible toxic gases.
- *Never* attempt to enter a closed building or room giving off grayish yellow smoke. To do so will cause a backdraft condition that immediately increases the intensity of the fire or causes an explosion.
- *Do not* enter a building unless others know that you are doing so. There

FIGURE 17–8.   If trapped by fire or smoke, stay low and crawl to safety.

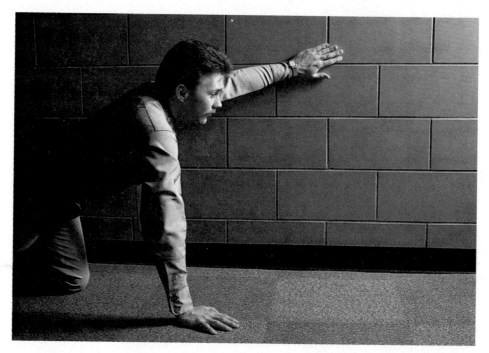

may be an undetected fire. When possible, do not work by yourself. Do as the fire service does and work with a partner or a team.

- *Never* open a door that is hot to your touch. Always feel the top of the door. If it is hot, *do not open the door.* (*Note:* Door knobs and handles also may be hot.) If the door is cool, open it with great caution and avoid standing in its path as it opens.
- *Never* use the elevator if there is the possibility of a fire in a building. The elevator shaft can act as a flue, pulling in flames, hot toxic gases, and smoke. Also, an electrical failure could trap you in the elevator. Keep in mind that some elevators have heat-activated call buttons. The elevator may take you to the fire floor, open, and expose you to lethal heat or toxic gases.
- If you find yourself in smoke, stay close to the floor and crawl to safety.

IMPORTANT: The best recommendation is this: if you lack fire fighting training, do not enter any building involved with fire or that may be on fire. If bystanders tell you there is a fire, do not enter, even if you do not see smoke or flames. Leave rescue and fire fighting to the fire service.

Electrical and Gas Hazards

The odor of natural gas at the scene of a motor vehicle accident is a rare occurrence. If you do find such a happening, move patients away from the apparent leak, keep bystanders away from the scene, and alert dispatch. The EMS System should be told about the gas so that they can activate other services and request that gas in the area be shut off or diverted.

1st The smell of natural gas in a building is a more likely possibility. If you find yourself in such a situation, leave the building and call dispatch. Report the odor of gas. If the gas is coming from a bottled source, do not try to turn off this source unless you have experience with this type of system, you can vent the area, and the gas odors around the tank are mild (this is very difficult to judge without specialized equipment). At your own risk, you may judge the odor of natural gas to be mild enough within a structure and enter to rescue a patient. Remember that there is always a danger of fire or explosion. Play it safe and request the help you will need.

WARNING: If you suspect a gas leak, do *not* turn lights on or off, use the doorbell, use any electrical equipment (including portable radios and flashlights), or use any open flames (matches, flares, and the like).

1st If electrical wires are down at a scene and block your pathway to a patient, or if they are lying across a car, do *not* attempt a rescue. Never assume that the lines are dead or that a "dead" line will stay dead. Do not be fooled by the surrounding area. Even if lights are off all around you, the wire blocking your path may be live or could be re-energized as you pass by. Call or have someone alert the dispatcher and request that the power be turned off. Even if you believe the power has been turned off, it is still best to wait for rescue personnel to arrive.

1st Patients in a car that is touching a downed wire or is near a downed wire should be told to stay in the vehicle and avoid touching its sides. If downed wires are touching the car and the patients have to leave the vehicle because of fire or other danger, you must tell them to jump clear of the car without touching it and the ground at the same time. If they touch both simultaneously, they will complete a circuit and may be electrocuted.

Hazardous Materials

There may be hazardous chemicals and other materials at the scene of an accident or medical emergency. If such materials are at the scene and you are told that there is a possible danger, or if you believe a possible danger exists, do *not* attempt a rescue or to provide First Responder care. No one should attempt a rescue unless he or she is trained to do so, has the needed equipment and personnel, and is in contact by radio or phone with hazardous materials experts.

The possibility of hazardous materials exists at every industrial scene and every farm, truck, train, ship, barge, and airplane accident. It should always be assumed that there are unsafe hazardous materials until their presence can be totally ruled out. When in doubt, stay clear.

As a First Responder in a hazardous materials situation, **protect yourself and call for the help you will need**.

If the scene has chemical transport tanks or containers, spilled liquids, leaking containers, gas cylinders, or bottles—stay clear! Do *not* think that a scene is safe simply because the substance has no apparent odor. Keep as far from the scene as is practical. Position yourself so that you are not downhill or downwind from the scene. Stay out of low spots where vapors may collect. Do not take a high point that may be contaminated with vapors should the wind shift. Avoid streams, drainage fields, sewers, and sewer openings.

Phone or radio the dispatcher. If the closest phone is at the scene, do not use it. Find a safe phone away from the scene. In localities that do not have a common dispatcher for all emergency services, it makes little difference if you phone the police, fire service, rescue squad, or hazardous materials team. Each can contact the other to coordinate a hazardous materials response.

If, for some reason, you cannot contact dispatch, phone 800-424-9300 (202-483-7616, collect, in the Washington, D.C. area). This will place you in contact with the Chemical Transportation Emergency Center (CHEMTREC), operated by the Chemical Manufacturers Association. Experts will provide you with the needed guidance.

CHEMTREC the Chemical Transportation Emergency Center that provides immediate expert information to emergency personnel at the scene of a hazardous materials incident.

Make certain that the dispatcher or CHEMTREC has your name and call back number. When possible, provide the following information:

1. The nature and location of the problem
2. An estimate of how many possible patients there are both in and out of the danger zone
3. Special problems at the scene such as fire, crowds, and traffic

Let the dispatcher know your position. Ask the dispatcher to find out if you are safe and if you should stay on the line. *Insist* that you be given this information from a hazardous materials expert. The dispatcher can reach this expert or patch you through. If this cannot be determined, you may have to move to another phone or radio location.

Be prepared to stay on the line and answer the following questions:

- What type of material is at the scene?—Experts need to know if the material is a gas, liquid, or dry chemical, a cooled chemical, or a radioactive solid, liquid, or gas.
- What is the name of the material, or does it have an identification number?—Look for labels or placards that are visible from your safe point. A pair of binoculars can be used to help in reading this information.
- Can you supply the name of the shipper or manufacturer?—From a safe point, look for names on railroad cars, trucks, or containers. Ask bystanders, drivers, or railroad or factory personnel.
- Can you describe the type of container?
- Is the material in a railcar, truck, open storage, covered storage, or housed storage?
- Can you estimate how much material is at the scene?
- What is the current state of the material?—You should report if its container is apparently still intact, or if you are dealing with a leaking

FIGURE 17–9. Hazardous materials placard.

liquid, an escaping gas, or a spilled powder. Report if the material appears stable or if it is in flames, vaporizing, or being blown into the air.

- Can you estimate how long the scene has been dangerous?
- Are other possible hazardous materials near the scene?
- What are the weather conditions?—Rain and wind are of major concern.

In most cases, it will not be possible for you to obtain and pass on most of this information. However, any information you supply can be of critical importance. Keep this in mind if you start feeling helpless because you cannot enter the scene and provide care. Calling and supplying any information will make a difference.

A major source of information at a hazardous material scene is the National Fire Protection Association (NFPA) or Department of Transportation materials, placard. This is a colored placard on the vehicle, tank, or railroad car. It has a four-digit identification number. Older placards have a "UN" or "UA" preceding the numbers. This number will give the dispatcher access to the name of the material.

Should a victim of a hazardous material incident leave the danger zone and be in need of help, limited First Responder care may be possible. If you have stayed in contact with the dispatcher, you can be given information as to what is safe for you to do. Without confirmation of your safety, you may have to shout directions to the victim or have victims care for each other. Even though it would be a rare incident, victims may have chemicals on their bodies and clothing that could be harmful to you. Initial care includes:

1. Flushing the skin, clothing, and eyes of anyone coming into contact with the hazardous substance. This should be done for at least 20 minutes with water, *unless* the material is dry lime(p. 337).
2. Contaminated clothing, shoes, and jewelry must be removed and the patient's skin should be flushed with water.
3. Blankets and protection from the enviornment must be used to maintain body temperature.

The victims may be able to wash themselves. If you decide to do the washing, it will have to be done by a small diameter hose from uphill and as far upwind as possible. Keep in mind that you would be doing so at your own risk.

Do *not* place yourself at risk by attempting mouth-to-mouth resuscitation of a contaminated victim. Resuscitation of contaminated patients requires equipment that will not "blow back" into the rescuer's mouth or face.

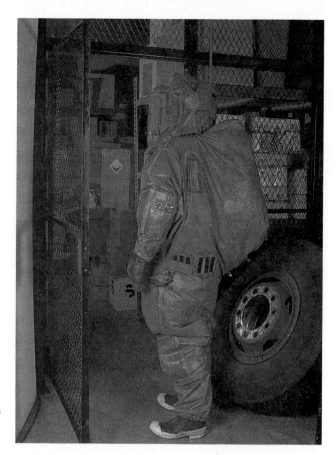

FIGURE 17–10. Special personnel and equipment are required at a hazardous materials incident.

REMEMBER: The best thing for you to do is to contact the experts and remain in a safe area.

NOTE: If you receive specialized training in the hazardous materials scene, you would do well to obtain Hazardous Materials, The Emergency Response Handbook, available from the Department of Transportation (DOT P 5800.2).

Radiation Accidents

1st First Responders should stay clear of accidents involving radioactive materials. Your first duty is to protect yourself from exposure. Your next step should be to call for assistance from a safe area away from the scene.

Be on the lookout for radiation hazard labels. Stay upwind from any containers having these labels. Follow the same basic rules as you would when dealing with any hazardous material. The greater the distance you are from the source and the more objects there are between you and the source (concrete, thick steel, earth banks, heavy vehicles, and the like), the safer you will be.

There are three types of radiation accident patients:

1. *Clean patient*—one who has received an external dose of radiation. In other words, the patient has been irradiated or exposed to the radiation without coming into contact with fallout and debris. Care can be provided for this type of patient, in a safe area, with no risk to the rescuer.
2. *Dirty patient, internal contamination*—one who has received an internal dose of radiation. The patient must be externally cleansed before care can be rendered.
3. *Dirty patient, external contamination*—one who must be decontaminated before contact and care are possible. If there are open wounds, these must be cleaned after external decontamination.

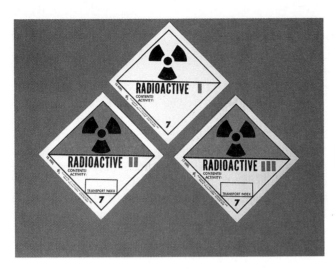

FIGURE 17–11. Radiation hazard labels.

If a victim leaving the danger zone requires care, you cannot provide direct care unless it is certain this is a clean patient. When there is the slightest doubt, treat this victim as a dirty patient. If additional help will be delayed in arriving, you can begin decontamination procedures at your own risk (you will probably not have a Geiger counter to determine radiation levels). This must be done outside the danger zone. A water wash and the removal of clothing, shoes, and jewelry with a continuous wash is recommended. It is best if this is done by the victim or other victims until help arrives. Whenever possible, have experts do the decontamination procedures. The contaminated clothing and wash water must be contained to prevent the spread of radiation.

SUMMARY

Part of your First Responder duties may include caring for patients at the scene of motor vehicle accidents. Your first priority is your own safety; your first duty, as a First Responder, will be patient care. However, you also may have to do your part to make the scene safe. **Evaluate the scene,** looking for hazards including: **traffic, fire, downed electrical lines, hazardous materials,** and **unstable vehicles.**

When evaluating the scene, make certain that you can **account for all victims** of the accident.

Always check to be certain that an upright vehicle will not roll forward or backward. Use wheel chocks, rocks, spare tires, or whatever is suitable at the scene to **stabilize vehicles** on inclines, tilts, or slippery surfaces. If one vehicle is stacked upon another, both vehicles must be stabilized.

Try to gain access to your patients by **opening doors.** If this is not possible, gain access **through a window.** If you must break the glass in a vehicle window, do so only if the vehicle is **stable** or has been stabilized. Your best choice is a rear or side window. Have the patients cover their faces or look away to protect themselves from flying glass.

Wear **gloves** and **eye protection** when you are breaking glass. If these items are not available at the scene, cover the glass and/or your face before trying to break the glass.

Do not use a blunt object when trying to break a tempered safety glass vehicle window. Use a **sharp tool** and **hammer,** with the tool positioned at a lower corner of the window. Start with light taps and increase the strength of each blow until the glass is broken.

First Responders should not attempt to work in and around overturned vehicles or try to right such vehicles.

When dealing with vehicles found on their sides, you must **stabilize** the vehicle before trying to reach the patients. Once this is done, do only what you are trained to do. For example, you might try to enter **through a door.** Be sure to tie open any door you use. If need be, enter by **breaking the rear window.**

First Responders should remove patients from vehicles only when there is danger or life-saving care requires such a move. Never try to remove patients trapped under a vehicle turned over on its roof. If the vehicle is upright or on its side and you have to free a person trapped by this vehicle, **have bystanders help.** Use a jack, pry bars and blocks, or all the bystanders needed to lift the vehicle. The vehicle must be **stabilized** and must be **shored up** as you lift.

When caring for a patient whose arm, leg, or head is thrown through a car window, protect the body part with dressing or some other covering. Carefully break or fold the glass away before moving the patient. Do not attempt this with glass impaled in the patient.

Patients jammed or trapped in wreckage often can be freed by **removing wreckage, adjusting** or **removing seats, removing shoes** or **cutting away clothing** or **seatbelts.**

Doors, then windows, are the best routes for gaining access to patients in buildings. If the doors are locked and you do not have a key, try the windows. If the windows are locked, **break glass** in a door or window, protecting yourself with gloves and goggles, or coverings over the glass and your face. Before breaking the glass, check to be sure that the **patient is safe** from being struck by the broken glass. Make certain that you are stepping onto a safe floor.

Leave fire fighting to those trained to do the job. Take great care at the scene of motor vehicle accidents if there is a fire. Do not approach a burning vehicle unless you have been trained to assess the hazard, evaluate and fight the fire, and have the needed protective and fire fighting equipment.

Building and other structural fires require actions to be taken by trained personnel. Do *not* enter a building that is on fire or may be on fire! Do *not* try to go through smoke or potentially toxic gases. Do *not* attempt to enter a building or room that has grayish-yellow smoke coming from the doors, windows, or other venting sources. **Always feel closed doors for heat. Do not open a door if it is hot.** Do *not* use elevators if there is the chance of a fire. If caught in a burning building, stay low and crawl to safety.

If you smell natural gas at the scene, stay clear and alert dispatch. If electrical hazards exist at the scene, *do not attempt a rescue.* Alert dispatch to have the power turned off. Shutting off gas or electricity should be done by trained personnel.

In cases of accidents where wires are touching a motor vehicle, stay clear and protect yourself. **Have the patients stay in the car.** If they must leave the car, warn them not to touch the car and the ground at the same time.

If the scene contains hazardous materials or radioactive materials that may pose a danger to you, stay in a safe area and phone for help. Be prepared to provide dispatch with essential information.

CHAPTER 18

Moving Patients

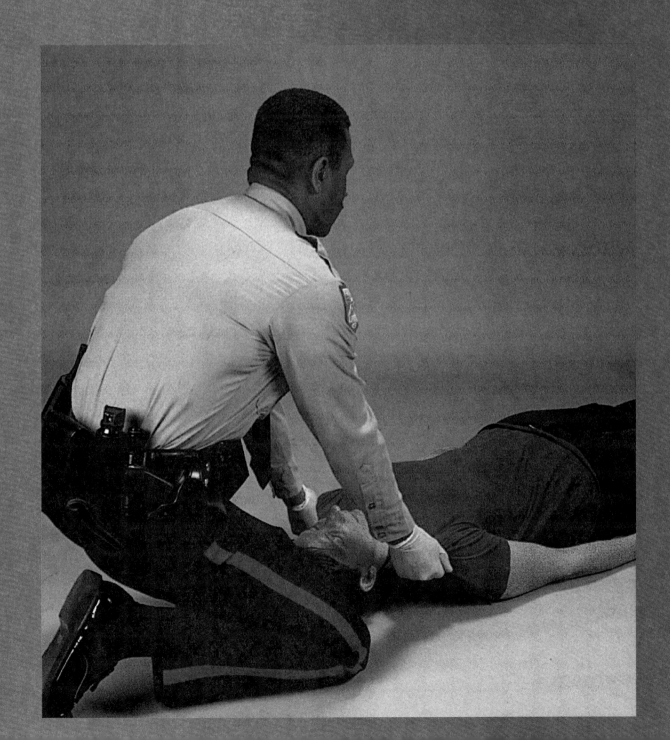

■ OBJECTIVES

By the end of this chapter, you should be able to:

1. Define emergency move and nonemergency move. (pp. 408–409)
2. State several reasons for moving a patient. (pp. 408–409)
3. Name the most common emergency moves to be used by First Responders. (pp. 410–417)
4. Name the most common moves used by First Responders in nonemergency situations. (pp. 417–419)

SKILLS

Upon completing this chapter and your class lectures and skills labs, you should be able to take situations presented by your instructor and:

1. Evaluate the situation and decide if the patient should be moved.
2. Select the best technique to use for moving a given patient.
3. Demonstrate the one-rescuer assist, the fire fighter's carry (optional), the pack strap carry, and at least one type of one-rescuer drag.
4. Working as a member of a team, demonstrate a direct ground lift for a patient with no neck or spinal injuries.
5. Working as a member of a team, demonstrate a direct ground lift for a patient with a suspected neck or spinal injury (if approved by your EMS System).
6. With one other student, demonstrate an extremity lift.

PRINCIPLES OF MOVING PATIENTS

When to Move a Patient

Whenever possible, you should not move a patient. First Responders should care for a patient, try to keep the patient stable, and wait for the EMTs to respond. This holds true even when the patient appears to be able to move about. Keeping the patient at rest is your best course of action. Remember, you may have missed the signs of an injury or a medical problem during your survey of the patient. Also, not all patients are honest in answering your questions during an interview. Some patients will deny injury or illness. **1st** There are times when you must move a patient. These situations call for emergency moves. An emergency move should take place when:

- **The scene is hazardous**—uncontrolled traffic, fire or threat of fire, possible explosions, impending structural collapse, possible electrical hazards, toxic gases, and other such dangers may make it necessary to move a patient quickly in order to protect both you and the patient.
- **Care requires repositioning**—you may have to move a patient to a hard, flat surface to provide CPR, or you may have to move a patient in order to reach a profusely bleeding wound.
- **You must gain access to other patients**—you may have to quickly move a patient with no neck or spinal injuries in order to reach another patient needing life-saving care. This is seen most often in motor vehicle accidents.

1st It may become necessary to perform a nonemergency move of a patient. Even though there is not immediate danger to yourself or to the patient, a nonemergency move could be justified because:

- *Factors at the scene cause patient decline*—if a patient's condition is *rapidly* declining due to heat or cold, moving may be necessary. If the patient is reacting strongly to something at the scene and may go into allergy shock, you may have to move the patient. These situations rarely call for emergency moves.
- *You must reach other patients*—when there are other patients at the scene, you must reach them to do a survey and to provide care. Care must be taken to avoid additional pain and injury to the patient being moved.
- *Care requires moving the patient*—this is usually seen in cases where there are no injuries or severe medical problems. Problems due to extreme heat or cold, such as heat cramps, heat exhaustion, hypothermia, and frostbite, are good examples. Reaching a source of water to provide washing in cases of serious chemical burns may be reason to move a patient.
- *The patient insists on being moved*—you are not allowed to restrain patients. If they will not listen to the reasons why they should not be moved and are trying to move on their own, you may have to assist them. Sometimes a patient becomes so upset that stress worsens the condition. If this type of patient can be moved, and the move is a short one, you may have to do so in order to keep the patient stable.

How to Move a Patient

There are a great number of techniques (called *moves*) to reposition or move a patient. In First Responder care, the best moves are done with the help of other trained personnel or bystanders. Unless you are alone, all nonemergency moves should be carried out with the help of others. More often than not, emergency moves will have to be made by yourself.

Moves a general term used to describe any organized procedure used to reposition or move a sick or injured person from one location to another.

Nonemergency moves should be carried out in such a way as to prevent additional injury to the patient. Care should be taken to avoid patient discomfort and pain. Emergency moves rarely provide any protection to patient injuries, and they may cause great pain for the patient. This is justified because of the reasons given for emergency moves. The situation is too dangerous for you and the patient, or life-saving care cannot be provided unless the patient is quickly moved.

1st The following rules are to be followed for a nonemergency move:

1. The patient should be conscious.
2. The patient survey should be completed.
3. Pulse and breathing rates and character should be stable, within normal ranges.
4. There shoud be no uncontrolled external bleeding or any indications of internal bleeding.
5. There must be *absolutely* no signs of neck or spinal injury, and the mechanism of injury should not point to possible neck or spinal injury.
6. All fractures must be immobilized or splinted.

Lifting Techniques

1st You must use the correct lifting techniques to avoid lower back and knee injuries. Utilizing the rules of correct lifting also will help you maintain your balance and help prevent a fall that could injure you and your patient. When you must lift a patient, you should:

1. Think through the move before attempting it. Know what you are going to do and how to prevent possible difficulties.
2. Do not attempt to lift or lower someone if you cannot handle and control the weight.

3. Always begin the move from a balanced position and stay aware of your balance. Losing your balance can cause serious injuries to you and the patient.
4. Make certain that you initially have good, firm footing and can maintain it throughout the lift.
5. Lift with your legs, not your back. Bend your knees, keeping one foot slightly in front of the other. Keep your back straight as you lift with your legs.
6. Stay aware of your breathing. You do not want to lift and carry a patient while holding your breath.
7. When possible, keep your back straight when carrying a patient.

EMERGENCY MOVES

1st The One-Rescuer Assist

You will find situations where a patient in a dangerous environment is able to walk alone or with a minimum of assistance. Always assist this type of patient. Keep in mind that the patient's condition could change rapidly.

Stand beside the patient and place the patient's arm closest to you around your neck. Keep hold of this arm by the wrist. Slip your free arm around the patient's waist. Walk the patient from the scene, moving as quickly as necessary, while still trying to adjust for the balance and speed of the patient. If this method proves too slow for the hazard you are trying to escape, you may have to use another method.

The one-rescuer assist is also an excellent way to move many minor injury patients during a nonemergency move.

The Fire Fighter's Carry

In extreme emergency situations, when fire or threat of explosion exists, the fire fighter's carry is a valuable technique to know and use. Typically, this move is used for patients who are unconscious or in a low state of awareness. As useful as the move may be, it is not considered to be part of many First Responder courses. Carrying out this technique requires strength, balance, and coordination that have been developed through prac-

FIGURE 18–1. The one-rescuer assist is useful in both emergency and nonemergency moves.

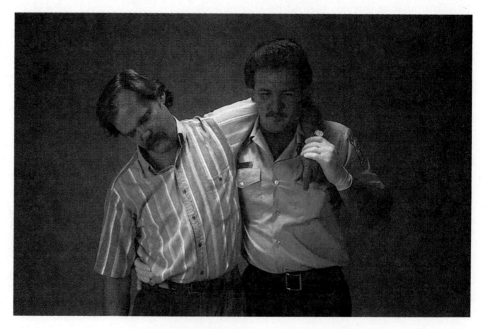

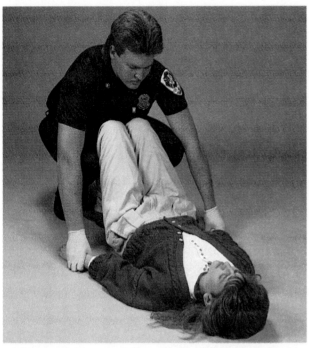

FIGURE 18–2.
Fire fighter's carry, step 1.

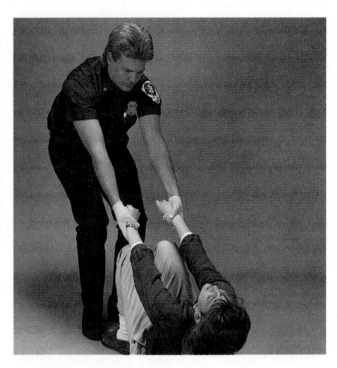

FIGURE 18–3.
Fire fighter's carry, step 2.

tice. Even when you know the move and are in good physical condition, *you may not be able to perform this carry because of the size of the patient.*

The fire fighter's carry requires you to lift the patient from ground level and carry the patient on your shoulder. You should begin the move with the patient lying face up. If conscious, have the patient bend the knees slightly, keeping the feet in a flat position. Since true emergencies seldom leave time for directions, you may find that it is best not to worry about the patient's knee and foot positions.

FIGURE 18–4.
Fire fighter's carry, step 3.

FIGURE 18–5.
Fire fighter's carry, final step.

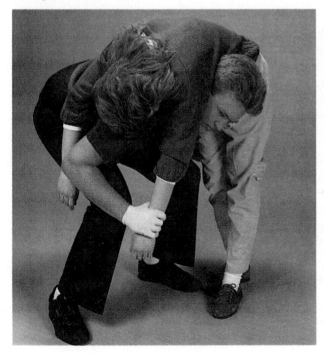

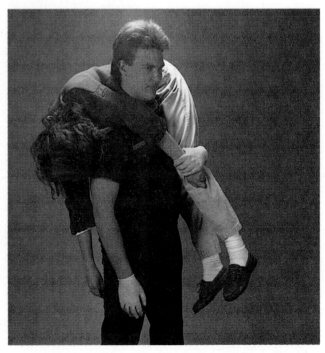

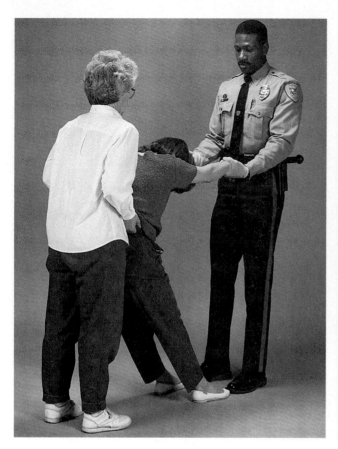
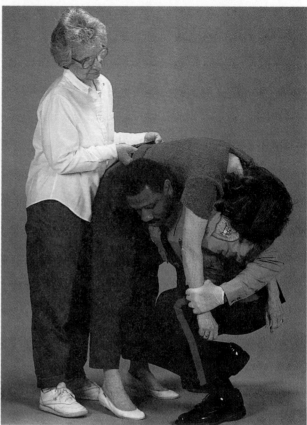

FIGURE 18–6A and 18–6B. The fire fighter's carry is more useful when you have someone to help you lift and position the patient.

Step close to the patient, taking hold of the patient's wrists. Balance yourself so that you can begin to pull the patient's upper body toward her knees. Place your feet against the patient's feet.

Pull the patient toward you, lifting her upper body. Bend at the waist and flex your knees to allow your shoulder to be in position to accept the patient's body at waist level.

Duck down and pull the patient across your shoulder, keeping hold of one of her wrists. With your free arm, reach between the patient's legs and grab hold of one thigh.

Let the weight of the patient fall onto your shoulders and stand, lifting with your legs, still holding onto the patient's wrist and thigh. Let go of your grip on the patient's thigh and transfer this grip to the patient's wrist. You should now have the patient on your shoulders, using one of your arms to hold the patient's wrist and leg. This will leave one of your hands free to help you maintain balance and to open doors or move obstructions.

1st The fire fighter's carry is much easier to perform if you have help in lifting the patient to your shoulders. Even though two rescuers are at the scene, the fire fighter's carry may prove to be quicker than both rescuers trying to lift and carry the patient by the extremities. When someone is on hand to help, and you are strong enough to carry the patient, have your helper assist in lifting and loading the patient onto your shoulders.

1st The Pack Strap Carry

Many people hear the phrase "pack strap carry" and think that this move requires some sort of equipment known as a pack strap. This is not true. The pack strap carry is performed with no equipment.

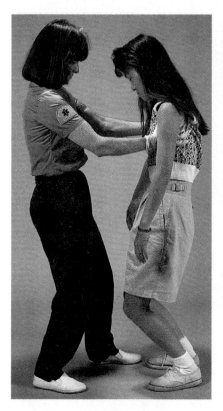 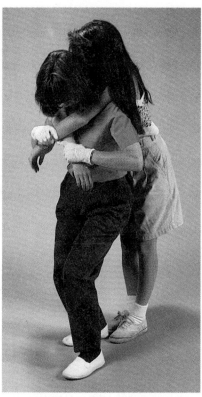 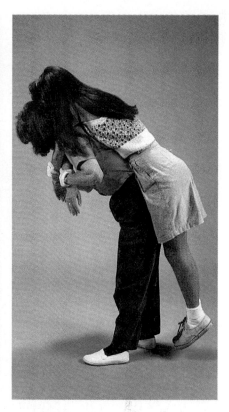

FIGURE 18–7. Beginning the pack strap carry.

FIGURE 18–8. The pack strap carry, step 2.

FIGURE 18–9. The pack strap carry, final step.

As a First Responder, you can easily use the pack strap carry for conscious patients. With assistance, this carry also can be used for unconscious patients. There are modifications of this technique that will allow you to work by yourself with the unconscious patient, but the nature of most emergencies seldom provides enough time to use these modifications. Your instructor may demonstrate how to use the pack strap carry when dealing with an unconscious patient.

Have the patient stand or have a helper hold the patient in a standing position.

Turn your back to the patient and bring his arms over your shoulders so that they cross your chest. Try to keep the patient's arms as straight as possible. Be sure that the armpits are over your shoulders.

While holding the patient's wrist, bend and pull the patient up onto your back. If possible, grasp both of the patient's wrists with one hand, leaving your other hand free for balance and to open doors and remove obstructions.

1st One-Rescuer Drags

There are a number of moves called drags. If you pull a patient to safety while grabbing the shoulders, this is a shoulder drag. If you pull by the foot, this is a foot drag. Pulling the patient by grasping hold of an article of clothing is a clothes drag. Drags are useful ways to move unconscious or heavy patients when you are working alone in a dangerous situation.

Never drag a patient sideways. *Always* drag in the direction of the length of the body. If possible, you should not bend, twist, or turn any part of the patient's body. When you are using a drag method and you have to take the patient down stairs or an incline, you should go first and use a shoulder drag to pull the patient head first by lifting at the armpits.

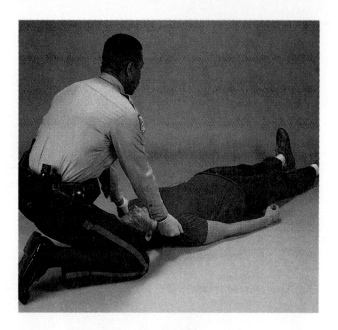

FIGURE 18–10. The clothes drag.

You may find that it is easier to drag a person on a blanket. This method offers some protection for the patient's neck and spine, but most of what is gained is lost by lifting or rolling the patient onto the blanket. Also, the blanket drag is time consuming. You may start to prepare the patient only to find that you must use a shoulder, foot, or clothes drag.

To carry out a blanket drag, position the patient face up. Lay an unfolded blanket next to the patient's side, gathering half of the material up against the patient.

Kneel on the opposite side of the patient. Take the patient's arm closest to you and place it in an outstretched position at the level of the patient's head. Reach across and roll the patient toward you, holding the patient against your knees with one hand. Use your free hand to push the gathered blanket material up against the patient's back.

With great care, roll the patient away from you so that the patient's back comes to rest on the blanket.

Fold the patient's arms over the body and then fold any excess blanket material over the patient. Grasp the blanket by both sides and pull the patient to safety, keeping the patient's head as low as possible.

FIGURE 18–11. Gather half of the blanket material up against the patient's side.

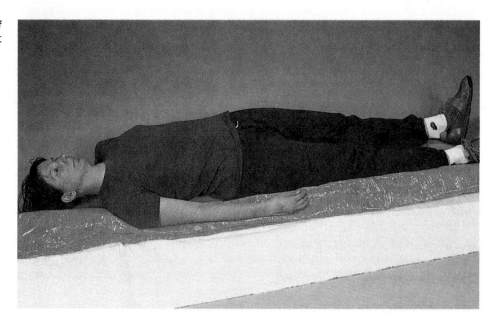

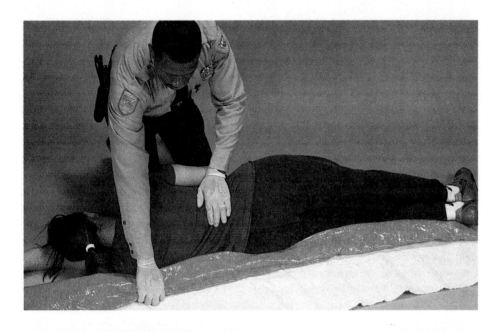

FIGURE 18–12. Roll the patient toward your knees so that you can place the blanket under the patient.

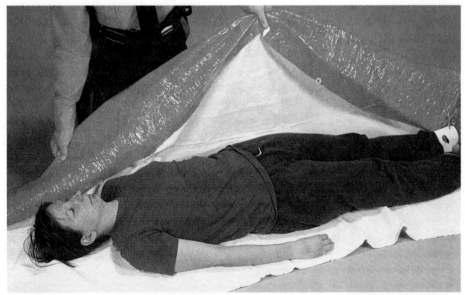

FIGURE 18–13. Gently roll the patient back onto the blanket.

FIGURE 18–14. When performing the blanket drag, keep the patient's head as low as possible.

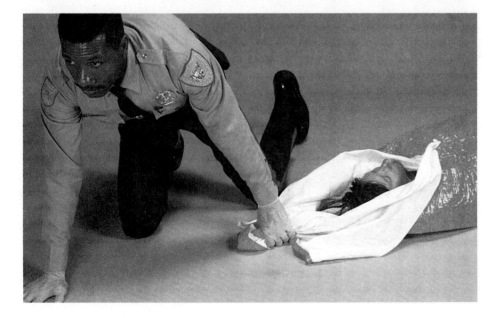

Direct Ground Lift—Spinal Injuries

In rare cases, you may find it necessary to make an emergency move of a patient with possible neck or spinal injuries, and you will have the time and help needed to lift and carry the patient. Usually, this occurs when fire or burning fuel is approaching the patient slowly enough to allow for an organized move. Unless there is imminent danger, you should not move a patient with possible neck or spinal injuries. Such moves require the application of rigid collars and spine boards. Since it is unlikely that you will have a spine board or the proper practice to use spine boards or scoop stretchers, you should not consider moving the patient with possible neck or spinal injuries unless you have no choice.

The procedures for carrying out a direct ground lift will be covered in this chapter under nonemergency moves. According to DOT guidelines, the only modification of this technique necessary for patients with neck or spinal injuries is the addition of one more rescuer to stabilize the patient's head and neck. This procedure is not recommended in this text. Use this procedure only if it is approved by your EMS System. When having bystanders assist you, you should be the person who applies this stabilization. In all cases, the person applying stabilization is in charge of the move. This person tells the others when to lift, when to stop lifting, and when to perform or stop any other move. You should have no less than three people help you with this move.

REMEMBER: A direct ground lift is considered a nonemergency move. Nonemergency moves are not to be done on patients with possible neck or spinal injuries. If you carry out a direct ground lift on a patient with possible neck or spinal injuries, it should be done only because the scene presents extreme danger for rescuers and patient. Never attempt a direct ground lift for patients with possible neck or spinal injuries unless you can apply stabilization for the head and neck.

FIGURE 18–15. There are many methods you can use during emergency moves.

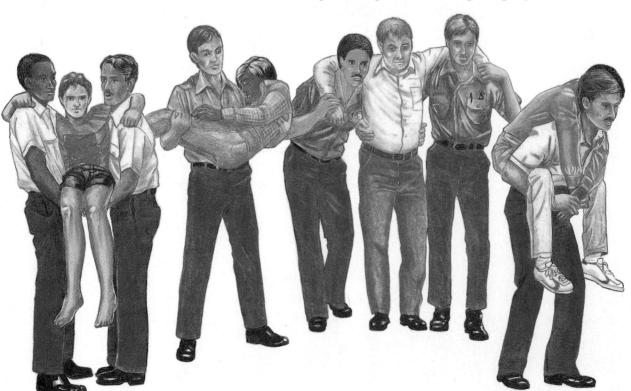

Other Emergency Moves

There are many other techniques that can be used to move a patient quickly. None of these moves protects the patient's neck or spine. Many of the emergency moves you carry out will have no special name. They will be combinations or variations of other moves used to remove a patient from a motor vehicle or from a scene having fire. In addition to the emergency moves described in this chapter, you may find yourself using a piggyback carry, cradling a patient in your arms, assisting a patient as part of a two-rescuer move, or even working with others to carry a patient who is sitting in a chair. Remember that an emergency move must be justified and that it should be carried out as quickly as possible.

NONEMERGENCY MOVES

1st The Extremity Lift

An extremity lift requires two people. This lift should not be performed if there is any possibility of head, neck, spine, shoulder, hip, or knee injuries, or any possible fractures to the upper or lower extremities that have not been immobilized. Ideally, the patient should not have any fractures or the fractures should be splinted. The patient should be conscious; otherwise, you may not have made a correct survey of neck and spinal injuries.

The patient should be placed face up, with knees flexed. You should kneel at the head of the patient, placing your hands under the patient's shoulders. Have your helper stand at the patient's feet and grasp the patient's wrist.

Direct your helper to pull the patient into a sitting position, while you push the patient from the shoulders. (Do *not* have your helper pull the patient by the arms if there are any signs of fractures to the bones of the arms or shoulders.) Slip your arms under the patient's armpits and grasp the wrists. Once the patient is in a semisitting position, have your helper crouch down and grasp the patient's legs behind the knees.

Direct your helper so that you both stand at the same time ("Ready? . . . lift") and move as a unit when carrying the patient. Try to walk out of step with your partner to avoid swinging the patient. Direct your helper as to when to stop the carry and when to place the patient down into a lying or seated position.

FIGURE 18–16.   The extremity lift, step 1.

FIGURE 18–17.   The extremity lift, step 2.

FIGURE 18–18.   The extremity lift, final step.

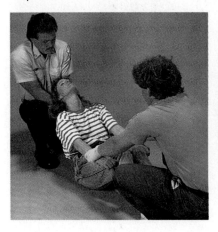

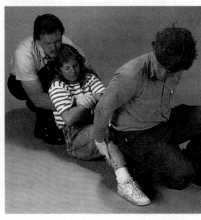

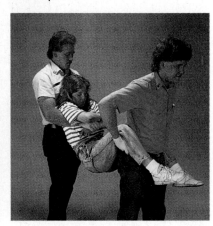

1st The Direct Ground Lift

The direct ground lift (three-rescuer lift) is a nonemergency move and is not recommended for use on patients with possible neck or spinal injuries. The procedure can be carried out by two people, but at least three are recommended. Additional rescuers can be used for the move by having them position themselves opposite the three main participants in the move.

To perform a direct ground lift, the patient should be lying face up and the arms should be placed on the chest. You and your helpers should line up on one side of the patient. You should be at the patient's head. Have one helper at the patient's midsection and the other helper at the patient's lower legs. Each of you should drop to one knee. This should be the knee closest to the patient's feet.

Place one arm under the patient's neck and grasp the far shoulder so you will be able to cradle the head. Your other arm should be placed under

FIGURE 18–19. The direct ground lift, step 1.

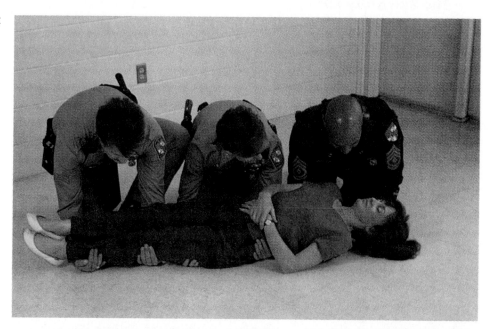

FIGURE 18–20. The direct ground lift, step 2.

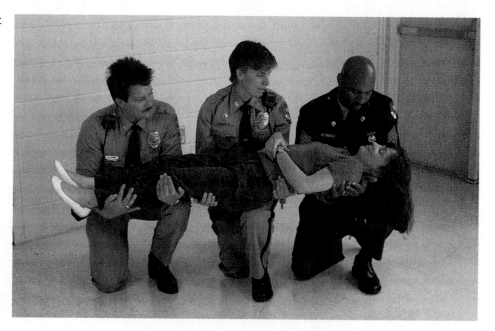

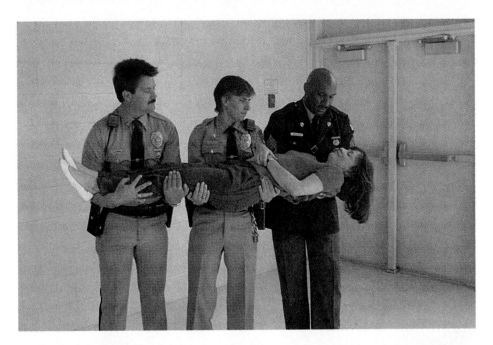

FIGURE 18–21. The direct ground lift, step 3.

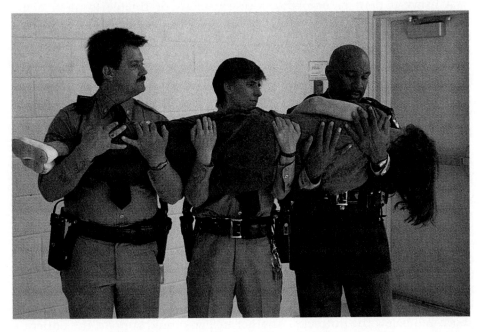

FIGURE 18–22. The direct ground lift, final step.

the patient's back, just above the waist. Your helper at the patient's midsection should place one arm above and one arm below the patient's buttocks. The helper at the patient's lower legs should place one arm under the patient's knees and the other arm under the patient's ankles.

On your signal, everyone should lift the patient up to the level of their knees.

On your signal, everyone should stand while holding the patient.

On your signal, everyone should roll the patient toward their chests. You can now move the patient, reversing the process when it is time to stop the move and place the patient back into a lying position.

NOTE: It is poor practice to use a two-rescuer ground lift. This procedure does not allow enough support for the patient and control during the move. If you must use this move and have only one helper, position this person at the patient's thigh so one arm can be placed on the patient's back above the patient's buttocks and one arm under the patient's knees.

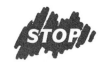

SUMMARY

Whenever possible, you should *not* move a patient. **Emergency moves** are carried out quickly when the scene is hazardous, care of the patient requires repositioning, or you must reach another patient needing life-saving care. **Nonemergency moves** can be carried out if there are factors at the scene causing the patient to decline, you must reach other patients, part of the care required forces you to move the patient, or the patient insists on being moved and tries to do so alone.

Nonemergency moves should be carried out only on **conscious patients.** You should have **completed** the **patient survey.** The patient should be **stable,** with normal rates and character for **breathing** and **pulse.** There should be **no serious bleeding** and **no signs of spinal injuries.** All **fractures** must be **immobilized** or **splinted.**

The **one-rescuer assist** is an easy method of helping a patient walk away from a dangerous scene. If you have to carry a conscious patient, you can do so by the procedures known as the **pack strap carry.** When you have a helper, the pack strap carry can be used for unconscious patients. A helper can also help you lift and position a patient for the **fire fighter's carry.**

A heavy patient or one who is unconscious or unable to move alone can be removed by using one of the **drag** methods. Always drag the patient in the **direction of the length of the body,** keeping the patient's head as low as possible.

The **direct ground lift** may be approved in your EMS System for use for patients with possible **spinal** or **neck injuries** who are found in dangerous situations, provided you **stabilize** the **head** and **neck** and have at least three other people to help you. In most cases, this move will not be practical at a dangerous emergency scene. The use of a drag may be more appropriate.

The **extremity lift** is a good move in **nonemergency** situations. This move should not be used if the patient has possible head, neck, or spinal injuries, is unconscious, or has injuries to the upper or lower extremities (including the shoulder and hip). This lift requires **two rescuers,** with you lifting the patient at the shoulders and your helper lifting the patient at the knees.

The **direct ground lift** is a **nonemergency move** that can be used for patients **with no neck** or **spinal injuries.** You should have two, three, or more people to help. The patient must be **supported** by the **head, neck, back,** and **knees.** Ideally, you should support the patient by the head and neck and by the lower back. A helper should control and support the patient above and below the buttocks. Another helper should support the patient's knees and ankles. When moving the patient, you should keep the patient rolled toward your chest.

CHAPTER 19

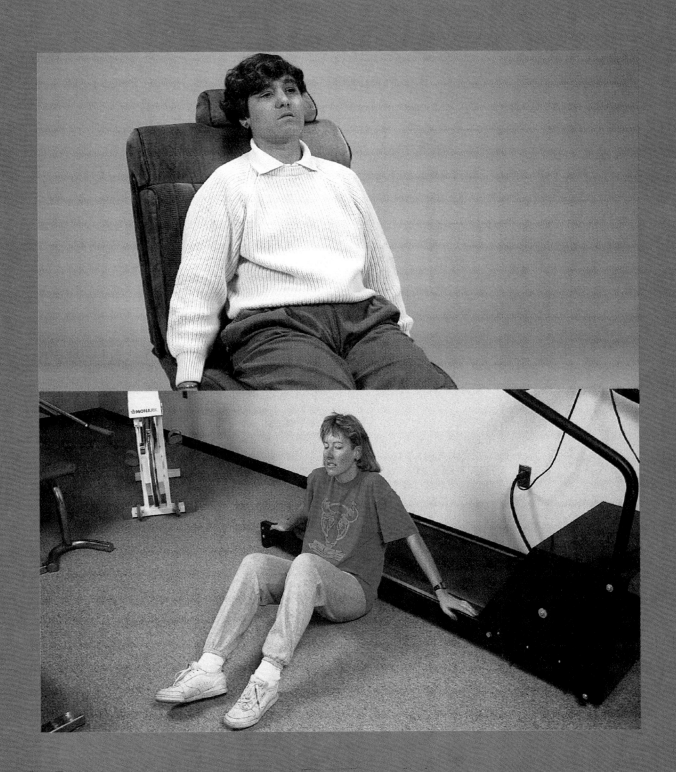

◼ OBJECTIVES

By the end of this chapter, you should be able to:

1. Define triage. (p. 422)
2. Classify given injuries in terms of their triage priority in accordance with the initial and standard systems of triage used in your locality. (pp. 423–426)
3. Relate given signs to specific injuries and illnesses. (pp. 426–427)
4. Describe First Responder responsibilities at:
   A. Motor vehicle accidents
   B. The fire scene
   C. The crime scene
   D. Cave-ins
   E. Declared emergencies and disasters (pp. 429–432)
5. List some of the more common injuries seen at:
   A. Motor vehicle accidents
   B. The fire scene
   C. The crime scene
   D. Cave-ins (pp. 429–432)

SKILLS

Upon completing this chapter and your class lectures and skills labs, you should be able to:

1. Work as a member of a team to carry out triage for a simulated multiple-victim accident.
2. Work as a member of a team to do complete patient assessments for a simulated multiple-victim accident.
3. Work as a member of a team to provide care to "patients" at the scene of a simulated multiple-victim accident.

TRIAGE

Priorities

Triage—a method of sorting patients for care and transport based on the severity of their injuries or illnesses.

1st Triage is the sorting of patients into categories of priority for care based on injuries and medical emergencies. This process is used at the scene of multiple-victim accidents and emergencies. When there are more victims than there are rescuers trained in emergency care, triage is essential. If triage is not performed, a patient with a minor wound could receive care while someone in respiratory arrest goes unnoticed.

Triage is also performed to determine the order of transport for patients. Heart attack, allergy shock, multiple-injury, and heat stroke patients cannot wait while patients with minor fractures are transported ahead of them.

Since First Responders are usually first on the scene, they must be able to conduct a triage of the patients and initiate care. When more highly trained personnel arrive, First Responders are called on to pass on information, help complete the triage, and help provide care. Remember, triage is not a waste of time. You cannot begin to treat patients randomly. You must begin treating those people who have the highest priority based on need for care.

Possibilities are very good that you will begin triage at the scene of an accident and then be relieved by EMTs before completing your triage. You will have to communicate the information you have gathered to EMTs when

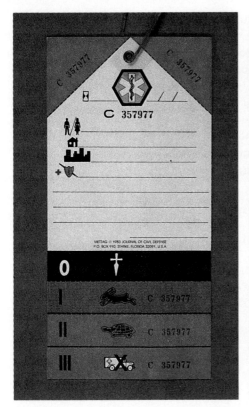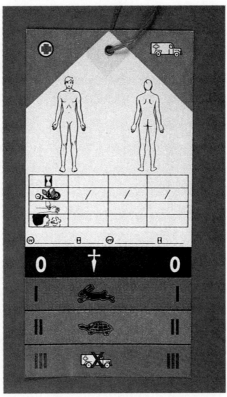

FIGURE 19–1.
An example of standard triage tags. (THE METTAG SYSTEM)

they arrive. It is a good idea to take notes while you are performing triage. Use one sheet of paper per patient. Leave your note attached to the patient so that others arriving at the scene can have immediate access to information. Do not delay care in order to make elaborate notes.

NOTE: Some localities have their First Responders use triage tags (see Figure 19–1). The use of these tags has been expanded by some systems to include every assessed patient at every incident. Even if you do not carry these tags, you should be familiar with them in case you are called on to help when others are using triage tags.

The typical triage process does not allow for assessment to pause or stop before all patients are evaluated. This means that you will not be able to stop triage for persons in need of immediate care, including patients who are in respiratory or cardiac arrest. If there are too many victims, they are too widely spread out, or simple visual observations do not give you the information you need, you will have to complete triage before beginning care. As more trained personnel arrive, care may begin for the serious patients while triage is in progress. Even with the arrival of additional rescuers, a patient in cardiac arrest (unwitnessed) may be given a low priority of care simply because there are too many patients needing lifesaving care. Instead of assigning a rescuer to this patient, the rescuer might be assigned to save the lives of several patients.

1st As a First Responder, you should use the classification for triage that has been adopted by your locality. At one time, patients were classified as highest, second, and lowest priority. Some systems still use this form of triage. Most jurisdictions now use a form of triage having four categories of patients. They classify patients as highest priority, second priority, delayed, and deceased. In some systems, highest priority is called class 1, severe, urgent, or immediate. Second priority is sometimes called class 2, moderate, emergent, or high priority. The low priority is sometimes called class 3, mild, nonemergent, or delayed priority. The final category, deceased, may be called class 4 or probable death in your EMS System.

The following is an example of a four-category triage:

1. *Highest priority* (number 1, immediate)
   - Respiratory arrest or airway obstruction
   - Cardiac arrest (witnessed)
   - Severed artery; severe bleeding (uncontrolled)
   - Cervical spine injury (stabilized)
   - Severe head injuries with unconsciousness
   - Open chest or abdominal wounds
   - Major or complicated burns
   - Severe shock
   - Burns of the respiratory tract
   - Closed chest wound—apparent punctured lung
   - Complications of medical problems (for example, obstetrical, cardiac disease, diabetes, seizures, hyperthermia, hypothermia, poisoning)
   - Unconsciousness
   - Fractures with no distal pulse
   - Fractured femur
   - Open eye wound

2. *Second priority* (number 2)
   - Back injuries with or without spinal cord damage
   - Moderate blood loss, usually less than 2 pints
   - Open or multiple fractures (major)
   - Stable abdominal injuries
   - Eye injuries (open wound makes it highest priority)
   - Serious head injuries (conscious)
   - Stable drug overdose
   - Moderate and minor burns

3. *Low priority* (number 3, hold/delayed)
   - Minor bleeding
   - Minor lacerations or soft tissue injuries
   - Minor or simple fractures
   - Sprains
   - Those who, because of the seriousness of their injuries, have little chance for survival (for example, patient unconscious from head injury and with brain exposed; severe burns of second and third degree over more than 40% of the body)

4. *Deceased* (*obvious death*)
   - Decapitation
   - No pulse for over 20 minutes (except with cold water drowning and extreme hypothermia)
   - Severed trunk
   - Fall from high places with multiple injuries and fractures, and not breathing
   - Incineration

NOTE: Your system may not have a deceased category. Instead, it might use a "Probable Death" category that includes obvious death, mortal wounds, and all injuries where death is considered to be certain under the conditions in which the rescue is taking place.

Not everyone agrees with the above classification. Variations do occur, but they tend to be minor. Your instructor will tell you of any variations for your area.

Various factors can change the priorities during triage. These factors include the type of incident, location of the incident, special weather conditions, number of patients, types of injuries, and number of rescuers. A major change in triage priorities is usually the result of limitations in what the EMS System can do in a given situation. As noted earlier, if there are many seriously injured victims and few rescuers, an unwitnessed cardiac arrest may be assigned a low priority. Even though this sounds objectionable, you must realize that this could be necessary if many patients could die while you tried to save the cardiac arrest victim. Triage has to be practical to save the most lives.

Remember that patients do not always remain stable. You may have to update your triage. You also will have to modify care procedures if you are dealing with a large number of patients. For example, an unconscious person may be classified as your highest priority. However, after checking vital signs and covering the patient, you may note that a patient classified as having moderate bleeding needs immediate care. You will have to come back to monitor the unconscious patient, but you cannot provide continuous monitoring while the other patient bleeds.

INITIAL TRIAGE—MULTIPLE-CASUALTY INCIDENT

There are multiple-casualty incidents (MCI) requiring a special form of triage. Usually such incidents involve a large number of casualties and a delay period before additional help will be on the scene. If the disaster is large enough or very remote, an hour or more may pass before there are enough rescuers present to render care for all the patients.

The modified triage system that is in most common use is the *START* plan (Table 19–1). The term *START* stands for simple triage and rapid treatment. The first rescuers on the scene begin the triage process. There are four major steps to the *START* plan. The patients are triaged into very broad categories that are based on the need for treatment and the chances of survival under the circumstances of the disaster.

The *START* plan allows the initial rescuers to quickly identify and separate out those patients who are probably the least injured and classify them as "delayed," tag the dead and the "nonsalvageable" as "dead," tag

START plan—a four-step simple triage and rapid treatment (care) program designed for use in multiple casualty incidents. It is usually employed when additional help will be delayed.

TABLE 19–1. TRIAGE—THE *START* PLAN

Immediate	Delayed	Dead
Respirations above 30/minute	Walking wounded	No respirations
Respirations below 30/minute; no radial pulse	Respirations below 30/minute; radial pulse	
Adequate respirations and perfusion; unable to follow directions	Adequate respirations and perfusion; able to follow directions	

those patients who are in most need of care as "immediate," and tag those patients who are in less need of care as "delayed." During the process of triage, the rescuers are able to take some basic actions to ensure an airway and control serious bleeding.

STEP ONE: Delayed Patients The rescuers direct all patients who can walk to go to an assigned area. These patients are now considered to be in the delayed category. The rescuers move to the closest patient who cannot walk and continue the triage.

STEP TWO: Respiration Check Each patient who cannot walk is assessed for respirations. Airway maintenance is accomplished by repositioning the patient's head to allow for hyperextension of the cervical spine. Patients who can walk might be able to assist to help keep the airway open for an unconscious patient. If this is not possible, items close at hand or debris can be used to position the patient to provide for an open airway and allow the rescuer to move on to the next patient. Respiration is used to classify the patients as:

- Dead/nonsalvageable (tagged)—no respirations
- Immediate (tagged)—respirations above 30 per minute
- Delayed (no tag)—respirations below 30 per minute

All respiratory rates are estimates based on quick observation. No actual rates are determined.

STEP THREE: Perfusion Assessment Patients who received a respiratory check and were classified as immediate or delayed are checked for adequate perfusion (the steady flow of blood through the vital organs). This is done on the basis of the presence or absence of a radial pulse. The presence of a radial pulse indicates a systolic blood pressure of at least 80 mm Hg (American College of Surgeons standard). Any patient with a radial pulse is assumed to have adequate perfusion and is considered to be "delayed" but is not yet tagged. Any patient without a radial pulse is assumed to have inadequate perfusion and is tagged "immediate."

During this third step, major bleeding can be discovered and direct pressure can be applied and then maintained by the patient or a "walking" patient. Any patient without a radial pulse should have the legs raised and held in this position with near-at-hand items or debris.

STEP FOUR: Brain Injury Assessment If a patient with adequate respirations and perfusion can follow simple directions (for example, open or close his eyes), the central nervous system is assumed to be intact and he is given a "normal mental status." This patient is tagged "delayed." Any patient with adequate respirations and perfusion who cannot follow the simple direction is tagged "immediate."
NOTE: The fourth step may be completed during the assessments for respiration and perfusion. If necessary, it can be done as a separate step for certain patients.

PATIENT ASSESMENT

Consideration of the mechanism of injury and the primary and secondary surveys (including the patient interview) are critical in determining the care and order of care when you have more than one patient. Vital signs and other highly signficant signs must be looked for and quickly related to possible problems, injuries, or illnesses.

1st As a First Responder, you must be able to apply the following information to the assessment and care of patients:

- *Pulse (vital sign)*
  Rapid, full: fear, overexertion, heat stroke, high blood pressure, early stages of internal bleeding
  Rapid, thready: shock, blood loss, heat exhaustion, diabetic coma, falling blood pressure
  Slow, full: stroke, skull fracture
  No pulse: carotid = cardiac arrest, distal = injury to the extremity (usually a fracture or dislocation)
- *Respiration (vital sign)*
  Rapid, shallow: shock, heart problems, heat exhaustion, insulin shock, congestive heart failure
  Deep, gasping, labored: airway obstruction, congestive heart failure, heart problems, lung disease, lung injury from excessive heat, chest injuries, diabetic coma
  Snoring: stroke, fractured skull, drug or alcohol abuse, airway obstruction
  Crowing: airway obstruction, airway injury due to excessive heat
  Gurgling: airway obstruction, lung disease, lung damage due to excessive heat
  Coughing blood: chest wound, rib fracture, internal injuries
- *Skin temperature (vital sign)*
  Cool, moist: shock, bleeding, body is losing heat, heat exhaustion
  Cool, dry: exposure to cold
  Cool, clammy: shock
  Hot, dry: heat stroke, high fever
  Hot, moist: infectious disease
- Skin color
  Red: high blood pressure, heart attack, heat stroke, diabetic coma, minor burn
  White, pale, ashen: shock, heart attack, excessive bleeding, heat exhaustion, fright, insulin shock
  Blue: Heart failure, airway obstruction, lung disease, certain poisonings, shock
- *Pupils of the eyes*
  Dilated, unresponsive to light: cardiac arrest, unconsciousness, shock, bleeding, heat stroke, certain types of drugs (LSD, uppers)
  Constricted: damage to the central nervous system, certain types of drugs (heroin, morphine, codeine)
  Unequal: stroke, head injury
  Dull (lackluster): shock, coma
- *State of consciousness*
  Confusion: fright, anxiety, illness, minor head injury, alcohol or drug abuse, mental illness, shock epilepsy
  Stupor: moderate to severe head injury, alcohol or drug abuse, stroke
  Brief unconsciousness: minor head injury, fainting, epilepsy
  Coma: stroke, allergy shock, severe head injury, poisoning, drug or alcohol abuse, diabetic coma, heat stroke, shock, heart attack
- *Paralysis or loss of sensation*
  One side of body: stroke, head injury
  Arms only: spinal injury in neck
  Legs only: spinal injury along back
  Arms and legs: spinal injury in neck and possibly along back
  No pain, obvious injury: spinal cord or brain damage, shock, hysteria, drug or alcohol abuse

All of this indicates some of the information you have learned during your First Responder course. This information will quickly fade unless you continue to study your notes and this text. It is a good idea to make a file of index cards with a different medical emergency or injury written on one side of each card and the corresponding symptoms and signs written on the opposite side of each card. Periodically, you can review injuries and illnesses and see if you can list the symptoms and signs for each. Then you can look at signs and symptoms and see if you can match an injury or illness to each set.

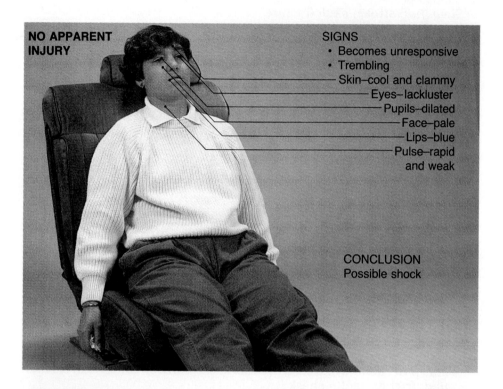

NO APPARENT INJURY

SIGNS
- Becomes unresponsive
- Trembling
- Skin–cool and clammy
- Eyes–lackluster
- Pupils–dilated
- Face–pale
- Lips–blue
- Pulse–rapid and weak

CONCLUSION
Possible shock

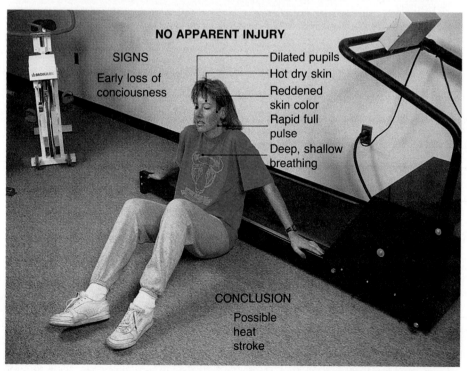

NO APPARENT INJURY

SIGNS

Early loss of conciousness

Dilated pupils
Hot dry skin
Reddened skin color
Rapid full pulse
Deep, shallow breathing

CONCLUSION
Possible heat stroke

FIGURE 19–2. First Responders must be able to relate signs to specific injuries and illnesses.

SPECIAL SITUATIONS

Motor Vehicle Accidents

First Responder duties at the scene of a motor vehicle accident were covered, in part, in Chapter 17. When the EMTs arrive, let them know that you are a First Responder and give them any information you have concerning the patients and mechanisms of injury. Tell the EMTs if you moved any patients and why you did so. Report clearly any care you have provided.

Depending on the situation, the EMTs may ask you to help them with triage, patient care, or moving patients. You may be asked to provide emotional support to families, bystanders, and children. Your help may be needed in moving equipment. Often, the EMTs will request help in controlling the scene. If you are a law enforcement officer or a member of the fire service, you may have duties to perform outside the realm of First Responder. If this is the case, then follow standard operating procedures. Since the EMTs may need your help with patient care, let them know where you will be at the scene and that you are willing to help when it is possible for you to do so.

Unless you are experienced in delivering care at the scene of a motor vehicle accident, you may miss injuries. The mechanisms of injury are very important when considering patient assessment at the motor vehicle accident scene. The type of accident and the type of damage to the vehicle can tell you a lot. For example, if a car is struck from behind, look for neck injuries to the patients in this car. If the steering wheel is damaged, look for chest injuries. Blood on the dashboard or windshield indicates that the patient on that side of the car should have open wounds. If the victims were not wearing their seat belts, look for injuries that could be caused by being thrown about inside the vehicle.

Take great care when trying to detect possible neck and spinal injuries. These injuries are often associated with motor vehicle accidents. So too are head injuries, with the incident of injury being highest for passengers not wearing seat belts. Chest injuries, particularly for the driver, are very common.

There can be differences in the types of injuries suffered by males and females because of differences in their centers of balance and muscle mass. Male patients may have fractures to the hips when they are involved in high-speed crashes. Female patients may have dislocated hips when involved in the same type of crash. Infants and children can suffer severe head and neck injury, even when all the adults in the vehicle are not injured. This is because their heads are larger in proportion to their bodies.

Always check those patients who are wearing lap belts for injuries to the abdomen and pelvis. Remember to check patients wearing shoulder belts for injuries to the collarbone (safety belt injuries are usually caused by wearing the belt too tightly, against the recommendations of the manufacturer).

Internal injuries and internal bleeding can be very hard to detect. If a patient has received a severe blow to the body during a motor vehicle accident, assume that there is internal bleeding until you can prove otherwise. Look for bruises to the sides of a patient's chest and waist. Sometimes patients are thrown against armrests, causing serious internal injuries. Internal injury can be on the side opposite the bruise.

Do not forget to consider medical problems. Heart attacks cause people to have accidents. Some individuals have a heart attack because of the stress of an accident. While you are doing patient surveys and interviews, be on the alert for symptoms and signs that may indicate a medical emergency.

Make a special effort to detect injuries to the bones and joints if your patient is elderly. Such patients often receive fractures during motor vehicle accidents, even when other passengers have no injuries. Detecting and caring for these fractures may prevent a long hospital stay.

The Fire Scene

The hazards of the fire scene and First Responder responsibilities were covered in Chapter 17. Remember, leave fire fighting to the fire service.

Your duties at the fire scene should center around providing care, if you can do so in a safe area. When the EMTs arrive, give them patient information and tell them what you have done. If you are in the fire service or are a law enforcement officer follow standard operating procedures. The EMTs will tell you if they need help with patients, moving equipment, or controlling the scene.

Once the EMTs take over responsibility for your patients, do not leave the scene. There may be victims yet to be discovered. Fire fighters may be injured. Your help could still be needed as long as there are activities at the fire scene.

Victims of fire may have burns, smoke inhalation, and injuries to soft tissues and bones due to falling objects or accidents occurring during an escape from the fire. The most common injuries to fire fighters include sprains and strains, cuts, smoke inhalation, burns, heat exhaustion, and fractures.

Heart attacks occur with high frequency at the fire scene. Heat, smoke, high humidity, and stress all combine to overwork a person's heart and lungs.

The Crime Scene

At a crime scene, your first priority is to make certain that the scene is safe before you try to reach the patient. Provide care for the patient, disturbing as little of the scene as possible. Do not break the chain of evidence by touching or moving items unless you must do so to provide care.

As additional help arrives, identify yourself as a First Responder. Do this for both the police and the EMTs. The EMTs will tell you if they need your assistance. You cannot leave the crime scene until you are given permission to do so by the police.

The violence associated with crime produces serious injuries. Head injuries are common. Puncture wounds, lacerations, fractures, and internal injuries occur with high frequency. Remember to look for both entrance and exit wounds in cases of shootings and stabbings.

Cave-ins

Cave-ins are associated with construction work, mining, and farming accidents. Away from the job site, many cave-ins involve children at play in unsafe surroundings. Cave-in rescue requires special skills, usually not part of First Responder training. Remember that your first priority is your own safety. Your primary action should be to make certain that dispatch is alerted. You should not take any actions unless the scene is obviously safe. If a pile of dirt shifted and trapped workers, you may be able to take some action. However, if a trench partially caves in, there is no way you can be certain that a second cave-in or collapse will not occur.

Take care in how you approach the cave-in site. Only a few rescuers at a time should approach the site since additional weight on the surface may set off another cave-in or compress the ground around trapped victims. Should you be able to reach a patient, uncover the body to the waist. If you only uncover the patient's head, pressure on the chest may be so great that it prevents breathing. In cases where digging is required, use hand tools, and proceed with great care. Do *not* try to use earth-moving equipment. Usually, when such equipment is used by those untrained in cave-in rescue, victims are seriously injured by the equipment.

As you uncover the patient, be on the alert for impaled objects. Do *not* try to pull victims free from their trapped position until they are completely uncovered. To do so might cause serious injury to the patient, especially if there are spinal injuries. The exception to this rule occurs when a scene becomes unsafe. Fire, the threat of falling objects, flooding, and possible new cave-ins may require an emergency patient move.

When EMTs arrive, give them patient information and state what you have done in terms of care. The EMTs will tell you what they would like to do at the scene.

Disasters and Complex Emergencies

The EMS System does not need First Responders reporting to every emergency scene. Except for major disasters, you should not respond to an emergency scene after dispatch is alerted (police and fire personnel should follow SOP). Your instructor can tell you what types of incidents will probably require your assistance. When in doubt, call your local EMS office and ask if you can be of help at the scene or at another location.

Certain types of emergencies automatically require a large number of personnel trained in emergency care. Large fires, severe storms, structural collapses, airplane crashes, train wrecks, and multiple-vehicle crashes usually place a heavy burden on the EMS System. First Responder help, even if it arrives after the EMTs are on the scene, is very important in these emergencies.

Those in the EMS System consider First Responders to be a part of the system. They expect you to respond to certain emergencies where help is sure to be needed. In disasters and emergencies, report to the scene and go directly to the command center. If you cannot find a command center, go to one of the EMTs to find out who is in charge of patient care. The individual in charge can tell you if help is needed, where, and what you can do to help. Should you be in law enforcement or the fire service, follow standard operating procedures for disasters and emergencies.

If you provide help at disasters and complex emergencies, beware of the stress that these events may place on you. Rescue workers have to keep a close watch on their emotions while they carry out their duties. Often they work to exhaustion, complicated by exposure to harsh environments. Stress is high and constant.

During disasters and complex emergencies, do not try to do too much. Obtain a work schedule from a supervisor and take needed break periods for rest, food, sleep and to escape the stress of the scene. During rest periods, converse with other rescuers. Talking with them about mutual problems and about topics unrelated to the scene will help reduce stress. Avoid "gallows humor" about the disaster or emergency. Such humor may seriously trouble some of your fellow workers and may bother you after the disaster is over.

It is not uncommon for rescue personnel to report emotional problems caused by certain types of disasters and emergencies. Injury, death, and destruction can produce serious emotional health problems. Sometimes the problem may surface shortly after the event. Other times the problem may delay showing itself, or it may become part of a series of problems related to other emergencies.

After an emergency, it helps to talk things over with others in the EMS System. During such conversations, it is important for you to discuss those events that upset you or made you feel uneasy. Your family can be of help, but it is very important that you share your feelings with other members of the EMS System. During your discussions with people outside the EMS System, remember to maintain patient confidentiality.

Remember, as a First Responder, you are part of the EMS System. Should you suffer problems that you feel are due to your activities at an emergency scene, contact your EMS System for assistance. Your system has people trained to help prevent you from becoming an emotional casualty of an emergency. Many EMS Systems hold Critical Incident Stress Debriefing (CISD) sessions. Do not be embarrassed to seek help.

Critical Incident Stress Debriefing (CISD)—sessions that are held after a disaster or emergency incident to address the needs of rescuers who may have been influenced by the scene and the stress generated in providing emergency care.

SUMMARY

Triage

Triage is the **sorting of patients** based on the severity of their injuries and illnesses (see page 424).

Immediate (highest) **priority** includes respiratory arrest, airway obstruction and severe breathing difficulties, cardiac arrest (witnessed), life-threatening bleeding, severe head injuries (unconscious patient), open chest and abdominal wounds, closed chest wounds with apparent punctured lung, severe shock, major burns and all burns involving the respiratory tract, severe medical problems, unconsciousness, possible fracture of the spine in the neck (cervical), fractured thigh (femur), and open wounds of the eye.

Secondary (high) **priority** includes moderate and minor burns, injuries to the spine, moderate bleeding, conscious patients with head injuries, multiple fractures, back injuries, and drug overdose (stable patient).

Delayed (low) **priority** includes minor bleeding, minor fractures and soft tissue injuries, sprains, and obvious mortal wounds beyond First Responder care. The fourth category is **deceased** (obvious death).

Patient assessment is very important during triage. Vital signs and other key signs are used. Pulse, respiration, skin temperature, skin color, pupils of the eyes, state of consciousness, paralysis, and loss of sensation are used in making initial assessments.

Special Situations

Motor vehicle accidents require that you consider the **mechanisms of injury** when evaluating patients. Injuries to the neck, spine, head, and chest are common. Internal injuries and internal bleeding may be difficult to detect.

Fires should be fought by the fire service. Do not place yourself in unnecessary danger. When caring for patients at the fire scene, pay close attention to detect burns, smoke inhalation, and heart attacks. Fire fighters often receive sprains, strains, cuts, smoke inhalation, burns, heat exhaustion, and broken bones.

Make certain that a crime scene is safe for you to provide care. Do *not* break the chain of evidence. You *must* report to the police before you can leave the crime scene.

Cave-in rescue requires special training. Do *not* attempt a rescue unless you *know* the scene is safe. Uncover victims to the waist to allow for breathing. Do not remove a patient from the cave-in until he or she is completely uncovered.

Disasters and complex emergencies require the EMS System to respond. As a First Responder, you are part of that system. Other personnel in the EMS System expect you to come to the scene and help with patient care.

Remember that the stress produced by working at the emergency scene can affect rescuers. Talk with others in the EMS System about problems you experience related to this stress.

Whenever you act as a First Responder, your main duty is to provide **patient care.** After the EMTs arrive, they may need your help with patient care or other duties. You not only turn patients over to the EMTs; you also turn over patient information and report what care you have provided.

■ SELF-TEST IV

This is a self-test. It has been designed for you to take on your own to evaluate your progress. After you have completed Chapters 16 to 19 and believe that you have met all the objectives listed for these chapters, take this test to see if you have any weaknesses in a specific area of study. Answers are listed at the end of the test. Page references are provided for each question so you can go back to the text to restudy any questions missed in the test.

If you wish to check your knowledge in more detail, note that the objectives listed at the beginning of each chapter can be read as questions and exercises. Go back to these objectives and see if you can list, describe, name, and so on, as directed in the objective statements.

Circle the letter of the best answer to each question.

1. Your primary course of action to take when dealing with a patient having an emotional emergency is to (p. 380)

   A. Talk to the patient and listen to what he is saying
   B. Call for police assistance and delay care
   C. Tell the patient you are trained to help people who are having an emotional emergency
   D. Tell the patient that everything is "OK"

2. A patient appears to be very confused and restless. His behavior approaches what you would consider to be insanity. You notice his hands are shaking, and there is an odor to his breath that is more like alcohol than the acetone you have noticed with diabetics. For this patient, the most obvious problem is likely to be (p. 381)

   A. Intoxication
   B. Insulin shock
   C. Alcohol withdrawal
   D. Congestive heart failure

3. You are caring for a patient who is intoxicated and in a state of stupor. You have the patient positioned so that his tongue is not blocking his airway. Now, the most likely cause of airway obstruction in this patient will be (p. 382)

   A. Swollen airway tissues
   B. Swollen tongue
   C. Dried mucus
   D. Vomit

4. A patient is "seeing things." He has no concept of time or his real environment. His pulse rate is fast, pupils are dilated, and the face is flushed. If this is a case of drug abuse, it is most likely due to (p. 383)

   A. Uppers
   B. Downers
   C. Mind-affecting drugs
   D. Narcotics

5. A drug abuse patient is very sluggish. His pulse and breathing rates are low. You decide to provide care for shock while waiting for the EMS System to respond. You must be prepared to render care for (p. 384)

   A. The patient trying to injure himself
   B. Violent behavior
   C. Respiratory arrest
   D. All of the above

6. A rape victim insists upon changing clothes. You should (p. 385)

   A. Say this is fine, since doing so will help the patient with the emotional crisis
   B. Encourage the patient not to do so in order to preserve the chain of evidence
   C. Stop the patient from doing so in order to preserve the chain of evidence
   D. Inform the patient that her changing clothes destroys evidence, meaning she will be breaking the law

7. You are trying to control the scene at a traffic accident on a straight, high-speed highway. Which of the following indicates the longest distance of your flare placement? (p. 389)

   A. 250 feet
   B. 300 feet
   C. 350 feet
   D. 400 feet

8. As a First Responder, your primary duty at the scene of a traffic accident is (p. 389)

   A. Crowd control
   B. Safely providing
   C. Traffic control
   D. Hazard control

9. A closed, upright vehicle contains accident victims. The vehicle is on a slightly inclined surface. You should (p. 391)

   A. Approach and begin care since such a vehicle has rolled to where it is stable
   B. Do nothing and wait for rescue personnel to arrive
   C. Control the scene and wait for rescue personnel to arrive
   D. Use wheel chocks or blocks to prevent vehicle movement

10. The doors to a vehicle which contains traffic accident victims are locked. The victims cannot help you unlock the door. You should protect yourself and then (p. 394)

    A. Try to punch through a door lock
    B. Use a sharp tool to strike through the lower edge of a side window
    C. Wait for rescue personnel to arrive
    D. Break through the windshield using a hammer

11. A vehicle containing traffic accident victims is on its side. After controlling the scene, you should (p. 396)

A. Gain immediate access through a door
B. Wait for rescue personnel to arrive
C. Go immediately to the rear window and break the glass in order to gain access
D. Stabilize the vehicle before making an attempt to enter

12. A victim in need of immediate care is pinned beneath stable wreckage. You should organize bystanders and (p. 397)

A. Lift the wreckage, shoring it as you work
B. Lift the wreckage and quickly pull the patient clear
C. Wait for rescue personnel to arrive
D. Use a bystander's vehicle to pull off the wreckage

13. A victim of a traffic accident has had his arm thrown through a window. The patient looks to you as if he is going into shock. You should (p. 397)

A. Wait for EMS response
B. Not move the patient, but treat for shock
C. Dress the arm, fold away the glass, and position the patient properly for care
D. Not waste time and quickly move the patient to prevent shock

14. You know that someone needing immediate care is in a locked building. There is no available key and all doors and windows are locked. You should (p. 398)

A. Wait for police before trying to enter
B. Wait for rescue personnel to arrive
C. Try to gain entry by breaking a window
D. Try to gain entry by breaking through a door

15. You are in a building. Someone tells you that a person needs emergency care. You arrive at the floor of the emergency to find a closed door. At the same time, you hear the building fire alarm sound. At your own risk, you decide not to leave until you can reach the person needing help. You should (p. 401)

A. Immediately look for fire fighting apparatus
B. Enter the room and move the patient as quickly as possible
C. Tell someone your location, enter the room, and begin care
D. Feel the top of the door to see if it is hot, enter if safe to do so, and move the patient in the safest way possible

16. You have no training in electrical hazards. All the lights at a traffic accident scene are out. An electrical line is down on a car containing people needing care. You should (p. 401)

A. Wait for rescue personnel to arrive
B. Have someone call the power company to turn off the line
C. Go to the car to provide care. The line is dead.
D. Use a long stick to remove the downed line

17. The only time you should move a patient with spinal injury is when (p. 408)

A. The scene is unsafe for you and the patient
B. You wish to make the patient more comfortable
C. You need to care for fractures
D. All of the above

18. The pack strap carry is best classified as a (p. 412)

A. Nonemergency move requiring no equipment
B. Nonemergency move requiring pack equipment
C. Emergency move requiring no equipment
D. Emergency move requiring pack equipment

19. You and an unconscious patient are in a dire emergency situation. You are acting alone and find the patient is too heavy for you to lift from the floor. You should try to use the (p. 413)

A. Pack strap carry
B. Direct ground lift
C. One-rescuer assist
D. Clothes drag

20. An extremity lift for a patient without spinal injury requires at least (p. 417)

A. 2 rescuers   C. 4 rescuers
B. 3 rescuers   D. 5 rescuers

21. Which of the following is the correct positioning for three rescuers beginning a direct ground lift? (p. 418)

A. One above patient's head and shoulders, one to the side of the waist, one below the feet
B. Two on one side at the head and knees and one on the opposite side at the waist
C. Two on opposite sides at the waist and one above the head
D. All three on one side, at the head, waist, and knees

22. In most triages, when there is an adequate number of rescuers, the top three priorities are (p. 424)

A. Respiratory arrest, cardiac arrest, severe shock
B. Severe shock, severe bleeding, spinal injuries
C. Respiratory arrest, cardiac arrest, severe bleeding
D. Cardiac arrest, respiratory arrest, severe shock

23. The third stage in the START plan is (p. 426)

A. Respiration check
B. Brain injury assessment
C. Sorting out delayed patients
D. Perfusion assessment

24. During patient assessment, vital signs in First Responder care include (p. 427)

A. Pulse, respirations, skin temperature
B. Respirations, skin temperature, skin color
C. Pulse, respirations, skin color
D. Pulse, respirations, pupils

25. A patient without head injury shows unequal

pupils. You should consider all signs and symptoms you have noted to see if they add up to the patient (p. 427)

A. Being on heroin
B. Having a stroke (CVA)
C. Having spinal injury
D. Having heat stroke

ANSWERS

Each question is worth 4 points

1.	A	4.	C	7.	A
2.	C	5.	D	8.	B
3.	D	6.	B	9.	D

10.	B	16.	B	22.	C
11.	D	17.	A	23.	D
12.	A	18.	C	24.	A
13.	C	19.	D	25.	B
14.	C	20.	A		
15.	D	21.	D		

Start with 100 points. Subtract four points for each wrong answer. If you scored below 70, you should see your instructor for additional help or new study methods. A score from 70 to 79 indicates you still need to do much more work on these chapters. You have done very well if you scored 80 or above; however, you should go over the text sections dealing with the questions that you missed.

CHAPTER 20

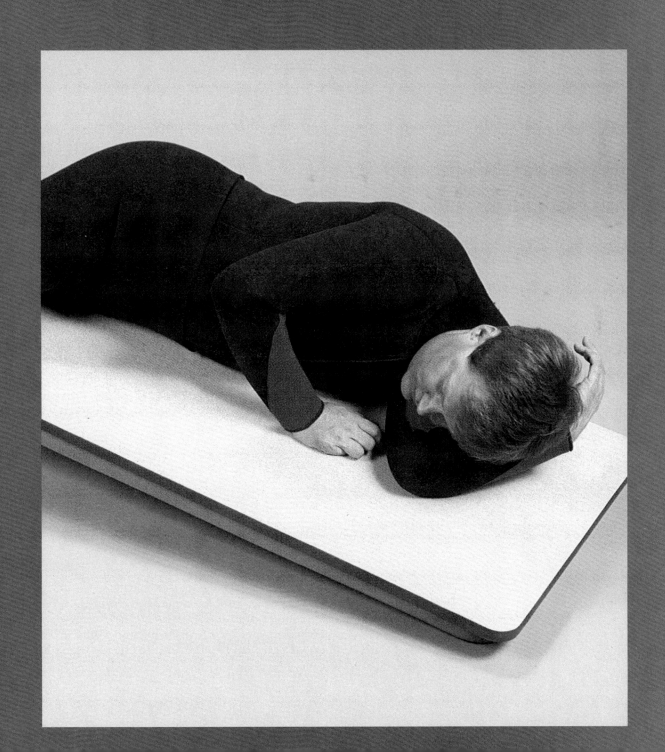

OBJECTIVES

By the end of this chapter, you should be able to:

1. List the common types of injuries associated with swimming and diving accidents. (p. 439)
2. Describe the types of problems faced when dealing with a simple water rescue procedure, and tell what the First Responder should do to solve these problems. (pp. 439–442)
3. State the First Responder care procedures for patients who are near-drowning victims. (pp. 442–444)
4. State the First Responder care procedures for victims of diving accidents who may have neck or spinal injury. (pp. 443–444)
5. Describe two special problems faced when providing care for scuba diving accident patients and state what the First Responder should do for each case. (pp. 446–448)
6. Describe basic ice rescue procedures. (p. 448–449)
7. Describe the activities a First Responder may be part of when helping EMTs at the scene of a swimming or diving accident. (p. 449)

NOTE: The amount of time spent on this subject in your First Responder course will depend upon the area in which you live and the length of your course. There are very few new procedures to learn about treating patients who have had swimming or diving accidents. Of key importance to you will be learning the types of injuries associated with water accidents and knowing the care skills used when the patient is a near-drowning victim. You also will have to know how to deal with the problems faced because of the water at the scene.

WARNING: Do *not* attempt a water rescue unless you have been trained to do so, you are a good swimmer, and others are on hand to help. Never attempt a water rescue by yourself. A personal flotation device (PFD) should be worn by all those involved in a water rescue. Except for shallow pools and open, shallow waters with uniform bottoms, the problems faced in water rescue are too great and too dangerous for the poor swimmer or untrained person to attempt. If this bothers you, having to stand by not being able to help, then take a course in water safety and rescue. Otherwise, you will probably become a victim yourself, rather than the person who rescues and provides care.

SKILLS

Upon completing this chapter and your class lectures and skills labs, you should be able to:

1. Demonstrate an evaluation of a patient who is the victim of a swimming or diving accident.
2. Demonstrate how you would solve problems faced in a water rescue situation and in an ice rescue situation.
3. Demonstrate how you would apply your knowledge and skills in emergency care to the near-drowning victim and to the patient who is a diving accident victim.

ACCIDENTS INVOLVING THE WATER

Types of Accidents

Most people, when they think of water-related accidents, tend to think only of drowning. There is no doubt that drowning must be the number one consideration, even if the first problem faced by a person in the water is an injury or a medical emergency.

Injuries occur on, in, and near the water. Boating, skiing, and diving accidents produce airway obstructions, fractures, bleeding, and soft tissue injuries. Other types of accidents, such as falls from bridges and motor vehicle accidents, also may involve the water. In these cases, the accident victims suffer the same type of injuries normally associated with the basic type of accident and the effects of the water hazard (drowning, hypothermia, delayed care because of complicated rescue, and so on.)

Sometimes, the accident or drowning may have been caused by a medical emergency that took place while someone was in the water or on a boat. Knowing how the accident occurred may give clues to detecting the medical emergency. As with all aspects of First Responder care, considering the mechanism of injury and doing the patient survey, complete with an interview, may be critical in deciding the procedures to be followed when caring for a patient.

Learn to associate the problems of drowning to scenes other than swimming pools and beaches. Remember, bathtub drownings do occur. Only a few inches of water are needed for an adult to drown. Even less is required for an infant.

1st As a First Responder, take particular care to look for the following when your patient is the victim of a water-related accident:

- **Airway obstruction**—this may be from water or foreign matter in the airway or swollen airway tissues (often seen if the neck is injured in a dive). Spasms along the airway are common in cases of near-drowning.
- **Cardiac arrest**—this is usually related to respiratory arrest.
- **Signs of heart attack**—through overexertion, the patient may have greater problems than the obvious near-drowning. Often, inexperienced rescuers are fooled into thinking that the chest pains reported by the patient are due to muscle cramps produced during swimming or the panic of a near-drowning situation.
- **Injuries to the head and neck**—these are to be expected in boating, skiing, and diving accidents, but they also occur in cases of near-drowning.
- **Internal injuries**—while doing the patient survey, be on the alert for fractures, soft tissue injuries, and internal bleeding. The fact that the patient is suffering from internal bleeding is often missed during the first stages of care because of the concern for other problems associated with near-drowning. Constantly monitor patients for the symptoms and signs of shock.
- **Hypothermia**—the water does not have to be very cold and the length of stay in the water does not have to be very long for hypothermia to occur (see Chapter 14).

Reaching the Victim

The U.S. Coast Guard, the American Red Cross, and the YMCA offer water safety and rescue courses. Unless you are a good swimmer and have been trained in water rescue, do *not* go into the water to save someone.

If the patient is responsive and close to shore or poolside, hold out an object to grab and **pull** the patient from the water. The best thing to use

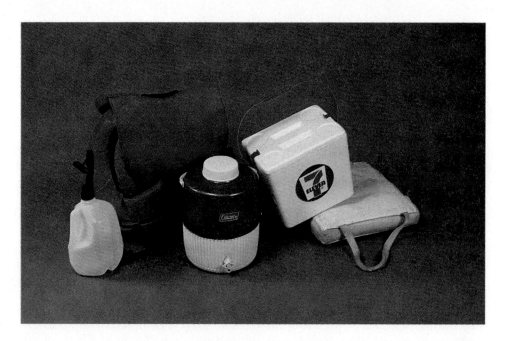

FIGURE 20–1. Throw the victim anything that will float.

for such a rescue is rope (line). If none is available, use a branch, fishing pole, oar, stick, or other such object. Keep in mind that a towel, shirt, or an article of your own clothing may work quite well. In cases where there is no object near at hand or conditions are such that you may only have one opportunity to grab the person (for example, strong currents), lie down flat on your stomach and extend your arm or leg (not recommended for the nonswimmer). In all cases, make sure that your position is secure and that you will not be pulled into the water. This is critical if you are extending an arm or leg to the person.

Should the person be alert, but too far away to be pulled from the water, then you must carefully **throw** an object that will float. A personal flotation device (lifejacket) or ring buoy (life preserver) is ideal, but these objects may not be at the scene. The best course of action is to throw anything that will float and to do this as soon as possible. Objects you might use include inflated automobile tires, foam cushions, plastic jugs, logs, boards, plastic picnic containers, surf boards, flat boards, large balls, and plastic toys. Two empty, capped plastic milk jugs can keep an adult afloat for hours. It is best to tie rope to the objects so that they can be retrieved if they do not land near the patient. You may have to add some water to lightweight plastic jugs so that you can throw them the required distance.

Once you are sure that the person has a flotation device or floating object to hold on to, try to find a way to **tow** the patient to shore. Throw the patient a line or another flotation device attached to a line. Make sure that your own position is a safe one. If conditions are safe and you are a strong swimmer, wade no deeper than your waist if you must reduce the distance for throwing the line.

You may find that the near-drowning victim is too far from shore to allow for throwing and towing, or the victim may be unconscious and unable to respond to your efforts. In such cases, if there is a boat at the scene, you may be able to take the boat to the patient. Do *not* go to the patient if you cannot swim. Even if you are a swimmer, you *must* wear a personal flotation device while you are in the boat. In cases where the patient is conscious, try to have the patient grab an oar or the stern (rear end) of the boat. Take great care in helping the person into the boat. This is a very tricky process in a canoe. Should the canoe or boat tip over, stay with the vessel, holding onto its bottom or side. It will almost certainly stay afloat.

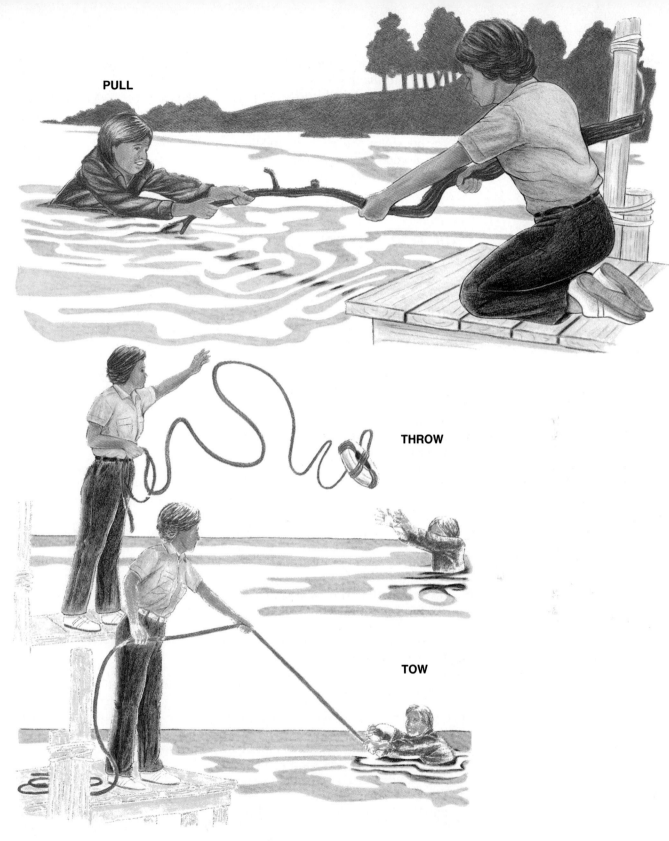

PULL

THROW

TOW

FIGURE 20–2.
If you can, *pull* the victim from the water. If this is not possible, *throw* him anything that will float and try to *tow* him from the water.

If you take a boat out and find that the patient is unconscious, assume that the patient has neck or spinal injury. Care for the patient will be discussed later in this chapter.

1st In water rescue situations, begin by trying to **pull** the patient from the water. If this cannot be done, **throw** objects that will float and try to **tow** the patient from the water. Do *not* try to take a boat to the victim if you cannot swim. Wear a personal flotation device while in the boat. Unless you are a good swimmer and trained in water rescue and lifesaving, **do not swim to the patient.**

CARE FOR THE PATIENT

The Patient with No Neck or Spinal Injuries

1st In all cases of water accidents, assume that the unconscious patient has neck and spinal injuries. If the patient can be removed quickly from the water or is out of the water when you arrive, you should:

1. Start your primary survey of the patient.
2. Provide mouth-to-mask resuscitation, if needed, as quickly as possible. Check for airway obstruction. If necessary, begin pulmonary resuscitation while the patient is still in the water. Mouth-to-mask techniques are usually not practical when the patient is in the water. You may use the mouth-to-mouth procedure, but know that this might expose you to infectious agents.
3. Provide CPR, if needed, as directed in Chapter 5. As in all such cases, make certain that someone alerts the EMS System dispatcher.
4. If the patient is breathing and has a pulse, check for bleeding and attempt to control any serious bleeding that you find.
5. If there is breathing and a pulse, cover the patient to conserve body heat and do a secondary survey. Uncover only those areas of the patient's body involved with your stage of the survey. Care for any problems you may find.
6. If the patient can be moved, take him or her to a warm place. Do *not* allow the near-drowning patient to walk. Handle the patient *gently* at all times.
7. Provide care for shock and make certain that the EMS System dispatcher has been alerted.

You may find more resistance than expected to your efforts to provide breaths to someone with water in the airway. Apply more force if necessary, once you are certain that no foreign objects are in the patient's airway. Watch the patient's chest rise and fall. Adjust your ventilations as needed to help prevent gastric distension. Remember, you must provide breaths to the patient's lungs as soon as possible.

Many times, a patient with water in the airway will also have water in the stomach. This may provide resistance to your efforts to resuscitate the patient. When this happens, you may find that some of the air from your breaths will go into the patient's stomach, even when you adjust your ventilations. Current AHA and ARC guidelines do *not* call for you to attempt to relieve water or air from the patient's stomach due to the risk of driving material from the stomach and possibly obstructing the patient's airway. When gastric distension occurs, reposition the patient's head, continue with your attempts at resuscitation, and adjust your breaths as required.

The AHA and ARC are considering whether they will approve the use of manual thrusts (see page 103) to clear the airway if the first attempt to provide rescue breathing fails. This maneuver may help clear the airway of water to allow effective rescue breathing. Your instructor will inform you if approval for the use of this technique has been allowed for First Responders in your state.

Human beings have something in common with many other mammals. This is called the mammalian diving reflex. When diving into cold water so that the face is submerged, the body sends more oxygenated blood to the brain and heart and the heart rate slows. The colder the water, the more oxygen is stored in these two locations. For this reason, a drowning victim *must* receive resuscitative care, even if the victim has not been breathing for 10 minutes or longer. Many such patients have been successfully resuscitated. Recent studies have shown that some patients have been resuscitated, without brain damage, after going over 20 minutes (for example, 45 minutes) without breathing. Infants and children can survive even longer than adults. The colder the water, the better the patient's chances for survival.

As a First Responder, you must be realistic when dealing with drownings. Many patients cannot be successfully resuscitated. The effects of water in the airway and the lack of oxygen to the brain may be too harsh for the body to endure. You may resuscitate some patients only to find out that they died within 48 hours due to pneumonia, lung damage, or brain damage. Even when you provide the best of care, some patients will die; however, you must give patients every opportunity for survival. You will not be able to tell which patient will survive. Provide resuscitation for all drowning victims.

Care for unconscious patients while they are still in the water is covered in the next section.

Mammalian diving reflex— when a person dives into cold water and submerges the face, breathing is inhibited, heart rate slows, and the major flow of blood is directed to the heart, lungs, and brain. Oxygen is diverted to the brain.

The Patient with Neck or Spinal Injuries

Injuries to the neck (cervical spine) and the rest of the spinal column occur during many water-related accidents. In First Responder care, you will not be expected to know how to use long spineboards and other floating, rigid devices for rescue situations. This does not mean that you cannot take certain actions to protect a patient's neck and spine during both rescue and care.

If a patient is unconscious, neck and spinal injuries may not be detected. In such a situation, assume that the patient has neck and spinal injuries and provide care accordingly. Whenever you survey a water-accident patient and find head injuries, assume there also are neck and spine injuries. Learn to quickly evaluate the patient for outward indications of possible neck and spinal injuries as described in Chapter 12. Remember, you will not have time to do a complete test for neck and spinal injuries for patients who are in the water. Likewise, a complete survey will not be possible for any patient you find in respiratory or cardiac arrest.

In cases when a patient with possible neck and spinal injuries is conscious and you are in shallow, warm water, stabilize the patient until the EMS System responds with personnel trained to remove the patient from the water. Simply keep the patient floating in a face-up position while you support the back and stabilize the head and neck. Seldom will this be the case. Too often, the water will be too cold or too deep, or there will be dangerous tides or currents. Often, the patient will need resuscitation and will have to be removed from the water as quickly as possible. Even though removal from the water may be dangerous in cases of spinal injury, it is better to have a live patient than a dead one.

1st Should you arrive at the scene and find the unconscious patient has already been removed from the water, have someone alert the EMS System dispatcher and begin your primary survey. Provide life-support care as needed, using the jaw-thrust technique rather than the head-tilt, chin-lift maneuver. After breathing and circulation are ensured, and bleeding is cared for, do a secondary survey, providing care as needed. Keep the patient warm and provide care for shock. Unless absolutely necessary, do not move the patient if there is any chance of neck or spinal injuries.

If the patient is still in the water, do not attempt a rescue unless you are a good swimmer, are trained to do so, and have others on hand who can help you. Make certain that someone alerts the EMS System dispatcher. This should be done immediately. Do not wait until after the rescue is attempted. Valuable time will be lost should the rescue fail. Providing care for the possible spinal injury patient still in the water requires you to:

1. Turn the patient face up in the water. This is best done while you are in the water, but it also can be done from a boat, poolside, or dockside. Wear a personal flotation device. To turn the patient, you should:
   a. Use one of your arms to keep the patient's neck and back in a straight line. Position this arm along the midline of your patient's back, keeping the head under your armpit.
   b. Use your free hand to grasp the patient at the armpit, as shown in Scansheet 20-1.
   c. Place the patient face up by gently rotating the body. This is done by pulling the patient up and over, while maintaining back and neck support. *Roll the patient as a unit.*
   d. Once the patient is face up, keep your arm in position to support the back and neck. Use your other hand to help stabilize the head.
2. If necessary, begin your primary survey while the patient is still in the water. Do not delay the detection of respiratory arrest.
3. If needed, provide pulmonary resuscitation as soon as possible. Use the jaw-thrust maneuver to protect the patient's neck and spine. Check for airway obstruction. If you are in shallow water, begin pulmonary resuscitation immediately. CPR will not be effective while the patient is in the water.
4. If someone is there to help you, have him or her support the patient along the midline of the back while you provide support to the patient's head and neck. Use the method described in Chapter 12. Float the patient to shore or lift from the water. Your job will be to keep the patient's head and neck as well-aligned as possible. Those helping you will have to lift the patient. NEVER pull the patient's neck during a lift from the water. If possible, provide two quick breaths to the patient in respiratory arrest before floating to shore or lifting into a boat.

   NOTE: If no one is on hand to help you and the patient must be removed from the water, lift the patient in any way you can, trying to provide some support to the head and neck. It will not be possible to provide support for the entire spine. Begin artificial ventilations as soon as possible.
5. Once the patient is out of the water, serious attempts at respiratory resuscitation can begin. Remember to check for a pulse to see if CPR should be started. If you are by yourself, rowing a cardiac arrest patient to shore, delay CPR until you have reached shore. You cannot row a boat and perform CPR. Also, CPR will be more effective once you are on shore. In some cases, depending on the stability of the boat and water conditions, you may be able to provide effective CPR in the boat until other rescuers arrive.
6. If the patient is breathing, check for and control all serious bleeding. Cover the patient to conserve body heat and perform a secondary survey, caring for any injuries you may find. Do not nove the patient if there are any signs of possible neck or spinal injuries.
7. Provide care for shock and make certain that the EMS System dispatcher has been alerted.

■ SCAN 20-1.

Water Rescue

WARNING:
DO ONLY WHAT YOU HAVE BEEN TRAINED TO DO. MAKE CERTAIN THAT YOU FOLLOW ALL LOCAL EMS PROTOCOLS.

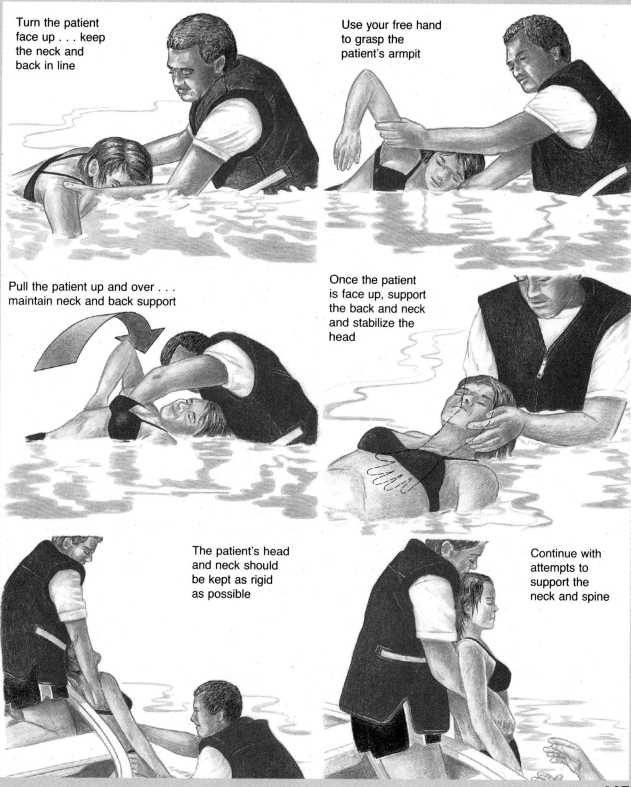

Turn the patient face up . . . keep the neck and back in line

Use your free hand to grasp the patient's armpit

Pull the patient up and over . . . maintain neck and back support

Once the patient is face up, support the back and neck and stabilize the head

The patient's head and neck should be kept as rigid as possible

Continue with attempts to support the neck and spine

DIVING ACCIDENTS

Diving Board Accidents

Each year, many people are injured as they attempt dives or enter the water from diving boards. These same injuries are seen in dives from poolsides, docks, boats, and the shore. A large number of such cases involve teenagers.

Most diving board accidents involve the head and neck. As a First Responder, you will also see injuries to the spine, hands, feet, and ribs occurring with great frequency. Any part of the body can be injured in these types of accidents, requiring complete primary and secondary surveys of all patients unless you are providing life-support measures. Remember, a medical emergency may have led to the diving accident.

Once the patient is out of the water, care for diving accident patients is the same as for any accident victim. Care provided in the water and in removing the patient from the water is the same as for any patient who may have neck and spine injuries. Remember, any unconscious or unresponsive patient is assumed to have possible neck and spinal injuries. If the patient is conscious, follow the procedures set down in Chapter 12 if you must deal with possible skull, neck, or spine injuries. Be sure to look for delayed reactions, particularly weakness, tingling sensations, or numbness in the limbs.

Scuba Diving Accidents

Scuba (SCUBA = self-contained underwater breathing apparatus) diving accidents have increased with the popularity of the sport and with inexperienced divers going into the water without the benefit of proper training. There are over two million people who scuba dive for sport or as part of their industrial or military employment. This number has been increasing at a rate of over 200,000 people each year.

Scuba diving accidents can produce body injuries or near-drownings. Medical problems can lead to scuba diving accidents. However, two special problems are seen in scuba diving accidents. They are gas bubbles in the diver's blood and the "bends."

Air embolism—gas bubbles in the blood. Gases leave a damaged lung and enter the bloodstream.

Gas bubbles in the blood (**air embolism**) occur when gases leave a diver's injured lung and enter the bloodstream. This can occur for many reasons, though it is most often associated with divers who hold their breath because of inadequate training, equipment failure, underwater emergency, or when trying to conserve air during a long dive. Air embolism can develop in the automobile accident victim who is trapped below water, as he takes gulps of air from air bubbles held inside the vehicle.

Air embolism can develop in both shallow and deep waters. The onset is rapid, with signs of personality changes and distorted senses sometimes giving the impression of drunkenness. The patient may have convulsions and rapidly lapse into unconsciousness. There may be signs of air outside of the lungs being trapped in the chest cavity.

You should suspect possible air embolism when the scuba diving accident victim has any of the following symptoms or signs:

- Personality changes
- Distorted senses (blurred vision is most common)
- Chest pains

- Numbness and tingling sensations in the arms and/or legs
- Total body weakness, or weakness of one or more limbs
- Frothy blood in the mouth or nose
- Convulsions

WARNING: Do *not* assume air embolism without first considering possible head injury or stroke.

The "bends" are really part of what is called **decompression sickness.** Patients with decompression sickness usually are those individuals who have come up too quickly from a deep, prolonged dive. When they do this, nitrogen gas is trapped in their tissues and may find its way into the bloodstream. The onset of the "bends" is usually slow for scuba divers, taking from 1 to 48 hours to appear. Because of this delay, the patient interview and reports from the patient's family and friends may be your only clue to relate the patient's problems to a dive.

NOTE: Scuba divers increase the risk of decompression sickness if they fly within 12 hours of the dive.

The symptoms and signs of decompression sickness include:

- Fatigue
- Deep pain to the muscles and joints (the "bends")
- Numbness or paralysis
- Choking, coughing, and/or labored breathing
- Chest pains
- Collapse that leads to unconsciousness
- Blotches on the skin (mottling). Sometimes, these rashes keep changing appearance.

If you think a patient has gas bubbles in the blood or decompression sickness due to a dive, be certain that the dispatcher is aware of the problem. The patient will need EMT transport to a medical facility as soon as possible. Dispatch may wish to direct the EMTs to take the patient to a special facility (hyperbaric trauma center).

While waiting for the EMTs to arrive, treat for shock and constantly monitor the patient. Respiratory and cardiac arrest are possible. Positioning of the patient is critical in order to avoid gas bubbles in the blood damaging the brain. Place the patient on the *left side* in a head down position. (This

> **Decompression sickness (the "bends")**—when a diver performs a quick ascent, nitrogen bubbles can be trapped in the body's tissues and later released into the bloodstream.

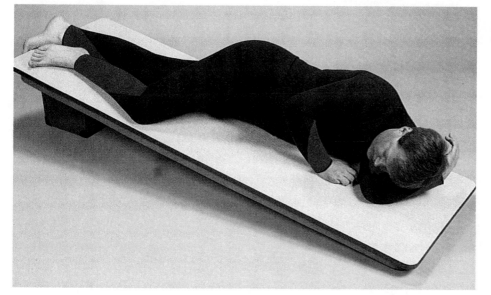

FIGURE 20–3. Positioning the patient after a scuba diving accident.

should not be tried if there are any signs of neck or spinal injuries.) Make certain that the patient's head is downward by slanting the entire body (about 15 degrees). Lifting the legs is not enough. Keeping an open airway may require slightly repositioning the patient.

ACCIDENTS INVOLVING ICE

Ice rescues require special training. Unless you are trained specifically to work on ice, do not attempt a rescue. If you cannot swim, you have no business going out onto the ice. You may walk on an undetected thin spot, fall through the ice, and quickly drown. All rescuers who are on or at the edge of the ice must wear personal flotation devices.

The major problem faced in ice rescue is reaching the victim. Never walk out to the person, or attempt to enter the water through a hole in the ice in order to find the victim. Never attempt an ice rescue by yourself unless you have some basic equipment, such as a personal flotation device and a ladder, and you are specifically trained in one-rescuer techniques. Never go onto ice that is rapidly breaking up. Your best course of action will be to work with others, from a safe ice surface or the shore.

Throwing a line to the victim or reaching out with a stick or a pole is your first choice of action. If the victim is not holding onto the ice, but trying to keep afloat in open water, throw anything that will float. Should you have to go onto the ice to get the patient, it is strongly recommended that you have help. Pushing a long ladder out onto the ice and then crawling along this ladder is a very effective method of safe rescue, providing someone is holding the ladder from a safe position. If enough people are on hand, a human chain can be formed to reach the victim.

One of the few methods of ice rescue that can be tried by the single rescuer is the use of a light boat. This craft can be moved along the ice

FIGURE 20–4. Work with others when attempting an ice rescue.

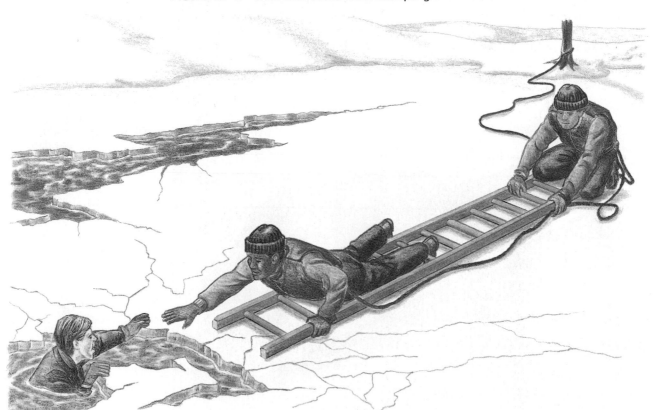

by riding inside of the boat and pushing the ice with your hands or with a stick or oar. This is often a very slow and awkward method, but if the ice cracks, at least you are safe in a boat.

Expect to find injuries with any patient who has fallen through the ice. Broken leg bones are common. Hypothermia may be a problem and should always be considered. **Do not attempt to rewarm the severe hypothermia patient** (see Chapter 14).

Alert the EMS System dispatcher for all patients who have had accidents on ice or have been in cold water. There may be injuries that are difficult to detect and problems due to the cold that may be delayed.

ASSISTING THE EMTs

You may be the first on the scene of a water or ice rescue and have the EMTs arrive during rescue or care. At other times, you may arrive at the scene after the EMTs. Some of the things you can do to help, if directed to do so, might be to:

- Interview bystanders—information gained could indicate the number of victims, a hidden medical emergency, or the cause of the accident.
- Crowd control—both the curiosity seeker and those wishing to help may come to the scene. Unless controlled, they may hinder rescue, fall into the water, or place too much weight on the ice surface.
- Find additional help—this is usual in cases of accidents involving ice.
- Find items used in rescue—you may have to look for a ladder or a boat.
- Help provide care—two-rescuer CPR, helping to position the patient, and helping to splint the patient may require your aid.
- Helping with a spineboard—if you are a good swimmer and have been trained in water rescue, the EMTs may need you in the water. Remember, a spineboard will float and will pop up very easily from below the surface of the water. If you are called upon to help place a spineboard under a patient who is still in the water, make sure of your position so as not to slip, and keep a firm grip on the board. If you have any doubts as to what the EMTs want you to do, ask questions.

SUMMARY

Do not attempt a water or ice rescue unless you can swim. Do not go into the water unless you are a good swimmer and have been trained in water rescue. Wear a personal flotation device.

Drowning is the number one problem faced in all water-related accidents. However, injuries of all types do occur and medical problems may have caused the accident to have taken place.

Often associated with water and ice accidents are **airway obstruction, cardiac arrest, heart attacks, head and neck injuries, internal injuries, and hypothermia.**

If the victim is in the water, try to **pull** him out, **throw** him something that will float, **tow** him from the water, or take a **boat** to him. If you go by boat to reach the person in the water, you should be wearing a personal flotation device.

Consider any **unconscious** patient to have **neck** and **spinal injuries.** Care for any patient already out of the water as required by your primary and secondary surveys and your interviews. Take special care to protect possible neck and spinal injuries.

When providing pulmonary resuscitation, use the **jaw-thrust** method to protect possible neck and spinal injuries.

If you are a good swimmer and have been trained in water rescue, you may be able to start artificial respirations while the patient is in the water. Never try to start CPR while the patient is in the water. If you are alone and must bring a cardiac arrest victim to shore, delay CPR and reach shore as quickly as possible in order to provide uninterrupted, effective CPR.

There are times when you should simply keep a patient floating until more help arrives. Do so only if you are both safe, the water is shallow, and it is not too cold. This should be done only if the patient is conscious and may have possible neck and spinal injuries.

Many patients in cardiac arrest can be resuscitated even after extended times in arrest. If the water is cold enough, they may last over 20 minutes before reaching biological death.

Always turn patients who are in the water into a face-up position. Remove the patient from the water as soon as possible. If life-support measures are needed, or if the scene becomes unsafe, you may have to disregard possible neck and spine injuries.

Whenever possible try to **support** the patient's **back** and keep the **neck supported** and in line with the midline of the back.

All patients who have been in water or ice accidents should receive care for shock. Keep them as warm as possible without overheating. Be alert for the symptoms and signs of hypothermia.

Do not allow the near-drowning victim to walk. Always alert dispatch for cases of near-drowning.

Diving board accidents usually produce head, neck, and spinal injuries. The hands, feet, and ribs are also frequently injured.

Scuba diving accidents may produce gas bubbles in the blood (air embolism) or decompression sickness. In cases of possible gas bubbles in the blood, look for unusual behavior, distorted senses, convulsions, and sudden loss of consciousness. For decompression sickness, expect a delayed reaction, difficult breathing, coughing, choking, chest pains, and changes in the appearance of the skin (blotches or changing rashes). Deep pains in the muscles and joints, known as the "bends," are typical signs in decompression sickness.

In cases of scuba diving accidents, if the possibility of gas bubbles in the blood exists, or if the patient is having the "bends," place the patient on the left side, tilting the entire body so that the head is in a slightly downward position.

If you must perform an ice rescue, have others help you. All rescuers should be wearing personal flotation devices. Try to throw a line to the victim or extend a pole to the victim. With the help of others, you may be able to reach the victim by crawling along a ladder or by forming a human chain out to the victim. When caring for the patient, be on guard against problems caused by **hypothermia.**

If requested, you can help EMTs at the water or ice accident scene by collecting information, going for more help, finding objects needed in the rescue, controlling the crowd, helping to provide care, and helping with spineboard procedures.

This is a posttest. It has been designed for you to take after you have completed the last unit in your First Responder course. This test is provided for self-evaluation so that you can see your weaknesses before taking a final exam. Page references are provided so that you can go back and restudy problem areas before final testing.

You may wish to study the situations provided in the appendix before taking this posttest. They will help you bring together what you have learned in various units and will challenge you to recall information. If you take the posttest before doing these situations, it is recommended that you go over the situations before your final exam and practical.

Since this is a posttest, you may take as much time as needed to complete the test. Your best approach would be to set aside 2 solid hours for the test. Try to do the first 50 questions in 60 minutes. Take a 10-minute break and try to do the last 50 questions in 50 minutes. Answers are provided so you can check your test and note the pages you need to reread and study.

For questions 1 to 5, match the letter from the list of diseases and conditions (A through E) to the description provided in the question.

A. Heat stroke   B. Shock   C. Heart attack
D. Diabetic coma   E. Stroke (CVA)

___ 1. Rapid and thready pulse; rapid and shallow breathing; cool, clammy, pale white skin; dilated pupils (p. 175)

___ 2. Rapid, full pulse; difficult, snoring respirations; unequal pupils; paralysis to one side (p. 307)

___ 3. Rapid and thready pulse; deep, gasping labored breathing; red skin; lackluster pupils (p. 313)

___ 4. Rapid, full pulse; deep, gasping labored breathing; hot, dry red skin; dilated pupils (p. 342)

___ 5. Rapid pulse; deep, gasping labored breathing; moist, blue skin; dilated pupils (p. 303)

Circle the letter of the best answer to each question.

6. An injured adult patient wants you to help him. He starts calling you "doctor." You should tell him you are a First Responder trained in emergency care so that his consent becomes (p. 14)

   A. Implied   C. Informed
   B. Actual   D. Limited

7. A penetrating wound to the medial right upper quadrant will probably lacerate (cut) the (p. 25)

   A. Spleen   C. Urinary bladder
   B. Liver   D. Appendix

8. You arrive at an emergency scene and find an unconscious patient who is not breathing. You should (p. 55)

   A. Ensure an open   C. Take a carotid
      airway   pulse
   B. Begin mouth-to-   D. Do a complete
      mask resuscitation   patient survey

9. During the secondary survey, checking for abdominal tenderness is done after checking for (p. 75)

   A. Back point   C. Pelvic injuries
      tenderness   D. Equal chest
   B. Abdominal   expansion
      penetrations

10. For the adult patient, the rate of providing breaths during mouth-to-mask resuscitation is (p. 93)

    A. 1 every 5 seconds   C. 2 every 5 seconds
    B. 1 every 15 seconds   D. 2 every 15 seconds

11. In one-rescuer CPR for the adult patient, compressions and ventilations are provided at a rate of (p. 129)

    A. 1 breath every 5 compressions at 60 compressions per minute
    B. 1 breath every 5 compressions at 80 compressions per minute
    C. 2 breaths every 15 compressions at 60 to 80 compressions per minute
    D. 2 breaths every 15 compressions at 80 to 100 compressions per minute

12. The order of care when trying to control profuse bleeding is (p. 158)

    A. Elevation, direct pressure, pressure points, tourniquet
    B. Tourniquet, pressure points, direct pressure, elevation
    C. Direct pressure, elevation, pressure points, tourniquet
    D. Pressure points, direct pressure, tourniquet, elevation

13. When caring for a patient without head or spinal injury who is developing shock, you should (p. 176)

    A. Elevate the head   C. Elevate the upper
    B. Elevate the feet   body
                           D. Leave in a flat
                              position

14. If you provide First Responder emergency care in good faith, to the best of your ability, you are protected in most states by the (p. 9)

    A. Actual Consent   C. Implied Consent
       Law   Law
    B. Good Samaritan   D. Applied Consent
       Law   Law

15. In two-rescuer CPR for the adult patient,

compressions and ventilations are delivered at a rate of (p. 147)

A. 1 breath every 5 compressions at a rate of 60 to 80 compressions per minute
B. 1 breath every 5 compressions at a rate of 80 to 100 compressions per minute
C. 2 breaths every 15 compressions at a rate of 60 to 80 compressions per minute
D. 2 breaths every 15 compressions at a rate of 80 to 100 compressions per minute

16. A patient has an object impaled in the globe of the eye. You should (p. 211)

A. Remove the object and apply direct pressure with a gauze pad
B. Remove the object and apply a loose dressing
C. Leave the object in place, pad around the eye, and place a cup or cone over the object
D. Leave the object in place, apply a pressure dressing around the object, and place a cup or cone over the object

17. An unconscious person is found in a field. The face is swollen and blotchy, respirations are labored with wheezings, and the pulse is very weak. You should suspect (p. 179)

A. Lung shock (respiratory shock)
B. Heart shock (cardiogenic shock)
C. Nerve shock (neurogenic shock)
D. Allergy shock (anaphylactic shock)

18. After repositioning the head of an unconscious adult patient and attempting to ventilate in order to clear the airway of a total obstruction, the correct order for efforts to clear the airway is (p. 107)

A. Finger sweeps, manual thrusts, ventilation
B. Manual thrusts, finger sweeps, ventilation
C. Back blows, finger sweeps, manual thrusts, ventilation
D. Manual thrusts, ventilation, finger sweeps

19. In the adult patient, the CPR compression site is (p. 124)

A. Directly between the nipples
B. Two finger widths below the collarbones, along the midline of the body
C. Two finger widths directly above the lower notch of the breastbone (sternum)
D. Three finger widths to the right of the left nipple

20. When providing CPR for a child patient, breaths and compressions are provided at a rate of (p. 137)

A. 1 breath every 5 compressions at 60 compressions per minute
B. 1 breath every 5 compressions at 80 to 100 compressions per minute
C. 2 breaths every 15 compressions at 60 to 100 compressions per minute
D. 2 breaths every 15 compressions at 80 compressions per minute

21. When providing emergency care, your best defense against most infectious diseases is to (p. 5)

A. Wear a gauze mask
B. Use occlusive dressings
C. Wear latex or vinyl gloves
D. Wash your hands with bleach after touching blood or body fluids

22. The best way to care for a simple nosebleed is to have the patient (p. 213)

A. Tilt his head back
B. Push gauze into his nose
C. Pinch his nostrils shut
D. Tilt his head forward

23. A patient has an open wound of the abdomen and his intestine has been exposed. You should (p. 219)

A. Apply an occlusive dressing
B. Push the intestine back into the abdominal cavity
C. Apply direct pressure
D. Lay a towel over the organ

24. The globe of a patient's eye is cut. You should (p. 209)

A. Let it bleed freely
B. Apply a loose dressing
C. Apply a pressure dressing
D. Apply direct pressure

25. A patient has clear fluids draining from his ear. You should (p. 212)

A. Pack the ear canal
B. Apply a pressure dressing
C. Do nothing
D. Apply a loose dressing

26. Part of a patient's ear has been torn off. After caring for the wound site, you should (p. 212)

A. Place the avulsed part in water
B. Place the avulsed part in ice
C. Wrap the avulsed part in cotton
D. Wrap the avulsed part in plastic

27. A patient is in shock and has a severe bruise on his abdomen twice the size of a man's fist. Internal blood loss probably equals about (p. 170)

A. 10%
B. 15%
C. 20%
D. 25%

28. When providing mouth-to-mask resuscitation for a patient having spinal injury, you should use the (p. 92)

A. Jaw thrust
B. Head tilt, neck lift
C. Head tilt, chin lift
D. Any of the above

29. Dark red blood is flowing from a wound to a patient's neck. You should first (p. 216)

A. Apply a pressure dressing
B. Use carotid artery pressure points
C. Apply an occlusive dressing
D. Apply a bulky dressing

30. As you approach the victim of a fall, you note that he is not responsive to bystanders around him. The patient is lying face up with both arms

extended above his head. You can begin to suspect (p. 282)

A. Severe internal bleeding   C. Pelvic fractures
B. Spinal injury   D. Hip dislocation

31. A large neck artery is severed. You cannot control the flow of blood using direct pressure applied with the palm of your gloved hand. You should (p. 215)

A. Use a roll of gauze and an occlusive dressing   C. Use a pressure dressing over a roll of gauze
B. Use pressure points   D. Pinch off the vessel

32. When caring for an open wound, your first step is to (p. 200)

A. Expose the wound   C. Control bleeding
B. Clean the site   D. Prevent contamination

33. When caring for an injured eye, you should (p. 210)

A. Apply direct pressure   C. Cover both eyes
B. Wash with flowing water   D. Leave both eyes open

34. An object is loosely impaled in the cheek. Its point has broken through the cheek wall into the mouth. You should (p. 208)

A. Remove the object and place packs between teeth and cheek wall
B. Not remove the object, but place packs between the teeth and the cheek wall
C. Simply remove the object
D. Leave the object in place

35. The victim of an automobile accident had his lap seat belt applied too tightly. During the accident, he had an organ ruptured because of this improper application. Most likely, the injured organ would be the (p. 29)

A. Liver   C. Spleen
B. Urinary bladder   D. Gallbladder

36. When breathing and circulation are arrested, lethal changes in the patient's brain begin in (p. 86)

A. 30 seconds   C. 4 to 6 minutes
B. 1 to 3 minutes   D. 10 to 15 minutes

37. A patient has an object impaled in the chest. You should (p. 293)

A. Do nothing to the site
B. Stabilize the object with pads of dressing
C. Remove the object and apply an occlusive dressing
D. Remove the object and apply a trauma dressing

38. When caring for a flail chest patient, you should (p. 290)

A. Apply tape around the entire chest

B. Apply cravats and a swathe
C. Position the patient face down
D. Secure pads over the flailed section

39. A patient has an obvious sucking chest wound. You should (p. 292)

A. Apply an occlusive dressing   C. Apply a trauma dressing
B. Apply a cravat   D. Wait for EMTs

40. You may correct slight angulations of fractures to the upper arm bone (humerus) in cases having (Chapter 11)

A. Shoulder dislocation   C. Closed fractures
B. Open fractures   D. Elbow fractures

Match the letter of the best procedure on the right to be used with each specific injury listed on the left. Page references will be given in the list of answers.

41. ___ Shoulder fracture   A. Wrist sling and swathe
42. ___ Shoulder anterior dislocation   B. Tie legs together
43. ___ Fractured ribs   C. Use 2 rigid splints
44. ___ Fractured upper arm (shaft)   D. Pillow, sling, and swathe
45. ___ Fractured wrist and hand   E. Wait for EMTs
    F. Single pillow splint
46. ___ Fractured pelvis   G. Standard sling and swathe
47. ___ Hip dislocation
48. ___ Knee   H. 2-pillow splint
49. ___ Fractured lower leg   I. Cravats and swathe
    J. Splint in position found
50. ___ Fractured foot

STOP NOW AND CONTINUE IN 10 MINUTES.

Circle the letter of the best answer to each question.

51. Facial bleeding is best controlled by (p. 208)

A. Pressure points   C. Occlusive dressing
B. Direct pressure   D. Loose dressing

52. A patient has received a skull fracture. You would expect his pupils to be (p. 278)

A. Dilated   C. Unequal
B. Constricted   D. Normal

53. A conscious patient has a mild closed head injury, with no indications of spinal injury. This patient should be positioned (p. 280)

A. As found   C. Face down
B. Legs elevated   D. Upper body elevated

54. A patient with severe spinal injuries is in cardiac arrest. You should (p. 283)

A. Begin CPR   C. Provide compressions only
B. Provide ventilations only   D. Fully stabilize the head and neck, then apply CPR

55. A patient is very restless and complains of pains in his chest. His breathing is very labored. You should suspect that the patient is having, or is about to have, a (p. 303)

    A. Stroke (CVA)
    B. Congestive heart failure
    C. Heart attack
    D. Epileptic seizure

56. A patient has slurred speech. His only complaint is a mild headache. You note that his pupils are slightly unequal. That patient slowly has a loss of consciousness and begins snoring. You can find no other indications of illness or injury. You should suspect (p. 307)

    A. Heart attack
    B. Stroke (CVA)
    C. Congestive heart failure
    D. Insulin shock

57. A patient has labored, rapid breathing. His ankles and abdomen are swollen. You note a blue coloration to his lips. The patient insists upon sitting up and supporting his upper body weight on his elbows. You should suspect (p. 304)

    A. Congestive heart failure
    B. Mild epilepsy
    C. Insulin shock
    D. Stroke (CVA)

58. A conscious patient has all the signs and symptoms of a stroke (CVA). He should be positioned (p. 307)

    A. Face down
    B. As found
    C. Legs elevated
    D. Head, shoulders, and back elevated

59. A patient has had a convulsive seizure. When you arrive, he acts somewhat confused and complains of a headache. You should suspect (p. 312)

    A. Diabetic coma
    B. Epilepsy
    C. Heart attack
    D. Insulin shock

60 A patient complains of dizziness. Breathing is normal and pulse is rapid and full. His skin is cool and clammy. The patient says that he is a diabetic and has been feeling well recently. There are no other signs. Highest on your list of suspected problems should be (p. 314)

    A. Insulin shock
    B. Diabetic coma
    C. Allergy shock
    D. Congestive heart failure

Fill in the blanks to complete each of the following statements.

61. If a patient is in insulin shock you should give _____. (p. 314)

62. Unless directed to do so, do not induce vomiting if a patient has ingested a strong acid, alkaline, or _____ product. (p. 320)

63. Burns to the eyes should be flooded with water for no less than _____ minutes. (p. 337)

64. When caring for a snakebite patient, you have only one constricting band. It should be placed between the bite and the patient's _____. (p. 324)

65. A burn patient has a painful, deep red burn with blistering. This is a _____ degree burn. (p. 331)

66. Before dressing a mild burn, the site should be _____. (p. 334)

67. Most of all, the patient in mild hypothermia requires _____. (p. 344)

68. In superficial frostbite, the skin appears waxy and _____. (p. 346)

69. The salted water given to heat cramp patients is made from one quart of cool water and _____ teaspoon(s) of salt. (p. 341)

70. A patient exposed to excess heat has pale and clammy skin. His pulse is weak and respirations are rapid and very shallow. If this is a heat-related problem, it is probably _____. (p. 341)

Circle the letter of the correct answer for each question.

71. When performing pulmonary resuscitation for an infant, breaths are delivered at the rate of (p. 96)

    A. 1 per second
    B. 1 per 3 seconds
    C. 1 per 9 seconds
    D. 2 per 15 seconds

72. A woman's first labor normally lasts (p. 354)

    A. 1 hour
    B. 4 hours
    C. 8 hours
    D. 16 hours

73. During a breech birth, the baby's head must deliver within 3 minutes of its buttocks and trunk. If delivery of the head does not occur in this time period, you should (p. 366)

    A. Transport immediately
    B. Wait 5 minutes as you massage the mother's abdomen
    C. Insert your fingers into the mother's vagina and create an airway for the baby
    D. Wait for EMTs to arrive

74. You have to tie an infant's umbilical cord. The distances from the infant's abdomen for tying are (p. 361)

    A. 10 and 7 inches
    B. 10 and 13 inches
    C. 1 and 5 inches
    D. 5 and 8 inches

75. To control normal postdelivery vaginal bleeding, you should place a sanitary napkin over the mother's vaginal opening, place her legs together, elevate her feet, and (p. 362)

    A. Massage her abdomen over the site of the uterus (womb)
    B. Apply direct pressure over the napkin
    C. Have her use her thighs in order to tighten and release pressure on the napkin
    D. Have her apply direct pressure over the napkin

76. To aid the mother in delivering her baby's upper shoulder, you should support the baby's head and gently (p. 357)

   A. Pull toward your waist
   B. Guide the baby's head upward
   C. Guide the baby's head downward
   D. Turn the baby's face toward the mother's thigh

77. If a newborn does not start breathing on its own in 30 seconds, you should (p. 360)

   A. Begin pulmonary resuscitation
   B. Snap your fingers on the soles of the baby's feet or vigorously rub his back
   C. Hold the baby up by its ankles and slap its buttocks
   D. Tie off the umbilical cord

78. When caring for a patient having dry lime burns, you should (p. 337)

   A. Soak the site in cold water for 5 minutes
   B. Wash the site in warm water for 15 minutes
   C. Apply a burn ointment
   D. Brush away the lime

79. A patient has a mild acid splashed into his eye. You arrive 1 minute after this happens. You should (p. 337)

   A. Apply moist dressings over the closed eyelids
   B. Flood the eyes with water for at least 5 minutes
   C. Flood the eyes with water for at least 15 minutes
   D. Not worry, the patient's tears have washed away the acid

80. A drug abuse patient is very sleepy. His pulse and breathing rates are dangerously low. You note that his pupils are constricted and he is sweating heavily. The patient has probably abused (p. 384)

   A. Uppers   C. Narcotics
   B. Downers   D. Volatile chemicals

81. The patient is in a coma. His pulse is rapid and weak, and respirations are deep and rapid. There is a fruity breath odor. The patient is probably (p. 313)

   A. In diabetic coma   C. On volatile
   B. In alcohol   chemicals
      withdrawal   D. Intoxicated on
                            alcohol

82. You are caring for a conscious patient who has ingested an unknown poison. You cannot call the poison control center. To begin care, you should (p. 320)

   A. Induce vomiting with syrup of ipecac
   B. Give the patient mineral oil to drink
   C. Induce vomiting with activated charcoal and water
   D. Dilute the poison by having the patient drink water or milk

83. You arrive at a cave-in and find a victim covered with soil. He is not breathing. Workmen at the scene tell you that it is safe to approach the patient.

You should (p. 431)

   A. Uncover the patient's head and neck and immediately begin resuscitation
   B. Uncover enough of the patient to pull him free from the soil and then begin resuscitation
   C. Uncover the patient's head, neck, and chest and then begin resuscitation
   D. Uncover the patient's entire body, move the patient, and then begin resuscitation

84. For patients having emotional emergencies, you should (p. 380)

   A. Tell them that everything is fine and not to worry
   B. Tell them they are to listen to you and do what you say because you are there to help
   C. Tell them that you are trained to care for people having emotional emergencies
   D. Talk to these patients and let them know that you are listening to what they tell you

85. Which of the following are listed in correct order in terms of the text example of triage priorities? (p. 324)

   A. Severe burns, moderate burns, heat stroke
   B. Open abdominal wounds, moderate bleeding, moderate burns
   C. Open chest wound, multiple fractures, heat stroke
   D. Heart attack, moderate burns, moderate bleeding

Fill in the blanks to complete the following statements.

86. You are the first to arrive at the scene of a traffic accident where there are injuries. Your first duties should be to _____. (p. 389)

87. To break into a side window of a locked automobile, you should place a sharp tool at a _____ corner of the window and strike the tool with a hammer. (p. 395)

88. Before trying to gain access to patients trapped in a vehicle that is on its side, you should _____ the vehicle. (p. 396)

89. For an emergency move of a patient who can walk, your best choice of procedure is the _____. (p. 410)

90. A patient having a medical emergency requires a nonemergency move. The patient has no injuries, but he cannot stand or walk. You have one person to help you with the move. Your best choice would be the _____ _____. (p. 417)

91. You cannot lift an unconscious patient who has to be moved. You should use a _____ (type of move). (p. 413)

92. You need to make a nonemergency move of a patient who cannot stand or walk. Two other people

are on hand to help. You should use the
_____. (p. 418)

93. You and the patient are in danger. The patient can stand, but he cannot walk. You should use the _____.
(p. 412)

94. At a crime scene, you must provide care for the patient and try not to _____.
(p. 430)

95. You have been providing care at an emergency scene. EMTs arrive to take over responsibilities. You need to turn over to them the patients, patients' possessions, and _____
_____. (p. 6)

96. A patient locked in a building needs immediate life-saving care. There is no key at the scene. You should _____
_____. (p. 398)

97. You are caring for a spinal injury patient when the scene becomes dangerous. You should _____
_____. (p. 408)

98. An electric line is down on a vehicle containing accident vcitims needing care. Before approaching the vehicle, you should _____
_____ .
(p. 401)

99. You are helping a patient out of a building. You believe there may be a fire on the other side of a door. Before opening the door, you should _____
_____. (p. 401)

100. You are performing triage at a multipatient scene. The first person you examine is an *unwitnessed* cardiac arrest. Unless directed otherwise by special triage protocols, you should
_____. (p. 423)

ANSWERS

1.	B	3.	D	5.	C
2.	E	4.	A	6.	C

7.	B	26.	D	45.	H (p. 242)
8.	A	27.	C		(D is possible)
9.	B	28.	A	46.	B (p. 245)
10.	A	29.	C	47.	E (p. 245)
11.	D	30.	B	48.	J (p. 265)
12.	C	31.	C	49.	C (p. 266)
13.	B	32.	A	50.	F (p. 247)
14.	B	33.	C	51.	B
15.	B	34.	A	52.	C
16.	C	35.	B	53.	D
17.	D	36.	C	54.	A
18.	B	37.	B	55.	C
19.	C	38.	D	56.	B
20.	B	39.	A	57.	A
21.	C	40.	C	58.	D
22.	C	41.	G (p. 236)	59.	B
23.	A	42.	D (p. 236)	60.	A
24.	B	43.	G (p. 288)		
25.	D	44.	A (p. 240)		

61. sugar 62. petroleum 63. 20 64. heart
65. second 66. exposed 67. external warmth
68. white 69. one 70. heat exhaustion

71.	B	76.	C	81.	A
72.	D	77.	B	82.	D
73.	C	78.	D	83.	C
74.	A	79.	B	84.	D
75.	A	80.	C	85.	B

86. make the scene safe without risking personal safety
87. lower 88. stabilize 89. one-rescuer assist
90. extremity lift 91. drag
92. direct ground lift
93. pack strap carry (or fire fighter's carry)
94. break the chain of evidence
95. patient information
96. break in (through window or door glass)
97. move the patient as quickly as possible
98. have someone call the electric company to turn off the power
99. feel the door at the top to see if it is hot
100. continue the triage

Let each question be worth 1 point. The lowest passing grade on this post-test is 70. It is hoped that you scored 80 points or higher. Regardless of your score, go back to the text and restudy any materials that you did not know or that you are unsure of.

APPENDIX 1

Study Problems: 25 Emergency Care Situations

These situations can be used with those supplied in the DOT lesson plans. They can be done on an individual basis or they may lend themselves well to classroom discussion or small group activities.

As part of your First Responder training, you will be given emergency care situations or simulated incidents to solve. Your instructor may make these problems a part of each unit, or they may be presented as part of a field training class held at the end of the course.

The situations you will be asked to solve are a very important part of your training. While learning to be a First Responder, information and procedures are presented in an orderly fashion. Often, only those materials dealing with a particular day's lesson are considered. When you finish your course and have to provide emergency care, you will frequently have to bring together knowledge and skills from several study units. Simulated emergency care situations help you to practice so that you may "bring together" many of the different things you have studied concerning First Responder emergency care.

The DOT has created practice situations for First Responder training. Since your instructor may wish to use these in class, or for testing, different situations are given in this appendix. You may use your text to help with the situations presented here. The best approach is to work with several fellow students. Have different members of the group take turns being the patient, First Responder, and bystanders. One student should serve as a judge of the First Responder's performance, using the text and classroom notes to check procedures. *Do not* try to create any "mock" accident scenes using real vehicles or hazards.

For each situation, be sure to correctly:

- Evaluate and control the scene
- Gain access
- Assess patients using surveys and interviews (the judge may have to provide you with signs and descriptions of the patients)
- Question and utilize bystanders
- Provide dispatch with all needed information
- Move patients when necessary
- Provide First Responder-level emergency care
- Turn patients and information over to more highly trained personnel

After completing the situations provided in this book, you and your fellow students may want to create additional situations for practice. Your instructor may be able to provide you with additional study problems and exercises.

SITUATIONS

1. During the summer, you respond to a private residence. The husband has been working under the house, in a crawl space foundation. You find him and his wife surrounded by neighbors. As you start to question the patient, he loses consciousness. His skin is hot, dry, and flushed. His pulse is rapid and weak, and his respirations are shallow.

2. Responding to the scene of a single vehicle accident, you find a victim seated in his car. The patient is conscious and has both arms folded over his chest. There are no signs of spinal injuries. The steering wheel is bent. The patient shows labored, painful breathing and says that he feels something moving in his chest when he breathes.

3. You arrive at a shopping center parking lot and find a young pregnant woman lying on the ground. She is unconscious and there is evidence of vaginal bleeding.

4. While walking down a street, you notice people looking in the window of a ranch-style house. You are asked if you can help. Looking through a window, you see an elderly woman lying on the floor. She is unresponsive and her lips are blue. The doors to the house are locked.

5. At the scene of an automobile accident, you find an unconscious patient who has been thrown through the windshield. The patient is breathing. Deep red blood is flowing from a wound in his neck.

6. At work, you see a blue flash coming from a utility pole. Outside, you find a worker who has fallen. He is on his back with his arms stretched above his head. There are burns on his hands. The patient is not responsive.

7. The scene is a shopping center. You find a middle-aged man walking around acting intoxicated. There is a sweet, "fruity" odor on his breath. Bystanders say that he has probably had too much wine.

8. At the scene of a vehicle accident, an occupant of one of the cars is walking around saying she is "OK." Suddenly, she falls to the ground and begins to have convulsions.

9. There is a disturbance around the door of a department store ladies' room. You find an expectant mother in great pain saying, "Something feels wrong." You find she is having a breech delivery.

10. A car and bike collide at an intersection. The bike rider is a young woman, lying face up in the street. She is conscious. You note that her right leg is rotated away from her body.

11. A victim of a vehicle accident has an open fracture of the left forearm and is bleeding profusely from the site.

12. The only victim of a traffic accident has a painful, swollen foot.

13. At a public park, you find a patient who has collapsed forward on a table. In front of the patient is a partially eaten sandwich. Bystanders are trying to perform what they believe to be mouth-to-mouth resuscitation.

14. A two-vehicle traffic accident takes place. In one car the driver is bleeding from the nose and part of his right ear is torn off. The passenger has an open fracture of the thigh bone (femur). In the other car you find one victim who is unconscious. There are bystanders at the scene.

15. At a self-service gas station you see a customer splash gasoline into his eyes.

16. A young boy is stabbed in the right side of his chest. He is still alert, lying on the sidewalk. His mother is frantic and keeps screaming for you not to touch her son. You notice that the boy has a sucking chest wound.

17. A passenger of a car involved in a traffic accident claims to be fine. After several minutes, she begins to hold her left upper abdomen and complains of pain.

18. While at a lunch counter, you notice a teenage girl who begins to breathe very heavily, making a wheezing sound. Her face begins to swell.

19. At a fire scene, an elderly neighbor falls to the ground. His wife says that he was having a headache. You find his speech slurred and his pupils unequal.

20. An industrial accident occurs and the victim's right arm is amputated above the elbow.

21. At a backyard cookout, a child receives burns of the right shoulder, arm, and hand. The burn sites are intense red and blistering. The child is in pain.

22. During a company softball game, a 40-year-old man complains of chest pains. He is very nervous and says that he will be fine if everyone leaves him alone. He wishes to jog in order to relax his chest muscles.

23. A 3-year-old child has swallowed bleach.

24. An accident victim is in the back seat of a car. He is not breathing. You strongly suspect spinal injuries have occurred.

25. You and two other First Responders arrive at the scene of a three-car accident. You see the following:
    a. In a car, a conscious woman with an open fracture of the upper arm bone (humerus).
    b. In the back seat, a conscious young woman lying on her right side, clutching her abdomen.
    c. In the driver's seat, a conscious man making gurgling sounds while in respiratory distress.
    d. Sitting against a guardrail, a child crying for help while bleeding from the face.
    e. On the pavement, a man with severe crush injuries to the skull. Portions of his brain are visible and there is complete deformity of his face. He is in a large pool of blood.
    f. In a car, an elderly man, not showing any signs of life.

Now that you have read the above, and perhaps tried to work out each situation, you must ask yourself if you have developed "tunnel vision." Did you find yourself worrying only about the major injury, sign, or symptom given? If so, you need to reread Chapter 3 and reconsider the roles of the First Responder.

In each situation, did you consider your own personal safety? Did you consider the importance of bystander interviews? What questions did you ask to gain as much information as quickly as possible?

Go back over each of the situations and:

1. Write out what you would report to the dispatcher.

2. List any tools, equipment, or supplies you would need.

3. Fill out a patient information sheet for each case. If First Responders do not use such

sheets in your EMS System, make out your own written reports. Exchange these with other students to compare assessments and the care provided for each patient.

The following pages in the text should be used as you evaluate your assessments and care for each situation:

APPENDIX 2

Blood Pressure Determination

It is best to follow AHA guidelines in regard to blood pressure determination unless your state EMS System recommends a different set of instructions.

In some localities, particularly those where First Responders work in isolated areas, a special training program for blood pressure determination is included in the standard First Responder course. If this is not part of your course, do not try to train yourself in the use of the blood pressure cuff. Do only what you have been trained to do.

INTRODUCTION

Blood pressure is a vital sign. A reading of blood pressure significantly above or below what is expected for a patient can be a valuable sign in determining what may be wrong with the patient and how the patient's condition might change (for example, shock). Blood pressure determination is a valuable method to check the patient's stability as you wait for the EMTs to arrive.

When the lower chamber on the left side of the heart (the left ventricle) **contracts,** it forces blood out of the heart to circulate throughout the body. This produces a pressure change in the arteries. The pressure created in the arteries due to this blood coming from the heart is called the **systolic** (sis-TOL-ik) blood pressure.

After the lower left chamber of the heart contracts, it **relaxes** and refills. While this is happening, the pressure in the arteries falls. This pressure is called the **diastolic** (di-as-TOL-ik) blood pressure.

Blood pressure is measured in specific units, millimeters of mercury (mm Hg). These are the units on the blood pressure gauge. Since this system of measurement is standard and known to the people receiving patient information from First Responders, you will not have to say "millimeters of mercury" after each reading. You will report the systolic pressure first and then the diastolic, as in 120 over 80 (120/80).

You will not know the normal blood pressure for a patient unless the person is alert, knows the information, and can tell you what it is. Blood pressure varies greatly among individuals; however, there is a general rule for estimating what a patient's blood pressure should be. This rule works for adults up to the age of 40. To estimate the systolic blood pressure of an adult male at rest, add his age to 100. To estimate the systolic blood pressure of an adult female at rest, add her age to 90.

Keep in mind that one blood pressure reading is often of little use. The first reading may be high because of the effects of stress produced by the emergency. You might find that a patient has a reading within normal range, but the condition may worsen. For example, a patient going into shock may have a rapid pulse and a normal blood pressure reading when you first arrive at the scene. A few minutes later, the blood pressure may fall dramatically. You will have to take several readings while you are providing care. Changes in blood pressure can be very significant.

Consider the patient to have a serious low blood pressure reading if the systolic pressure is below 90 mm Hg. Any drop of blood pressure to 90/60 or below may indicate that the patient is probably going into shock. High blood pressure would be any reading above 140/90. The problem with high-blood pressure readings is that many individuals show a short-term rise in blood pressure at the emergency scene. You will need more than one reading to confirm high blood pressure.

Use the following guidelines at the emergency scene:

ADULTS

- Systolic above 180—serious
- Systolic below 90—serious

- Diastolic above 106—serious
- Diastolic below 60—serious

CHILDREN: Ages 1 to 5

- Systolic above 120—serious
- Systolic below 70—serious
- Diastolic above 76—serious
- Diastolic below 50—serious

CHILDREN: Ages 5 to 12

- Systolic above 150—serious
- Systolic below 90—serious
- Diastolic above 86—serious
- Diastolic below 60—serious

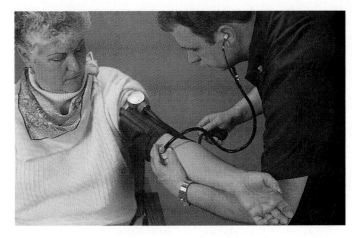

FIGURE A2–2.   Positions for taking blood pressure.

MEASURING BLOOD PRESSURE

There are two common techniques used to measure blood pressure in emergency field situations. They are:

1. **Auscultation** (os-skul-TAY-shun)—using a blood pressure cuff and a stethoscope to listen for characteristic sounds
2. **Palpation**—using a blood pressure cuff and feeling the patient's radial pulse

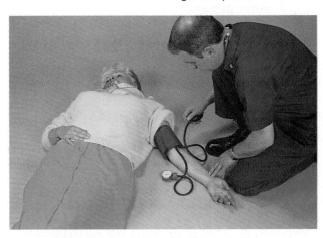

Determining Blood Pressure by Auscultation

To determine blood pressure using a blood pressure cuff and a stethoscope, you should:

1. Have the patient sitting or lying down. Cut away or remove clothing over the arm. Support the arm at the level of the heart.

FIGURE A2–1.   Blood pressure determination equipment.

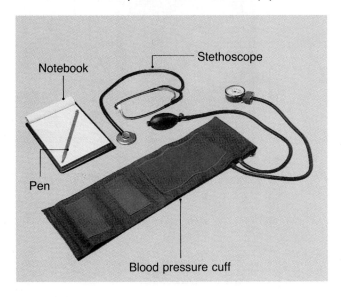

WARNING: Do *not* move the patient's arm if there is any possibility of spinal injury. Make certain that the arm to be used has not been injured.

2. Select the correct-size blood pressure cuff. Do not try to use an adult-size cuff on a child.
3. Wrap the cuff around the patient's upper arm. The lower border of the cuff should be about 1 inch above the crease in the patient's elbow. The center of the cuff must be placed over the major artery in the upper arm, the brachial (BRAY-key-al) artery.
   NOTE: Some cuffs have a marker to tell you how to line up the cuff in relation to the brachial artery. Know your equipment. Some cuffs have no markers, while others have inaccurate markers. The tubes entering the bladder in the cuff may not be in the correct location. The AHA recommends that you find the bladder center and line this up over the medial surface of the arm.
4. Apply the cuff securely but not too tightly. You should be able to place one finger under the bottom edge of the cuff.
5. Place the ends of the stethoscope in your ears.
6. Use your fingertips to locate the brachial artery at the crease in the elbow.

Stress the importance of an adequate cuff width in order to provide the required pressure to the artery. First Responders should use cuffs that are supplied or recommended by their local EMS Systems.

7. Position the diaphragm or bell of the stethoscope over the brachial artery pulse site. Do *not* touch the cuff. This will give sounds that may cause false readings.

8. Close the bulb valve and inflate the cuff. As you do this, listen to the pulse sounds through the stethoscope. At a certain point, you will not be able to hear the pulse sounds.

9. Keep inflating the cuff to a point 30 mm Hg higher than the point where the pulse sounds stopped.

10. Open the bulb valve *slowly* to release pressure from the cuff. It should fall at a smooth rate of 2 to 3 mm Hg per second.

11. Listen carefully for and note the start of clicking or tapping sounds. This is the systolic pressure.

12. Let the cuff continue to deflate. Listen for and note when the clicking or tapping sounds fade (not when they stop). When the sound turns dull or soft, this is the diastolic pressure.

13. Let the rest of the air out of the cuff quickly. If practical, leave the cuff in place so you can make additional readings.

14. Record the time, the arm used, the position of the patient (lying down, sitting), and the patient's pressure. Round off the readings to the next highest number. For example, 145 mm Hg should be recorded as 146 mm Hg.

NOTE: Some EMS Systems have First Responders use the point where the sounds stop as the diastolic pressure.

Some people cannot find the brachial artery, or they cannot hear the pulse sounds when they

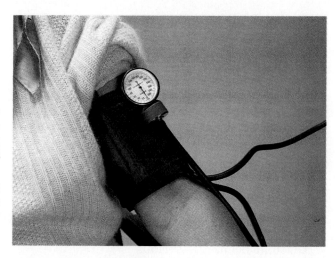

FIGURE A2–4. Positioning the blood pressure cuff.

inflate the cuff, but they can hear the sounds when they deflate the cuff. If you have this problem, use your fingertips to find the radial pulse in the wrist of the arm to which you have applied the cuff. Inflate the cuff until you can no longer feel the radial pulse. Continue to inflate the cuff to a point 30 mm Hg higher than where the pulse stopped. The rest of the procedure is the same.

FIGURE A2–5. Graphic of blood pressure sounds.

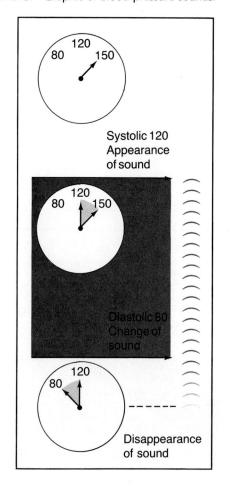

Systolic 120
Appearance of sound

Diastolic 80
Change of sound

Disappearance of sound

FIGURE A2–3. The brachial artery. A pulse can be felt in the position indicated.

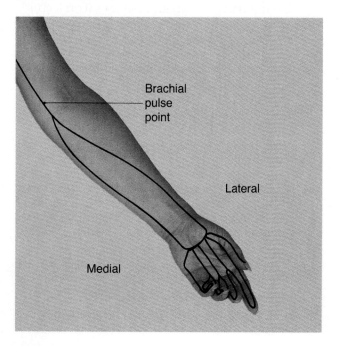

Brachial pulse point

Lateral

Medial

If you are not certain of a reading, be sure the cuff is totally deflated and wait 1 or 2 minutes and try again, or use the other arm. Should you try the same arm too soon, you may get false high readings.

Sometimes patients with high systolic readings will have the sounds disappear as you deflate the cuff, only to reappear again. This can lead to both false systolic and diastolic readings. Whenever you have a high diastolic reading, wait 1 or 2 minutes and take a second reading. For this reading, feel for the disappearance of the radial pulse as you inflate the cuff (this will ensure that you did not measure a false systolic pressure) and listen as you deflate the cuff down into the normal range. Use the last fade of sound as the diastolic pressure.

Determining Blood Pressure by Palpation

Using palpation (feeling the radial pulse) is not a very accurate method. It will provide you with one reading, an approximate **systolic pressure.** The method is used when there is too much noise around to use a stethoscope, or when there are too many patients for the number of rescuers at the scene. To determine blood pressure by palpation, place the cuff the same as you would for auscultation and:

1. Find the radial pulse on the arm to which you have applied the cuff.
2. Close the valve and inflate the cuff until you can no longer feel the pulse.
3. Continue to inflate the bulb to a point 30 mm Hg above the point where the pulse disappeared.

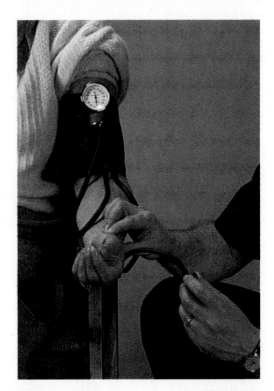

FIGURE A2–6. Measuring blood pressure by palpation.

4. Slowly deflate the bulb and note the reading when you feel the pulse returns.
5. Record the time, the arm used, the position of the patient, and the systolic pressure, and note that the reading was done by palpation. If you give this information orally to someone, make sure that they know the reading was by palpation, as in, "Blood pressure is 146 by palpation."

■ SCAN A2-1.

Measuring Blood Pressure—Auscultation

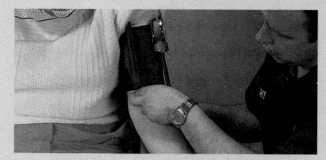

1 Position Cuff and Find Pulse Site

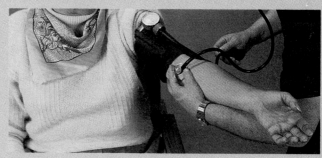

2 Set Bell or Diaphragm Over Pulse Site

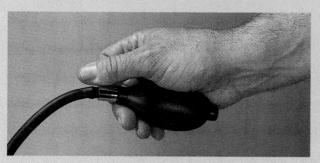

3 Close Valve and Inflate Cuff

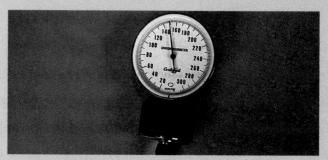

4 Listen for Sound to Disappear—Inflate 30 mm Hg Beyond this point

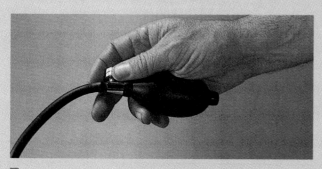

5 Open Valve to Deflate 2–3 mm Hg/sec

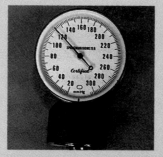

6 Listen for Start of Sound—Systolic
Listen for Sound to Fade—Diastolic

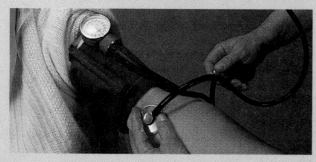

7 Deflate Cuff Completely

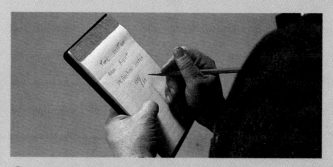

8 Record Results

APPENDIX 3

Breathing Aids and Oxygen Therapy

The approach for teaching First Responders the use of breathing aids and oxygen therapy must be very similar to the one used to train EMT-A personnel. Since oxygen is a medication, little information in terms of assessment and care can be deleted. Certain aspects of medical terminology can be modified to simpler terms without harm; however, the same basic step-by-step procedures must be presented to both levels of learner for the pocket face mask with one-way valve, the bag-valve-mask unit, and standard oxygen delivery systems.

THE FIRST RESPONDER'S ROLE

The vast majority of First Responders will not be trained in the use of aids for breathing and oxygen therapy. However, in some localities special training programs have been established to meet community needs. The use of aids to ventilation and oxygen administration may be part of your course, especially if you are to perform your First Responder duties in an isolated area. Keep in mind that you cannot train yourself to use this equipment to administer oxygen. Do only what you have been trained to do.

Basic life support is possible without equipment and should never be delayed while you locate, retrieve, and set up equipment. There is no doubt that the prompt and efficient use of certain pieces of equipment will allow you to provide more effective emergency care in terms of maintaining an open airway, assisting with ventilation, and providing more oxygen to the patient. However, improper care may be provided if you delay care, use faulty equipment, or use the wrong equipment.

New responsibilities come with the use of equipment in basic life support. You *must*:

- Be sure that the equipment is clean and operational before a situation occurs requiring its use.
- Select the proper equipment for the patient.
- Monitor the patient more closely once you begin to use any device or delivery system.
- Make certain that the equipment is properly discarded, cleaned, or tested after its use.
- Stay current with the equipment being used and keep your skills to the level needed to provide efficient emergency care.

The administration of oxygen may require orders from a physician in your locality. This is be-cause **oxygen is a medication.** As a First Responder, you may be able to initiate the use of oxygen by radio communications with a medical facility, or you may be able to begin oxygen administration without such orders in very specific situations. Your instructor will give you the guidelines for your locality. You may only be allowed to work with certain devices or administer oxygen while assisting EMTs.

VENTILATION-ASSIST DEVICES

In Chapter 4A, we discussed the oropharyngeal airway and the pocket face mask with one-way valve, and how these devices could be used to assist in the delivery of ventilations. One other device, the bag-valve-mask ventilator, can also be used to assist with ventilation.

The Bag-Valve-Mask Ventilator

NOTE: Most EMS Systems recommend that an oropharyngeal airway be inserted before attempting to ventilate the patient with a bag-valve-mask ventilator.

The bag-valve-mask ventilator is one of the most commonly used field devices for cases requiring a rescuer to ventilate a nonbreathing patient. This hand-held resuscitator is commonly called a bag-mask unit. Some EMS Systems also use the bag-valve-mask unit to ventilate patients with shallow failing respirations (for example, in drug overdose). This device comes in pediatric and adult sizes.

When providing atmospheric air to the patient's lungs, the bag-valve-mask unit delivers 21% oxygen. The unit can be connected to an oxygen supply source to deliver 50% to nearly 100% oxygen. More will be said later in regard to using oxygen sources with a bag-valve-mask unit.

REMEMBER: When providing mouth-to-mask ventilations, you are delivering 16% oxygen to the patient. The bag-valve-mask unit will deliver 21% oxygen from the atmosphere and from 50% up to nearly 100% oxygen from an oxygen delivery source.

Numerous types of this ventilator are available; however, all have the same basic parts. There is a self-refilling bag, valves that control the flow of air, and a face mask to apply to the patient's face. The face mask *must* have a transparent facepiece so that the rescuer can see the patient's mouth in order to detect vomiting and to note lip color changes.

The principle behind the bag-valve-mask ventilator is not complicated. When you squeeze the bag, air is delivered to the patient's airway through a one-way valve. The valve that allows atmospheric air to enter the bag is closed during delivery. When you release the bag, air can flow from the patient's lungs out into the atmosphere. The exhaled air does not go back into the bag. While the patient is exhaling, air from the atmosphere refills the bag.

The above appears to be very simple; however, the bag-valve-mask unit can be very difficult to operate. This is especially true if you do not use it on a regular basis. If you are assigned a bag-valve-mask ventilator for use in the field, you must practice using this device in the classroom until you can use it effectively. Then you must continue to develop and maintain your skills. Many EMS Systems have decided that there are too many problems with this device and have selected the pocket face mask as the ventilation assist device of choice for First Responders.

When using the bag-valve-mask ventilator, you should:

1. Position yourself at the patient's head and provide an open airway. Clear the airway if necessary.
2. Insert an oropharyngeal airway (see p. 115).
3. **Be certain** to use the correct-size mask for the patient. The apex or top of the triangular mask should be over the bridge of the nose. The base of the mask should rest between the patient's lower lip and the projection of the chin.
4. **Be certain** to hold the mask **firmly** in position, with:
   - The thumb holding the upper part of the mask
   - The index finger between the valve and the lower cushion
   - The third, fourth, and fifth fingers on the lower jaw, between the chin and ear
5. With your other hand, squeeze the bag **once every 5 seconds.** The squeeze should be a full one, causing the patient's chest to rise.

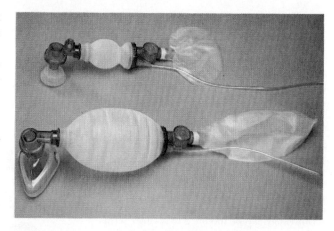

FIGURE A3–1. Pediatric and adult bag-valve-mask ventilators.

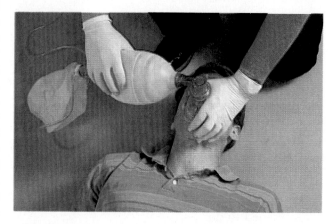

FIGURE A3–2. Hand positioning for using the bag-valve-mask.

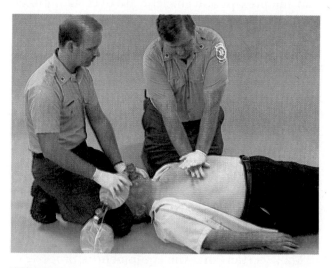

FIGURE A3–3. Two-rescuer CPR using a bag-valve-mask ventilator.

6. Release pressure on the bag and let the patient passively exhale and the bag refill from the atmosphere.

There are times when the bag-valve-mask unit will not deliver air to the patient's lungs. Sometimes the problem is due to an airway obstruction that must be cleared. More often, the problem is caused by an improper seal between the patient's face and the mask. It should be rare for the bag, valves, or mask to be the problem, provided you have kept the unit clean and in working order.

The bag-valve-mask ventilator can be used very effectively during two-rescuer CPR by a skilled operator. The ventilator squeezes the bag on the compressor's fifth upstroke.

OXYGEN THERAPY

The Importance of Oxygen

A patient may require oxygen for a variety of reasons, including respiratory arrest, cardiac arrest, major blood loss (there is a reduction in the number of red blood cells required to carry oxygen), heart attack or heart failure, lung disease, injury to the lungs or the chest, airway obstruction, stroke (remember that the brain requires a constant supply of oxygen), and shock.

Atmospheric air can provide no more than 21% oxygen to the patient. This is far more than the patient needs, providing the airway is open, the exchange surfaces of the lungs are working properly, there is enough oxygen being picked up by the blood, and the patient's heart and blood vessels are properly circulating blood to all the body tissues. When any of these factors is not present, or fails, a higher concentration of oxygen must be delivered to the patient's lungs so that the required level of oxygen reaches the body's tissues.

If you provide oxygen to the nonbreathing patient by mouth-to-mask techniques, you are delivering 16% oxygen. This will be enough to keep the patient alive. When providing CPR, interposed ventilations provided by mouth-to-mask techniques only deliver 16% oxygen to the patient's lungs. The efficiency of CPR to circulate the blood is less than a third that of a healthy, beating heart. Body tissues do not receive any more than the minimum oxygen they require for short-term survival. Oxygen therapy can allow up to nearly 100% oxygen to reach the lungs. With more oxygen in the patient's blood, some of this inefficiency is improved and the patient has a better chance for survival.

REMEMBER: **Oxygen is a medication.** The use of oxygen is a special responsibility that can be given only to someone of professional status.

Disadvantages of Oxygen Therapy

There are certain hazards associated with the administration of oxygen, including:

1. Oxygen used in emergency care is stored under **pressure** (2000 pounds per square inch or greater). If the tank is punctured, or if a valve breaks off, the supply tank can become a missile.
2. Oxygen supports **combustion,** causing fire to burn more rapidly. It can saturate towels, sheets, and clothing, causing them to burn very rapidly.
3. Under pressure, **oxygen and oil do not mix.** When they come into contact with one another, there will be a severe reaction, causing an explosion. This can easily occur if you try to lubricate a delivery system or gauge with petroleum products.
4. Long-term use of high concentrations of oxygen can result in medical dangers. They include the destruction of lung tissue (oxygen toxicity), lung collapse, eye damage in premature infants, and respiratory arrest in patients with chronic obstructive pulmonary disease (COPD), including emphysema, chronic bronchitis, and black lung. With the exception of the problems seen with COPD patients and the potential hazard of providing a high concentration of oxygen to premature newborns, these events are not field problems because of the short duration of administration.

You should not attempt to administer oxygen directly to newborn infants unless ordered to do so by a physician. When oxygen is required (difficult delivery, infant is very weak, premature birth, or other emergency), it should be provided into a foil tent formed over the infant's head, neck, and shoulders. If this is not practical, an adult mask can be placed near the infant's mouth and nose.

In cases of known chronic obstructive pulmonary disease, too high a dosage of oxygen (above 28%) may cause these patients to go into respiratory arrest. In most cases, the patient will have to be in distress before this will happen. Most EMS System guidelines call for no more than 24% oxygen to be delivered initially to the COPD patient unless the patient is developing shock, has respiratory distress not related to COPD, or is already in respiratory arrest.

REMEMBER: Never withhold the concentration of oxygen that is appropriate for the patient. If you are in doubt as to how much oxygen to deliver, radio or phone the emergency department for advice.

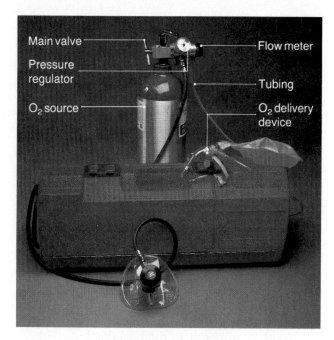

FIGURE A3–4. An oxygen delivery system.

EQUIPMENT AND SUPPLIES FOR OXYGEN THERAPY

An oxygen delivery system for the breathing patient includes a source, pressure regulator, flowmeter, and a delivery device (face mask or cannula). When possible, a humifidier should be added to provide moisture to the dry oxygen if the patient will be on the system for more than 30 minutes. (Some EMS Systems will not allow the use of humidifiers because of improper storage and contamination.) The delivery system is the same for a nonbreathing patient, but a device must be added to allow the rescuer to force oxygen into the patient's lungs. This is known as *positive pressure ventilation.* As a First Responder, you will probably use a bag-valve-mask resuscitator connected to 100% oxygen when administering oxygen to the nonbreathing patient.

Oxygen Cylinders

When providing oxygen in the field, the standard source of oxygen is a seamless steel or lightweight alloy cylinder filled with oxygen under pressure. The pressure is equal to 2000 to 2200 pounds per square inch (psi). Cylinders come in various sizes, identified by letters. The smaller sizes practical for the First Responder include:

- D cylinder—contains about 350 liters of oxygen
- E cylinder—contains about 625 liters of oxygen

You cannot tell if an oxygen cylinder is full, partially full, or empty by lifting or moving the cylinder. Part of your duty as a First Responder is to make certain that the oxygen cylinders you will use are full and ready before they are needed in providing care. The length of time that you can use an oxygen cylinder depends on the pressure in the cylinder and the flow rate. The method of calculating cylinder duration is shown in Table A3–1. Oxygen cylinders should **never** be allowed to empty below the **safe residual.** The safe residual for an oxygen cylinder is determined when the pressure gauge reads 200 psi. At this point, you must switch to a fresh cylinder.

Safety is of prime importance when working with oxygen cylinders. You should:

- *Never* allow a cylinder to drop or fall against any object. The cylinder must be well secured, preferably in an upright position. *Never* let a cylinder stand by itself.
- *Never* allow smoking around oxygen equipment. Carry and use signs to clearly mark the area of oxygen use. The signs should read, "OXYGEN—NO SMOKING."
- *Never* use oxygen equipment around open flame or sparks.
- *Never* use grease or oil on devices that will be attached to an oxygen supply cylinder. Do *not* handle these devices when your hands are greasy.
- *Never* put tape on the cylinder outlet or use tape to mark or label any oxygen cylinder or oxygen delivery equipment. The oxygen can react with the adhesive and produce a fire.

FIGURE A3–5. Left, D size cylinder; right, E size cylinder.

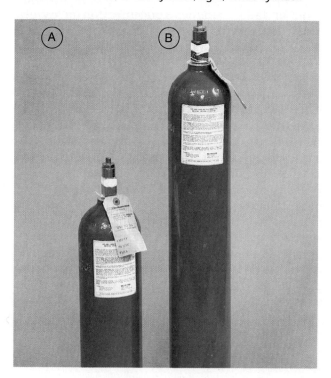

TABLE A3–1. DURATION OF FLOW FORMULA

SIMPLE FORMULA

$$\frac{\text{Gauge pressure in psi} - \text{residual pressure} \times \text{constant}}{\text{Flow rate in liters/minute}} = \text{the safe duration of flow in minutes}$$

RESIDUAL PRESSURE = 200 psi

CYLINDER CONSTANT

D = 0.16	G = 2.41
E = 0.28	H = 3.14
M = 1.56	K = 3.14

Determine the life of a D cylinder that has a pressure of 2000 psi and a flow rate of 10 liters/minute.

$$\frac{(2000 - 200) \times 0.16}{10} = \frac{288}{10} = 28.8 \text{ minutes}$$

- *Never* try to move an oxygen cylinder by rolling it on its side or bottom.
- *Never* store a cylinder near high heat or in a closed vehicle that is parked in the sun.
- *Always* use the pressure gauges and regulators that are intended for use with oxygen and the equipment you are using.
- *Always* ensure that valve seat inserts and gaskets are in good working order. This will help prevent dangerous leaks.
- *Always* use medical-grade oxygen (USP). There are impurities in industrial-grade oxygen. The cylinder's label should state, "OXYGEN U.S.P."
- *Always* fully open the valve of an oxygen cylinder; then close it half a turn when it is in use. This will serve as a safety measure should someone else think the valve is closed and try to force it open.
- *Always* store reserve oxygen cylinders in a cool, ventilated room as approved by your EMS System.
- *Always* have oxygen cylinders hydrostatically tested. This should be done every **five years** (three years for aluminum cylinders). The date for retesting should be stamped on the cylinder.

Pressure Regulators

The safe working pressure for oxygen administration is 30 to 70 pounds per square inch (psi). This means that the pressure in an oxygen cylinder is too high to be used directly from the cylinder. A pressure regulator must be connected to the oxygen cylinder before it can be used to deliver oxygen to a patient.

On cylinders of the E size or smaller, a yoke assembly is used to secure the pressure regulator to the cylinder valve assembly. The yoke has pins that *must* mate with the corresponding holes found in the valve assembly. This is called a *pin-index safety system*. The position of the pins varies for

different gases to prevent an oxygen delivery system from being connected to a cylinder of another gas.

Cylinder pressure can be reduced in either one or two steps. For a one-step reduction, a single-

FIGURE A3–6. (A) Single-stage regulator. (B) Two-stage regulator for D and E size cylinders.

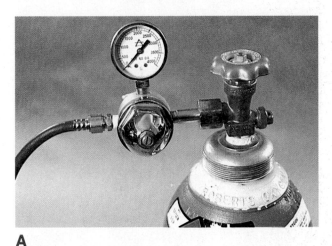

A

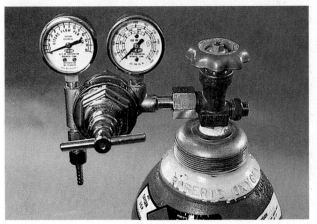

B

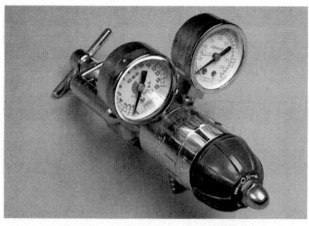

A

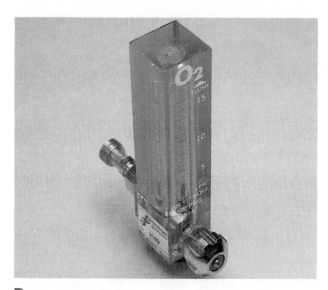

B

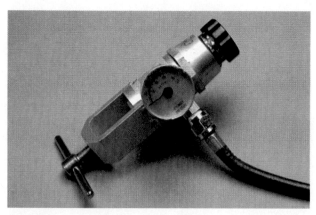

C

FIGURE A3–7. A. Bourdon gauge flowmeter (pressure gauge). B. Pressure-compensated flowmeter. C. Constant flow selector valve.

stage pressure regulator is used. A two-step reduction requires a two-stage regulator. Most regulators used in emergency care are of the single-stage variety.

Before connecting the pressure regulator to an oxygen supply cylinder, *open the cylinder valve* slightly for just a second to clear dirt and dust out of the delivery port or threaded outlet. This is called "cracking" the cylinder valve.

Flowmeters

A flowmeter is connected to the pressure regulator to give the user control over the flow of oxygen in liters per minute. Three types of flowmeters are available. In emergency care use in the field, the pressure compensated flowmeter is considered superior to the bourdon gauge flowmeter; however, it is more delicate than the bourdon gauge and must be in an upright position for proper operation. For these reasons, most EMS Systems employ the bourdon gauge for field use. The constant flow selector valve is a new type of flowmeter that is gaining in popularity.

- *Bourdon gauge flowmeter*—This flowmeter is a pressure gauge calibrated to indicate flow of gas in liters per minute. It is inaccurate at low flow rates and has been criticized for being unstable. This device will not compensate for back pressure. A partial obstruction (as from a kinked hose) will produce a reading higher than the actual flow. The gauge may read 4 liters/minute and be delivering only 1 liter/minute. False high readings also can be produced when the filter in the gauge becomes clogged. The bourdon gauge is fairly sturdy and will operate in any position.

- *Pressure compensated flowmeter*—This is a gravity-dependent meter that must be in an upright position to deliver accurate readings. It has an upright, calibrated glass tube containing a ball float. The float will rise and fall according to the amount of gas passing through the tube. Its readings indicate the *actual flow* of the gas at all times. This is true even when there is a partial obstruction to gas flow (as from a kinked delivery tube). Should the delivery tubing collapse, the ball will drop to indicate the lowered delivery rate.

- *Constant flow selector valve*—This device has no gauge. It allows for the adjustment of flow in liters per minute in stepped increments (2, 4, 6, 8, . . . 15 liters per minute). When using this type of flowmeter, *make certain* that it is properly adjusted for the desired flow and monitor the meter to make certain that it stays properly adjusted. This type of meter should be tested for accuracy as recommended by the manufacturer.

Oxygen Delivery Devices: Breathing Patients

The nasal cannula and four types of face masks are the five oxygen delivery devices in common use for the field administration of oxygen to *breathing patients*. Many EMS Systems use the nasal cannual to start oxygen therapy on medical emergency patients who are breathing (the exception is the COPD patients in distress). If shock appears to be a problem, or if the patient is very cyanotic (blue or gray facial skin, blue lips, blue nail beds), or has very labored breathing, they will begin with a face mask. These same systems use one of the four types of face masks to begin oxygen therapy for breathing trauma patients. As a First Responder, you will probably be issued a simple face mask and/or a nasal cannula.

There is a simple rule that can be used to determine the percentage of oxygen being delivered to a patient. This rule states: *For every 1 liter per minute increase in oxygen flow, you deliver a 4% increase in the concentration of oxygen.* If a particular device will give 24% oxygen at 4 liters per minute, an increase to 5 liters per minute will deliver a concentration of 28% oxygen.

The five major oxygen delivery devices for breathing patients are covered in Table A3–2. The major devices in use include:

- *Nasal cannula*—A nasal cannula delivers oxygen into the patient's nostrils by way of two small plastic prongs. Its efficiency is greatly reduced by nasal injuries, colds, and other types of nasal airway obstruction. In common usage, a flow rate of 4 to 6 liters per minute will provide the patient with 32% to 44% oxygen. The relationship of oxygen concentration to liter per minute flow is:

1 liter/minute	24% oxygen
2 liters/minute	28% oxygen
3 liters/minute	32% oxygen
4 liters/minute	36% oxygen
5 liters/minute	40% oxygen
6 liters/minute	44% oxygen

At 4 liters per minute and above, the patient's breathing patterns may prevent the delivery of the stated percentages. At 5 liters per minute, rapid drying of the nasal membranes is possible. After 6 liters per minute, the device does not deliver any higher concentration of oxygen and proves to be very uncomfortable for most patients.

NOTE: The Venturi mask is the delivery device of choice for COPD patients in a hospital setting; however, the nasal cannula is often used in field emergency care. Follow your local guidelines. The nasal cannula can be used for COPD patients if a flow rate no greater than 1 to 2 liters per minute is maintained.

There are two types of nasal cannula. The older model has an elastic band for holding the device in place, while the newer design has a slip loop to be secured around the patient's ears and chin.

- *Simple face mask*—This soft, clear plastic mask conforms to the contours of the patient's face. The small perforations in the mask allow atmospheric air to enter and the patient's exhaled air to escape. The mask may be used

TABLE A3–2. OXYGEN DELIVERY DEVICES

Oxygen Delivery Device	Flow Rate	% Oxygen Delivered	Special Use
Nasal cannula	1 to 6 liter per minute	24% to 44%	Most medical patients and COPD at low concentrations
Simple face mask	Start at 6 LPM . . . can go as high as 15 LPM, but 8 LPM more practical	35% to 60%	Preferred on trauma patients
Partial rebreathing mask	6 to 10 LPM	35% to 60%	Trauma patients
Nonrebreathing mask	Start with 8 LPM, practical high is 12 LPM	80% to 95%	Good for severe non-COPD and shock patients. Provides high oxygen concentrations
Venturi mask	4 to 8 LPM	24% to 40% (delivers as indicated on adaptor)	COPD patients and long-term use

to deliver moderate concentrations of oxygen (35% to 60%) with a flow rate of 6 to 8 liters per minute. The practical maximum flow is considered to be 12 liters per minute.

CAUTION: Always start with 6 liters per minute flow when using this mask. If you start with less, carbon dioxide can build up in the mask. At a flow of 1 liter per minute, the patient is getting less oxygen than she would from atmospheric air.

- *Venturi mask*—This mask is used when low concentrations of oxygen (24% to 44%) are required. The oxygen is delivered into the mask by way of a jet that pulls in atmospheric air to mix with the oxygen. The flow is rapid enough to flush carbon dioxide that tends to accumulate in a face mask. Various size adaptors can be attached to the device to control the liter of oxygen flow to the patient. Standard sizes include 3-, 4-, and 6-liters-per-minute adaptors. If a 4-liter adaptor is in place and you try to deliver 8 liters of oxygen per minute, the jet will draw in more atmospheric air to mix with the oxygen. This "Venturi effect" draws in enough air so that only 4 liters of oxygen per minute reaches the patient.

NOTE: The Venturi face mask is recommended for COPD patients who are free of trauma or other serious medical emergencies (see page xxx). Delivery concentrations should be 24%.

- *Nonrebreathing mask*—This device is used to deliver high concentrations of oxygen (see Table A3–2). Make certain that you inflate the reservoir bag before placing the mask on the patient's face. This is done by using your finger to cover the exhaust portal or the connection between the mask and the reservoir. Care must be taken to ensure a proper seal with the patient's face. The reservoir must not deflate by more than one-third when the patient takes his deepest inspiration. This volume can be maintained by the proper flow of oxygen. Note that the patient's exhaled air does not return to the reservoir. The minimum flow rate when using this mask is 8 liters per minute.

FIGURE A3–8. A loop-type nasal cannula.

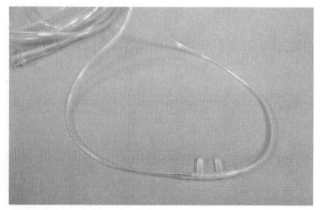

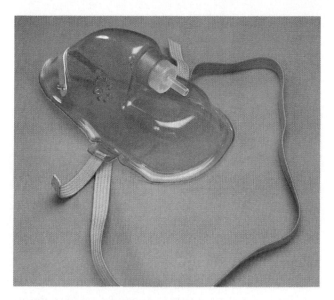

FIGURE A3–9. A simple face mask.

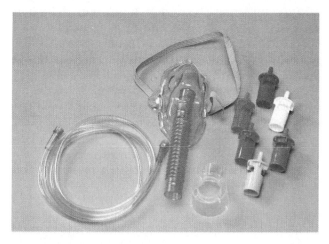

FIGURE A3–10. A Venturi mask.

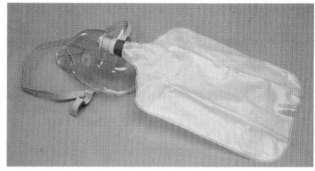

FIGURE A3–11. A nonrebreathing mask.

ADMINISTERING OXYGEN

Scansheet A3-1 will take you step by step through the process of administering oxygen and discontinuing the administration of oxygen.

■ SCAN A3-1A.

Preparing the O₂ Delivery System

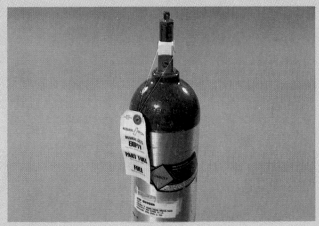

1 Select Desired Cylinder. Check Label, "Oxygen U.S.P."

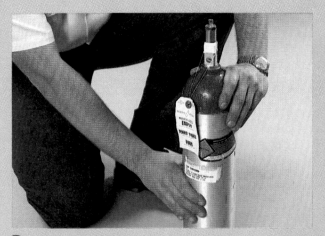

2 Place the Cylinder in an Upright Position and Stand to One Side.

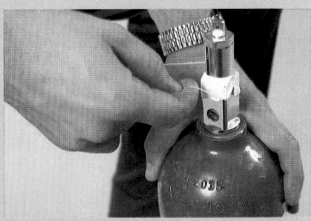

3 Remove the Plastic Wrapper or Cap Protecting the Cylinder Outlet. Do Not Use Adhesive Tape.

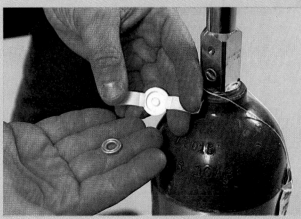

4 Keep the Plastic Washer (Some Set-Ups).

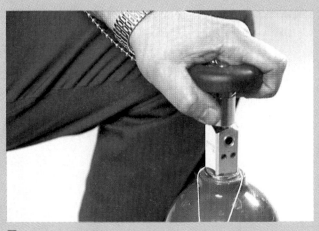

5 "Crack" the Main Valve for One Second.

PIN **DISS**

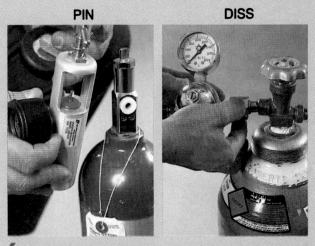

6 Select the Correct Pressure Regulator and Flowmeter.

The O₂ Delivery System (cont'd)

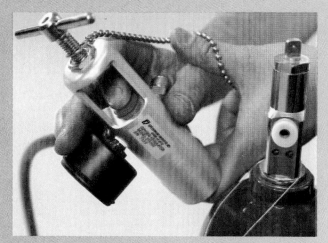

7 Place Cylinder Valve Gasket on Regulator Oxygen Port.

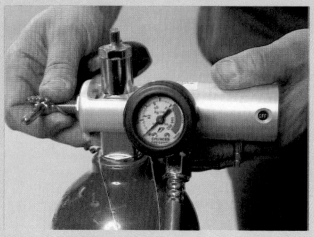

8 Make Certain That the Pressure Regulator Is Closed.

PIN   **DISS**

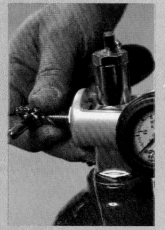
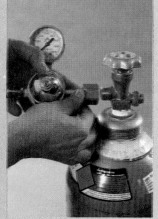

9 Align Pins. For Diss, Thread by Hand.

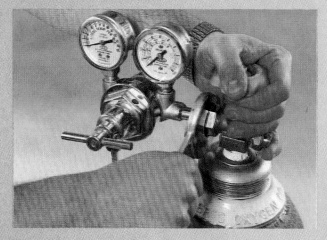

Tighten with a Wrench for Diss.

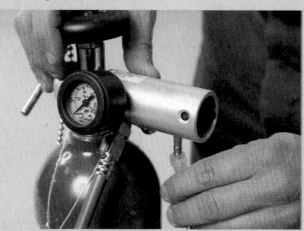

10 Tighten T-Screw for Pin-Index.

11 Attach Tubing and Delivery Device.

■ SCAN A3-2.

Administering Oxygen

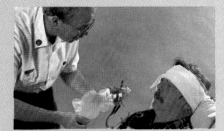

1 Explain to Patient the Need for Oxygen

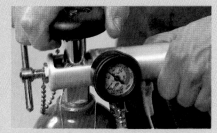

2 Open Main Valve—Adjust Flowmeter

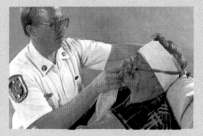

3 Place Oxygen Delivery Device

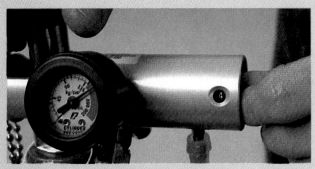

4 Adjust Flowmeter

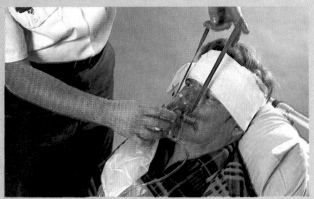

5 Secure During Transfer

Discontinuing Oxygen

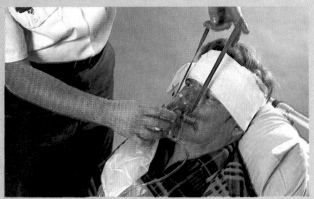

1 Remove Delivery Device

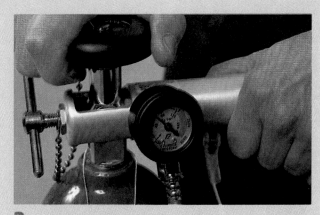

2 Close Main Valve

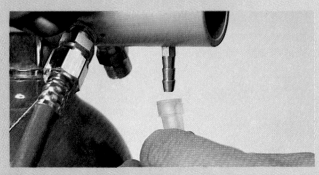

3 Remove Delivery Tubing

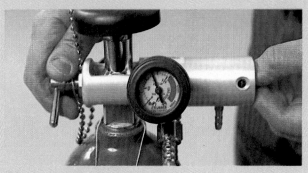

4 Bleed Flowmeter

ADMINISTRATION OF OXYGEN TO A NONBREATHING PATIENT

The pocket face mask (see Chapter 4A) with oxygen inlet and your own breath can be combined to deliver oxygen to a nonbreathing patient. The bag-valve-mask resuscitator with 100% oxygen under pressure and the demand valve resuscitator with 100% oxygen under pressure can be used in ventilating the nonbreathing patient. The demand valve resuscitator is considered an EMT-level device. You may receive training with this device so that you can assist EMTs.

NOTE: When using either of these two devices, an oropharyngeal airway should be inserted.

WARNING: Both of these devices can be used for two-rescuer CPR. They should *not* be employed for one-rescuer CPR. The face mask will not remain in place and keep a tight seal, even when face straps are used. When these devices are used, there is too great a delay between compressions and properly interposed ventilations for one-rescuer CPR.

Bag-Valve-Mask Ventilator and Oxygen

Oxygen tubing can be connected to the outlet of the flowmeter and the oxygen inlet of the bag-valve-mask unit to deliver 100% oxygen to the patient's airway. Preferred devices have an oxygen reservoir attached to the bag to improve efficiency. The bag-valve-mask device used with oxygen will deliver 100% oxygen for pulmonary resuscitation and for interposed ventilations during two-rescuer CPR. Maintain a tight mask-to-face seal, squeeze the bag to deliver oxygen, and release the bag to allow for a passive expiration. There is no need to remove the mask when the patient exhales.

This device can also be used to assist the breathing efforts of a patient who has failing respirations (as in drug overdose).

OXYGEN THERAPY

The following dosages of oxygen are recommended according to the nature of the patient's problem. The standing orders for oxygen vary slightly in different EMS Systems. Follow your local guidelines.

NOTE: When 50% to 100% by mask is recommended and you only have a nasal cannula, provide oxygen by the cannula at a rate of 6 liters per minute.

Accidents

Except for minor scratches, scrapes, and cuts, possible minor fractures (finger, toe, rib), strains, sprains, and possible minor dislocations (finger, toe), provide 50% to 100% oxygen by mask. If the

FIGURE A3–12. A. A pocket face mask with one-way valve set to deliver supplemental oxygen. B. A bag-valve-mask ventilator connected to an oxygen supply.

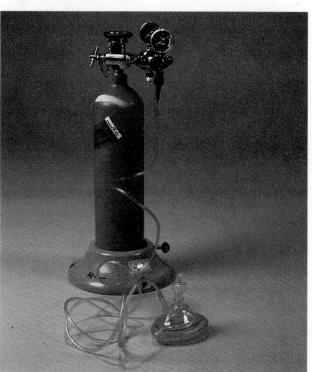
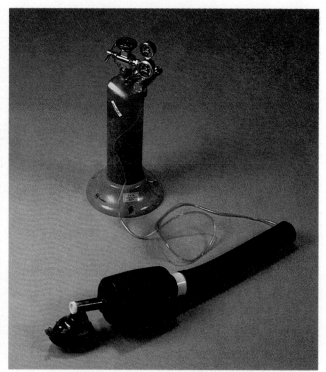

patient is developing shock, provide 50% to 100% oxygen by mask.

Childbirth

Mother

Predelivery bleeding, excessive postdelivery bleeding, during breech birth, miscarriage or induced abortion that has excessive bleeding, ectopic pregnancy, toxemia (eclampsia)—50% to 100% by mask.

Newborn

Premature, difficult breech birth, bleeding from umbilical cord, appears weak, has lasting blue color (cyanosis) other than hands and feet—deliver oxygen to tent over infant's head and shoulders.

Environmental Emergencies

Allergy (anaphylactic) shock—50% to 100% by mask

Burns—50% to 100% by mask

Drug overdose—50% to 100% by mask (pocket face mask with oxygen, or bag-valve-mask with oxygen to assist ventilations)

Near-drowning—50% to 100% by mask (pocket face mask with oxygen, or bag-valve mask with oxygen to assist ventilations)

Poisonings—50% to 100% by mask (pocket face mask with oxygen, or bag-valve mask with oxygen to assist ventilations; 100% recommended for carbon monoxide poisoning and most other inhaled poisons)

SCUBA accidents—50% to 100% oxygen by mask

Medical Emergencies

Angina—50% to 100% oxygen by mask

Asthma—24% oxygen by Venturi or nasal cannula

Black lung—24% oxygen by Venturi or nasal cannula

Chronic bronchitis—24% by Venturi or nasal cannula

Congestive heart failure (no COPD)—50% to 100% by mask

COPD (unknown)—24% oxygen by Venturi or nasal cannula

Diabetic emergencies—50% to 100% oxygen by mask

Difficult breathing (no COPD)—50% to 100% by mask

Emphysema—24% by Venturi or nasal cannula

Heart attack—50% to 100% by mask

Pneumonia—50% to 100% by mask

Stroke (CVA)—50% to 100% by mask

APPENDIX 4

First Responder Automated Defibrillation

NOTE: This appendix is designed to aid First Responders who are being trained to assist with or perform automated defibrillation. It is meant to be part of a formal training program that leads to approval for assisting EMTs or special defibrillation certification. This program and First Responder defibrillation must be under the direction of a physician. The information presented here conforms to the guidelines and standards being developed by the National Council of State EMS Training Coordinators. For more information on defibrillation and the procedures used with defibrillators, see J. R. Graves, D. Austin, Jr., and R. Cummins, *Rapidzap Automated Defibrillation* (Englewood Cliffs, N.J.: Brady/Prentice Hall, 1989) and K. Stults, *EMT-D Prehospital Defibrillation* (Englewood Cliffs, N.J.: Brady/Prentice Hall, 1986).

INTRODUCTION

Each year over 400,000 people die suddenly of heart attacks. There is little warning for most of these victims. Nearly 25% of these sudden cardiac deaths occur to persons who have had no history of heart problems.

The fact that most sudden cardiac deaths occur away from hospitals is the reason why there are EMS personnel and citizen-level cardiopulmonary resuscitation (CPR) programs. There are two problems with an approach that depends solely on CPR. The first problem is the delay in starting CPR. In all but a few cases, CPR must be started as soon as possible after cardiac arrest begins. Ideally, CPR should be started before EMS personnel reach the scene. Training more citizens may help correct this problem.

The second problem with a program limited to CPR is that many heart attacks will be fatal no matter how soon the procedure is started. These deaths are often related to lethal heart rhythms that must be corrected as soon as possible if the patients are to survive. The special procedure needed to save some of these patients can now be done in the prehospital setting. It is called **defibrillation.** Understanding how this procedure helps to save lives requires some knowledge of the heart's electrical system.

The heart is a cone-shaped, hollow muscular organ that is roughly the size of the individual's clinched fist (see the anatomy plate on page 36). Its muscular walls are called myocardium (mi-o-KAR-de-um). Most of this myocardium is cardiac muscle that is involved with maintaining the heart's shape and contracting to pump blood. Some of this myocardium becomes modified to produce what is known as the **conduction system.** These modified cells are involved with the heart's electrical activity.

The heartbeat originates at a small region of modified tissue called the pacemaker or sinoatrial (si-no-A-tre-al) or SA node. The electrical wave that is sent out from this site will occur about every 0.8 second in the at-rest adult's heart. It spreads to the heart's upper chambers (atria) and then is delayed slightly and sent on to the lower chambers (ventricles). This delay and transfer take place at a second node called the atrioventricular (a-tre-o-ven-TRIK-u-lar) or AV node.

The impulse that is sent to the lower chambers first travels the septum* that separates the two lower chambers. The routes taken are known as the right and left bundle branches. The wave continues out to the muscular walls by way of the Purkinje (pur-KIN-je) fibers.

The conduction system initiates the heartbeat, giving time for the upper chambers to ready for

---

* A septum divides two chambers. An easy to see septum is the one in your nose that separates the two nostrils.

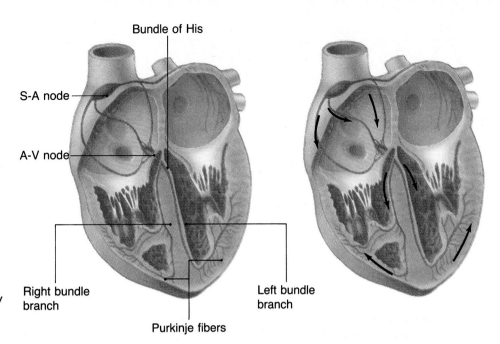

Bundle of His

S-A node

A-V node

Right bundle branch

Left bundle branch

Purkinje fibers

FIGURE A4–1.
The conduction system of the heart. Note the flow of energy from the pacemaker to the muscular walls.

contraction and then contract with a delay built in before the lower chambers contract. This allows for proper chamber filling, contraction, relaxation, and preparation for the next contraction. Any disease of or damage to the heart muscle may also damage the conduction system. This could lead to an interruption of the heart's rhythm that could stop circulation.

Automated Defibrillation

Defibrillators are designed to deliver an electrical shock that will disrupt the diseased heart's electrical activity. This process is not intended to start a dead heart, but will stop certain lethal rhythms and then give the heart a chance to spontaneously develop an effective rhythm on its own. The entire process is called defibrillation.

The use of manual defibrillators requires very special training to determine if a shock should be delivered and to perform the skills to properly deliver the shock. These demands are so extensive that the manual defibrillator is not practical for First Responders. There are special implanted automated defibrillators that do not require the help of a rescuer; however, the most promising of these devices is now in experimental form. The answer to the problem of field defibrillation lies in the use of **automated defibrillators.**

Currently, EMS Systems are using automated external defibrillators. These devices are usually referred to as automated defibrillators or AEDs. They are relatively easy to operate and are becoming a part of more EMT and First Responder programs. The use of automated defibrillators means that the EMS System can now propose effective emergency cardiac care for many individuals who would certainly die without the AED program.

AEDs can recognize a heart rhythm that requires a shock, charge up, and deliver the shock or advise the rescuer to press an indicated button to deliver the shock. The limit of usefulness for these devices is related to the nature of the heart problem. The major heart problems that must be considered in a prehospital setting include, but are not limited to:

- *Disorganized rhythm*—this is called **ventricular fibrillation** (ven-TRIK-u-lar fib-bre-LAY-shun) or VF. It is the state of totally disorganized heart activity in the lower pumping chambers (see Figure A4–2). If there is not an organized rhythm in these chambers, the heart cannot pump blood. It is believed that 50% to 60% of all cardiac arrest patients are in ventricular fibrillation (VF) when EMS personnel arrive. Many cases of VF can be corrected by defibrillator shock. The time that the patient is in cardiac arrest is a big factor. The sooner defibrillation shock is delivered, the better the patient's chances are for survival.

- *Organized rhythm, very rapid heart rate*—this is called **ventricular tachycardia** (ven-TRIK-u-lar tack-e-KAR-de-ah), in which a very fast lower chamber heart rate is observed. In some cases, the rate is so rapid that the heart cannot pump blood. Less than 10% of the prehospital cardiac arrest cases have this problem. Defibrillation may help these patients.

- *Organized rhythm, very slow heart rate*—this can become **electromechanical dissociation,** a condition in which the electrical activity of the heart is within normal range, but the heart

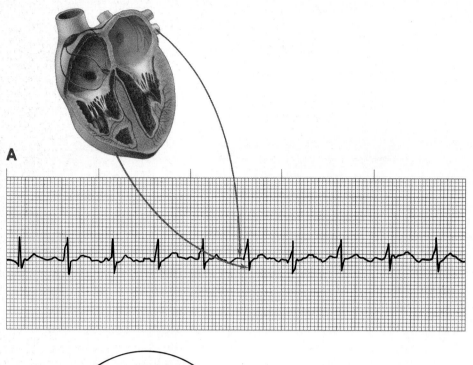

A

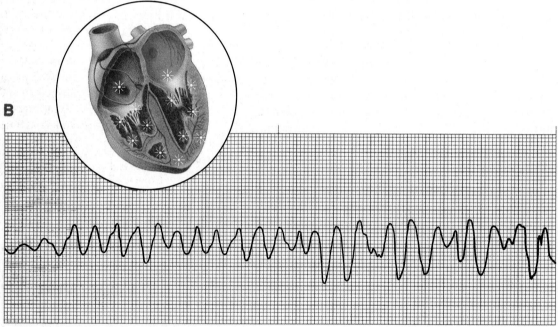

B

FIGURE A4–2.
A. Normal heart rhythm (normal sinus rhythm). B. Ventricular fibrillation. Note the many false "pacemaker" sites.

muscle is too sick to pump blood. Thus, the electrical activity of the heart is separated (dissociated) from the pumping (mechanical) activity. Between 10% and 20% of all cardiac arrest patients have this problem. It cannot be helped by defibrillation.

- *No electrical impulses*—this is known as **asystole** (a-SIS-to-le). Without electrical impulses, the heart muscle is not stimulated to contract. Defibrillation will not help this problem.

THE EMS SYSTEM'S ROLE

The time that elapses from the moment a person collapses until the defibrillation shock is delivered is a critical factor. This time can be divided into four segments:

1. *EMS access time*—the time from collapse until the EMS System is alerted.
2. *Dispatch time*—the time from the dispatcher

receipt of the call until the person or crew who will defibrillate the patient is alerted.

3. *Response time*—the time it takes for the alerted person or crew to arrive and reach the patient.

4. *Shock time*—the time it takes from reaching the patient until the defibrillation shock is delivered.

The goal of every EMS System is to reduce the time involved with each stage of the process. In particular, the time from dispatch to the arrival of the defibrillator is being shortened by having rescuers with defibrillators available 24 hours a day. If the patient can receive the first shock within 6 minutes of collapse, survival is more likely. Table A4–1 shows the ideal time components for a defibrillation. It is believed that reaching the goals stated in this table will improve witnessed cardiac arrest with VF survival rate by 25%.

USING AUTOMATED DEFIBRILLATORS

First Responder defibrillation may be done with either fully automatic or semiautomatic defibrillators. The physician advisory board for your EMS System may have approved one or both of these devices. The operation of both will be covered in this text.

A defibrillator must be ready for use at any given moment. Make certain that you follow all your EMS and manufacturer guidelines to ensure that the defibrillators you will use are in working order and prepared for use. Always carry fully charged spare batteries.

Basic Warnings

Certain warnings must be noted when working with automated defibrillators, regardless of type. These basic warnings include:

- Follow the same precautions that you would for operating any electrical device.
- *Do not* defibrillate a patient who is not in cardiac arrest.
- *Do not* defibrillate a patient who is in contact with rescuers, bystanders, or other patients.
- *Do not* assess or shock a patient who is moving or when the defibrillator or its leads are being moved.
- *Do not* defibrillate a patient in a moving ambulance or other motor vehicle.
- *Do not* defibrillate a patient who has an obstructed airway. The patient who is in respiratory arrest, but not cardiac arrest (assess pulse), does not need defibrillation.
- *Do not* defibrillate a patient who is in water.
- *Do not* defibrillate a patient who is lying on a metal surface that may transfer the electrical shock to others.
- *Do not* defibrillate a child who is less than 12 years of age or weighs under 30 kilograms (under 80 pounds) unless directed to do so by a physician. It is recommended that you phone or radio the emergency department physician or medical command for all cases involving children as patients.

TABLE A4.1 AUTOMATED DEFIBRILLATION TIME GOALS

Time Component	Objective	Goal	Method
EMS access time	To minimize the time from collapse until someone places a call for help	1 min	An increased community awareness to the need for quickly calling for an ambulance; more public CPR programs
Dispatch time	To minimize the time it takes for an EMS dispatcher to elicit information from a caller and get a defibrillator-equipped unit on the road	0.5 min	Better dispatcher training, improved call handling procedures
Response time	To minimize the time it takes to get a trained defibrillator team to the patient	3.0 min	Strategic placement of automated defibrillators with first-response personnel
Shock time	To minimize the time it takes to deliver the first shock	1.5 min	Use automated defibrillators; continually practice to maintain peak efficiency

Information provided by Kenneth R. Stults, M.S., Director of the University of Iowa Hospitals and Clinics Emergency Medical Services Learning Resource Center. New data suggest that a higher rate of success occurs with patients who receive CPR with oxygenation prior to the first shock. Follow your EMS Systems' guidelines.

The policy of defibrillating trauma victims is established at the state level. Follow your EMS System's protocols. Basically, a determination has to be made as to whether the accident was caused by the heart problem, the accident set off a preexisting heart problem, or the heart problem was a direct result of the injury. If you are not certain as to what you are to do, phone or radio the emergency department physician or EMS medical command.

First Responder Care

The use of a defibrillator must follow other procedures of care and assessment. You must do a primary survey to confirm the fact that the patient is in cardiac arrest. If an EMT trained in difibrillation is at the scene, you will probably begin CPR using the mouth-to-mask method or the procedure used in your EMS System. This will allow the EMT to prepare and attach the defibrillator and operate the device. Make certain that you are clear of the patient before a shock is given.

If there is no EMT or more highly trained personnel at the scene and you are with a partner or someone else trained in basic life support, have this person begin CPR while you prepare and attach the defibrillator. Make certain that both of you are clear of the patient before a shock is given. **NOTE:** In all cases, make certain that dispatch is informed of the emergency, that the patient is in cardiac arrest, and that defibrillation is being done.

Attaching the Defibrillator

The procedure for attaching the defibrillator to a patient is the same for both fully and semiautomatic systems. Electrodes in the form of self-adhesive pads will have to be properly placed on the patient's bare chest to monitor heart rhythm and deliver the electrical shock. It is recommended that the defibrillation device be placed on the left side of the patient, close to his or her head. The operator should work from the left side of the patient.

While someone performs CPR, the defibrillator operator should:

1. Bare the patient's chest. If the patient's chest is wet, it should be quickly wiped dry.
2. Remove two pads from their protective packages.
3. Remove the plastic backing from the first pad and place it adhesive-side down on the patient's upper right chest. (If you are using color-coded pads, this should be the white pad.) The top of the pad should touch the skin over the top of the clavicle (collarbone), while the medial edge should be on the skin next to the sternum. The pad should not be placed over the top of the patient's sternum (see Figure A4–3).
4. Press the adhesive zone of the pad so that it

FIGURE A4–3. The correct placement of the defibrillator pads.

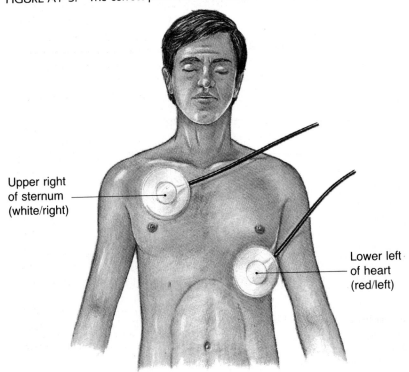

Upper right of sternum (white/right)

Lower left of heart (red/left)

makes full contact with the patient's skin. *Do not* press on the center of the pad if it has a sponge center. Pressing in this region might force gel onto the adhesive or skin and prevent proper contact.

5. Remove the adhesive backing from the second pad and place it on the patient's skin below and left of the nipple. (If you are using color-coded pads, this is the red pad.) This placement is over the apex of the heart. Ensure good adhesive contact.

6. Tightly connect the lead cables from the AED to the pads. Follow the manufacturer's instructions. If the cables are color coded, they should be placed with the white cable attached to the upper right pad and the red cable attached to the lower left (apex) pad. This placement will allow for the correct input of the patient's electrocardiogram (ECG) signal into the monitor circuitry.

Automatic defibrillators will not function unless the pads are fully adhered to the patient's chest and the cables are tightly secured. If either of these problems exist, the "no contact" signal or error message will usually appear.

Operating the Fully Automatic Defibrillator

NOTE: The following is an example of the operational procedures for an automatic defibrillator. Be aware that various defibrillator models are available. Follow the manufacturer's manual and your EMS System's guidelines for the defibrillator you will be using. Be aware that when three shocks are given the energy level of the third shock is usually greater than the first two. You may have to set the defibrillator for this higher level. This is not necessary with the newer models.

Once attached to the patient and turned on, the latest models of fully automated defibrillators will automatically assess the patient's heart rhythm, sense if a shock should be delivered, charge to the preset energy level, and deliver the shock to the patient. These defibrillators have voice synthesizers to alert the rescuer and give instructions that typically include "Stop CPR," "Stand back," and "Check breathing and pulse." Should this voice system fail, the rescuer is expected to know what to do and how to ensure personal safety.

To operate a fully automatic defibrillator, you should:

1. Assess the patient to determine cardiac arrest.
2. Have your partner or someone trained in basic life support begin CPR. If you are acting alone, ready the defibrillator, attach the pads to the patient, and connect the cables.* After this is done, begin CPR and continue for one full minute or for the time designated by your EMS medical advisory board.

3. Make certain that you, your partner, and all other persons at the scene are not in contact with the patient.

4. Press the defibrillator ON button and remain clear of the patient. Note the time this was done. The defibrillator voice synthesizer should state, "Stop CPR." At this time, the defibrillator will perform an analysis of the patient's heart rhythm. If the patient is to be shocked, the voice synthesizer will announce, "Stand back." Make certain that you do not touch or move the patient or the defibrillator. The defibrillator will charge to 200 joules of energy and deliver the shock.

5. Stay clear of the patient and allow the defibrillator to reassess the patient's heart rhythm. If a second shock is required, the voice synthesizer will state, "Stand back," and the defibrillator will again charge (usually to 200 joules) and deliver the second shock.

6. Continue to stay clear of the patient. A third shock may be required. If three shocks have been delivered, the voice synthesizer will announce, "Check breathing and pulse."

7. Assess the patient's breathing and pulse.
   - **If there is a pulse,** leave the defibrillator attached to monitor the patient. Maintain an open airway and continue life-support procedures. The patient would benefit from oxygen therapy and, if necessary, assisted ventilations. *Do only what you have been trained to do.*
   - **If there is no pulse,** leave the defibrillator attached to the patient and continue CPR.

8. After 60 seconds, the defibrillator will state, "Stop CPR," and do another analysis of the patient's heart rhythm. If a shock is to be delivered, the voice synthesizer will state, "Stand back," and deliver from one to three more electrical shocks.

9. If no more shocks are indicated or if all three additional shocks have been delivered, the voice synthesizer will state, "Check breathing and pulse." You should take the same course of action as stated in step 7.

The defibrillator will enter a **perpetual monitoring mode,** allowing it to continue to assess the patient's heart rhythm. It will not be able to deliver additional shocks without rescuer assistance. Instead, it will announce, "Check breathing and

* Each EMS System has its own protocols for First Responders acting alone. You may be required to perform CPR for one full minute before you ready and attach the defibrillator or perform some other step before readying the defibrillator. Follow your local protocols.

pulse." If the patient is still in cardiac arrest, you will have to make certain that you are not touching the patient and then clear everyone away. Press the ON button, note the time that this was done, and continue with steps 4 through 9.

Operating the Semiautomatic Defibrillator

NOTE: The following is an example of the operational procedures for a semiautomatic defibrillator. Various defibrillator models are available. Follow the instructions given in the manufacturer's manual and your EMS System's guidelines for the defibrillator that you will be using.

Semiautomatic defibrillators are also called shock advisory defibrillators. They will automatically monitor and assess the patient's heart rhythm and determine if a shock should be given and, if necessary, charge to a preset level. They will not automatically deliver the shock. The rescuer must push a button to do this.

The same basic assessment and safety procedures that apply to the fully automatic defibrillator also apply to the operation of the semiautomatic defibrillator. Some models do not have a voice synthesizer. They all require the rescuer to push a button to deliver the shock. For these reasons, all standard operating procedures for safety must be given extra consideration during semiautomatic defibrillator use.

To operate a semiautomatic defibrillator, you should:

1. Assess the patient to determine cardiac arrest.
2. Have your partner or someone trained in basic life support begin CPR. If you are acting alone, ready the defibrillator, attach the pads to the patient, and connect the cables (see page 482). After this is completed, begin CPR and continue for one full minute or for the time designated by your EMS medical advisory board.
3. Turn on the defibrillator by lifting open the display model or as directed by the manufacturer. The message screen should show the command "PRESS TO ANALYZE" with an arrow pointing to the button you need to depress. Do not allow anyone to touch or move the patient or defibrillator. Press the indicated button and allow the defibrillator to analyze the patient's heart rhythm. If the patient is to be shocked, the defibrillator will automatically charge to 200 joules of energy. A prompt will appear on the message screen telling you to "STAND BACK." Your defibrillator may also have a voice synthesizer command that gives the same message.
4. Make certain that you, your partner, and all other persons are clear of the patient.

5. Press the button indicated by the "READY PRESS TO SHOCK" prompt on the message screen. Note the time that this was done.
6. After the shock is delivered, press the analyze button.
   - **Shock indicated**—Repeat the procedure to deliver a second shock. Press the analyze button to determine if a third shock is necessary. If a third shock is to be delivered, increase the energy level to 360 joules of energy by pressing the indicated button as the defibrillator charges (see note below). Press the appropriate button when the defibrillator is ready to shock the patient.
   - **No shock indicated**—Assess both respirations and pulse. If they are absent, resume CPR. If they are present, provide appropriate care and ready the patient for transport. Continue to monitor the patient.

NOTE: The number of shocks allowed to be delivered to a patient and the joules of energy delivered for each of these shocks is part of your EMS System's **physician-determined standing orders.** If you are in doubt as to what to do, phone or radio the emergency department physician or medical command.

FIGURE A4–4.
Operating a semiautomatic defibrillator. Before the shock is applied, make certain that everyone, including yourself, is clear of the patient.

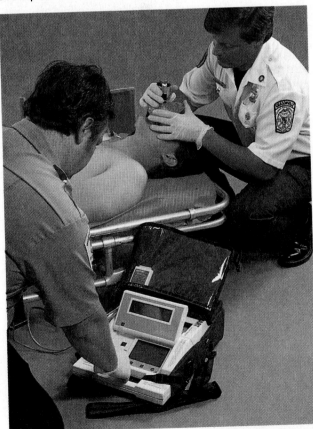

■ Scan A4-1

Automated Defibrillation—The Automatic Defibrillator

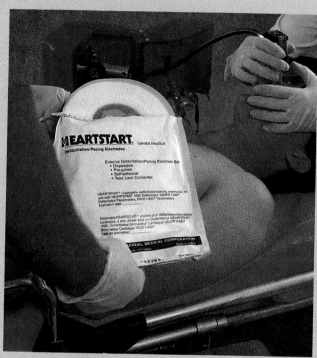

A The Patient's Chest is Exposed and the Pads Are Removed from the Protective Covering.

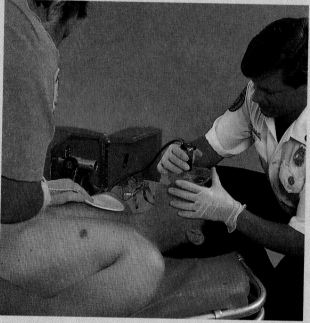

B The Plastic Backing is Removed from the First Pad and the Pad is Placed on the Chest.

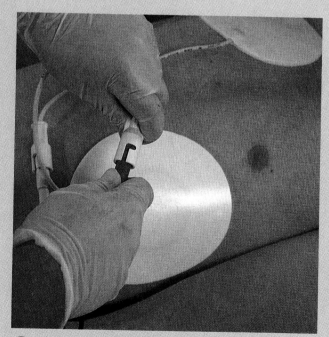

C The Second Pad is Placed on the Patient's Chest and the Cables Are Connected.

Turn on the device and follow the defibillator prompts:

- Stop CPR.
- Stand back.
- Check breathing and pulse.
  Pulse—follow prompts.
  No pulse—begin CPR and follow prompts.

Problems Operating a Defibrillator

Most of the problems with defibrillator operations that can be corrected by the rescuer involve the attachment of the pads and/or cables. Usually, making certain that the pads are in full contact and the cables are tightly connected will be all that is needed to correct most problems.

There may be times when you cannot secure the pads fully to the patient's chest. The patient's chest should be dry and free of anything in contact with its surface. Make certain that you remove any dressings and nitroglycerin patches that are on the pad placement sites. Wipe off any nitropaste found on the patient's chest (your hands should be gloved). If necessary, you may have to shave the pad placement areas of the patient's chest. Use the disposable safety razor provided for this procedure.

The defibrillators used by First Responders have error message modes. These messages can be audio, visual, or a combination of both. You must be knowledgeable of the error messages that apply to your defibrillator and what you should do in response to each message.

ASSESSMENT AND QUALITY ASSURANCE

A prehospital defibrillation program needs a continuous process design to evaluate its effectiveness and to correct any problems. This assessment and quality assurance program must consider specific situations as they relate to standard operating procedures and physician-directed standing orders, the care delivered by the rescuers, the performance of the equipment, and the effectiveness of training programs. Changes in any aspect of the program must be the result of physician evaluation and orders.

All automated defibrillators have a recording device that will provide a record of the resuscitation and defibrillation incident. Since defibrillation incidents are very complex situations and the rescuer must render care without a physician at the scene, certain medical assessments must be made after the fact. The event and how the various aspects of the defibrillation program performed can be evaluated by a physician to help improve patient care. Part of this evaluation will include rescuer performance. You should view this as a helping process, designed to aid you as you improve your skills as a First Responder. This is part of the professional approach needed for modern patient care.

Be certain to complete your EMS System's records and keep your own notes for each defibrillation incident. Your notes should include when you determined cardiac arrest, how many shocks were delivered, when they were delivered, and the energy level for each shock.

Part of your equipment inspection and assessment should include the operation of your defibrillator recording device. Audiotape devices have caused some field problems. Follow the manufacturer's instruction manual and your EMS System's recommendations to correct any problems before the unit is needed.

■ Glossary

A

Abandonment to leave an injured or sick patient before more highly trained EMS personnel arrive. Leaving the scene without giving patient information may be viewed as a form of abandonment.

ABC method the sequence of operations required in cardiopulmonary resuscitation. A stands for airway, B stands for breathe, and C stands for circulate.

Abdomen (AB-do-men) the region of the body between the diaphragm and pelvis.

Abdominal cavity the anterior body cavity that is located between the diaphragm and the bones of the ring of the pelvis. It houses and protects the abdominal organs, glands, major blood vessels, and nerves.

Abdominal quadrants the four zones that are assigned to the anterior abdominal wall. These zones are used for quick reference for the location of structures, injuries, and pain.

Abdominal thrusts manual thrusts that are delivered to the midline of the abdomen, between the xiphoid process and the navel, to create pressure to help expel an airway obstruction. See *Manual thrusts.*

Abdominopelvic (AB-dom-i-no-PEL-vik) the front (anterior) cavity below (inferior to) the diaphragm.

Abduction movement of a limb away from the midline of the body.

Abortion (ah-BOR-shun) the spontaneous (miscarriage) or induced delivery of the fetus and placenta before the 28th week of pregnancy.

Abrasion (ab-RAY-zhun) a scratch.

Abscess (AB-ses) a contained or otherwise limited structure that collects the pus associated with tissue death and infection.

Acetone breath a sweet breath with a fruitlike odor. This is a sign of diabetic coma.

Achilles (ah-KEL-ez) **tendon** the common term for the tendon that connects the posterior leg muscles to the heel. The calcaneal (kal-KA-ne-al) tendon.

Acid being acidic, as opposed to being neutral or basic (alkaline). Associated with free hydrogen ions.

Acquired immune deficiency syndrome (AIDS) a contagious disease that is usually fatal. The infectious agent is the HIV virus. This agent may be passed from person to person by sexual contact, blood transfusion, sharing needles, or across the placenta from mother to fetus (unborn child). The virus is found in blood, body fluids, and wastes. It is also associated with mucous membranes. Even though it is found in saliva, there is no clear evidence of the disease being transmitted in this substance.

Actual consent consent by the rational adult patient, usually in oral form, accepting emergency care. This must be informed consent.

Acute to have a rapid onset. Sometimes the term is used to mean severe.

Acute abdomen inflammation in the abdominal cavity, often producing sudden, intense pain.

Acute myocardial infarction (AMI) (my-o-KARD-e-al in-FARK-shun) a heart attack. The sudden death of heart muscle due to oxygen starvation. Usually caused by a narrowing or blockage of one of the blood vessels (coronary arteries) supplying the heart muscle.

Adduction movement of an extremity toward the midline of the body.

Advanced Cardiac Life Support (ACLS) prehospital emergency care that involves the use of intravenous fluids, drug infusions, cardiac monitoring, defibrillation, intubations, and other advanced procedures. See *Basic life support.*

Afterbirth the placenta, part of the umbilical cord, and some tissues of the womb's lining that are delivered after the birth of the baby.

AIDS see *Acquired immune deficiency syndrome.*

Air embolism gas bubbles in the bloodstream.

Air sacs the microscopic parts of the lung where gas exchange takes place. The medical term is alveoli (al-VE-o-li).

Air splint see *Inflatable splint.*

Airway the passageway for air from the nose and mouth to the exchange levels of the lungs. The term can also be used to mean artificial airways, such as an oropharyngeal airway.

Airway adjunct a device that is placed in the patient's mouth or nose to help maintain an open airway. Oral airway adjuncts may help to hold the tongue clear of the airway.

Alkali a substance that is basic, as opposed to being acid or neutral.

Allergen (AL-er-jin) any substance that can cause an allergic response.

Allergy shock the most severe type of allergic reaction, in which a person goes into shock when he comes into contact with a substance to which he is allergic. Also called anaphylactic (an-ah-fi-LAK-tik) shock.

Alveoli (al-VE-o-li) see *Air sacs.*

Ambulance a vehicle that is specifically designed for patient transport and emergency care. It has a driver compartment and a patient compartment and carries all the equipment and supplies needed to provide EMT-level care at the scene and en route to the medical facility.

Amnesia the short- or long-term loss of memory. This loss usually has a sudden onset.

Amniotic sac see *Bag of waters*.

Amputation the surgical or traumatic removal of a body part. The most common usage applies to the traumatic amputation of an extremity or one of its parts.

Analgesic a pain reliever.

Anaphylactic shock (an-ah-fi-LAK-tik) see *Allergy shock*.

Anatomical position the standard reference position for the body in the study of anatomy. The body is standing erect, facing the observer. The arms are down at the sides and the palms of the hands face forward.

Anesthetic to be free of pain and feeling. Commonly used to mean a substance that will block pain or feeling.

Aneurysm (AN-u-riz′m) The dilated or weakened section of an arterial wall. A blood-filled sac formed by the localized dilation of an artery or vein.

Angina pectoris (an-JIN-ah or an-JI-nah PEK-to-ris) the chest pains often caused by an insufficient blood supply to the heart muscle. This is not a heart attack as defined by the average patient.

Angulation the angle formed above and below a break in a bone. The fracture changes the straight line of a bone into an angle.

Ankle bones the tarsals (TAR-sals).

Anterior the front.

Antiseptic a substance that will stop the growth of or prevent the activities of germs (microorganisms).

Anus (A-nus) the outlet of the large intestine.

Aorta (a-OR-tah) the major artery that carries blood from the heart out to the body.

Apical pulse the heartbeat felt over the lower portion of the heart.

Apnea (ap-NE-ah) the temporary cessation of breathing.

Apoplexy (AP-o-plek-see) the loss of consciousness, movement, and awareness of sensation that is caused by a stroke (CVA).

Appendicular skeleton (AP-pen-dik-u-ler) collarbones, shoulder blades, and the bones of the arms, forearms, wrists, hands, pelvis, thighs, legs, ankles, and feet. The bones of the upper and lower extremities.

Arm the body part from shoulder to elbow.

Arrhythmia (ah-RITH-me-ah) disturbance of heart rate and rhythm. Sometimes the term dysrhythmia is used to mean the same thing.

Arterial bleeding the loss of bright red blood from an artery. The flow may be rapid, spurting as the heart beats. See *Capillary bleeding* and *Venous bleeding*.

Arteriosclerosis (ar-TE-re-o-skle-RO-sis) "hardening of the arteries" caused by calcium deposits. See also *Atherosclerosis*.

Artery any blood vessel carrying blood away from the heart.

Articulate to join together. To unite to form a joint.

Ascites (a-SI-tez) the noticeable distention of the abdomen caused by an accumulation of excessive fluids.

Aseptic clean, free of particles of dirt and debris. This does not mean sterile.

Asphyxia (As-FIK-si-ah) suffocation resulting in the loss of consciousness caused by too little oxygen reaching the brain. The functions of the brain, heart, and lungs will cease.

Aspiration to inhale materials into the lungs. Often used to describe the breathing in of vomitus.

Asthma (AS-mah) the condition in which the bronchioles constrict, causing a reduction of airflow and creating congestion. Air usually will enter to the level of the air sacs (alveoli), but it cannot be exhaled easily.

Asystole (a-SIS-to-le) when the heart stops beating. This is cardiac standstill.

Atelectasis (at-i-LEK-tah-sis) the partial or complete collapse of the air sacs (alveoli) of the lungs.

Atherosclerosis (ATH-er-o-skle-RO-sis) the buildup of fatty deposits on the inner wall of an artery. This buildup is called plaque. If calcium is deposited in the plaque, the arterial wall will become hard and stiff.

Atrium (A-tree-um), **Atria** (A-tree-ah) a superior chamber of the heart. The heart has a right and left atrium.

Auscultation (os-skul-TAY-shun) listening to sounds that occur within the body.

Avulsion (Ah-VUL-shun) a piece of tissue or skin that is torn loose or pulled off by injury.

Axial skeleton (AK-si-al) the skull, spine, breastbone (sternum), and ribs.

Axilla (ak-SIL-ah) the armpit.

B

Bag of waters the fluid-filled sac that surrounds the fetus. The medical term is amniotic sac.

Bag-valve-mask ventilator an aid for artificial ventilation. It has a face mask, a self-inflating bag, and a valve that allows the bag to refill while the patient exhales. It can be attached to an oxygen line.

Bandage an item, such as gauze or tape, that can be used to hold a dressing in place.

Basic Life Support (BLS) the ABCs of emergency care. Those events related to the findings of the primary survey. See *ABC method*.

Bilateral existing on both sides of the body.

Bile fluid formed in the liver and sent to the small intestine. It may be stored in the gallbladder. Bile has many functions, including changing the speed at which the intestine moves things along (intestinal motility) and helping to digest fatty foods.

Biological death when the patient has stopped lung and heart activity and his brain cells die. Lethal changes usually begin to take place in the brain within 4 to 6 minutes after breathing stops. This process may be delayed by cold temperatures.

Bladder usually referring to the urinary bladder located in the pelvic cavity.

Blanch to become pale or to turn white.

Bleeding shock caused by the loss of blood or plasma. Also known as hemorrhagic (HEM-or-RIJ-ic) shock.

Blood pressure the pressure caused by blood exerting a force on the walls of blood vessels. Usually, arterial blood pressure is measured.

Bloodstream shock caused by infection-producing poisons that are released into the blood. The blood vessel dilates, producing too great a volume to be filled by the body's blood. Also called septic shock.

Body fluid shock caused by the loss of body fluids, as in cases of severe vomiting or diarrhea. Also called metabolic shock.

Bolus a mass of chewed or partially chewed moistened food that is swallowed.

Bourdon (bore-DON) **gauge** a gauged flowmeter that indicates the flow of a gas in liters per minute.

Bowel the intestine.

Brachial (BRAY-ke-al) **artery pressure point** the pressure point used to help control bleeding from the upper limb.

Brachial pulse (BRAY-key-al) the pulse measured by compressing the major artery of the upper arm. This pulse is used to detect heart action and circulation in infants.

Bradycardia (bray-de-KAR-de-ah) an abnormal condition where the heart rate is slow. The pulse rate will be below 50 beats per minute.

Breastbone the sternum.

Breech birth a delivery where the buttocks or both legs of the baby are born first.

Bronchiole (BRONG-key-ol) the small branches of the airway that carry air to and from the air sacs of the lungs.

Bronchus (BRON-kus) the portion of the airway connecting the trachea to the lungs (plural is bronchi).

Bruise a contusion. The simplest form of closed wound; blood flows between tissues causing a discoloration.

Burns see *Major burns* and *Minor burns*.

C

Capillary a microscopic blood vessel through which exchange takes place between the bloodstream and the body tissues.

Capillary bleeding the slow oozing of blood from a capillary bed. See *Arterial bleeding* and *Venous bleeding*.

Cardiac (KAR-de-ak) in reference to the heart.

Cardiac arrest when the heart stops beating.

Cardiogenic shock (KAR-de-o-JEN-ik) see *Heart shock*.

Cardiopulmonary resuscitation (KAR-de-o-PUL-mo-ner-e re-SUS-ci-TA-shun) CPR. Heart—lung resuscitation where there is a combined effort to artificially restore or maintain respiration and circulation.

Carotid artery (kah-ROT-id) the large neck artery. One is found on each side of the neck. Its pulse is of great importance in the primary survey and CPR.

Carpals (KAR-pals) the wrist bones.

Catheter a flexible tube passed through a body channel (such as the urethra or a blood vessel) to allow for drainage or the withdrawal of fluids.

Central nervous system (CNS) the brain and spinal cord.

Cephalic (ce-FAL-ik) in reference to the head.

Cerebrospinal fluid (ser-e-bro-SPI-nal) the clear, watery fluid that helps to protect the brain and spinal cord.

Cerebrovascular accident (CVA) see *Stroke*.

Cervical (SER-ve-kal) relating to the neck or to the lower (inferior) end of the uterus (womb).

Cervix (SER-vicks) the lower (inferior) portion of the uterus (womb), where it enters the vagina (birth canal).

CHEMTREC the Chemical Transportation Emergency Center that provides immediate expert information to emergency personnel at the scene of a hazardous materials incident.

Child abuse assault of an infant or child that produces physical and/or emotional injuries. Sexual assault is included as a form of child abuse. The victim of physical assault is called a battered child.

Chronic the opposite of acute. It can be used to mean long and drawn out or recurring.

Chronic heart failure see *Congestive heart failure*.

Chronic obstructive pulmonary disease (COPD) a group of diseases and conditions in which there is a progressive decline of the lungs in their ability to exchange gases. COPD includes chronic bronchitis, emphysema, and miner's black lung disease.

Clavicle (KLAV-i-kul) the collarbone.

Clinical death the state reached by a patient when breathing and heart action cease.

Closed fracture a simple fracture where the skin is not broken by the fractured bones. The fracture site is not exposed to the outside world.

Closed wound an injury where the skin is not broken, as in the case of a bruise (contusion).

Clot the formation composed of fibrin and entangled blood cells that acts to help stop the bleeding from a wound. See *Fibrin*.

Coccyx (KOK-siks) the lowermost bones of the spinal column. They are fused into one bone in the adult.

Collarbone the clavicle (KLAV-i-kul).

Coma the state of complete unconsciousness. The depth of unconsciousness may vary.

Comminuted fracture (KOM-i-nu-ted) a fracture where the bone is fragmented or turned to powder.

Concussion caused by a blow to the head, often producing a mild state of stupor or temporary unconsciousness. There is no laceration to or detectable bleeding in the brain.

Condyles (KON-dials) the large, rounded projections at the distal end of the thigh bone (femur) and the proximal end of the medial leg bone (tibia). Most people refer to these structures as the sides of their knees.

Congestive heart failure associated with lung conditions and diseases, or heart disease. Excessive fluid buildup occurs in the lungs and/or body organs. The heart fails in its efforts to properly circulate blood and the lungs fail to exchange gases properly.

Constant flow selector valve a meterless device that allows the user to adjust the flow of supplemental oxygen by selecting the flow in stepped increments (2, 4, 6, 8, . . . , 15 liters per minute).

Constricting band used to restrict the flow of venom.

Contraindicated any condition, sign, symptom, or existing treatment that makes a particular course of treatment or care procedure inadvisable.

Contusion (kun-TU-zhun) a bruise.

Convulsion uncontrolled skeletal muscle spasm, often violent.

COPD see *Chronic obstructive pulmonary disease.*

Core temperature the body temperature measured at a central point, such as within the rectum.

Cornea (KOR-ne-ah) the transparent tissue covering that lies over top of the iris and pupil of the eye.

Coronary (KOR-o-nar-e) in reference to the blood vessels that supply blood to the heart muscle (myocardium). Many people use this term to mean heart attack.

Coronary artery disease the narrowing of one or more places in the coronary arteries brought about by atherosclerosis. Blockage (occlusion) will eventually occur in many cases.

CPR cardiopulmonary resuscitation.

CPR compression site the mid-breastbone (mid-sternal) point found by placing the hand approximately two fingerwidths above (superior to) the substernal notch. During CPR of adults and children, compressions are delivered to this site. For the infant, compressions are delivered with two or three fingertips placed one fingerwidth below an imaginary line drawn directly between the nipples.

Cranial (KRAY-ne-al) pertaining to the braincase of the skull.

Cranium KRAY-ne-um) the braincase of the skull. Many people use the term skull when they mean cranium.

Cravat a piece of cloth material that can be used to secure a dressing or splint.

Crepitus (KREP-i-tus) a grating noise or the sensation felt caused by the movement of broken bone ends as they rub together.

Crisis any event that is seen as a crucial moment or turning point in the patient's life.

Critical Incident Stress Debriefing (CISD) sessions that are held after a disaster or emergency incident to address the needs of rescuers who may have been influenced by the scene and the stress generated in providing emergency care.

Croup (Kroop) a general term for a group of viral diseases that produce swelling of the larynx.

Crowing an atypical sound made when a patient breathes. It usually indicates airway obstruction.

Crowning when the presenting part of the baby first bulges out of the vaginal opening. It is usually in reference to a normal head-first delivery.

Cut an open wound with smooth edges (incision) or jagged edges (laceration).

Cyanosis (sigh-ah-NO-sis) when the skin color changes to blue or gray because of too little oxygen in the blood.

D

Debridement the surgical removal of dead, injured, or infectious materials from around a wound or burn.

Decompression sickness the "bends." In most cases, this involves SCUBA divers who have surfaced too rapidly. Nitrogen is trapped in body tissues and may find its way into the divers' bloodstreams.

Deep frostbite see *Freezing.*

Defibrillation to apply an electric shock to a patient's heart in an attempt to disrupt a lethal rhythm and allow the heart to spontaneously reestablish a normal rhythm. This is done with a defibrillator.

Delerium tremens (DTs) a severe, possibly life-threatening reaction related to alcohol withdrawal. The patient's hands tremble, hallucinations may be present, behavior may be unusual, and convulsions may occur.

Dermis (DER-mis) the inner (second) layer of the skin. It is the layer that is rich in blood vessels and nerves found below the epidermis.

Diabetes (di-ah-BE-teez) a disease caused by the inadequate production of insulin.

Diabetic coma the result of an inadequate insulin supply that leads to unconsciousness, coma, and eventually death unless treated.

Diaphoresis (DI-ah-fo-RE-sis) profuse perspiration. The patient is said to be diaphoretic (DI-ah-fo-RET-ik).

Diaphragm (DI-ah-fram) a dome-shaped muscle that separates the chest cavity (thorax) from the abdominal cavity (abdominopelvic cavity). It is the major muscle of respiration.

Diaphragmatic (DI-ah-FRAG-mat-ik) **breathing** weak and rapid respirations with little or no chest movement. There may be slight movement of the abdomen. The patient's attempt to breathe with the diaphragm alone.

Diastolic (di-as-TOL-ik) **pressure** the pressure exerted on the internal walls of the arteries when the heart is relaxing.

Dilation to enlarge, having expanded in diameter.

Direct pressure the quickest, most effective way to control most external bleeding. Pressure is applied directly over the wound site.

Dislocation the displacement (pulling or pushing out) of a bone end that forms part of a joint.

Distal away from a point of reference, such as the shoulder or the hip joint. When used with the word proximal (closer to), distal means more distant to.

Distended inflated, stretched, or swollen.

Downer a substance that affects the central nervous system to relax the user. A depressant.

Dressing a protective covering for a wound that will aid in the stoppage of bleeding and helps to prevent contamination.

Duodenum (du-o-DE-num or du-OD-e-num) the first portion of the small intestine, connected to the stomach.

It is more rigid than the other portions, causing it to suffer greater injury in accidents.

Dyspnea (disp-NE-ah) difficult or labored breathing.

E

Ecchymosis (EK-i-MO-sis) the discoloration of the skin due to internal bleeding. Typically, a "black and blue" mark.

Eclampsia (e-KLAM-se-ah) a life-threatening complication of pregnancy that produces convulsions and may result in coma or death. See *Preeclampsia*.

-ectomy (EK-toe-me) a word ending meaning surgical removal.

Ectopic (ek-TOP-ik) **pregnancy** when the embryo implants somewhere other than in the body of the uterus. Ectopic implantation can take place in the oviducts (fallopian tubes), cervix, or abdominopelvic cavity.

Edema (e-DE-mah) swelling due to the accumulation of fluids in the tissues.

Embolism (EM-bo-liz-m) movement and lodgement of a blood clot or foreign body (fat or air bubble) inside a blood vessel. The clot or foreign body is called an embolus (EM-bo-lus).

Emergency care the prehospital assessment and basic care provided for the sick or injured patient. The care is started at the emergency scene and is continued through transport and transfer at the medical facility. During this care, both the physical and emotional needs of the patient are considered.

Emergency Medical Services System (EMS System) a chain of services linked together to provide care for the patient at the scene, during transport to the hospital, and upon entry at the hospital.

Emergency Medical Technician (EMT) a professional-level provider of emergency care, trained above the level of the First Responder. This individual has received formal training equal to or greater than the standard DOT emergency medical technician training program and is state certified.

Emesis (EM-e-sis) vomiting.

Emotional emergency when a patient's behavior is not considered to be typical for the occasion. Often, this behavior is not socially acceptable. The patient's emotions are strongly evident, interfering with his or her thoughts and behavior.

Emphysema (EM-fi-SEE-mah) a chronic disease in which the lungs suffer a progressive loss of elasticity. See *Chronic obstructive pulmonary disease*.

Epidermis (ep-i-DER-mis) the outer layer of skin.

Epiglottis (EP-i-GLOT-is) a flap of cartilage and other tissues that is at the top of the voice box (larynx). It closes off the airway and diverts solids and liquids down the esophagus.

Epilepsy (EP-i-lep-see) a medical disorder characterized by attacks of unconsciousness, with or without convulsions.

Episodic a medical problem that affects the patient at regular intervals.

Epistaxis (ep-e-STAK-sis) a nosebleed.

Esophageal obturator airway (EOA) a breathing tube that is inserted partway into the esophagus. It has vents in its tube that will deliver air into the larynx. Typically, this device is used by EMTs.

Esophagus (e-SOF-ah-gus) the muscular food tube leading from the throat to the stomach.

Evisceration (e-VIS-er-a-shun) usually applies to the intestine protruding through an incision or wound.

Expiration breathing out. To exhale.

External auditory canal the opening of the external ear and its pathway to the middle ear.

Extrication any actions that disentangle and free from entrapment.

Extruded when an organ, bone, or vessel is pushed out of position.

F

Fainting the simplest form of shock, occurring when the patient has a temporary, self-correcting loss of consciousness caused by a reduced supply of blood to the brain. Also called psychogenic (SI-ko-JEN-ic) shock.

False motion movement where there should be none. This term is used to describe the movement seen at the point of an extremity fracture.

Febrile feverish

Femoral artery (FEM-o-ral) the main artery of the upper leg (thigh). It is a major pulse location and pressure point site.

Femoral (FEM-o-ral) **artery pressure point** the pressure point in the thigh that can be used to help control bleeding from the lower limb.

Femur (FE-mer) the thigh bone.

Fetus (FE-tus) the developing unborn child. It is an embryo until the third month, when it becomes a fetus until birth.

Fibrillation uncoordinated contractions of the heart muscle (myocardium) that are produced from independent individual muscle fiber activity. The totally disorganized activity of heart muscle. See *Ventricular fibrillation* and *Defibrillation*.

Fibrin (FI-brin) fibrous protein material that is formed and used to produce blood clots.

Fibula (FIB-yo-lah) the lateral lower leg bone.

Finger bones the phalanges (fah-LAN-jez).

Finger sweeps a procedure used to clear the mouth of airway obstructions. The rescuer's gloved fingers are used to sweep and lift away objects, clots, and debris. When used on infants and children, the object must be visible. Blind finger sweeps should not be used on these patients.

First-degree burn a mild partial-thickness burn, involving only the outer layer of skin.

First Responder an individual who has received training in emergency care in order to provide for the patient before EMTs arrive. The level of training allows this individual to assist EMTs at the emergency scene.

Flail chest the condition where the ribs and/or the breastbone are fractured in such a way as to produce a loose section of the chest wall that will not move with the rest of the wall during breathing.

Flexion to lessen an angle of a joint. To bend, as in bending the knee or bending at the elbow.

Flowmeter a Bourdon, pressure-compensated, or constant flow selector valve device used to indicate supplemental oxygen flow in liters per minute.

Foot bones the metatarsals (meta-TAR-sals).

Forearm bones the ulna and radius.

Formed elements red blood cells, white blood cells, and platelets. The blood minus its plasma.

Fracture a break, crack, split or crumbling of a bone.

Freezing deep frostbite. An injury due to cold involving the skin and the layers below the skin. Deep structures such as bone and muscle may be involved.

Frostbite superficial frostbite. The skin is frozen, but the layers below it are still soft and have their normal bounce. See *Freezing*.

Frostnip incipient frostbite. Very minor damage to the outer layer of skin caused by exposure to cold. See *Frostbite*.

G

Gallbladder an organ attached to the lower back of the liver. It stores bile.

Gastro- (GAS-tro) used as a beginning of words in reference to the stomach.

Genitalia (jen-i-TA-le-ah) the external reproductive organs.

Good Samaritan laws a series of laws written to protect emergency care personnel. These laws require a standard of care to be provided in good faith, to the level of training, and to the best of ability.

Grand mal a severe epileptic seizure.

Greenstick fracture a split along the length of a bone, giving the bone the appearance of a green stick that is bent to its breaking point.

Gurgling an atypical sound of breathing made by patients having airway obstruction, lung disease, or lung injury due to heat.

H

Hallucinogen a mind-affecting drug that acts on the central nervous system to excite the user or distort his or her perception of the surroundings.

Hand bones the bones of the palm of the hand, known as the metacarpals (meta-KAR-pals)

Handoff the orderly transfer of the patient, patient information, and patient valuables to more highly trained personnel.

heart attack usually the sudden blockage of a coronary vessel that can cause death to the heart muscle.

Heart shock caused by the heart failing to pump enough blood to all parts of the body. Also known as cardiogenic (KAR-de-o-JEN-ic) shock.

Heat cramps a condition brought about by the loss of body fluids and possibly salts. It usually occurs in people working in hot environments. Muscle cramps occur in the legs and abdomen.

Heat exhaustion a form of shock that is caused by the loss of fluids and salts. This is heat prostration.

Heat stroke a true emergency caused by the failure of the body's heat-regulating mechanisms. The patient cannot cool his overheated body.

Hematemesis (HEM-ah-TEM-e-sis) vomiting bright red blood.

Hematoma (hem-ah-TO-mah) the collection of blood under the skin or in tissues as a result of an injured blood vessel.

Hematuria (HEM-ah-TU-ri-ah) passing blood in the urine.

Hemorrhage (HEM-o-rej) internal or external bleeding.

Hemorrhagic shock (HEM-o-RIJ-ic) see *Bleeding shock*.

Hemothorax (he-mo-THO-raks) the condition of blood and bloody fluids in the area between the lungs and the walls of the chest cavity.

Hip the joint made between the pelvis and the thigh bone (femur). Some people use this term to refer to the upper portion of the thigh bone.

Hives slightly elevated red or pale areas of the skin that may be produced as a reaction to certain foods, drugs, infections, or stress. Often there is an itching sensation associated with hives. See *Wheal*.

Humerus (HU-mer-us) the upper arm bone.

Humidifier a device that is attached to a supplemental oxygen delivery system to add moisture to the dry oxygen coming from the cylinder.

Hyperextension the overextension of a limb or body part.

Hyperglycemia (hi-per-gli-SEE-me-ah) an excess of sugar in the blood.

Hyperventilation an increased rate and depth of breathing. This may occur as a condition brought on by stress or it may be a sign of a more serious problem (for example, allergy shock, impending heart attack, respiratory distress).

Hypoglycemia (hi-po-gli-SEE-me-ah) too little sugar in the blood.

Hypothermia a general cooling of the body.

Hypovolemic shock (HI-po-vo-LE-mik) the state of shock that develops due to an excessive loss of whole blood or plasma. See *Hemorrhagic shock*.

Hypoxia (hi-POK-se-ah) an inadequate supply of oxygen to the body tissues.

I

Ileum (IL-e-um) the upper portions of the pelvis that form the wings of the pelvis.

Iliac (IL-e-ak) **crest** the upper, curved boundary of the wings of the pelvis. See *Ileum*.

Implied consent a legal position that assumes an unconscious patient (or one so badly injured or ill that he cannot respond) would consent to receiving emergency care. Implied consent may apply to children, the developmentally disabled, or emotionally or mentally disturbed patients when parents or guardians are not at the scene.

Incipient frostbite see *Frostnip*.

Incision see *Cut*.

Infarction (in-FARK-shun) localized tissue death due to the discontinuation of its blood supply. Sometimes used to mean a myocardial (heart muscle) infarction.

Infectious disease any disease produced by an infectious agent such as a bacterium or virus.

Inferior away from the top of the body. Usually compared with another structure that is closer to the top (superior).

Inflammation the pain, heat, redness, and swelling of tissues as they react to infection, irritation, or injury.

Inflatable splint a soft plastic splint that can be inflated with air to become rigid enough to help immobilize a fractured extremity.

Informed consent actual consent given after the patient knows your level of training and what you are going to do.

Inguinal (IN-gwin-al) **canal** the passageway from the scrotum into the pelvic cavity that carries the blood vessels, nerves, and cord of the testis.

Inspirations to breathe in. To inhale.

Insulin (IN-su-lin) a hormone produced in the pancreas that is needed to move sugar (glucose) from the blood into cells.

Insulin shock a state of shock resulting from too much insulin in the blood, causing low sugar levels for the brain and nervous system. See *Hypoglycemia*.

Intercostal (in-ter-KOS-tal) **muscles** the muscles found between the ribs. These muscles contract during an inspiration, lifting the ribs. This helps to increase the volume of the chest (thoracic) cavity.

Intermammary line an imaginary line that is drawn to connect the nipples.

Interposed ventilations the artificial ventilations provided during CPR.

Intravenous (IV) into a vein.

Iris the colored portion of the anterior eye. It adjusts the size of the pupil.

Ischemia (is-KE-me-ah) a decreased blood supply to an organ, part of an organ, or one of its specific tissues. Often used as an adjective (ischemic) to describe the state of the heart muscle in coronary artery disease.

Ischium (IS-ke-em) the lower, posterior portions of the pelvis.

-itis (I-tis) a word ending used to mean inflammation.

J

Jaundice (JON-dis) the yellowing of the skin, usually associated with liver or bile apparatus (gallbladder and bile ducts) injury or disease.

Jaw-thrust a method of opening the airway without lifting the neck or tilting the head.

Jugular veins (JUG-u-ler) the large veins in the neck that drain blood from the head.

K

Ketoacidosis (KE-to-as-i-DO-sis) a condition that occurs when a diabetic breaks down too many fats trying to obtain energy. Toxic ketone bodies form in the blood and the blood becomes acid.

Kidneys excretory organs located high in the back of the abdominal region. They are behind the abdominal cavity.

Kneecap the patella (pah-TEL-lah).

L

Labor the three stages of childbirth, including the beginning of contractions, delivery of the child, and delivery of the afterbirth (placenta, umbilical cord, and some of the lining tissues of the uterus).

Laceration see *Cut*.

Lacrimal (LAK-ri-mal) **gland** tear gland.

Laryngectomy (lar-in-JEK-toe-me) the total or partial removal of the voice box (larynx). The patient is called a neck-breather or a laryngectomee.

Larynx (LAR-inks) the airway between the throat and the windpipe. It contains the voice box.

Lateral to the side, away from the midline of the body.

Ligament fibrous tissue that connects bone to bone.

Liter (LE-ter), **Litre** the metric measurement of liquid volume that is equal to 1.057 quarts. One pint is almost equal to one-half liter.

Liver the largest gland in the body, having many functions. Located in the upper-right abdominal region, extending over to the central abdominal region.

Lumbar (LUM-bar) **spine** the five bones (vertebrae) of the lower back.

Lung shock caused by too little oxygen in the blood due to some sort of lung failure. Also called respiratory shock.

M

Major burn any third-degree burn; a second-degree burn involving an entire body area, joint, or crucial area; a first-degree burn that covers a large area; any burn to the face (other than simple sunburn); or any burn that involves the respiratory system. See *Minor burn*.

Mammalian diving reflex a reaction that occurs when a person dives into cold water and submerges the face. Breathing is inhibited, heart rate slows, and the major blood flow is directed to the heart, lungs, and brain. Oxygen is diverted to the brain.

Mandible (MAN-di-bl) the lower jaw bone.

Manual thrusts abdominal or chest thrusts provided to expel an object causing an airway obstruction.

Mechanisms of injury forces that caused the injury. Consideration is given to the type of force, its intensity and direction, and the body part it affects.

Medial toward the vertical midline of the body.

Mediastinum (me-de-as-TI-num or me-de-ah-STI-num) the central portion of the chest cavity (thoracic cavity) containing the heart, its greater vessels, part of the esophagus (food tube), and part of the trachea (windpipe).

Medical Practices Act requiring an individual to be licensed or certified in order to practice medicine or to provide certain levels of care.

Meninges (me-NIN-jez) the three membranes surrounding the brain and spinal cord.

Metabolic shock see *Body fluid shock.*

Metacarpals (meta-KAR-pals) hand bones.

Metatarsals (meta-TAR-sals) foot bones.

Midline an imaginary vertical line drawn down the center of the body, dividing it into right and left halves.

Minor burn a first- or second-degree burn that involves a small portion of the body with no damage to the respiratory system, face, hands, feet, groin, buttocks, or major joints. See *Major burn.*

Minor's consent a form of implied consent used when a minor is seriously ill or injured and the parents or guardians cannot be reached quickly.

Moves a general term used to describe any organized procedure that is employed to reposition or move a sick or injured person from one location to another.

Myocardium (mi-o-KAR-de-um) heart muscle. The cardiac muscle that makes up the walls of the heart.

N

Narcotic a class of drugs that affects the central nervous system for the relief of pain. Illicit use is to provide an intense state of relaxation.

Negligence at the First Responder level, this usually is the failure to provide the expected standard of care, leading to additional injury of the patient.

Nerve shock caused when the nervous system fails to control the diameter of the blood vessels. The vessels remain widely dilated, providing too great a volume to be filled by available blood. Also called neurogenic (NU-ro-jen-ic) shock.

O

Objective examination the hands-on survey of the patient during which vital signs are determined and a head-to-toe examination is given. This is part of the secondary survey.

Occlusion blockage. A blocked artery has an occlusion. It is occluded.

Occlusive dressing covering a wound and forming an airtight seal.

Open fracture when a bone is broken and bone ends or fragments cut through the skin. Also called a compound fracture. If a wound opens the fracture site to the outside world (for example, gunshot wound), the fracture is classified as an open fracture.

Open wound when the skin is broken.

Oropharyngeal airway (or-o-fah-RIN-jee-al) a curved breathing tube inserted into the patient's mouth. It will hold the base of the tongue forward.

P

Packaging part of the procedure of preparation for removal of the patient at an accident scene. It may involve applying splints and dressings, neck and spine immobilization, and stabilizing impaled objects.

Palpate, Palpation to feel a part of the body as to palpate the abdomen or palpate a radial pulse. To use a blood pressure cuff while feeling the radial pulse in order to determine the approximate systolic blood pressure.

Pancreas (PAN-cre-as) the gland in the back of the upper portion of the abdominal cavity, behind the stomach. It produces insulin and digestive juices.

Paradoxical motion (movement) when a loose segment of an injured chest wall moves in the opposite direction to the rest of the wall during breathing movements. This is associated with flail chest.

Paralysis complete or partial loss of the ability to move a body part. Sensation in the area may also be lost.

Patella (pah-TEL-lah) the kneecap.

Patient assessment the systematic gathering of information through interviews and a physical examination in order to determine the possible nature of a patient's injury or illness.

Pedal pulse a foot pulse.

Pelvic cavity the lower anterior body cavity that is surrounded by the bones of the pelvis.

Penetrating wound a puncture wound with only an entrance wound.

Perineum (per-i-NE-um) the region of the body located between the genitalia and the anus.

Perforating wound a puncture wound having an entrance and an exit wound.

Perfusion the constant flow of blood through the capillaries.

Pericardium (per-e-KAR-de-um) the sac that surrounds the heart.

Peritoneum (per-i-toe-NE-um) the membrane that lines the abdominal cavity.

Personal interaction a way of acting in a calm professional manner to talk with and listen to a patient. During this process, emotional support may be accepted by the patient.

Petit mal the minor epileptic attack that is noted by a momentary loss of awareness, with no major convulsive seizures.

Phalanges (fah-LAN-jez) the bones of the toes and fingers.

Pharynx (FAR-inks) the throat.

Pinna (PIN-ah) the external ear. It is also called the auricle (AW-re-kal).

Placenta (plah-SEN-tah) an organ made of both maternal and fetal tissues to allow for exchange between the circulatory systems of the mother and fetus without having a mixing of blood.

Plasma (PLAZ-mah) the fluid portion of the blood. It is the blood minus the blood cells and other structures.

Platelet (PLATE-let) those formed elements of the blood that release factors needed to produce blood clots.

Pleura (PLOOR-ah) a double-membrane sac. The outer layer lines the chest wall and the inner layer covers the outside of the lungs.

Pleural (PLOOR-al) **cavities** the right and left portions of the chest cavity (thorax) that contain the lungs and the pleura membranes.

Pneumothorax (NU-mo-THO-raks) the collection of air in the chest cavity to the outside of the lungs, caused by punctures to the chest wall or the lungs.

Pocket face mask a device designed to aid the delivery of ventilations and mouth-to-mask resuscitations. The mask prevents rescuer contact with the patient's mouth. A one-way valve must be part of the mask to protect the rescuer from blood, body fluids, and vomitus.

Posterior the back.

Preeclampsia (pre-e-KLAMP-se-ah) a complication of pregnancy. This is the early stages of toxemia of pregnancy. Usually there is swelling of the face, hands, and feet and an elevation of blood pressure. Sometimes this condition is called pregnancy-induced hypertension (PIH). See *Eclampsia*.

Premature infant any newborn weighing less than 5.5 pounds or being born before the thirty-seventh week of pregnancy.

Pressure regulator a device that is connected to an oxygen cylinder to reduce the cylinder pressure to a safe working level, thus providing a safe pressure for delivery to the patient.

Priapism (PRE-ah-pizm) persistent erection associated with spinal damage in the male patient.

Primary survey the first examination of a patient to detect life-threatening problems dealing with level of awareness, breathing, heart action, and profuse bleeding.

Prolapsed cord abnormal delivery where the umbilical cord is presented first.

Prone lying face down.

Proximal close to a point of reference such as the shoulder or hip joint. Used with distal, meaning away from.

Psychogenic shock (SI-ko-JEN-ic) see *Fainting*.

Pubic (PYOO-bik), **Pubis** (PYOO-bis) the middle, anterior region of the pelvis. The region associated with the external genitalia.

Pulmonary (PUL-mo-ner-e) applies to the lungs.

Pulmonary (PUL-mo-ner-e) **resuscitation** (re-SUS-ci-TAY-shun) providing rescue breaths (ventilations) to a patient in an attempt to artificially restore lung function.

Pulse the alternate expansion and contraction of artery walls as the heart pumps blood.

Puncture wound an open wound tearing through the skin and destroying tissue in a straight line. See *Penetrating wound* and *Perforating wound*.

R

Radial pulse the wrist pulse.

Radius the lateral forearm bone.

Rectum (REK-tum) the lower portion of the large intestine, ending with the anus.

Red blood cells (RBCs) the circulating blood cells that carry oxygen to the tissues and return carbon dioxide to the lungs. The erythrocytes (e-RITH-ro-sites).

Referred pain the pain felt in a region of the body other than where the source or cause of the pain is located. For example, pain in the gallbladder may be felt over the right shoulder blade (scapula).

Respiratory arrest the cessation of breathing.

Respiratory shock see *Lung shock*.

Resuscitation (re-SUS-ci-TA-shun) any effort to restore or provide normal heart and/or lung function artificially.

Rule of nines a system used for estimating the amount of skin surface that is burned. The body is divided into 12 regions. Each of 11 regions equals 9% of the body surface and the genital region is classified as 1%.

S

Sacrum (SA-krum) the fused bones (vertebrae) of the lower back that are immediately inferior to the lumbar spine.

Sanitize a rigid standard of cleaning, often to the point of practical sterilization.

Scapula (SKAP-u-lah) the shoulder blade.

Sclera (SKLE-rah) the "whites of the eyes."

Scratch an abrasion (ab-RAY-shun). An open wound that damages the surface of skin without breaking all the skin layers.

Secondary survey the patient interview and the physical examination performed after the primary survey. This is done to detect problems that may become life-threatening if allowed to go untreated.

Second-degree burn a partial-thickness burn where the outer layer of skin (epidermis) is burned through and the second layer (dermis) is damaged.

Septic shock see *Bloodstream shock*.

Shock the failure of the circulatory system to provide an adequate blood supply to all the vital organs of the body. The failure of perfusion.

Shoulder blade the scapula (SKAP-u-lah).

Sign any observed evidence of injury or illness.

Sling a large triangular bandage or other cloth device that is applied as a soft splint to immobilize possible fractures and dislocations of the shoulder girdle and upper extremity.

Sphygmomanometer (SFIG-mo-mah-NOM-e-ter) an instrument used to measure blood pressure. This is commonly called a blood pressure cuff.

Spinal cavity the area within the spinal column that contains the spinal cord and its coverings, the meninges (me-NIN-jez).

Spleen an organ located to the left of the upper abdominal cavity, behind the stomach. It stores blood and destroys old blood cells.

Splint any device that will immobilize a fracture.

Sprain an injury in which ligaments are partially torn.

Standard of care the minimum accepted level of emergency care. It is set forth by law, administrative orders, guidelines published by medical and emergency care organizations and societies, local protocols and practices, and precedent (what has been accepted).

START plan a four-step simple triage and rapid treatment (care) program designed for use in multiple casualty incidents. It is usually employed by the First Responder when additional help will be late in arriving.

Sterile free of all life forms.

Sternum (STER-num) the breastbone.

Stethoscope an instrument used to amplify body sounds.

Stoma (STO-mah) applied to the opening in the neck of a neck-breather.

Strain injuries to muscles caused by overexertion.

Stroke the result of blockage or damage to an artery supplying oxygenated blood to the brain. Headache, confusion, paralysis (often to one side only), impaired vision, impaired speech, unequal pupil size, and many other signs and symptoms are possible. This is a cerebrovascular accident or CVA.

Subcutaneous (SUB-ku-TA-ne-us) beneath the skin. It refers to the fats and connective tissues found immediately below the dermis.

Subjective interview the gathering of bystander and patient information obtained by asking specific questions. It is part of the secondary survey, usually preceding the physical examination. The process may continue during physical assessment and care.

Substernal notch referring to the area of the lower breastbone to which the ribs attach.

Sucking chest wound an open chest wound into which air is sucked through the wound and into the chest cavity each time the patient breathes.

Superficial frostbite see *Frostbite*.

Superior toward the top of the body. Often used in reference with inferior, meaning away from the top of the body.

Supine lying flat on the back.

Swathe a large cravat, usually make of cloth. It is used to secure a sling or rigid splint and sling to the body. It may be used to hold an upper limb to the chest.

Sympathetic eye movement the coordinated movement of both eyes in the same direction. If one eye moves, the other eye will carry out the same movement.

Symptom evidence of injury or illness told to you by the patient.

Syrup of ipecac (IP-e-kak) a compound used to induce vomiting in certain conscious poisoning patients. Its use must be approved by the EMS System medical advisory board and be directed for use by the poison control center or medical command for each case unless otherwise stated in local protocols.

Systemic (sis-TEM-ik) referring to the entire body.

Systolic (sis-TOL-ik) **blood pressure** the force exerted on the artery walls when the heart is contracting.

T

Tachycardia (tak-e-KAR-de-ah) rapid heartbeat, usually 100 or more beats per minute.

Tarsals (TAR-sals) the ankle bones.

Tendon fibrous tissue that connects muscle to bone.

Thigh bone the femur (FE-mur).

Third-degree burn a full-thickness burn, where all layers of the skin are damaged. Deep structures may also be burned.

Thoracic cavity (tho-RAS-ik) the anterior body cavity above (superior to) the diaphragm. It protects the heart and lungs.

Thorax (THO-raks) the chest.

Tibia (TIB-e-ah) the medial lower leg bone.

Toe bones the phalanges (fah-LAN-jez).

Tongue jaw lift a procedure used to open the mouth of an unconscious patient. The rescuer grasps the tongue and lower jaw between thumb and fingers to move the tongue away from the back of the throat.

Tourniquet the last resort used to control bleeding. A band or belt is used to constrict blood vessels to stop the flow of blood.

Trachea (TRA-ke-ah) the windpipe.

Tracheostomy (TRA-ke-OS-to-me) a surgical opening made in the anterior neck that enters into the windpipe (trachea).

Traction a part of the action taken to pull gently along the length of the limb to stabilize a broken bone to prevent any additional injury.

Transient ischemic attack (TIA) an attack of short duration that is due to a reduced flow of blood to an area of the brain. Dizziness, numbness, general weakness, vision problems, and unconsciousness may occur.

Trauma an injury caused by violence, shock, or pressure.

Triage a method of sorting patients according to the severity of their injuries.

Tympanic (tim-PAN-ik) **membrane** the eardrum.

U

Ulna (UL-nah) the medial lower arm bone.

Umbilical cord (um-BIL-i-kal) the structure that connects the body of the fetus to the placenta.

Umbilicus (um-bi-LIK-us or um-BIL-i-kus) the navel.

Universal precautions recommendations from the Centers for Disease Control for medical and emergency care personnel to wear latex or vinyl gloves, eye protection, masks, and gowns to avoid contact with the patient's blood, body fluids, wastes, and mucous membranes. Pocket face masks with one-way valves or other approved methods of resuscitation are recommended to prevent infectious diseases resulting from resuscitative efforts.

Upper a stimulant that will affect the central nervous system to excite the user.

Uterus (U-ter-us) the muscular structure in which the fetus develops. The womb.

V

Vagina (vah-JI-nah) the birth canal.

Vascular referring to the blood vessels.

Vein   any blood vessel that returns blood to the heart.

Venae (VE-ne) **cavae** (KA-ve)   the superior and inferior vena cava. The two major veins that return blood from the body into the heart.

Venous bleeding   the loss of blood from a vein. It is dark red to maroon in color. Loss is as a steady flow and can be very heavy.

Ventilation   supplying air to the lungs.

Ventral   front of the body. See *anterior*.

Ventricle   one of the two lower chambers of the heart. Ventricles pump blood from the heart.

Ventricular fibrillation   the totally disorganized contractions of the myocardium of the lower heart chambers. See *Defibrillation*.

Vertebra (VER-te-brah)   each individual bone of the spinal column.

Vial of Life   a program designed to aid emergency care personnel by having certain patients place information and medications in special vials in their refrigerators. A "Vial of Life" sticker is placed on the main outside door, closest window to the main door, or refrigerator door.

Viscera (VIS-er-ah)   the internal organs. Usually refers to the abdominal organs.

Vital signs   in First Responder care, these are pulse rate and character, breathing rate and character, and relative skin temperature.

Vitreous (VIT-re-us) **fluid**   transparent, jellylike substance that fills the posterior cavity of the eye.

Volatile chemicals   vaporizing chemicals that will cause excitement or produce a "high" when breathed in by the abuser.

Vulva (VUL-vah)   the external female genitalia.

W

Wheal   The localized collection of fluid under the skin that may be accompanied by itching and a change in skin coloration. A hive.

Wheeze   a whistling breathing sound. This sound is often associated with asthma when air is trapped in the air sacs and cannot be expired easily.

White blood cells (WBCs)   the blood cells that destroy microorganisms and produce antibodies to help fight off infection. The leukocytes (LU-co-sites).

Womb   see *Uterus*.

X

Xiphoid (ZI-foyd)   the lower process of the breastbone (sternum).

Z

Zygomatic (zi-go-MAT-ik) **bone**   the cheek bone; also called the malar (MA-lar).

■ Index